McCracken's

Removable Partial Prosthodontics

Dear Uma
wishing you all luck
[illegible]
6/05

McCracken's

Removable Partial Prosthodontics

Eleventh Edition

Alan B. Carr, DMD, MS, FACP
Professor, Department of Dental Specialties
Mayo Clinic
Rochester, Minnesota

Glen P. McGivney, DDS, FACD
Adjunct Professor, Department of Prosthodontics
University of North Carolina
School of Dentistry
Chapel Hill, North Carolina

David T. Brown, DDS, MS
Vice Chair, Department of Restorative Dentistry
Indiana University
School of Dentistry
Indianapolis, Indiana

Selected illustrations by Donald O'Connor

with 807 illustrations

MOSBY
An imprint of Elsevier

McCracken's Removable Partial Prosthodontics, 11/ed
Carr, et al.

MOSBY
An Imprint of Elsevier
11830, Westline Industrial Drive
St. Louis, Missouri 63146

Original ISBN: 0-323-02628-1

First Indian Reprint 2005

Indian Reprint ISBN: 81-8147-532-1

This edition is manufactured in India and is authorized for sale only in India, Bangladesh, Bhutan, Maldives, Nepal, Pakistan, Sri Lanka and any other country as authorized by the publisher.

Published by Elsevier, a division of Reed Elsevier India Private Limited, 17-A/1, Main Ring Road, Lajpat Nagar-IV, New Delhi-110 024.

Printed and bound by Replika Press Pvt. Ltd., India.

PREFACE

The opportunity to continue the tradition of a textbook, such as *McCracken's Removable Partial Prosthodontics*, is both an honor and a significant responsibility. Many talented and knowledgeable individuals have helped produce this text to guide students and clinicians over the last 10 editions spanning 44 years. Although dental practice in the year 2005 is not as practice was when the early editions were printed, the basic principles guiding the practice of removable partial dentures remain. This point is evident in the comment made by W.L. McCracken in the preface to the first edition.

> "Unless a partial denture is made with adequate abutment support, with optimal base support, and with harmonious and functional occlusion, it should be clear to all concerned that such a denture should be considered only a temporary treatment. . . ."

It is appropriate that an important focus of this statement is support, as it is a critical requirement associated with functional stability. In light of this early emphasis and its relationship to stability, it is compelling to note that a recent large population study* found that 65% of the removable partial dentures worn exhibited lack of stability. Recognizing that this finding potentially reflects both clinician application of design principles and maintenance procedures, it provides food for thought for anyone considering educational issues for removable partial dentures (teaching quality and quantity, and materials).

This edition of *McCracken's Removable Partial Prosthodontics* will make an attempt to address the above findings without losing any emphasis on basic principles. The authors have tried to present the material as it applies to the focus of the patient-based outcome, functional stability. The importance of this relates to the realization that prosthodontics is an elective oral health pursuit of our patients. They present with unique reasons for and expectation of treatment. Our task is to carefully match the best treatment option to their specific needs and expectations. Compared to the natural dentition, these options can vary significantly relative to the anticipated functional stability. This text provides information to help clinicians understand and optimize removable partial denture functional stability.

This edition has undergone changes in part as a response to a perception that learning needs of students are evolving. The challenge has been in determining how best to meet those needs without losing an appropriate emphasis on important principles and concepts. Changes to this edition of the text include a brief introduction to the overall concept of tooth loss and the place for removable partial dentures in practice. Another change is the addition of color. A great deal of effort was put into both the line art and photographs, which were updated with color where possible. There has been an increase in information on implant considerations, especially where it was considered to be appropriate to contrast alternative treatment considerations, and as a means to use them in controlling functional movement of removable partial dentures. Lastly, the maxillofacial chapter has been rewritten and color photographs were added. The reader will notice that some black and white photographs were retained. The reasons for this are that often a new series of photographs, showing procedures and examples, are difficult to produce because they are difficult to find. Another reason is that when new examples are found they may not illustrate the principles and concepts as well as the original picture or series.

Input from users of the text has suggested that although the text provides a broad representation of the topic, both at the graduate and undergraduate level, it can be difficult to separate basic level material from that which is an extension of the basic understanding. Because of this, the authors decided to

*Hummel SK, Wilson MA, Marker VA, Nunn ME: Quality of removable partial dentures worn by the adult U.S. population. J Prosthet Dent Jul;88(1):37-43, 2002.

try and make the distinction to facilitate both the first-time learner and the more experienced clinician. The convention used was to separate the advanced level material by adding a colored background to the text. This was accomplished with the full understanding that such a distinction is not always clear, and that some readers will object to how certain material was classified. Our hope is that it will help clarify the material for the majority of readers.

ACKNOWLEDGMENTS

We would like to express our gratitude to many who contributed to this text in a variety of ways. A contribution to the text was provided by Dr. Vanchit John who updated the periodontal information in Chapter 12. We also would like to acknowledge the following contributors to the clinical images: Drs. Ned van Roekel, James Taylor, Miguel Alfaro, and Carl Andres. We also acknowledge the helpful work of a dedicated group of laboratory technicians who contributed to the updates of many laboratory procedure images: Mr. Joe Bly, Mr. Albert Evans, Mr. Gerry Hensley, Mr. Rick Lee, and Mr. Richard Kerkhof. The clerical assistance of Mrs. Melanie Budihas, who helped arrange and organize much of this work, is also greatly appreciated.

A final note of sincere appreciation goes to one of the authors, Dr. Glen McGivney, who has decided that this will be the final *McCracken's* edition to which he will contribute. It has been a pleasure to work with someone of his clinical expertise, educational experience, and scholarly background. His contributions to prosthodontics have been both numerous and significant, with this textbook being a lasting example of his impact. We are grateful for the opportunity we have had to work with him, and his contributions will be missed.

Alan B. Carr
Glen P. McGivney
David T. Brown

PREFACE TO THE FIRST EDITION

Although I welcomed the invitation to author a textbook on the subject of partial denture construction, I realized from the outset that such a book would follow closely in the wake of several excellent textbooks on this subject. I therefore approached the task with a sense of great responsibility. However, I would not have accepted the challenge had I not felt sincerely that I could add something to what had already been written and thus produce a text in this field which is sorely needed and which provides the dental student, the dental practitioner, and the dental laboratory technician with the information necessary to produce a partial denture that is in itself a definitive restorative entity. It is my sincere hope that this textbook will be used not only by teachers of prosthetic dentistry but also by practicing dentists and dental technicians, and that in this book the dentist and dental technician may find a common meeting ground for better solution of the problems associated with the partially edentulous patient.

I am deeply grateful for the opportunities that I have had to combine private practice with teaching and for the knowledge that has evolved from this experience. Although I have attempted to present various philosophies and techniques in order that the reader may select that which to him seems most applicable, it is inevitable that certain preferences will be obvious. These are based upon convictions evolved through experience both in private practice and in the teaching of clinical prosthodontics. It is only logical, then, that I should therefore state my own personal beliefs which are as follows:

1. I believe that the practice of prosthetic dentistry must forever remain in the hands of the dentist and that he must therefore be totally competent to render this service. In the fabrication of a partial denture restoration, the dentist must be competent to render a comprehensive diagnosis of the partially edentulous mouth and, utilizing all of the mechanical aids necessary, plan every detail of treatment. He must either personally accomplish whatever mouth preparations are necessary or delegate to his colleagues such specialized services as surgical, periodontal, and endodontic treatment. In any case, primary responsibility for adequate mouth preparations remains his alone. He must undertake whatever impression procedures are necessary and must be primarily responsible for the accuracy of any casts of the mouth upon which work is to be fabricated. He must provide the laboratory technician with an adequate prescription in the form of diagrams and written instructions and with a master cast which has been completely surveyed with a specific design outlined upon it. He must be solely responsible for the accuracy and adequacy of any jaw relation records and must specify all materials and, in many instances, the exact method by which occlusion is to be established on the finished restoration. Finally, he must be competent to judge the excellence of the finished restoration or recognize its inadequacies and must assume the responsibility for demanding a degree of excellence from the technician that will continually raise rather than lower the standards of dental laboratory service.
2. I believe that the dental laboratory technician has a responsibility to his profession to demand a quality of leadership from the dentist which he can respect and follow without question. The responsibility for providing adequate prosthetic dentistry service to the patient must be shared by both dentist and technician, and each has not only a right to expect that the other do his part competently but also an obligation to demand a quality of service from the other that will not jeopardize the finished product. The technician therefore would do dentistry a great service if he would reject inadequate material from the dentist and respectfully suggest whatever improvements are necessary for him to produce an acceptable piece of work. As long as the technician accepts inadequate material from the dentist and the dentist is willing to place an inadequate product in the patient's mouth, the quality of removable prosthetic appliances will continue to be, as it all too frequently is, a far poorer service than the

dentist and technician together are capable of rendering.

I believe also that dental laboratories should always be willing to adopt newer techniques and philosophies developed by the dental profession and being taught to dental graduates. Too often the commercial dental laboratory insists upon using stereotyped techniques that suite its production methods and actively attempts to discourage the recent graduate from putting into practice modern methods and techniques that were painstakingly taught in dental school by instructors whose knowledge of the subject far exceeds that of the laboratory technician who deprecates it.

3. I believe that any free-end partial denture must have been the best possible support from the underlying edentulous ridge and that the design of the abutment retainers must apply a minimum of torque to the adjacent abutment teeth. I believe that some kind of secondary impression is necessary to obtain adequate support for the denture base, both through tissue placement and from the broadest possible coverage compatible with biologic requirements and limitations.
4. I believe in the functional, or dynamic, registration of occlusal relationships rather than in relying upon intraoral adjustment of an established centric occlusion or upon the ability of an instrument to simulate articulatory movements. I believe that the occlusion on a partial denture, be it fixed or removable, should be made to harmonize with the existing adjusted natural occlusion and that this can best be accomplished by the registration of functional occlusal paths. For this to be done adequately, occlusion on the partial denture must be established upon either the final denture base(s) or upon an accurate substitute for the final base(s). The practice of attempting to submit jaw-relation records to the technician prior to the fabrication of the denture framework is therefore, with few exceptions, strongly condemned.
5. I believe that a partial denture, when properly designed, carefully made, and serviced when needed, can be an entirely satisfactory restoration and can serve as a means of preserving remaining oral structures, as well as restoring missing dentition. Unless a partial denture is made with adequate abutment support, with optimal base support, and with harmonious and functional occlusion, it should be clear to all concerned that such a denture should be considered only a temporary treatment, or interim denture rather than a restoration representative of the best that modern prosthetic dentistry has to offer.

W.L. McCracken

CONTENTS

Part II Clinical and Laboratory, 187

McCracken's

Removable Partial Prosthodontics

I

General Concepts/ Treatment Planning

1

PARTIALLY EDENTULOUS EPIDEMIOLOGY, PHYSIOLOGY, AND TERMINOLOGY

This textbook focuses on what the clinician should know about partially edentulous patients to appropriately provide comfortable and useful tooth replacements in the form of removable partial dentures. Removable partial dentures are a component of prosthodontics, which denotes the branch of dentistry pertaining to the restoration and maintenance of oral functions, comfort, appearance, and health of the patient by the restoration of natural teeth and/or the replacement of missing teeth and craniofacial tissues with artificial substitutes.

Current practice in the management of partial tooth loss involves consideration of various types of prostheses (Figure 1-1). Each type of prosthesis requires use of various remaining teeth and/or tissues, and consequently demands appropriate application of knowledge and critical thinking to ensure the best possible outcome given the patient needs and desires. Although more than one prosthesis could serve the needs of a patient, any prosthesis should meet the basic objectives of prosthodontic treatment, which includes: (1) the elimination of oral disease to the greatest extent possible; (2) the preservation of the health and relationships of the teeth and the health of oral and paraoral structures, *which will enhance the removable partial denture design*; and (3) the restoration of oral functions that are comfortable, esthetically pleasing, and do not interfere with the patient's speech. It is critically important to emphasize that the preservation of health requires proper maintenance of removable partial dentures. To provide a perspective for understanding the impact of removable partial denture prosthodontics, a review of tooth loss and its sequelae, functional restoration with prostheses, and prosthesis use and outcomes is in order.

TOOTH LOSS AND AGE

It should come as no surprise that tooth loss and age are linked. It has been documented that there is a specific tooth loss relationship with increasing age because some teeth are retained longer than others. It has been suggested that there is an interarch difference in tooth loss, with the maxillary teeth lost before mandibular teeth. It has also been suggested that there is an intraarch difference, with posterior teeth lost before anterior teeth. Frequently the last remaining teeth in the mouth are the mandibular anterior teeth, especially the mandibular canines, and it is a common finding to see an edentulous maxilla opposing mandibular anterior teeth.

If one accepts that tooth loss and age are linked, how will this impact current and future dental

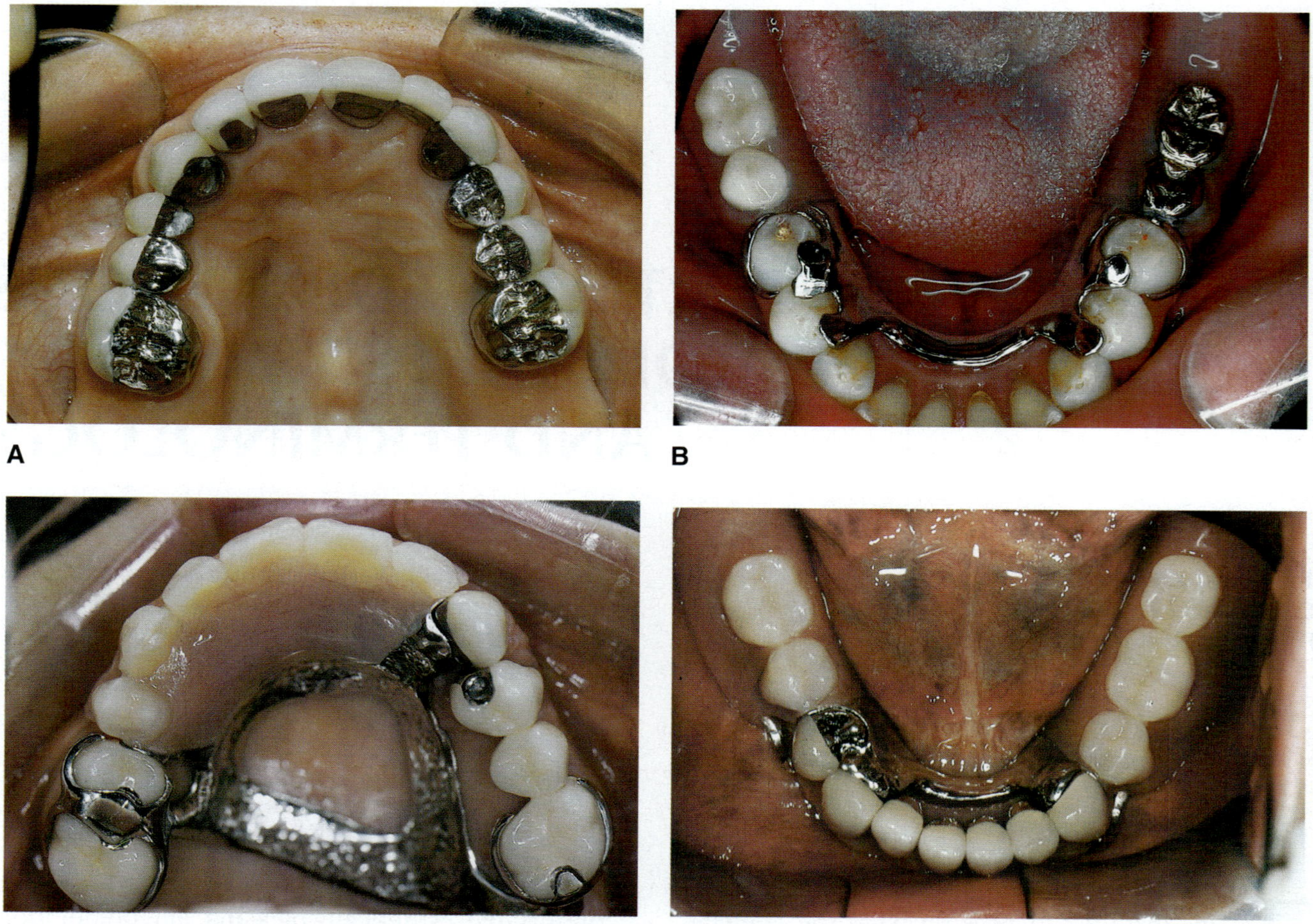

A B C D

Figure 1-1 **A,** Fixed partial dentures that restore missing anterior (#10) and posterior (#5, 13) teeth. Teeth bounding edentulous spaces are used as abutments. **B,** Clasp-type removable partial denture restoring missing posterior teeth. Teeth adjacent to edentulous spaces serve as abutments. **C,** Tooth-supported removable partial denture restoring missing anterior and posterior teeth. Teeth bounding edentulous spaces provide support, retention, and stability for restoration. **D,** Mandibular bilateral distal extension removable partial denture restoring missing premolars and molars. Support, retention, and stability are shared by abutment teeth and residual ridges.

practice? Replacement of missing teeth is a common patient need and patients will demand it well into their elderly years. Current population estimates show that 13% of the United States population is 65 years of age or older. By the year 2030 this percentage is expected to double, with a significant increase also expected worldwide. These individuals are expected to be in better health, and health care strategies for this group should focus on maintenance of active and productive lives. Oral health care is expected to be a highly sought after and significant component of their overall health care.

Tooth loss patterns associated with age are also evolving. The proportion of edentulous adults has been reported to be decreasing, although this varies widely by state. However, it has been reported that the absolute number of edentulous patients needing care is actually increasing. More pertinent to this text, estimates suggest the need for restoration of partially edentulous conditions will also be increasing. An explanation for this is presented in an argument that 62% of Americans of the "baby boomer" generation and younger have benefited from fluoridated water. The result of such exposure has been a decrease in caries-associated tooth loss. In addition, current estimates suggest patients are keeping more teeth longer, demonstrated by the fact that 71.5% of 65- to 74-year-old individuals are partially edentulous (mean number of retained teeth = 18.9). It has been suggested that partially edentulous conditions are more common in the maxillary arch, and that the most commonly missing teeth are first and second molars.

CONSEQUENCES OF TOOTH LOSS

With the loss of teeth the residual ridge no longer benefits from the functional stimulus it once experienced. Because of this, a loss of ridge volume—both height and width—can be expected. This finding is not predictable for all individuals with tooth loss, as the change in anatomy has been reported to be variable across patient groups. In general, bone loss is greater in the mandible than the maxilla, more pronounced posteriorly than anteriorly, and it produces a broader mandibular arch while constricting the maxillary arch. These anatomical changes can present challenges to prosthesis fabrication, including implant-supported prostheses and removable partial dentures. Associated with this loss of bone is the accompanying alteration in the oral mucosa. The attached gingiva of the alveolar bone can be replaced with less keratinized oral mucosa, which is more readily traumatized.

The esthetic impact of tooth loss can be highly significant and may be more of a concern to a patient than loss of function. It is generally perceived that in today's society, loss of visible teeth, especially in the anterior region of the mouth, carries with it a significant social stigma. With the loss of teeth and diminishing residual ridge, facial features can change secondary to altered lip support and/or reduced facial height as a result of a reduction in occlusal vertical dimension. Restoring facial esthetics in a manner that maintains an appropriate appearance can be a challenge, and is a major factor in the restoration and maintenance decisions for various prosthetic treatments.

FUNCTIONAL RESTORATION WITH PROSTHESES

Individuals with a full complement of teeth report some variation in their levels of masticatory function. The loss of teeth can lead a patient to seek care for functional reasons as they notice a diminished function to a level that is unacceptable to them. The level at which a patient finds function to be unacceptable varies among individuals. This variability increases with accelerating tooth loss. These variables may be confusing to clinicians, who perceived that they have provided prostheses of equal quality to different patients with the same tooth loss patterns and yet achieve different patient reports of success.

An understanding of these variations among individuals with a full complement of teeth and those with prostheses can help clinicians formulate realistic treatment goals that can be communicated to the patient. A review of oral function, especially mastication, may help interested clinicians better understand issues related to the impact of removable partial denture function.

Mastication

Though functionally considered as a separate act, mastication as part of the feeding continuum precedes swallowing and is not an end to itself. The interaction of the two distinct but coordinated aspects of feeding suggests some judgment of mastication termination or completeness precedes the initiation of swallowing. Though the mastication-swallowing sequence is obvious, the interaction of the two functions is not widely understood and may be important to prosthesis use when removable partial dentures are considered.

Mastication involves two discrete but well-synchronized activities: subdivision of food by applied force, and selective manipulation by the tongue and cheeks to sort out coarse particles and bring them to the occlusal surfaces of teeth for further breakdown. The initial subdivision or comminution phase involves the processes of selection, which is the chance that a particle is placed between the teeth in position to be broken, and breakage, which is the degree of fragmentation of a particle once selected. The size, shape, and texture of the food particles provide the sensory input that influences the configuration and area of each chewing stroke. The larger particles are selectively reduced in size more rapidly than fine particles in efficient mastication. The process of mastication is therefore greatly influenced by factors that impact the physical ability to reduce food and to monitor the reduction process by neurosensory means.

Food Reduction

Teeth or prostheses serve the role of reducing food to a point ready for swallowing. An index of food reduction is described as masticatory efficiency, or the ability to reduce food to a certain size in a given time frame. It has been shown that there is a strong correlation between masticatory efficiency and the number of occluding teeth in dentate individuals, which would suggest variability of particle selection related to contacting teeth. Performance measures reveal a great deal of functional variability in patients with similar numbers of contacting teeth, and an even greater variability is seen within populations with greater loss of teeth (increasing degrees of edentulousness).

Since occlusal contact area is highly correlated with masticatory performance, the loss of molar teeth would be expected to have a greater impact on measures of performance since the molar has a larger occlusal contact area. This effect has been demonstrated in individuals with missing molars who reveal a greater number of chewing strokes required and a greater mean particle size before swallowing. The point at which an individual is prepared to swallow the food bolus is another measure of performance and is described as the swallowing threshold. Superior masticatory ability that is highly correlated with occlusal contact area also achieves greater food reduction at the swallowing threshold. Conversely, a diminished ability to chew is reflected in larger particles at the swallowing threshold.

These objective measures, which show a benefit to molar contact in dentate individuals, are in conflict with some subjective measures from patients who express no perceived functional problems associated with having only premolar occlusion. This shortened dental arch concept has highlighted that patient perceptions of both functional compromise, as well as benefit, should be considered when deciding whether to replace missing molars. When the loss of posterior teeth results in an unstable tooth position, such as distal or labial migration, tooth replacement should be carefully considered and is a separate situation from the shortened dental arch concept.

It has been reported that prosthetic replacement of teeth provides function that is often less than that seen in the complete, natural dentition state. Functional measures are closest to the natural state when replacements are fixed partial dentures rigidly supported by teeth or implants, intermediate in function when replacements are removable and supported by teeth, lower in function when replacements are removable and supported by teeth and edentulous ridges, and lowest in function when replacements are removable and supported by edentulous ridges alone.

Objective and subjective measures of a patient's oral function are often not in agreement. It has been shown that subjective measures of masticatory ability are often overrated compared with objective functional tests, and that for complete denture wearers the subjective criteria may be more appropriate in monitoring perceived outcomes. Some literature reports that removable partial dentures can be described by patients as adding very little benefit over no prostheses. However, these findings could relate to a number of factors, including the lack of maintenance of the occluding tooth relationships, the limitations of this form of dental prosthesis for patient populations that may be unreliable in maintaining follow-up visits, and the intrinsic variation in patient response to prostheses.

Food reduction is also influenced by the ability to monitor the process that is required to determine the point at which swallowing is initiated. As mentioned earlier, the size, shape, and texture of food are monitored during mastication to allow modification in mandibular movement for efficient food reduction. This has been demonstrated in dentate individuals, given food particles of varying size and concentration suspended in yogurt, who revealed that increased concentrations and particle size required more time to prepare for swallowing (i.e., greater swallowing threshold). These findings suggest that the oral mucosa has a critical role in detecting characteristics necessary for efficient mastication. The influence of the removable partial denture on the ability of the mucosa to perform this role in mastication is not known.

CURRENT REMOVABLE PARTIAL DENTURE USE

Given an understanding of the relationship between tooth loss and age, the consequences of tooth loss, and our ability to restore function with removable partial prostheses, what do we know about current prosthesis use for these conditions, and what are some common clinical outcomes? A recent study estimated 21.4% prosthesis use among individuals aged 15 to 74. In the 55- to 64-year-old group, 22.2% were found to wear a removable partial denture. This age group has the highest use of removable partial dentures among those reviewed. It has been suggested that the use of removable partial dentures among individuals aged 55 years or older is even greater.

Analysis of this study provides some useful information for consideration. Partially edentulous individuals not wearing a prosthesis were 6 times more likely to have missing mandibular teeth (19.4%) than missing maxillary teeth (2.2%). This might suggest more difficulty in the use of a mandibular prosthesis. The distribution of prostheses used in this large patient group is shown in Box 1-1. The prostheses in this large study were evaluated based on five technical quality characteristics: integrity, excessive wear of posterior denture teeth, presence of temporary reline material or tissue conditioner or adhesive, stability, and retention. As seen in Table 1-1, a lack of stability was the most common characteristic noted. In the maxilla, lack of stability was seven times more prevalent than lack of retention. In the mandible, lack of stability was 1.8 times more prevalent than lack of retention. In another study, rest form, denture base extension, stress distribution, and framework fit were identified as being common flaws associated with poor removable partial dentures. These

BOX 1-1 Distribution of Prostheses

Removable partial dentures	RPD/RPD 9.0%,	RPD/−15.3%, −/RPD 4.5%
Complete dentures	CU/CL 3.8%,	CU/−20.7%
Combination	CU/RPD 11.5%,	RPD/CL 0.3%

RPD, Removable partial denture; CU, complete upper denture; CL, complete lower denture. Natural teeth denoted with dash (–).

TABLE 1-1. Technical Quality Concerns for Removable Partial Dentures

	Lacks Stability	Lacks Integrity	Lacks Retention	Reline/Adhesive	Excessive Wear
Maxillary RPD	43.9%	24.3%	6.2%	3.9%	21.6%
Mandibular RPD	38.2%	13.2%	21.2%	21.6%	7.1%

characteristics are directly related to functional stability of prostheses.

NEED FOR REMOVABLE PARTIAL DENTURES

What does all this information mean to us today? It means a number of things that are important to consider. The need for partially edentulous care will be increasing. Patient use of removable partial dentures has been high in the past and is expected to continue in the future. Some patients who are given the choice between an implant-supported prosthesis and a removable partial denture are not able to pursue implant care. This contributes to higher use of removable partial dentures.

Finally, these findings suggest that we should strive to understand how to maximize the opportunity for providing and maintaining stable prostheses because this is the most frequently deficient aspect of removable partial denture service. Consequently, throughout this text the basic principles of diagnosis, mouth preparation, prosthesis design, fabrication, placement, and maintenance will be reinforced to improve an understanding of removable partial denture prostheses care.

TERMINOLOGY

Although familiarity with accepted prosthodontic terminology would help in the understanding of the material in this and other dental textbooks, it is unrealistic to expect a working knowledge of terminology to develop without clinical examples to reinforce learning. Consequently, prosthodontic terms are introduced at this point in time and will be reinforced with clinical examples throughout the text (Figures 1-2 and 1-3).

Additional terminology can be reviewed in *The Glossary of Prosthodontic Terms*[1] and a glossary of accepted terms in all disciplines of dentistry—*Mosby's Dental Dictionary*.[2] Both are excellent resources for spoken and written communication in prosthodontics.

Although the following is not meant to be a complete glossary of removable partial prosthodontic terminology, the definitions given are considered basic and are used throughout the text. The format of presentation is not alphabetical, and it is hoped that this creates only a minor inconvenience.

The term **appliance** is correctly applied only to devices (such as splints, orthodontic appliances, and space maintainers) worn by the patient in the course

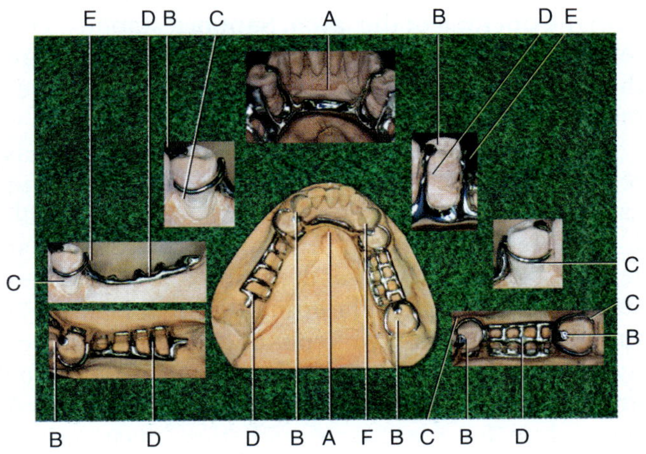

Figure 1-2 Mandibular framework designed for a partially edentulous arch with a Kennedy Classification II, modification 1 (see Chapter 3). Various component parts of the framework are labeled for identification. Subsequent chapters will describe their function, fabrication, and use. **A,** Major connector. **B,** Rests. **C,** Direct retainer. **D,** Minor connector. **E,** Guide plane. **F,** Indirect retainer.

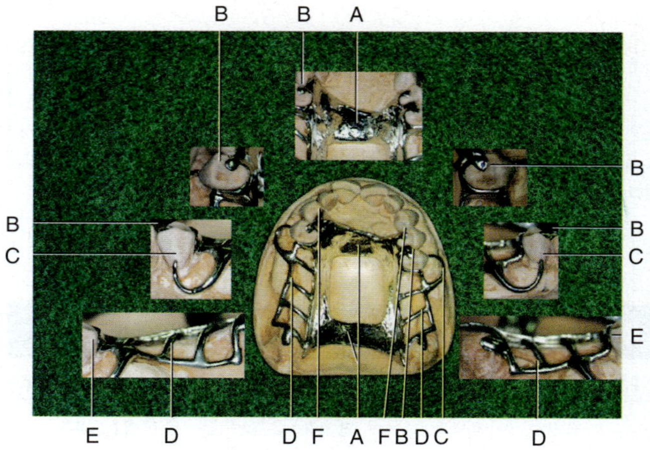

Figure 1-3 Maxillary framework designed for a partially edentulous arch with a Kennedy Classification I (see Chapter 3). As in Fig. 1-2, component parts are labeled for identification. **A,** Major connector. **B,** Rests. **C,** Direct retainer. **D,** Minor connector. **E,** Guide plane. **F,** Indirect retainer.

of treatment. A denture, an obturator, a fixed partial denture, or a crown is properly called a **prosthesis**. The terms *prosthesis, restoration,* and *denture* are equally acceptable terms and are used synonymously in this book.

Support is defined as the foundation on which a dental prosthesis rests, or to hold up and serve as a foundation. **Stability** is defined as the quality of a prosthesis to be firm, stable, or constant and to resist displacement by functional, horizontal, or rotational stresses. **Retention** is spoken of as that quality inherent in the denture that resists the vertical forces of dislodgment (e.g., the force of gravity, the adhesiveness of foods, or the forces associated with the opening of the jaws). Support, stability, and retention become more meaningful when they are thought of in terms of providing resistance to movement of a removable partial denture.

A **removable partial denture** is a prosthesis that replaces some teeth in a partially dentate arch, and can be removed from the mouth and replaced at will. A **complete denture** is a dental prosthesis that replaces all of the natural dentition and associated structures of the maxilla or mandible. It is entirely supported by tissues (mucous membrane, connective tissues, and underlying bone). An **interim,** or **provisional, denture** is a dental prosthesis used for a short time for reasons of esthetics, mastication, occlusal support, or convenience, or for conditioning the patient to accept an artificial substitute for missing natural teeth until a more definite prosthetic dental treatment can be provided.

An **abutment** is a tooth, a portion of a tooth, or a portion of an implant that serves to support and/or retain a prosthesis. The term **height of contour** is defined as a line encircling a tooth, designating its greatest circumference at a selected position determined by a dental surveyor. The term **undercut**, when used in reference to an abutment tooth, is that portion of a tooth that lies between the height of contour and the gingiva; when it is used in reference to other oral structures, undercut means the contour or cross section of a residual ridge or dental arch that would prevent the placement of a denture. The **angle of cervical convergence** is an angle viewed between a vertical rod contacting an abutment tooth and the axial surface of the abutment cervical to the height of contour.

Two or more vertically parallel surfaces of abutment teeth shaped to direct a prosthesis during placement and removal are called **guiding planes.** Guiding plane surfaces are parallel to the path of the placement and parallel to each other; preferably these surfaces are made parallel to the long axes of abutment teeth.

In a description of the various components of the partial denture, conflicting terminology must be recognized and the preferred terms defined. A **retainer** is defined as any type of clasp, attachment, device, etc., used for the fixation, stabilization, or retention of a prosthesis. A retainer may be either intracoronal or extracoronal and can be used as a means of retaining either a removable or a fixed restoration. A **direct retainer** is that component of a removable partial denture used to retain or prevent dislodgment. It consists of a clasp assembly or precision attachment. A **clasp assembly** is the part of a removable partial denture that acts as a direct retainer and/or stabilizer for a prosthesis by partially encompassing or contacting an abutment. A **clasp** (direct retainer) is the component of the clasp assembly that engages a portion of the tooth surface and either enters an undercut for retention or remains entirely above the height of contour to act as a reciprocating element. Generally it is used to stabilize or retain a removable prosthesis.

A **bar clasp** is a type of extracoronal retainer that originates from the denture base or framework, traverses soft tissue, and approaches the tooth undercut area from a gingival direction. In contrast, the term **circumferential clasp** is used to designate a clasp arm that originates above the height of contour and approaches the tooth undercut from an occlusal direction. Both types of clasp arms terminate in the area from the undercut to the height of contour, and both types provide retention through the resistance of metal to deformation rather than frictional resistance created by the contact of the clasp arm to the tooth.

The current *Glossary of Prosthodontic Terms* replaces the term **internal attachment** with the term **precision attachment**, which refers to an interlocking device, one component of which is fixed to an abutment or abutments, while the other is integrated into a removable prosthesis to stabilize and/or retain it. A **semiprecision rest** is a rigid metallic extension of a fixed or removable partial denture that fits into an intracoronal preparation in a cast restoration.

The term **indirect retainer** denotes a part of a removable partial denture that assists the direct retainers in preventing displacement of distal extension denture bases by resisting lever action from the opposite side of the fulcrum line.

A **major connector** is the part of a removable partial denture that connects the components on one side of the arch to the components on the opposite side of the arch. A **lingual bar connector** is a component of the partial denture framework located lingual to the dental arch and above the moving tissues of the floor of the mouth but as far below the gingival tissues as possible. In the mandible, when the lingual bar major connector is attached to a thin, contoured apron adjacent to the lingual surfaces of the anterior teeth, it is designated a **linguoplate**.

Any thin, broad palatal coverage that is used as a major connector is called a **palatal major connector**, or if it is of lesser width (less than 8 mm), it is called a **palatal bar**. A palatal major connector may be further described according to its anteroposterior location on the palatal surface, for example, as an anterior palatal major connector or a posterior palatal bar. The differentiation between a palatal bar and a **palatal strap** is somewhat subjective. A palatal strap is proportionally thinner and broader than a palatal bar. In this textbook a palatal major connector component that is less than 8 mm in width is referred to as a **bar**.

The term **rest** is used to designate any component of the partial denture that is placed on an abutment tooth, ideally in a prepared rest seat, so that it limits movement of the denture in a gingival direction and transmits functional forces to the tooth. When a rest is placed on the occlusal surface of a posterior tooth, it is designated an **occlusal rest**. If the rest occupies a position on the lingual surface of an anterior tooth, it is referred to as a **lingual rest**. A rest placed on the incisal edge of an anterior abutment tooth is called an **incisal rest**.

The residual bone, with its soft tissue that covers the underlying area of the denture base, is referred to as the **residual ridge** or **edentulous ridge**. The exact character of the soft tissue covering may vary, but it includes the mucous membrane and the underlying fibrous connective tissue. The oral tissues and structures of the residual ridge supporting a denture base are referred to as the **basal seat** or **denture foundation area. Denture base** is used to designate the part of a denture (whether it is metal or is made of a resinous material) that rests on the residual bone covered by soft tissue and to which the teeth are attached. Resurfacing of a denture base with new material to make it fit the underlying tissue more accurately is spoken of as **relining**. **Rebasing** refers to a process that goes beyond relining and involves the refitting of a denture by the replacement of the entire denture base with new material without changing the occlusal relations of the teeth.

The terms **functional impression** and **functional ridge form** are used to describe an impression and the resulting cast of the supporting form of the edentulous ridge. These terms have been accepted as meaning the form of the edentulous ridge when it is supporting a denture base. It is artificially created by means of a specially molded (individualized) impression tray or an impression material, or both, that displaces those tissues that can be readily displaced and that would be incapable of rendering support to the denture base when it is supporting functional load. Firm areas are not displaced because of the flow characteristics of the impression material, thus the tissues are recorded more nearly in the form they will assume when supporting a functional load. In contrast, the **static form** of the edentulous ridge, as often recorded in a soft impression material—such as hydrocolloid or metallic oxide impression paste, is referred to as the **anatomic ridge form** and results when an impression tray is uniformly relieved. This is the surface form of the edentulous ridge when at rest or when not supporting a functional load.

Perhaps no other terms in prosthodontics have been associated with more controversy than have **centric jaw relation** and **centric occlusion**. The use of these terms in this text will follow the definitions in the seventh edition of *The Glossary of Prosthodontic Terms.*

For complete dentures, centric occlusion is the occlusion that should be made to coincide with centric relation for that particular patient. In an adjustment of natural occlusion the objective may be to establish harmony between centric relation and centric occlusion. With removable partial dentures, the objective is to make the artificial occlusion coincide and be in harmony with the remaining natural occlusion. Ideally the natural occlusion will have been adjusted to harmonious contact in centric relation and be free of eccentric interference before occlusal relationships are established on the partial denture.

Balanced occlusion is a term that describes the contact of opposing teeth. It is defined as the simultaneous contacting of maxillary and mandibular teeth on the right and left in the anterior and posterior occlusal areas in centric or any eccentric position within the functional range.

Functional occlusal registration is sufficiently descriptive and is used to designate a dynamic registration of opposing dentition rather than the recording of a static relationship of one jaw to another. Though centric position is found somewhere in a functional occlusal registration, eccentric positions are also recorded, and the created occlusion is made to harmonize with all the gliding and chewing movements that the patient is capable of making.

Cast is used most frequently in this text as a noun to designate an accurate and positive reproduction of a maxillary or mandibular dental arch made from an impression of that arch. It is further designated according to the purpose for which it is made, such as *diagnostic cast, master cast,* or *investment cast.* The word *cast* is preferable to the term *model,* which should be used only to designate a reproduction for display or demonstration purposes.

The word **cast** may be used as an infinitive (to cast) or as an adjective (cast framework, or cast metal base). An **investment cast** also may be referred to as a **refractory cast** because it is compounded to withstand high temperatures without disintegrating and, incidentally, to perform certain functions relative to the burnout and expansion of the mold. A **refractory investment** is an investment material that can withstand the high temperatures of casting or soldering. Plaster of Paris and artificial stone also may be considered investment if either is used to invest any part of a dental restoration for processing. Use of the term **mold** is also incorrect when referring to a reproduction of a dental arch or a portion thereof. The word mold is used to indicate either the cavity into which a casting is made or the shape of an artificial tooth.

A **wax pattern** is converted to a casting by the elimination of the pattern by heat, leaving a mold into which the molten metal is forced by centrifugal force or other means. **Casting** is therefore used most frequently as a noun, meaning a metal object shaped by being poured into a mold to harden. It is used primarily to designate the cast metal framework of a partial denture but also may be used to describe a molded metal denture base that is actually cast into a mold.

Dental stones are used to form an artificial stone reproduction from an impression, and they are used as an investment or for mounting purposes. All dental stones are gypsum products. Use of the word **stone** in dentistry should be applied only to those gypsum materials that are employed for their hardness, accuracy, or abrasion resistance.

A **dental cast surveyor** is an instrument used to determine the relative parallelism of two or more axial surfaces of teeth or other parts of a cast of a dental arch. This instrument is used to locate and delineate the contours and relative positions of abutment teeth and associated structures.

Some controversy exists over the use of the terms **x-ray, radiograph**, and **roentgenogram** in dentistry. Examination of several recent textbooks on dental subjects finds usage divided between all three terms. However, in deference to the terminology preferred by the American Academy of Oral Roentgenology, the terms roentgenogram, roentgenographic survey, and roentgenographic interpretation are used herein.

Use of the term **acrylic** as a noun is avoided. Instead it is used only as an adjective, such as **acrylic resin**. The word **plastic** may be used either as an adjective or a noun. In the latter sense, it refers to any of various substances that harden and retain their shape after being molded. The term **resin** is used broadly for substances named according to their chemical composition, physical structure, and means for activation or curing, such as acrylic resin.

REFERENCES

1. Glossary of prosthodontic terms, J Prosthet Dent; 81: 41-110, 1999.
2. Mosby's dental dictionary, St. Louis, 2004, Mosby.

2

CLASP-RETAINED PARTIAL DENTURE

POINTS OF VIEW

In Chapter 1 we introduced some of the basic differences between removable partial dentures and other types of prostheses. In this chapter we will highlight differences between the major categories of removable partial dentures by referencing the natural dentition and fixed partial dentures.

Considering tooth replacement prostheses from a patient's perspective, the desire is to replace teeth that serve functional and social roles in their everyday life. In considering how well various types of prostheses may meet their specific needs, it is helpful to consider what features of the original dentition—the gold standard in this instance—we strive to duplicate in the replacement. Although it is common to find that the existing oral condition(s) does not easily allow complete restoration to the state of a fully dentate patient, considering the respective strengths and weaknesses of the prosthodontic options (compared with this "gold standard") helps identify realistic expectations.

In this text the focus will be on a type of replacement prosthesis for patients with some, but not all, missing teeth. The replacement prosthesis ideally should provide the function and a level of comfort as equivalent as possible to a normal dentition. To do this, stability while chewing is a primary focus of attention, and we should strive to determine what is required to ensure it. If the prosthesis will be visible during casual speaking, smiling, and/or laughing, it is obvious that the replacement should look as natural as the surrounding environment. In summary, tooth replacement prostheses should provide a combination of several features found with natural teeth: socially acceptable in appearance, comfortable and stable in function, and these should be maintained throughout their serviceable lifetime at a reasonable cost.

Tooth-Supported

For partially edentulous patients the prosthetic options available include natural tooth-supported fixed partial dentures, removable partial dentures, and implant-supported fixed partial dentures. How well these options restore and maintain the features of natural teeth mentioned above depends to a large extent on the numbers and location of the missing teeth. The major categories of partial tooth loss (see Chapter 3) are those (1) with teeth anterior and posterior to the space (a tooth-supported space) and (2) those with teeth either anterior or posterior to the space (a tooth- and tissue-supported space). All of the prosthetic options listed are available for the tooth-bound space (though not necessarily are they all indicated for every clinical situation), but only removable partial dentures and implant-supported prostheses are available for the distal extension.

Removable partial dentures can be designed in various ways to use abutment teeth and supporting tissue for stability, support, and retention of the prosthesis. When dealing with the tooth-bound spaces the removable partial denture in some respects is like a fixed partial denture because natural teeth alone provide direct resistance to functional forces. Because natural teeth support the prosthesis, it should not move under these functional forces. In this condition the interface between or relationship of the removable partial denture framework and abutment teeth should be designed to take advantage of the tooth support—similar to the relationship between a fixed partial denture retainer and prepared tooth. This means providing positive vertical support (rest preparations) and a restrictive angle of dislodgment (opposing guide planes). Put another way, when the removable partial denture is selected for a tooth-bound situation, stability under functional load should be as well controlled as that seen when a fixed partial denture is used if appropriate tooth preparation is provided. Since the removable partial denture clasps do not completely encircle the tooth as a fixed partial denture retainer, they must be designed to engage more than half the circumference to allow the prosthesis to maintain position under the influence of horizontal chewing loads. It should be obvious that careful planning and execution of the necessary natural tooth contour modifications are required to assure movement control and functional stability for removable partial dentures supported by teeth. The similarities between the prosthesis-tooth interface for fixed partial dentures and removable partial dentures are highlighted to emphasize the modification principles required to assure stability for movement control in removable partial dentures. Over time the natural tooth support can be maintained like the fixed partial denture. Chapter 14 helps explain how this is accomplished when producing natural tooth modifications or surveyed crowns.

Tooth- and Tissue-Supported

For removable partial dentures that do not have the benefit of natural tooth support at each end of the replacement teeth (the extension base removable partial denture), it is necessary that the residual ridge be used to assist in the functional stability of the prosthesis. When a removable partial denture is selected for a tooth-tissue-supported arch, the prosthesis must be designed to allow functional movement of the base to the extent expected by the residual ridge mucosa. This mucosa movement "extent" is variable, but for healthy residual ridge (masticatory) mucosa, movement from 1 to 3 mm can be expected. Consequently, unlike the tooth-bound space, tooth modification for the tooth-tissue-supported prosthesis must be designed with the dual goal of framework tooth contact to allow appropriate functional stability from the tooth but with allowance for the anticipated vertical and/or horizontal movement of the extension base. This introduces the concept of anticipated movement with a prosthesis and suggests our role in designing prostheses to appropriately control the movement. Additionally, since the tissue support in the tooth-tissue removable partial denture predictably changes with time, to continue to maintain movement control we must carefully monitor our patients to maintain support and assure maximum prosthetic function.

The clasp-retained partial denture, with extracoronal direct retainers, is probably used a hundred times more than is the precision attachment partial denture (Figure 2-1). Although the clasp-retained partial denture has disadvantages, for reasons of cost and time devoted to fabrication, it will continue to be widely used because it is capable of providing physiologically sound treatment for most patients needing partial denture restorations. The following are some of the possible disadvantages of a clasp-retained partial denture:

1. Strain on the abutment teeth often is caused by improper tooth preparation, clasp design, and/or loss of tissue support under distal extension partial denture bases.
2. Clasps can be unesthetic, particularly when they are placed on visible tooth surfaces.
3. Caries may develop beneath clasp components, especially if the patient fails to keep the prosthesis and the abutments clean.

Despite these disadvantages, the use of removable prostheses may be preferred whenever tooth-bounded edentulous spaces are too large to be restored safely with fixed prostheses or when cross-arch stabilization and wider distribution of forces to supporting teeth and tissues are desirable. Fixed partial dentures, however, should always be considered and used when indicated.

The removable partial denture retained by internal attachments eliminates some of the disadvantages of clasps, but it also has other disadvantages—one of which is too great a cost for a large percentage of patients needing partial dentures. However, when the alignment of the abutment teeth is favorable, the periodontal health and bone support are adequate, the clinical crown is of sufficient length, the pulp morphology can accommodate the required tooth preparation, and the economic status of the patient permits, an internal attachment prosthesis is unquestionably preferable for esthetic reasons. In most instances, if the extracoronal clasp-retained partial denture is designed properly, the only advantage of the internal attachment denture is esthetics because abutment protection and stabilizing components should be used with both internal and external retainers. However, economics permitting, esthetics

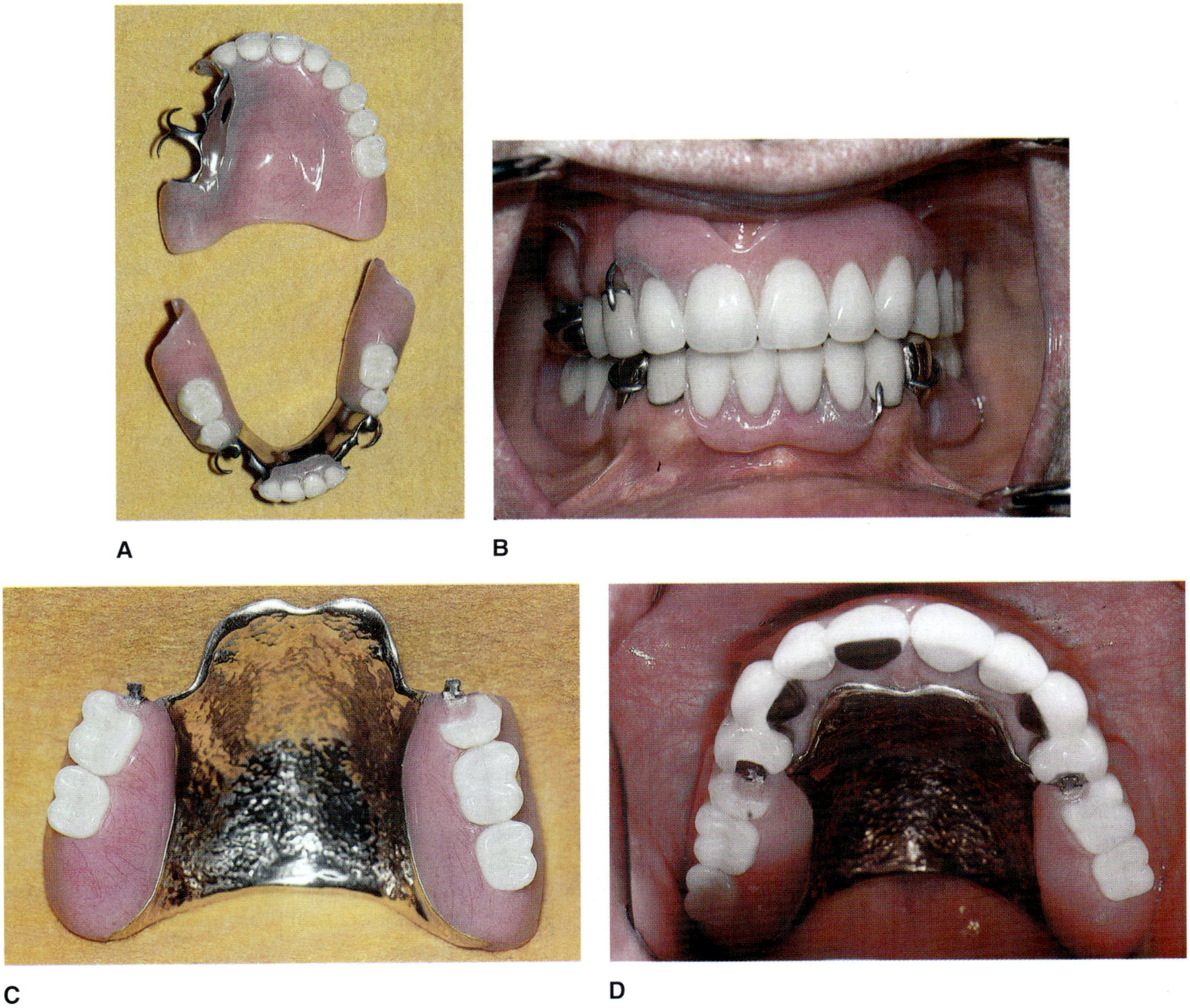

Figure 2-1 **A,** Maxillary and mandibular clasp-retained removable partial dentures. All clasps are extracoronal retainers (clasps) on abutments. **B,** Prostheses from **(A)** shown intraorally in occlusion. **C,** Maxillary prosthesis using intracoronal retainers and full palatal coverage. The male portions of the attachments are shown at the mesial position of the artificial teeth and will fit into intracoronal rests. **D,** Internal attachment prosthesis in the patient's mouth. Note the precise fit of male and female portions of the attachments.

alone may justify the use of internal attachment retainers. Injudicious use of internal attachments can lead to excessive torsional load on the abutments supporting distal extension removable partial dentures, especially in the mandible.

The use of hinges or other types of stress breakers is discouraged in these situations. It is not that they are ineffective, but they are frequently misused. As an example, in the mandibular arch, a stress-broken distal extension partial denture does not provide for cross-arch stabilization and frequently subjects the edentulous ridge to excessive trauma from horizontal and torquing forces. Therefore a rigid design is preferred, and some type of extracoronal clasp retainer is still the most logical and frequently used. It seems likely that its use will continue until a more widely acceptable retainer is devised.

As reviewed in Chapter 1, the most commonly cited problem associated with removable partial dentures was instability. Healthy natural teeth should not move when used, therefore, we should strive to provide and maintain as stable a prosthesis as possible given the means available. How do we assure functional stability? By understanding that a removable partial denture can move under function (since it is not cemented to teeth like a fixed partial denture).

We should take steps to prescribe the necessary prosthetic fit to teeth (and tissue) to control the movement as much as possible. This entails providing appropriate natural tooth mouth preparations, ensuring an accurate frame fit at tooth and tissue, providing a simultaneous contacting relationship between natural and prosthetic opposing teeth, and providing and maintaining optimum support from the soft tissue and teeth.

As we will review in Chapter 4 , control of the anticipated movement of your prosthesis is addressed by assigning the appropriate component part of the prosthesis to contact/engage the tooth or tissue in a manner that allows movement **and** removal of the prostheses. Are there movements that we should control for that are more important than others? Of course we need to resist movement away from the teeth and tissue to prevent prostheses falling out of mouths. However, the most damaging forces are those from functional closure while chewing (and in some patients parafunction). Consequently, control of combined vertical (tissue wound) and horizontal movement is most critical and places a premium on tooth modifications (rest and stabilizing component preparations) and verifying adequate fitting of the frame to the teeth.

SIX PHASES OF PARTIAL DENTURE SERVICE

Partial denture service may be logically divided into six phases. The first phase is related to patient education. The second phase includes diagnosis, treatment planning, design of the partial denture framework, treatment sequencing, and execution of mouth preparations. The third phase is the provision of adequate support for the distal extension denture base. The fourth phase is establishment and verification of harmonious occlusal relationships and tooth relationships with opposing and remaining natural teeth. The fifth phase involves initial placement procedures, including adjustments to the contours and bearing surfaces of denture bases, adjustments to ensure occlusal harmony, and a review of instructions given the patient to optimally maintain oral structures and the provided restorations. The sixth and final phase of partial denture service is follow-up services by the dentist through recall appointments for periodic evaluation of the responses of oral tissue to restorations and of the acceptance of the restorations by the patient. The following is an overview of these phases. The context of each phase is discussed in greater detail in the respective chapters of this book.

Education of Patient

The term *patient education* is described in *Mosby's Dental Dictionary* as "the process of informing a patient about a health matter to secure informed consent, patient cooperation, and a high level of patient compliance."

The dentist and the patient share responsibility for the ultimate success of a removable partial denture. It is folly to assume that a patient will have an understanding of the benefits of a removable partial denture unless he or she is so informed. It is also unlikely that the patient will have the knowledge to avoid misuse of the restoration or be able to provide the required oral care and maintenance procedures to ensure the success of the partial denture unless he or she is adequately advised.

The finest biologically oriented removable partial denture is often doomed to limited success if the patient fails to exercise proper oral hygiene habits or ignores recall appointments. Preservation of the oral structures, one of the primary objectives of prosthodontic treatment, will be compromised without the patient's cooperation in oral hygiene and regular maintenance visits.

Patient education should begin at the initial contact with the patient and continue throughout treatment. This educational procedure is especially important when the treatment plan and prognosis are discussed with the patient. The limitations imposed on the success of treatment through failure of the patient to accept responsibility must be explained before definitive treatment is undertaken. A patient will not usually retain all the information presented in the oral educational instructions. For this reason, patients should be given written suggestions to reinforce the oral presentations.

Diagnosis, Treatment Planning, Design, Treatment Sequencing, and Mouth Preparation

Treatment planning and design begin with thorough medical and dental histories. The complete oral examination must include both clinical and radiographic interpretation of (1) caries, (2) the condition of existing restorations, (3) periodontal conditions, (4) responses of teeth (especially abutment teeth) and residual ridges to previous stress, and (5) the vitality of remaining teeth. Additionally, evaluation of the occlusal plane, the arch form, and the occlusal relations of the remaining teeth must be meticulously accomplished by clinical visual evaluation and diagnostic mounting. After a complete diagnostic examination has been accomplished and a removable partial denture has been selected as the treatment of choice, a treatment plan is sequenced and a partial denture design is developed based on the support available.

The dental cast surveyor (Figure 2-2) is an absolute necessity in any dental office in which patients are being treated with removable partial dentures. The surveyor is instrumental in diagnosing and guiding

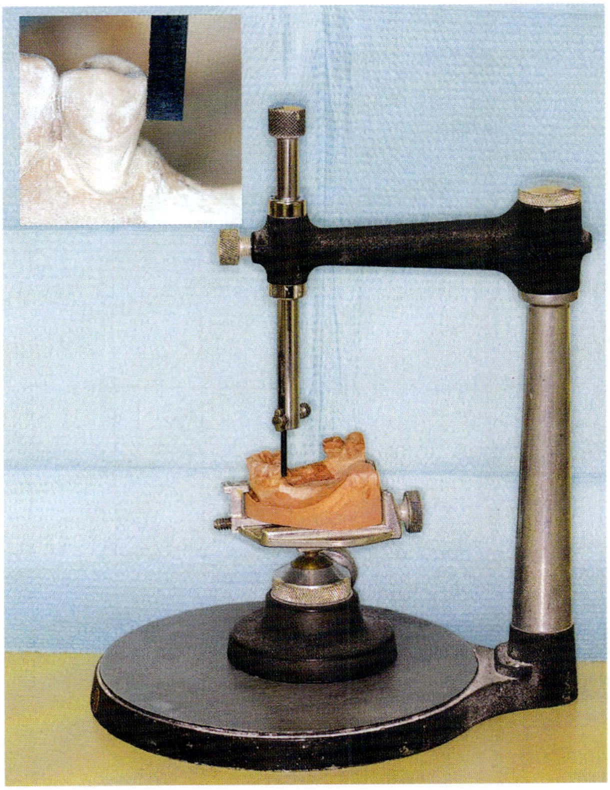

Figure 2-2 Dental cast surveyor facilitates the design of a removable partial denture. It is an instrument by which parallelism or lack of parallelism of abutment teeth and other oral structures, on a stone cast, can be determined (magnified view shows parallel guide plane surface). Use of the surveyor is covered in succeeding chapters.

the appropriate tooth preparation and verifying that the mouth preparation has been performed correctly. There is no more reason to justify its omission from a dentist's armamentarium than there is to ignore the need for roentgenographic equipment, the mouth mirror and explorer, or the periodontal probe used for diagnostic purposes.

Several moderately priced surveyors that adequately accomplish the diagnostic procedures necessary for designing the partial denture are available. In many dental offices, this most important phase of dental diagnosis is delegated to the commercial dental laboratory because this invaluable diagnostic tool is absent or because the dentist is apathetic. This situation places the technician in the role of diagnostician. Any clinical treatment based on the diagnosis of the technician remains the responsibility of the dentist. This makes no more sense than relying on the technician to interpret roentgenograms and to render a diagnosis.

After treatment planning, a predetermined sequence of mouth preparations can be performed with a definite goal in mind. It is mandatory that the treatment plan be reviewed to ensure the mouth preparation necessary to accommodate the removable partial denture design has been properly sequenced. Mouth preparations, in the appropriate sequence, should be oriented toward the goal of providing adequate support, stability, retention, and a harmonious occlusion for the partial denture. Placing a crown or restoring a tooth out of sequence may result in the need to restore teeth that were not planned for restoration, or it may necessitate remaking a restoration or even seriously jeopardizing the success of the removable partial denture. Through the aid of diagnostic casts on which the tentative design of the partial denture has been outlined and the mouth preparations have been indicated in colored pencil, occlusal adjustments, abutment restorations, and abutment modifications can be accomplished.

Support for Distal Extension Denture Bases

The third of the six phases in the treatment of a patient with a partial denture is obtaining adequate support for distal extension bases. Therefore it does not apply to tooth-supported removable partial dentures. In the latter, support comes entirely from the abutment teeth through the use of rests.

For the distal extension partial denture, however, a base made to fit the anatomic ridge form does not provide adequate support under occlusal loading (Figure 2-3). Neither does it provide for maximum border extension nor accurate border detail. Therefore some type of corrected impression is necessary. This may be accomplished by several means, any of which satisfy the requirements for support of any distal extension partial denture base.

Foremost is the requirement that certain soft tissue in the primary supporting area should be recorded or related under some loading so that the base may be made to fit the form of the ridge when under function. This provides support and ensures the maintenance of that support for the longest possible time. This requirement makes the distal extension partial denture unique in that the support from the tissue underlying the distal extension base must be made as equal to and compatible with the tooth support as possible.

A complete denture is entirely tissue supported, and the entire denture can move toward the tissue under function. In contrast, any movement of a partial denture base is inevitably a rotational movement that, if toward the tissue, may result in undesirable torquing forces to the abutment teeth and loss of planned occlusal contacts. Therefore every effort must be made to provide the best possible support for the distal extension base to minimize these forces.

Usually no single impression technique can adequately record the anatomic form of the teeth and adjacent structures and at the same time record the supporting form of the mandibular edentulous ridge.

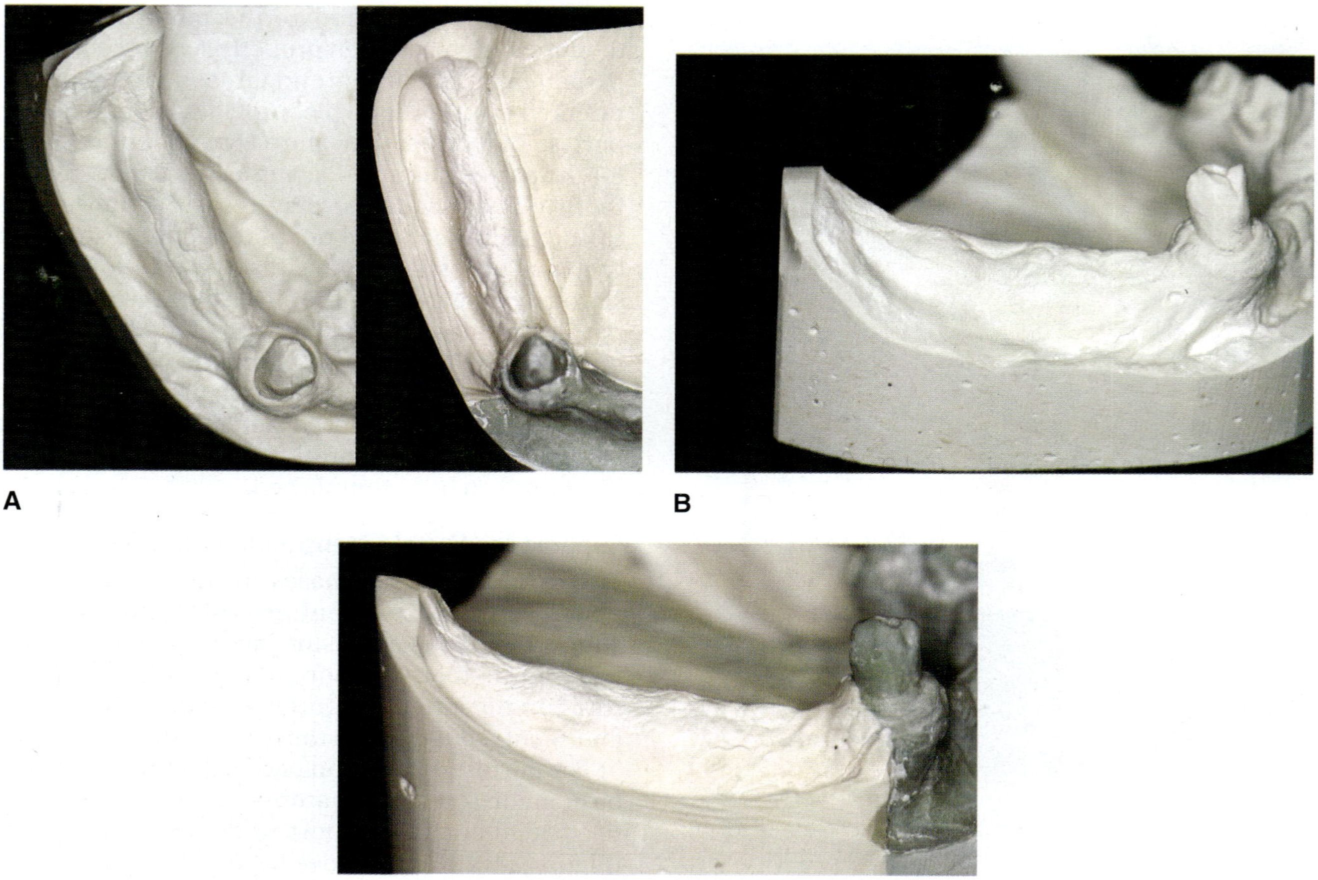

A

B

C

Figure 2-3 **A,** Occlusal view of a cast from a preliminary impression, which produced an anatomic ridge form *(left)*, and an altered cast of the same ridge showing a functional or supportive form *(right)*. The altered cast impression selectively placed pressure to the buccal shelf region, which is the primary stress-bearing area of the mandibular posterior residual ridge. **B,** Buccal view of anatomic ridge form. **C,** Buccal view of functional or supportive ridge form. Note that the supportive form of the ridge clearly delineates the extent of coverage available for a denture base and is most different from the anatomic form when the mucosa is easily displaced.

A method should be used that can record these tissues either in their supporting form or in a supporting relationship to the rest of the denture (see Figure 2-3). This may be accomplished by one of several methods that will be discussed in Chapter 16.

Establishment and Verification of Occlusal Relations and Tooth Arrangements

Whether the partial denture is tooth supported or has one or more distal extension bases, the recording and verification of occlusal relationships and tooth arrangement are important steps in the construction of a partial denture. For the tooth-supported partial denture, ridge form is of less significance than it is for the tooth- and tissue-supported prosthesis, because the ridge is not called on to support the prosthesis. For the distal extension base, however, jaw relation records should be made only after obtaining the best possible support for the denture base. This necessitates the making of a base or bases that will provide the same support as the finished denture. Therefore the final jaw relations should not be recorded until after the denture framework has been returned to the dentist, the fit of the framework to the abutment teeth and opposing occlusion has been verified and corrected, and a corrected impression has been made. Then either a new resin base or a corrected base must be used to record jaw relations.

Occlusal records for a removable partial denture may be made by the various methods described in Chapter 17.

Initial Placement Procedures

The fifth phase of treatment occurs when the patient is given possession of the removable prosthesis.

Inevitably it seems that minute changes in the planned occlusal relationships occur during processing of the dentures. Not only must occlusal harmony be ensured before the patient is given possession of the dentures, but also the processed bases must be reasonably perfected to fit the basal seats. It must also be ascertained that the patient understands the suggestions and recommendations given by the dentist for care of the dentures and oral structures and understands about expectations in the adjustment phases and use of the restorations. These facets of treatment are discussed in detail in Chapter 20.

Periodic Recall

Initial placement and adjustment of the prosthesis is certainly not the end of treatment for the partially edentulous patient. Periodic reevaluation of the patient is critical for early recognition of changes in the oral structures to allow steps to be taken to maintain oral health. These examinations must monitor the condition of the oral tissue, the response to the tooth restorations, the prosthesis, the patient's acceptance, and the patient's commitment to maintain oral hygiene. Although a 6-month recall period is adequate for most patients, a more frequent evaluation may be required for some. Chapter 20 contains some suggestions concerning this sixth phase of treatment.

REASONS FOR FAILURE OF CLASP-RETAINED PARTIAL DENTURES

Experience with the clasp-retained partial denture made by the methods outlined has proved its merit and justifies its continued use. The occasional objection to the visibility of retentive clasps can be minimized through the use of wrought-wire clasp arms. There are few contraindications for use of a properly designed clasp-retained partial denture. Practically all objections to this type of denture can be eliminated by pointing to deficiencies in mouth preparation, denture design and fabrication, and patient education. These include the following:

Diagnosis and treatment planning

1. Inadequate diagnosis
2. Failure to use a surveyor or to use a surveyor properly during treatment planning

Mouth preparation procedures

1. Failure to properly sequence mouth preparation procedures
2. Inadequate mouth preparations, usually resulting from insufficient planning of the design of the partial denture or failure to determine that mouth preparations have been properly accomplished
3. Failure to return supporting tissue to optimum health before impression procedures
4. Inadequate impressions of hard and soft tissue

Design of the framework

1. Failure to use properly located and sized rests
2. Flexible or incorrectly located major and minor connectors
3. Incorrect use of clasp designs
4. Use of cast clasps that have too little flexibility, are too broad in tooth coverage, and have too little consideration for esthetics

Laboratory procedures

1. Problems in master cast preparation
   a. Inaccurate impression
   b. Poor cast-forming procedures
   c. Incompatible impression materials and gypsum products
2. Failure to provide the technician with a specific design and necessary information to enable the technician to execute the design
3. Failure of the technician to follow the design and written instructions

Support for denture bases

1. Inadequate coverage of basal seat tissue
2. Failure to record basal seat tissue in a supporting form

Occlusion

1. Failure to develop a harmonious occlusion
2. Failure to use compatible materials for opposing occlusal surfaces

Patient-dentist relationship

1. Failure of the dentist to provide adequate dental health care information, including care and use of prosthesis
2. Failure of the dentist to provide recall opportunities on a periodic basis
3. Failure of the patient to exercise a dental health care regimen and respond to recall

A removable partial denture designed and fabricated so that it avoids the errors and deficiencies listed is one that proves the clasp-type of partial denture can be made functional, esthetically pleasing, and long lasting without damage to the supporting structures. The proof of the merit of this type of restoration lies in the knowledge that (1) it permits treatment for the largest number of patients at a reasonable cost; (2) it provides restorations that are comfortable and efficient over a long period of time, with adequate support and maintenance of occlusal contact relations; (3) it can provide for healthy abutments, free of caries and periodontal disease; (4) it can provide for the continued health of restored, healthy tissue of the basal seats; and (5) it makes possible a partial denture service that is definitive and not merely an interim treatment.

Removable partial dentures thus made will contribute to a concept of prosthetic dentistry that has as its goal the promotion of oral health, the restoration of partially edentulous mouths, and the elimination of the ultimate need for complete dentures.

SELF-ASSESSMENT AIDS

1. In chronological order of accomplishment, give the six sequential, correlated phases in treating a partially edentulous patient with removable prostheses.
2. If the dentist and the patient share responsibility for the success of treatment, what must be undertaken to prepare patients to accept their responsibility?
3. Because treatment planning is the sole responsibility of the dentist, which if any of the following may be omitted as noncontributory to total treatment: (1) a complete health history, (2) a history of past dental experiences, (3) an oral examination, (4) a radiographic examination, (5) an evaluation of occlusal relations of remaining teeth, (6) a survey of diagnostic casts, (7) cost, or (8) patient desires?
4. A specific design of the removable restoration must be planned before mouth preparation procedures. The dentist (*can—should not*) delegate the responsibility for the design to a dental laboratory technician.
5. Stability in a removable restoration (*is—is not*) desirable to help maintain the health of oral structures. A tooth-supported restoration usually (*can—cannot*) be made more stable than a restoration supported by teeth and residual ridges.
6. In the fifth phase of treatment (initial placement of the restorations), three things are done before the patient is given possession of the denture(s). Two of these are (1) correction of denture base contours and occlusal discrepancies that may have resulted from processing and (2) review of patient education, including adjustment expectations. What other step must be accomplished during the appointment?
7. What is the purpose of periodic recall of patients treated with removable partial dentures?
8. What is the one predominant reason why the clasp-type of partial denture is used more often in most practices than is the internal attachment type of prosthesis?
9. Deficiencies in design and fabrication and those related to patient education are the culprits of limited success in treatment with removable prostheses. Avoiding these deficiencies will make the goal of prosthetic dentistry obtainable. This goal is to ______, ______, and ______.

3

CLASSIFICATION OF PARTIALLY EDENTULOUS ARCHES

Even though recent reports have shown a consistent decline in the prevalence of tooth loss during the past few decades, there remains significant variation in tooth loss distribution. It would be most helpful to consider which combinations of tooth loss are most common and to classify these for the purpose of assisting our management of partially edentulous patients. Several classifications of partially edentulous arches have been proposed and are in use. This variety has led to some confusion and disagreement concerning which classification best describes all possible configurations and should be adopted.

The most familiar classifications are those originally proposed by Kennedy, Cummer, and Bailyn. Beckett, Godfrey, Swenson, Friedman, Wilson, Skinner, Applegate, Avant, Miller, and others have also proposed classifications. It is evident that an attempt should be made to combine the best features of all classifications so that a universal classification can be adopted.

A recent classification has been proposed for partial edentulism that is based on diagnostic criteria.[1] The purpose of this system of classification is to facilitate treatment decisions based on treatment complexity. Complexity is determined from four broad diagnostic categories that include: location and extent of the edentulous areas, condition of the abutments, occlusal characteristics and requirements, and residual ridge characteristics. The advantage of this classification system over those in standard use has yet to be documented.

The Kennedy method of classification is probably the most widely accepted classification of partially edentulous arches today. In an attempt to simplify the problem and encourage more universal use of a classification and in the interest of adequate communication, the Kennedy classification will be used in this textbook. The student can refer to the Selected Reading Resources section for information relative to other classifications.

Although classifications are actually descriptive of the partially edentulous arches, the removable partial denture restoring a particular class of arch is described as a denture of that class. For example, we speak of a Class III or Class I removable partial denture. It is simpler to say "a Class II partial denture" than it is to say "a partial denture restoring a Class II partially edentulous arch."

REQUIREMENTS OF AN ACCEPTABLE METHOD OF CLASSIFICATION

The classification of a partially edentulous arch should satisfy the following requirements:

1. It should permit immediate visualization of the type of partially edentulous arch that is being considered.
2. It should permit immediate differentiation between the tooth-supported and the tooth- and tissue-supported removable partial denture.
3. It should be universally acceptable.

KENNEDY CLASSIFICATION

The Kennedy method of classification was originally proposed by Dr. Edward Kennedy in 1925. Like the Bailyn and Skinner classifications, it attempts to classify the partially edentulous arch in a manner that suggests certain principles of design for a given situation (Figure 3-1).

Kennedy divided all partially edentulous arches into four basic classes. Edentulous areas other than those determining the basic classes were designated as modification spaces (Figure 3-2).

The following is the Kennedy classification:

Class I Bilateral edentulous areas located posterior to the natural teeth

Class II A unilateral edentulous area located posterior to the remaining natural teeth

Class III A unilateral edentulous area with natural teeth remaining both anterior and posterior to it

Class IV A single, but bilateral (crossing the midline), edentulous area located anterior to the remaining natural teeth

One of the principal advantages of the Kennedy method is that it permits immediate visualization of the partially edentulous arch and allows easy distinction between tooth-supported versus tooth- and tissue-supported prostheses. Those schooled in its use and in the principles of partial denture design can readily relate the arch configuration design to be used in the basic partial denture. This method permits a logical approach to the problems of design. It makes possible the application of sound principles of partial denture design and is therefore a logical method of classification. However, a classification

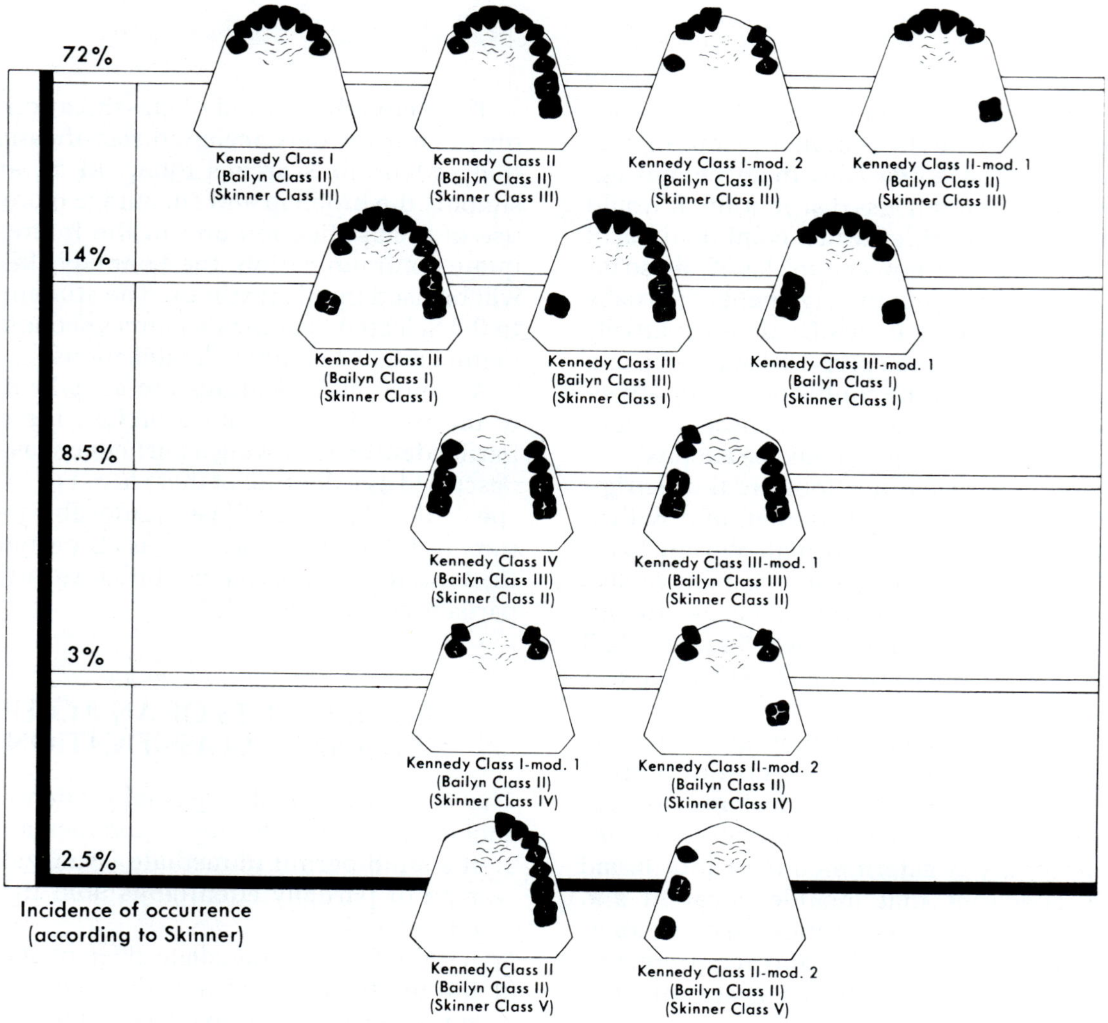

Figure 3-1 Representative examples of partially edentulous arches classified by the Kennedy, Bailyn, and Skinner methods.

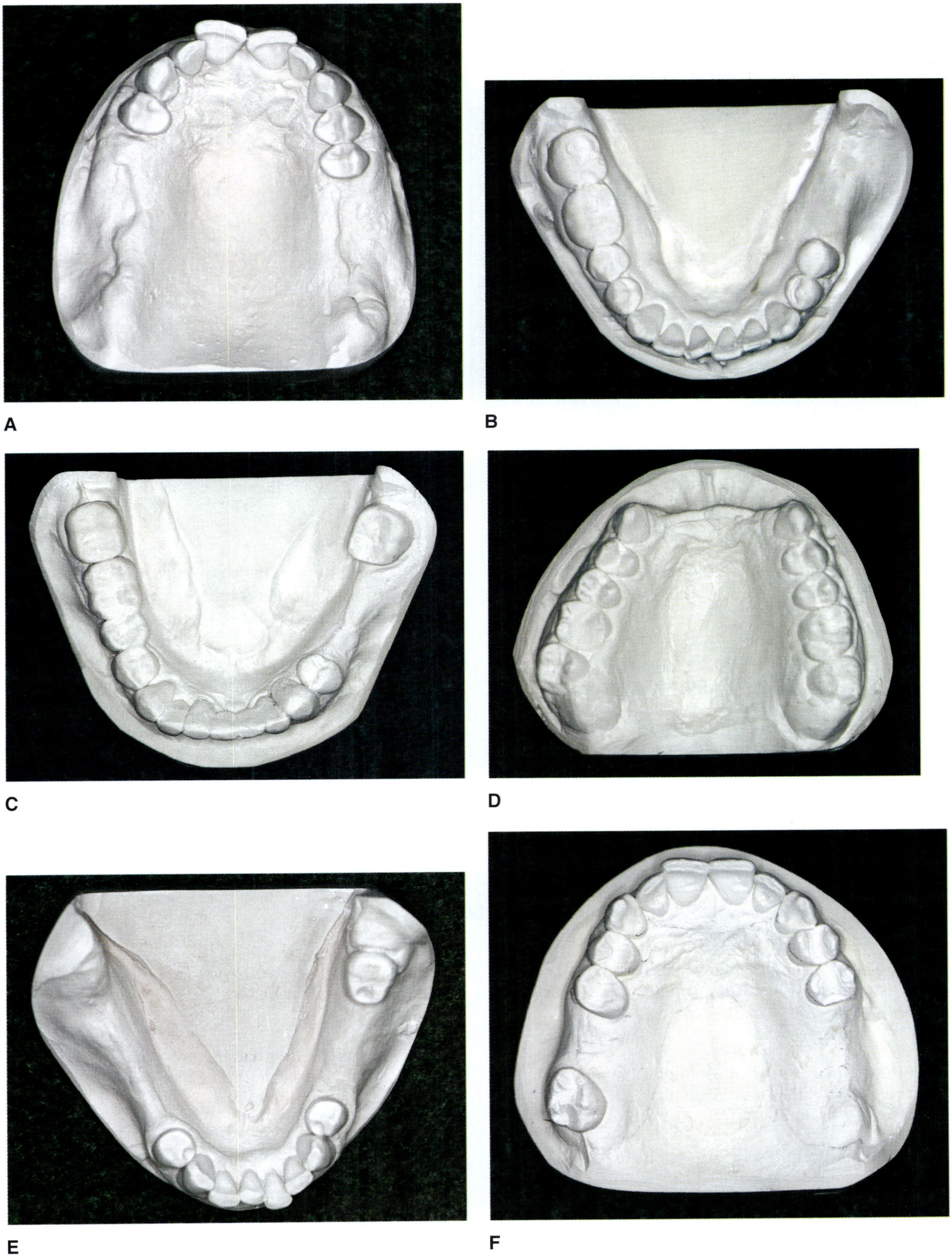

Figure 3-2 Kennedy classification with examples of modifications. **A,** Class I maxillary arch. **B,** Class II mandibular arch. **C,** Class III mandibular arch. **D,** Class IV maxillary arch. **E,** Class II, modification 1 mandibular arch. **F,** Class II, modification 1 maxillary arch.

Continued

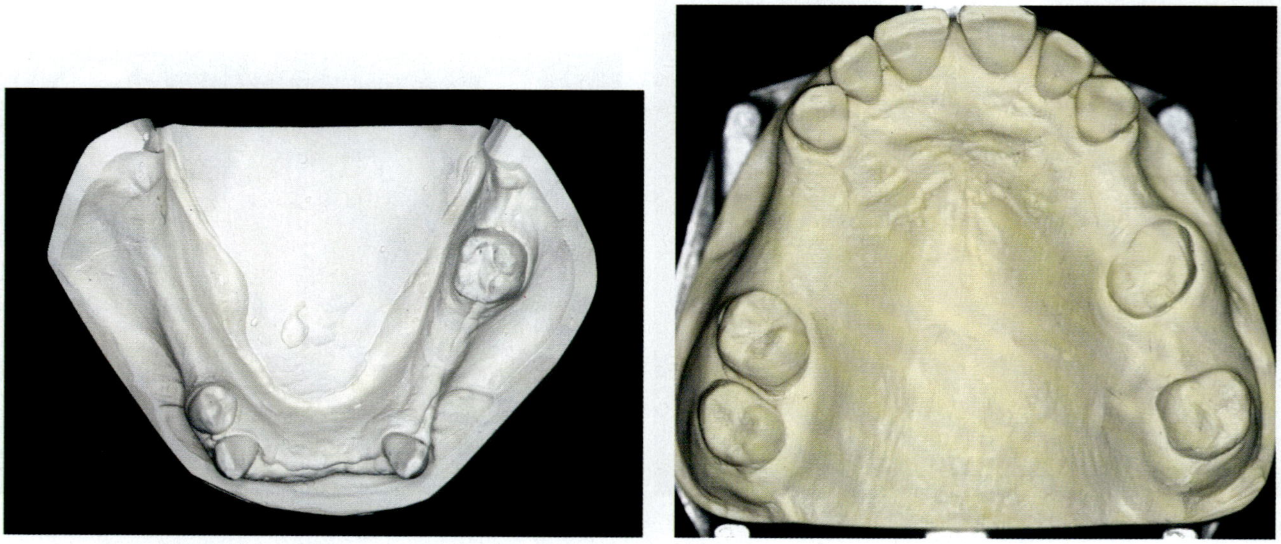

G H

Figure 3-2 Cont'd **G,** Class II, modification 2 mandibular arch. **H,** Class III, modification 2 maxillary arch.

system should not be used to stereotype or limit the concepts of design.

APPLEGATE'S RULES FOR APPLYING THE KENNEDY CLASSIFICATION

The Kennedy classification would be difficult to apply to every situation without certain rules for application. Applegate provided eight rules governing the application of the Kennedy method (Box 3-1).

Although there may be some confusion initially as to why Class I should refer to two edentulous areas and Class II should refer to one, the principles of design make this distinction logical. Kennedy placed the Class II unilateral distal extension type between the Class I bilateral distal extension type and the Class III tooth-supported classification because the Class II partial denture must embody features of both, especially when tooth-supported modifications are present. Because it has a tissue-supported extension base, it must be designed similarly to a Class I partial denture. Often, however, there is a

BOX 3-1 Rules Governing the Application of the Kennedy Method

Rule 1

Classification should follow rather than precede any extractions of teeth that might alter the original classification.

Rule 2

If a third molar is missing and not to be replaced, it is not considered in the classification.

Rule 3

If a third molar is present and is to be used as an abutment, it is considered in the classification.

Rule 4

If a second molar is missing and is not to be replaced, it is not considered in the classification (e.g., if the opposing second molar is likewise missing and is not to be replaced).

Rule 5

The most posterior edentulous area (or areas) always determines the classification.

Rule 6

Edentulous areas other than those determining the classification are referred to as *modifications* and are designated by their number.

Rule 7

The extent of the modification is not considered, only the number of additional edentulous areas.

Rule 8

There can be no modification areas in Class IV arches. (Other edentulous areas lying posterior to the single bilateral areas crossing the midline would instead determine the classification; see Rule 5.)

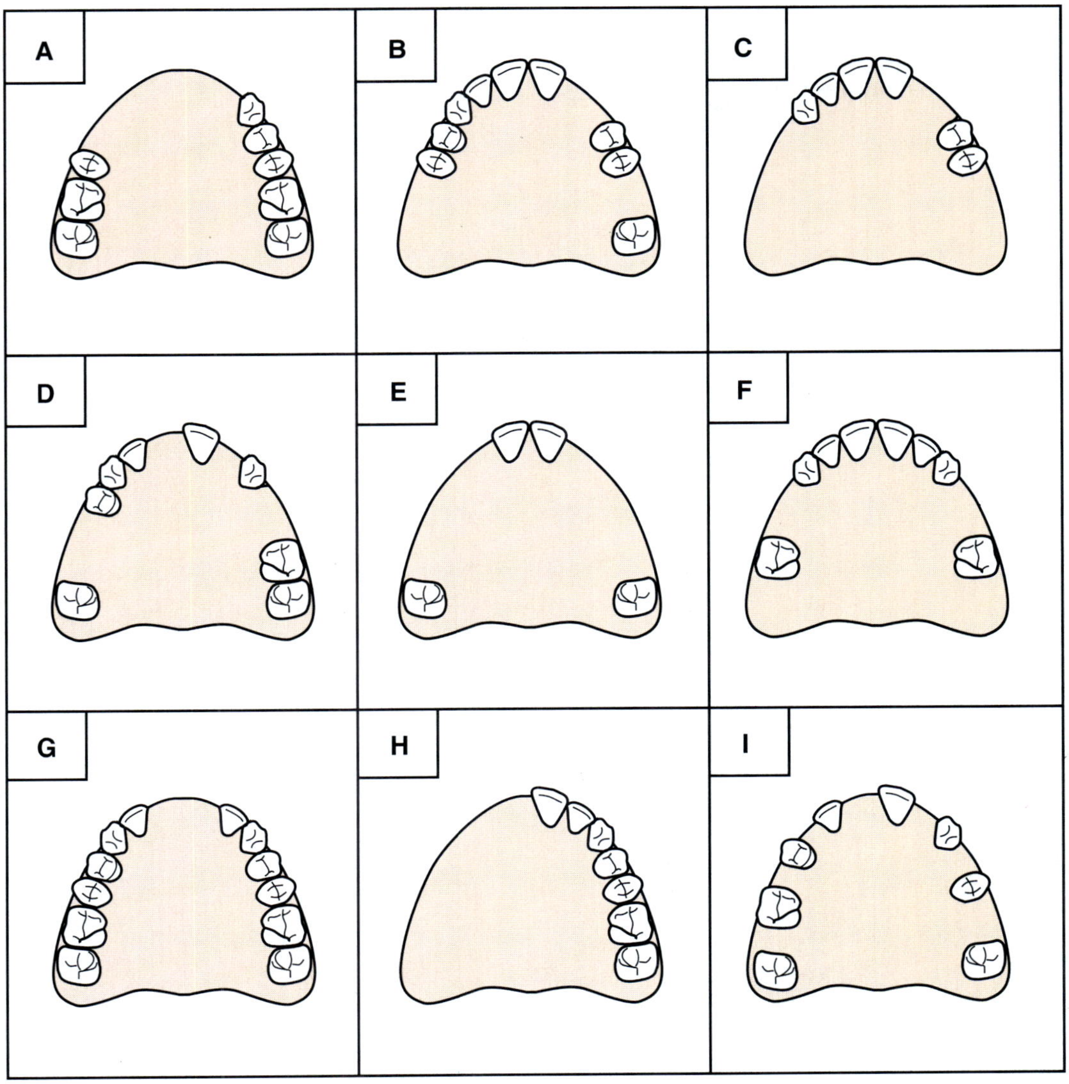

Figure 3-3 Nine partially edentulous arch configurations.

tooth-supported, or a Class III, component elsewhere in the arch. Thus the Class II partial denture rightly falls between the Class I and the Class III, because it embodies design features common to both. In keeping with the principle that design is based on the classification, the application of such principles of design is simplified by retaining the original classification of Kennedy.

SELF-ASSESSMENT AIDS

1. Would you agree that the primary purpose of a classification is to enhance communication among dentists? Support your answer.
2. Many classification systems have been proposed; however, the most widely accepted system in the United States is the one proposed by ______ in 1925.
3. A classification of partially edentulous arches should satisfy at least three requirements. List them.
4. Kennedy divided all partially edentulous arches into ______ main types.
5. What is meant by a modification space?
6. Which two classes of partially edentulous arches have the greatest incidence of occurrence according to Skinner?
7. Dr. O.C. Applegate contributed greatly to the application of the original Kennedy classification system. What was this contribution?
8. Classify the partially edentulous arches illustrated in Figure 3-3.

REFERENCE

1. McGarry TJ, Nimmo A, Skiba JF, et al: Classification system for partial edentulism, J Prosthodont 11(3): 181-193, 2002.

4

BIOMECHANICS OF REMOVABLE PARTIAL DENTURES

As stated in Chapter 1, the goal is to provide useful, functional removable partial denture prostheses by striving to understand how to maximize every opportunity for providing and maintaining a stable prosthesis. Since removable partial dentures are not rigidly attached to teeth, the control of potential movement under functional load is critical to providing the best chance for stability. The consequence of prosthesis movement under load is an application of stress to the teeth and tissue that are contacting the prosthesis. It is important that the stress not exceed the level of physiological tolerance, which is a range of mechanical stimulus that a system can resist without disruption or traumatic consequences. In the terminology of engineering mechanics, the prosthesis induces stress in the tissue equal to the force applied across the area of contact with the teeth and/or tissue. This same stress acts to produce strain in the supporting tissue, which results in a load displacement in the teeth and tissue. The understanding of how these mechanical phenomena act within a biological environment that is unique to each patient can be discussed in terms of biomechanics. In designing removable partial dentures, with a focus on the goal of providing and maintaining stable prostheses, consideration of basic biomechanical principles associated with the unique features of each mouth is essential. Oral hygiene and appropriate prosthesis maintenance procedures are required for continued benefit of optimal biomechanical principles.

BIOMECHANICS AND DESIGN SOLUTIONS

Removable partial dentures by design are intended to be placed into and removed from the mouth. Because of this, they cannot be rigidly connected to the teeth or tissue. This makes them subject to movement in response to functional loads, such as those created by mastication. It is important for clinicians providing removable partial denture service to understand the possible movements in response to function and to be able to logically design the component parts of the removable partial denture to help control these movements. Just how this is accomplished in a logical manner may not be clear to a clinician new to this exercise. One method to help organize design thought is to consider it as an exercise in creating a design solution.

Designing a removable partial denture can be considered similar to the classic, multifaceted design problem in conventional engineering, which is characterized by being open ended and ill structured. *Open ended* means that the problems typically have more than one solution, and *ill structured* means that the solutions are not the result of standard mathematical formulas in some structured manner. The design process is a series of steps that lead toward a solution of the problem and includes: identifying a need, definition of the problem, setting design objectives, searching for background information and data, developing a design rationale,

BOX 4-1 Design Process for Removable Partial Dentures

Need
Tooth replacement

Definition of problem
Provision of stable removable prosthesis

Objectives
Limited functional movement within tooth-tissue tolerance

Background information
Forces of occlusion, tissue "load-displacement" character and potential for movement, biomechanical principles applied to specific features of this unique mouth, removable partial denture component parts assigned to control movement

Choice of a solution (among alternatives) for application
Based on prior experience, principles and concepts learned from school and textbooks, applicable clinical research

devising and evaluating alternative solutions, and providing the solution (i.e., decision making and communication of solutions) (Box 4-1).

The rationale for design should logically develop from the analysis of the unique oral condition of each mouth under consideration. However, it is possible that alternative design "solutions" could be applied, and it is the evaluation of the perceived merits of these various designs that seems most confusing to clinicians.

The following biomechanical considerations provide a background regarding principles of the potential movement associated with removable partial dentures, and the subsequent chapters covering the various component parts describe how these components are applied in designs to control the resultant movements of the prostheses.

BIOMECHANICAL CONSIDERATIONS

As Maxfield states, "Common observation clearly indicates that the ability of living things to tolerate force is largely dependent upon the magnitude or intensity of the force." The supporting structures for removable partial dentures (abutment teeth and residual ridges) are living things and are subjected to forces. Whether the supporting structures are capable of resisting the applied forces depends upon the following questions: What are the typical forces requiring resistance? What are the duration and intensity of these forces? What is the capacity of the teeth and/or mucosae to resist the forces? How does material use and application influence this teeth-tissue resistance? Does the resistance change over time?

Consideration of the forces inherent in the oral cavity is critical. This includes the direction, duration, frequency, and magnitude of the force. In the final analysis, it is bone that provides the support for a removable prosthesis (i.e., the alveolar bone by way of the periodontal ligament and the residual ridge bone through its soft tissue covering). If potentially destructive forces can be minimized, then the physiological tolerances of the supporting structures are not exceeded and pathological change does not occur. The forces occurring with removable prosthesis function can be widely distributed and directed, and their effect minimized by appropriate design of the removable partial denture. An appropriate design includes the selection and location of components in conjunction with a harmonious occlusion.

Unquestionably the design of removable partial dentures necessitates mechanical and biological considerations. Most dentists are capable of applying simple mechanical principles to the design of a removable partial denture. For example, the lid of a paint can is more easily removed with a screwdriver than with a half dollar. The longer the handle, the less effort (force) it takes. This is a simple application of the mechanics of leverage. By the same token, a lever system represented by a distal extension removable partial denture could magnify the applied force of occlusion to the terminal abutments, which would be undesirable.

Tylman states, "Great caution and reserve are essential whenever an attempt is made to interpret biological phenomena entirely by mathematical computation." However, an understanding of simple machines applied to the design of removable partial dentures helps to accomplish the objective of preservation of oral structures. Without such understanding, a removable partial denture can be inadvertently designed as a destructive machine.

Machines may be classified into two general categories: simple and complex. Complex machines are combinations of many simple machines. The six simple machines are lever, wedge, screw, wheel and axle, pulley, and inclined plane (Figure 4-1). Of the simple machines, the lever and the inclined plane should be avoided in designing removable partial dentures.

In its simplest form, a lever is a rigid bar supported somewhere along its length. It may rest on the support or may be supported from above. The support point of the lever is called the *fulcrum*, and the lever can move around the fulcrum (Figure 4-2).

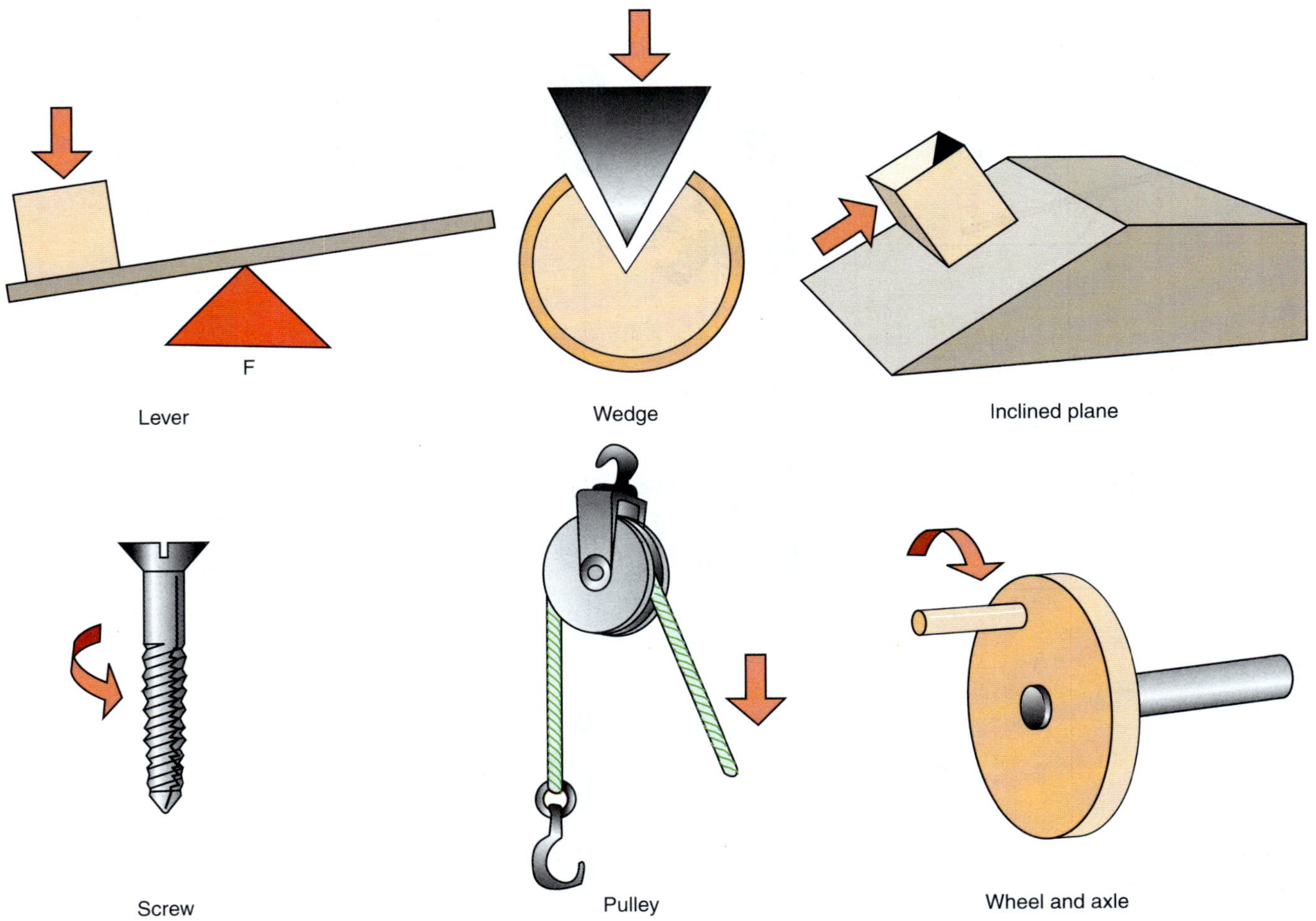

Figure 4-1 The six simple machines: lever, wedge, inclined plane, screw, pulley, and wheel and axle. The fulcrum, wedge, and inclined plane are concerns in removable partial denture designs because of the potential for harm if not appropriately controlled. *F*, Fulcrum.

The rotational movement of an extension base type of removable partial denture, when a force is placed on the denture base, is illustrated in Figure 4-3. It will rotate in relation to the three cranial planes because of differences in the support characteristics of the abutment teeth and the soft tissue covering the residual ridge. Even though the actual movement of the denture may be small, a lever force may be imposed on abutment teeth. This is especially detrimental when prosthesis maintenance is neglected. There are three types of levers: first, second, and third class (see Figure 4-2). The potential of a lever system to magnify a force is illustrated in Figure 4-4. A cantilever is a beam supported at one end and can act as a first-class lever (Figure 4-5). A cantilever design should be avoided (Figure 4-6). Examples of other lever designs and suggestions for alternative designs to avoid or to minimize their destructive potential are illustrated in Figures 4-7 and 4-8.

A tooth is apparently better able to tolerate vertically directed forces than nonvertical, torquing, or horizontal forces. This characteristic is observed clinically and it seems rational that more periodontal fibers are activated to resist the application of vertical forces to teeth than are activated to resist the application of nonvertical forces (Figure 4-9).

Again a distal extension removable partial denture rotates when forces are applied to the artificial teeth attached to the extension base. Because it can be assumed that this rotation must create predominantly nonvertical forces, location of stabilizing and retentive components in relation to the horizontal axis of rotation of the abutment becomes extremely important. An abutment tooth will better tolerate nonvertical forces if these forces are applied as near as possible to the horizontal axis of rotation of the abutment (Figure 4-10). The axial surface contours of abutment teeth must be altered

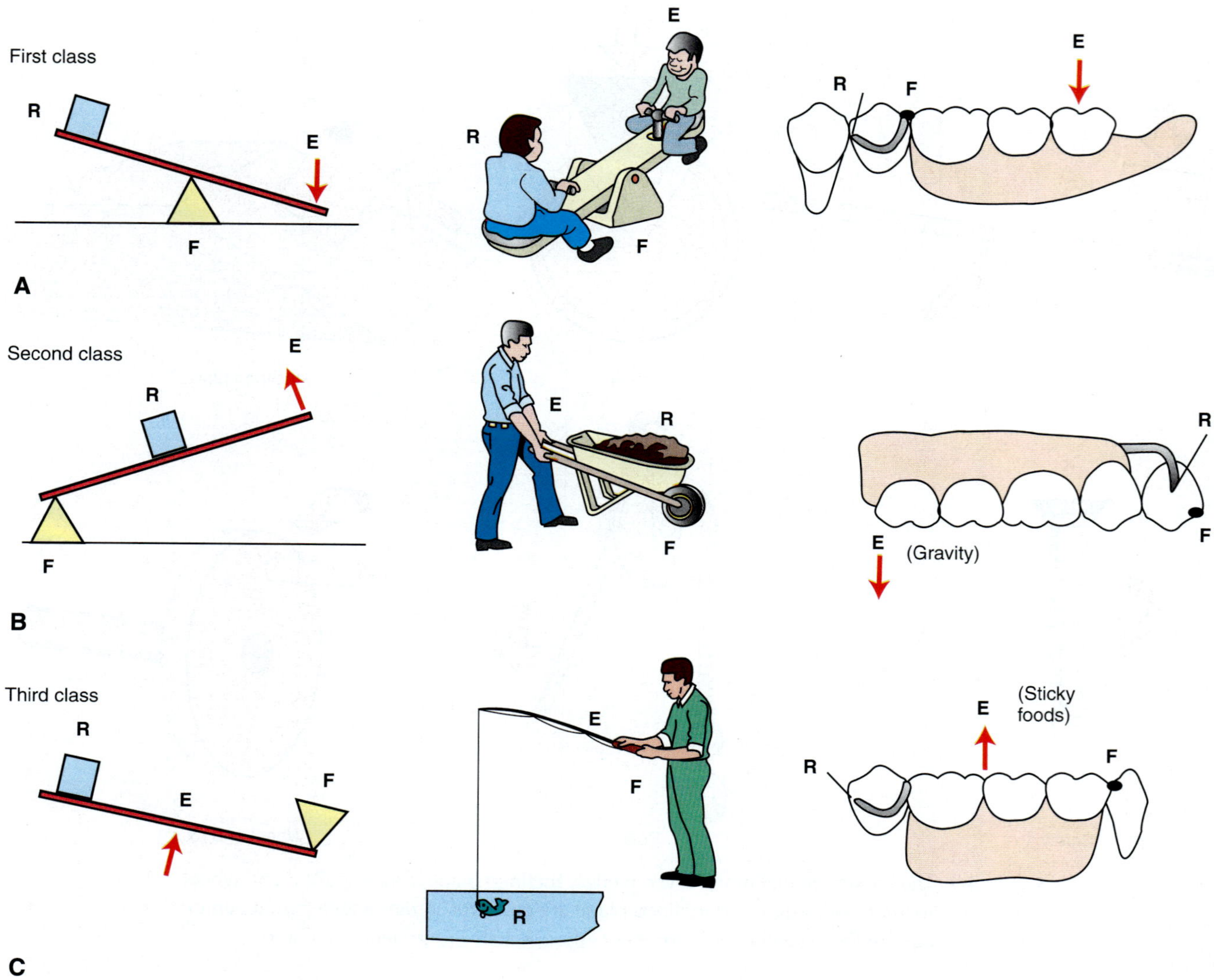

Figure 4-2 A-C, The three classes of levers. Classification is based on location of fulcrum *(F)*, resistance *(R)*, and direction of effort (force) *(E)*. In dental terms, *E* can represent either the force of occlusion or gravity; *F* can be a tooth surface such as an occlusal rest; and *R* is the resistance provided by a direct retainer or a guide plane surface.

to locate components of clasp assemblies more favorably in relation to the abutment's horizontal axis (Figure 4-11).

POSSIBLE MOVEMENTS OF PARTIAL DENTURE

Presuming that direct retainers are functioning to minimize vertical displacement, rotational movement will occur about some axis as the distal extension base or bases move either toward, away, or horizontally across the underlying tissue. Unfortunately, these possible movements do not occur singularly or independently but tend to be dynamic, and all occur at the same time. The greatest movement possible is found in the tooth-tissue-supported prosthesis, because of the reliance on the distal extension supporting tissue to share the functional loads with the teeth. Movement of a distal extension base toward the ridge tissue will be proportionate to the quality of that tissue, the accuracy and extent of the denture base, and the applied total functional load. A review of prosthesis rotational movement that is possible around various axes in the mouth provides some understanding of how component parts of removable partial dentures should be prescribed to control prosthesis movement.

One movement is rotation about an axis through the most posterior abutments. This axis may be through occlusal rests or any other rigid portion of a direct retainer assembly located occlusally or incisally to the height of contour of the primary abutments (see Figures 4-6 and 4-7). This axis,

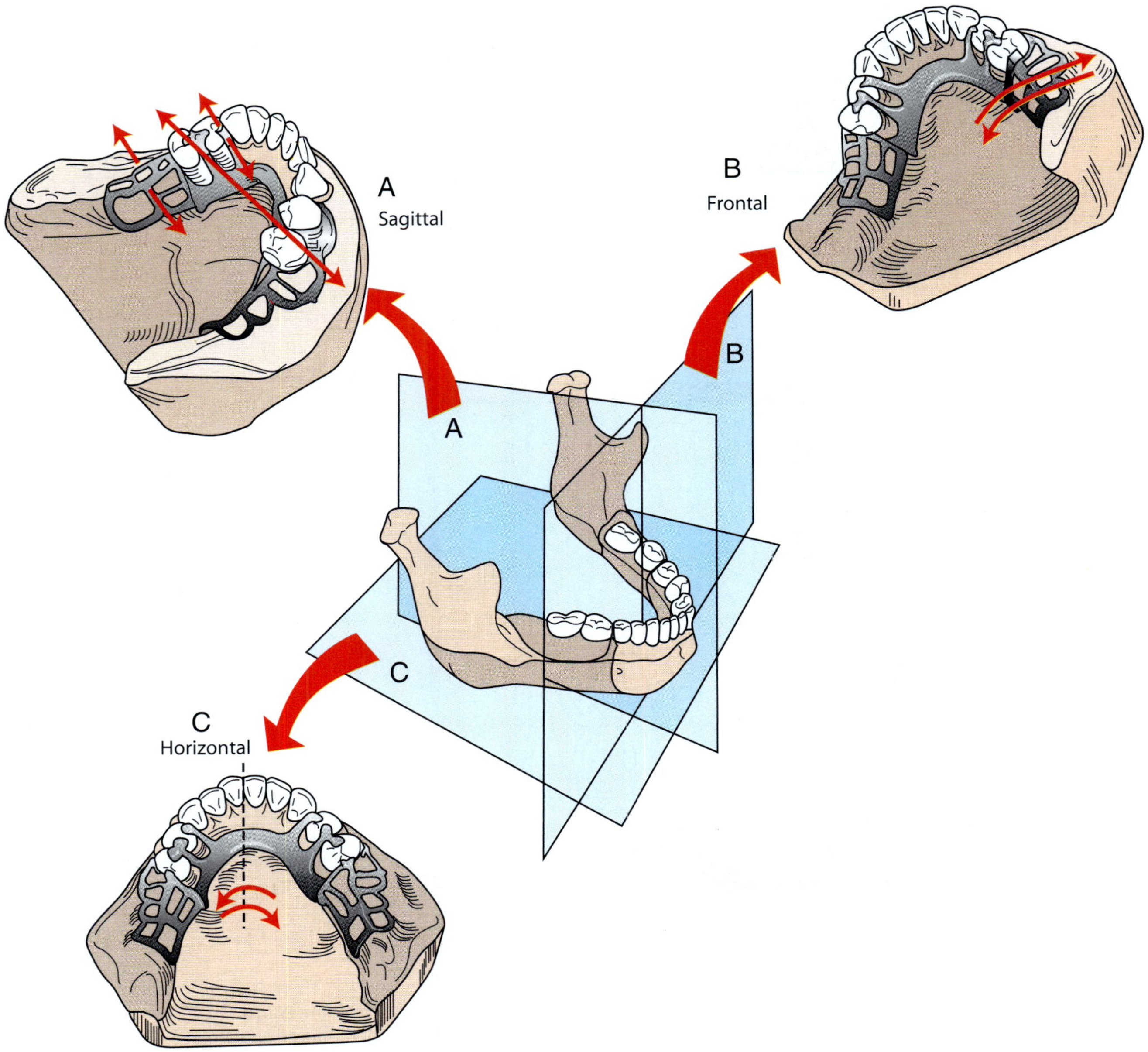

Figure 4-3 Distal extension removable partial dentures will rotate when force is directed on the denture base. Differences in displaceability of the periodontal ligament of the supporting abutment teeth and soft tissue covering the residual ridge permit this rotation. It would seem that rotation of the prosthesis is in a combination of directions rather than unidirectional. The three possible movements of distal extension partial dentures are **A,** rotation around a fulcrum line passing through the most posterior abutments when the denture base moves vertically toward or away from the supporting residual ridges; **B,** rotation around a longitudinal axis formed by the crest of the residual ridge; and **C,** rotation around a vertical axis located near the center of the arch.

known as the *fulcrum line*, is the center of rotation as the distal extension base moves toward the supporting tissue when an occlusal load is applied. The axis of rotation may shift toward more anteriorly placed components, occlusal or incisal to the height of contour of the abutment, as the base moves away from the supporting tissue when vertical dislodging forces act on the partial denture. These dislodging forces result from the vertical pull of food between opposing tooth surfaces, the effect of moving border tissue, and the forces of gravity against a maxillary partial denture. Presuming that the direct retainers are functional and that the supportive anterior components remain seated, rotation—rather than total displacement—should occur. Vertical tissueward movement of the denture base is resisted by the

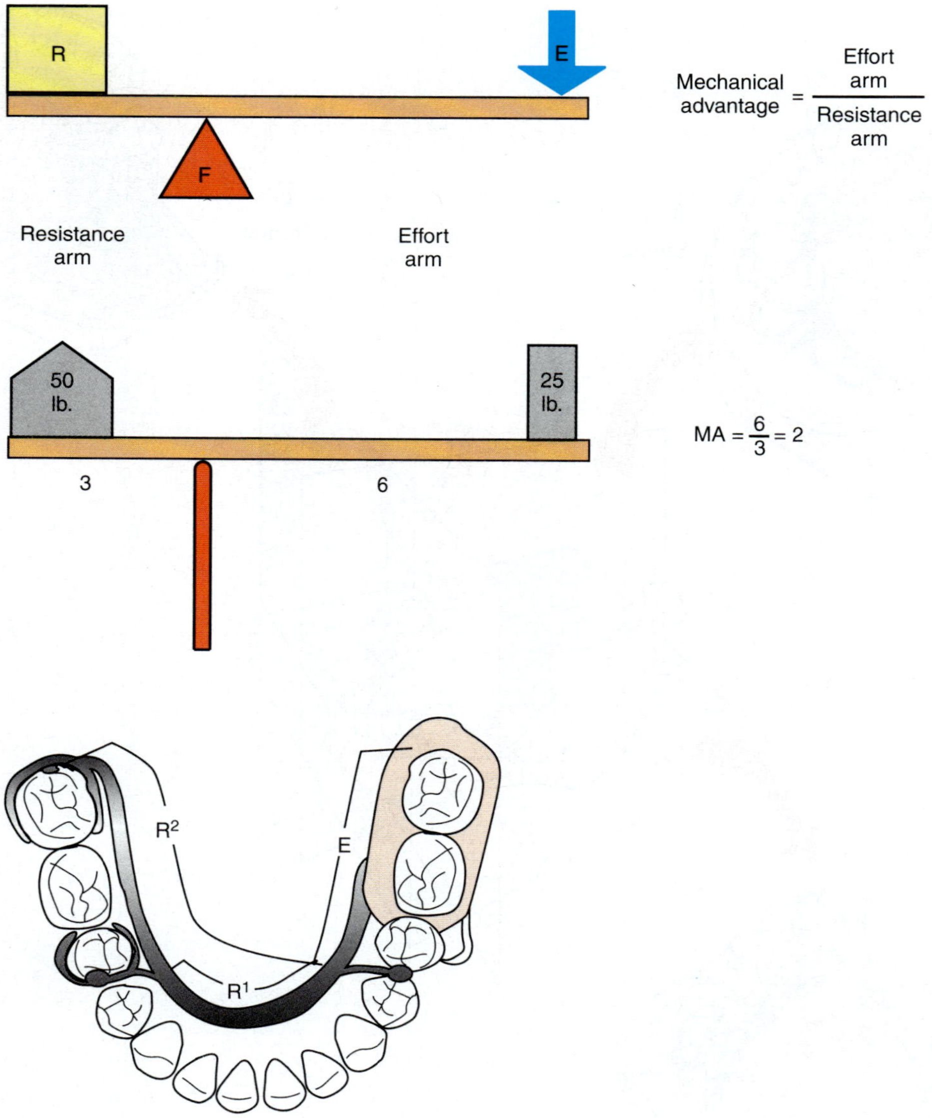

Figure 4-4 Length of lever from fulcrum *(F)* to resistance *(R)* is called *resistance arm.* That portion of lever from fulcrum to point of application of force *(E)* is called *effort arm.* Whenever effort arm is longer than resistance arm, mechanical advantage is in favor of effort arm, proportional to difference in length of the two arms. In other words, when effort arm is twice the length of the resistance arm, a 25-lb weight on effort arm will balance a 50-lb weight at end of resistance arm. The opposite is also true and helps illustrate cross-arch stabilization. When the resistance arm is lengthened (cross-arch clasp assembly placed on a second molar versus a second premolar) the effort arm is more efficiently counteracted.

tissue of the residual ridge in proportion to the supporting quality of that tissue, the accuracy of the fit of the denture base, and the total amount of occlusal load applied. Movement of the base in the opposite direction is resisted by the action of the retentive clasp arms on terminal abutments and the action of stabilizing minor connectors in conjunction with seated, vertical support elements of the framework anterior to the terminal abutments acting as indirect retainers. Indirect retainers should be placed as far as possible from the distal extension base, affording the best possible leverage against the lifting of the distal extension base.

A second movement is rotation about a longitudinal axis as the distal extension base moves in a rotary direction about the residual ridge (see Figure 4-3). This movement is resisted primarily by the rigidity of the major and minor connectors and their ability to resist torque. If the connectors are not rigid or if a stress-breaker exists between the distal extension base and the major connector, this rotation about a longitudinal axis either applies undue stress to the

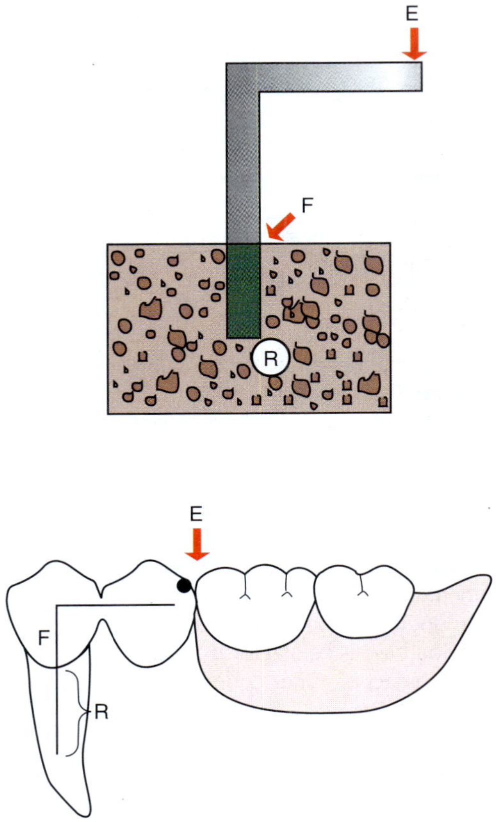

Figure 4-5 Cantilever can be described as a rigid beam supported only at one end. When force is directed against unsupported end of beam (as in this rest placed on a cantilevered pontic), cantilever can act as a first-class lever. Mechanical advantage in this illustration is in favor of the effort arm.

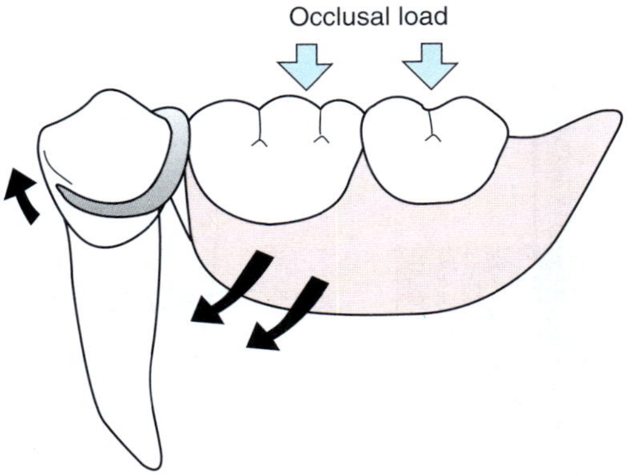

Figure 4-6 Design often seen for distal extension removable partial denture. Cast circumferential direct retainer engages mesiobuccal undercut and is supported by distocclusal rest. If rigidly attached to the abutment tooth, this could be considered a cantilever design, and it may impart detrimental first-class lever force to abutment if tissue support under extension base allows excessive vertical movement toward the residual ridge.

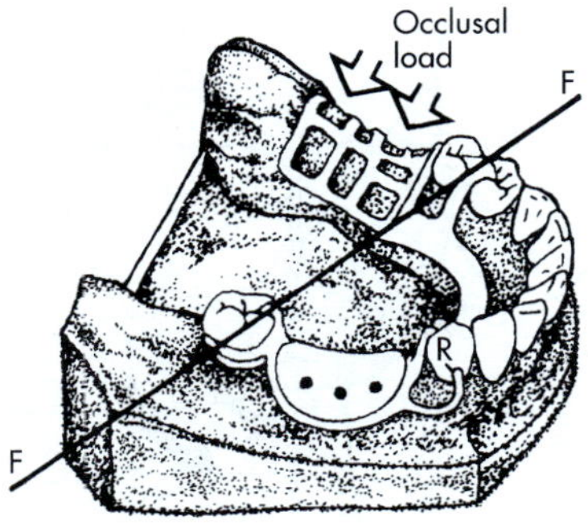

Figure 4-7 As shown in Figure 4-6, the potential for first-class lever action can also exist in Class II, modification 1 designs for removable partial denture frameworks. If cast circumferential direct retainer with a mesiobuccal undercut on right first premolar were used, force placed on denture base could impart upward and posteriorly moving force on premolar, resulting in loss of contact between premolar and canine. Tissue support from extension base area is most important to minimize lever action of clasp. Retainer design could help accommodate more of an anteriorly directed force during rotation of the denture base in an attempt to maintain tooth contact. Other alternatives to first premolar design of direct retainer would be tapered wrought-wire retentive arm that uses mesiobuccal undercut or just has buccal stabilizing arm above height of contour.

sides of the supporting ridge or causes horizontal shifting of the denture base.

A third movement is rotation about an imaginary vertical axis located near the center of the dental arch (see Figure 4-4). This movement occurs under function because diagonal and horizontal occlusal forces are brought to bear on the partial denture. It is resisted by stabilizing components, such as reciprocal clasp arms and minor connectors that are in contact with vertical tooth surfaces. Such stabilizing components are essential to any partial denture design regardless of the manner of support and the type of direct retention employed. Stabilizing components on one side of the arch act to stabilize the partial denture against horizontal forces applied from the opposite side. It is obvious that rigid connectors must be used to make this effect possible.

Horizontal forces always will exist to some degree because of lateral stresses occurring during mastication, bruxism, clenching, and other patient habits. These forces are accentuated by failure to consider the orientation of the occlusal plane, the influence of malpositioned teeth in the arch, and the effect of abnormal jaw relationships. Fabricating an occlusion that is in harmony with the opposing dentition and that is free of lateral interference during eccentric jaw movements may minimize the magnitude of lateral stress. The amount of horizontal movement occurring in the partial denture therefore depends on the magnitude of the lateral forces that are applied and on the effectiveness of the stabilizing components.

In a tooth-supported partial denture, movement of the base toward the edentulous ridge is prevented primarily by the rests on the abutment teeth and to

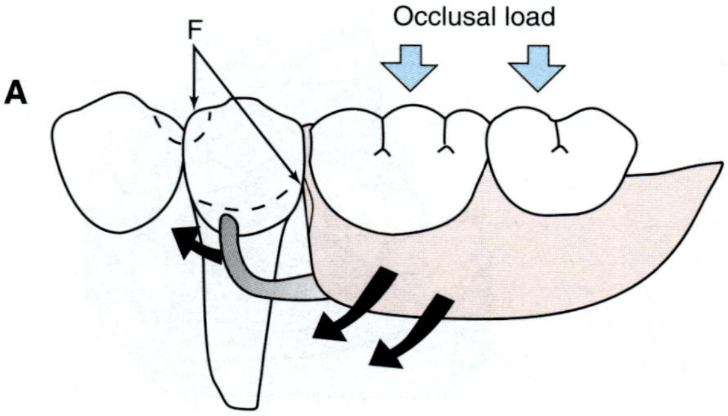

Figure 4-8 Mesial rest concept for distal extension removable partial dentures. Recognizing that clasp movement occurs with functional displacement of the distal extension base, the primary aim of a mesial rest is to alter the fulcrum position and the resultant clasp movement, disallowing harmful engagement of the abutment tooth. **A,** Bar type of retainer, minor connector contacting guiding plane on distal surface of premolar, and mesio-occlusal rest used to reduce cantilever or first-class lever force when and if denture rotates toward residual ridge. **B,** Tapered wrought-wire retentive arm, minor connector contacting guiding plane on distal surface of premolar, and mesio-occlusal rest. This design is applicable when distobuccal undercut cannot be found or created or when tissue undercut contraindicates placing bar-type retentive arm. This design would be kinder to periodontal ligament than would a cast, half-round retentive arm. Again, tissue support of extension base is key factor in reducing lever action of clasp arm. *Note*: Depending on amount of contact of minor connector proximal plate with guiding plane, fulcrum point will change.

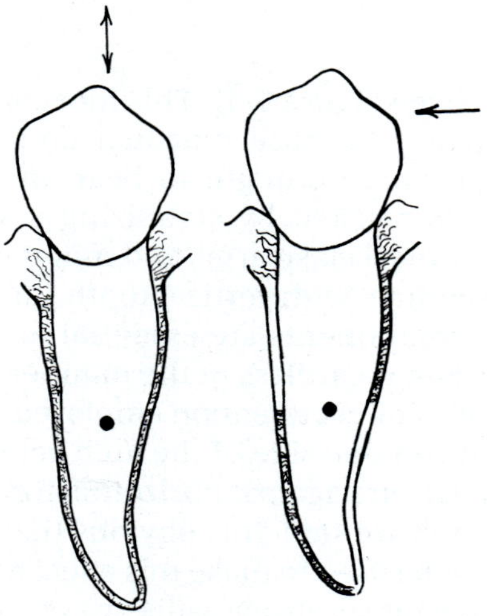

Figure 4-9 More periodontal fibers are activated to resist forces directed vertically on tooth than are activated to resist horizontally (off-vertical) directed force. Horizontal axis of rotation is located somewhere in root of tooth.

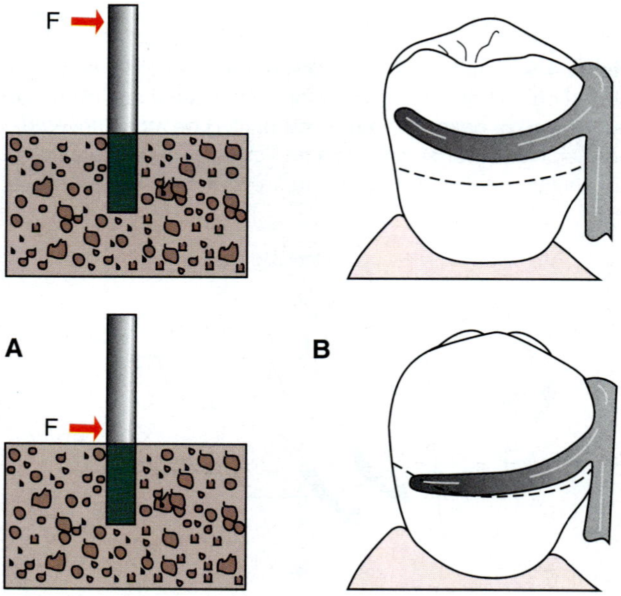

Figure 4-10 **A,** Fence post is more efficiently removed by applying force *(F)* farther from the support. Force placed closer to the support reduces the effort arm. **B,** Clasps placed closer to the occlusal/incisal surface have a greater likelihood of imparting tipping forces to abutments. This represents similar effect of force application shown in **A,** *top image*.

some degree by any rigid portion of the framework located occlusal to the height of contour. Movement away from the edentulous ridge is prevented by the action of direct retainers on the abutments that are situated at each end of each edentulous space and by the rigid, minor connector stabilizing components. Therefore the first of the three possible movements can be controlled in the tooth-supported denture. The second possible movement, which is along a longitudinal axis, is prevented by the rigid components of the direct retainers on the abutment teeth and by the ability of the major connector to resist torque. This movement is much less in the tooth-supported denture because of the presence of

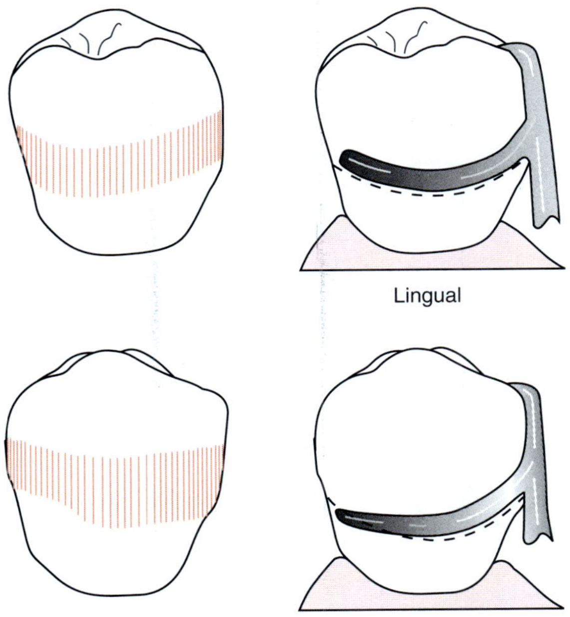

Figure 4-11 Abutment has been contoured (see hatched region) to allow rather favorable location of retentive and reciprocal stabilizing components *(mirror view)*. This is similar to Figure 4-10 *A, bottom image.*

posterior abutments. The third possible movement occurs in all partial dentures. Therefore stabilizing components against horizontal movement must be incorporated into any partial denture design.

For prostheses capable of movement in three planes, occlusal rests should only provide occlusal support to resist tissueward movement. All movements of the partial denture other than those in a tissueward direction should be resisted by components other than occlusal rests. For the occlusal rest to enter into a stabilizing function would result in a direct transfer of torque to the abutment tooth. Because movements around three different axes are possible in a distal extension partial denture, an occlusal rest for such a partial denture should not have steep vertical walls or locking dovetails, which could possibly cause horizontal and torquing forces to be applied intracoronally to the abutment tooth.

In the tooth-supported denture, the only movements of any significance are horizontal, and these may be resisted by the stabilizing effect of components placed on the axial surfaces of the abutments. Therefore in the tooth-supported denture, the use of *intracoronal rests* is permissible. In these instances the rests provide not only occlusal support but also notable horizontal stabilization.

In contrast, all Class I and Class II partial dentures, having one or more distal extension bases, are not totally tooth supported. Neither are they completely retained by bounding abutments. Any extensive Class III or Class IV partial denture that does not have adequate abutment support falls into the same category. These latter dentures may derive some support from the edentulous ridge and therefore may have a composite support from both teeth and ridge tissue.

SELF-ASSESSMENT AIDS

1. What elements prevent movement of the base(s) of a tooth-supported denture toward the basal seats?
2. Movement of a distal extension base away from basal seats will occur as a rotational movement or as ______.
3. What is the difference between fulcrum line and axis of rotation?
4. Identify the fulcrum line on a Class I arch; a Class II, modification 1; and a Class IV.
5. In the treatment planning and design phase of partial denture service, the functional movements of removable partial dentures should be considered when designing the individual ______ ______ of the prosthesis.
6. Forces are transmitted to abutment teeth and residual ridges by removable partial dentures. One of the factors of a force is its magnitude. List the other three factors of a force that a dentist must consider in designing removable partial dentures.
7. The design of a removable restoration necessitates consideration of mechanics and biological considerations. True or false?
8. Of the simple machines, which two are more likely to be encountered in the design of removable partial dentures?
9. What is a lever? A cantilever?
10. Name the three classes of levers and give an example of each.
11. Of the three classes of lever systems, which two are most likely to be encountered in removable partial prosthodontics?
12. Explain how one would figure the mechanical advantage of a lever system given dimensions of effort and resistance arms.
13. What class lever system is most likely to be encountered with a restoration on a Class II, modification 1 arch when a force is placed on the extension base?
14. What factor permits a distal extension denture to rotate when the denture base is forced toward the basal seat?
15. Is an abutment tooth better able to resist a force directed apically or horizontally? Why?
16. Where is the location of the horizontal (tipping) axis of an abutment tooth?
17. Why should components of a direct retainer assembly be located as close as possible to the tipping axis of a tooth?

5

MAJOR AND MINOR CONNECTORS

Components of a typical removable partial denture are illustrated in Figure 5-1.

1. Major connectors
2. Minor connectors
3. Rests
4. Direct retainers
5. Stabilizing or reciprocal components (as parts of a clasp assembly)
6. Indirect retainers (if the prosthesis has distal extension bases)
7. One or more bases, each supporting one to several replacement teeth (see Figure 5-1)

When using a prosthesis that can be removed from the mouth, the prosthesis must extend to both sides of the arch. This enables direction of functional forces to supporting teeth and tissue for optimum stability. It is through this cross-arch tooth contact, which is at some distance from the functional force, that optimum resistance can be achieved. This is most effective when a rigid major connector joins the portion of the prosthesis receiving the function to selected regions throughout the arch.

The chief functions of a major connector include unification of the major parts of the prosthesis, distribution of the applied force throughout the arch to selected teeth and tissue, and minimization of torque to the teeth. A properly designed rigid major connector effectively distributes forces throughout the arch and acts to reduce the load to any one area while effectively controlling prosthesis movement.

The principle of leverage is connected with this component part. A rigid major connector will limit movement possibilities by acting as a counteracting lever. This phenomenon is referred to as *cross-arch stability*. Cross-arch stability becomes more important in situations associated with a high potential for greater prosthesis movement (i.e., distal extensions).

In this chapter, major and minor connectors are considered separately as to their function, location, and design criteria. Other components are presented in designated chapters.

MAJOR CONNECTORS

A major connector is the component of the partial denture that connects the parts of the prosthesis located on one side of the arch with those on the opposite side. It is that unit of the partial denture to which all other parts are directly or indirectly attached (Figure 5-2). This component also provides the cross-arch stability to help resist displacement by functional stresses.

The major connector may be compared with the frame of an automobile or with the foundation of a building. It is through the major connector that other components of the partial denture become unified and effective. If the major connector is flexible, the ineffectiveness of connected components jeopardizes the supporting oral structures and can be a detriment to the comfort of the patient. Failure of the major connector to provide rigidity may be manifest

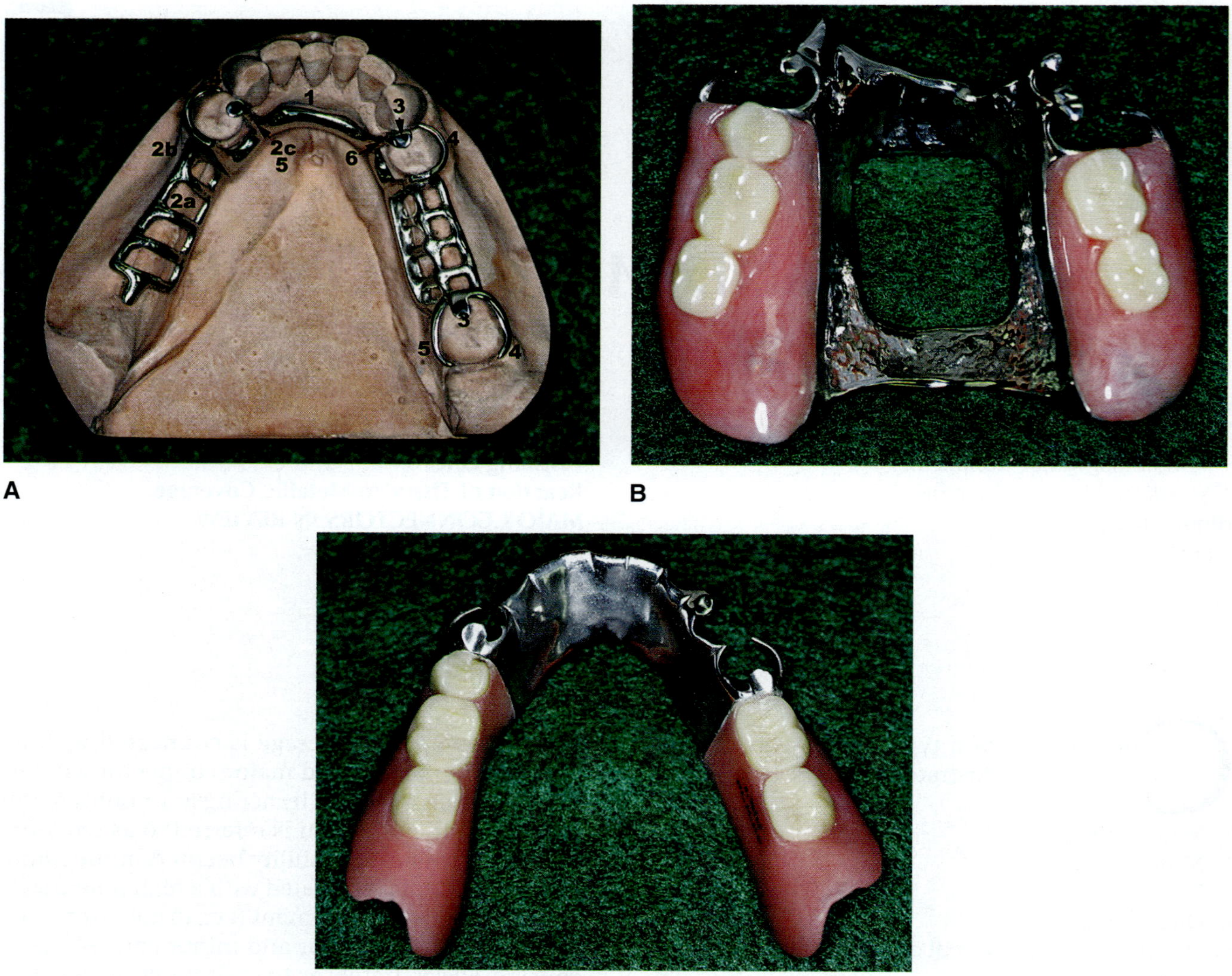

A B C

Figure 5-1 **A,** Framework for mandibular removable partial denture with the following components: *1,* lingual bar major connector; *2a,* minor connector by which the resin denture base will be attached; *2b,* minor connector, proximal plate, which is part of clasp assembly; *2c,* minor connector used to connect rests to major connectors; *3,* occlusal rests; *4,* direct retainer arm, which is part of the total clasp assembly; *5,* stabilizing or reciprocal components of clasp assembly (includes minor connectors); and *6,* an indirect retainer consisting of a minor connector and an occlusal rest. **B,** Maxillary removable partial denture with resin denture bases supporting artificial posterior teeth. Bases are attached to metal framework by ladderlike minor connectors similar to those seen in *2a.* **C,** Mandibular bilateral distal extension removable partial denture with resin denture bases supporting artificial posterior teeth.

by traumatic damage to periodontal support of abutment teeth, injury to residual ridges, or impingement of underlying tissue. It is the dentist's responsibility to ensure that the appropriate design and fabrication of the major connector are accomplished.

Location

Major connectors should be designed and located with the following guidelines in mind:

1. Major connectors should be free of movable tissue.
2. Impingement of gingival tissue should be avoided.
3. Bony and soft tissue prominences should be avoided during placement and removal.
4. Relief should be provided beneath a major connector to prevent its settling into areas of possible interference, such as inoperable tori or elevated median palatal sutures.

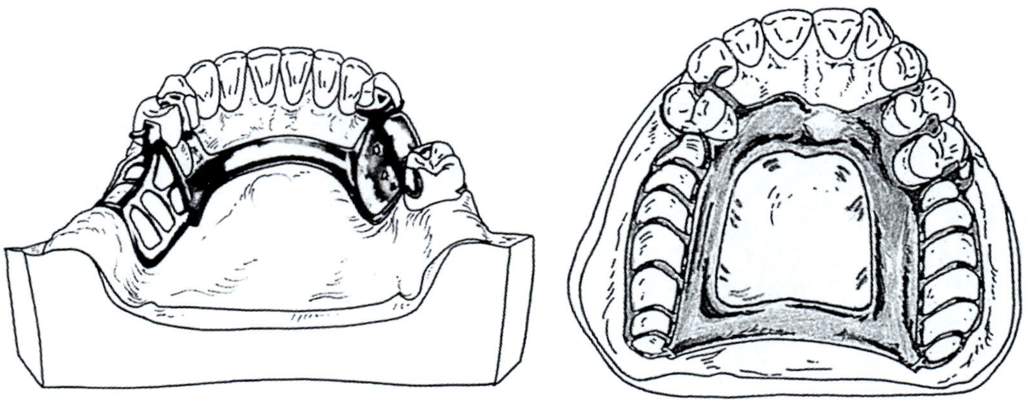

A B

Figure 5-2 **A,** Lingual bar major connector for mandibular removable partial denture framework. It rigidly joins the tooth-stabilized cast base on right across the arch to the framework components on the opposite side. **B,** Anterior-posterior strap maxillary major connector for a Kennedy Class I partially edentulous arch. This is a rigid type of major connector and covers only a small portion of palatal tissue.

5. Major connectors should be located and/or relieved to prevent impingement of tissue because the distal extension denture rotates in function.

Appropriate relief beneath the major connector avoids the need for its adjustment after tissue damage has occurred. In addition to being time consuming, grinding to provide relief from impingement may seriously weaken the major connector, which can result in flexibility or possibly fracture. Major connectors should be carefully designed for proper shape, thickness, and location. Alteration of these dimensions by grinding can only be detrimental. Relief is covered at the end of this chapter and expanded in Chapter 11.

Margins of major connectors adjacent to gingival tissue should be located far enough from the tissue to avoid any possible impingement. To accomplish this, it is recommended that the superior border of a lingual bar connector be located a minimum of 4 mm below the gingival margin(s) (Figure 5-3). At the inferior border of the lingual bar connector the limiting factor is the height of the moving tissue in the floor of the mouth. Because the connector must have sufficient width and bulk to provide rigidity, a linguoplate is commonly used when there is insufficient space for a lingual bar.

In the maxillary arch, because there is no moving tissue in the palate as in the floor of the mouth, the borders of the major connector may be placed well away from gingival tissue. Structurally the tissue covering the palate is well suited for placement of the connector because of the presence of firm submucosal connective tissue and an adequate, deep blood supply. However, when soft tissue covering the midline of the palate is less displaceable than the tissue covering the residual ridge, varying amounts of relief under the connectors must be provided to avoid impingement of tissue. The amount of relief required is directly proportional to the difference in displaceability of the tissue covering the midline of the palate and the tissue covering the residual ridges. The gingival tissue, on the other hand, must have an unrestricted superficial blood supply to remain healthy. To accomplish this, it is recommended that the borders of the palatal connector be placed a minimum of 6 mm away from and parallel to the gingival margins. Minor connectors that must cross gingival tissue should do so abruptly, joining the major connector at nearly a right angle (Figure 5-4). In this way the maximal freedom is ensured for gingival tissue.

Except for a palatal torus or prominent median palatal suture area, palatal connectors ordinarily require no relief. Intimate contact between the connector and the supporting tissue adds much to the support, stability, and retention of the denture. Except for gingival areas, intimacy of contact elsewhere in the palate is not detrimental to the health of the tissue if rests are provided on abutment teeth to prevent tissueward movement.

An anterior palatal strap or the anterior border of a palatal plate also should be located as far as possible posteriorly to avoid interference with the tongue in the rugae area. It should be uniformly thin and its anterior border should be located to follow the contours between the crests of the rugae. The anterior border of such palatal major connectors will therefore be irregular in outline as it follows the contours between the rugae. The tongue may then pass from one ruga prominence to another without encountering the border of the connector. When the connector

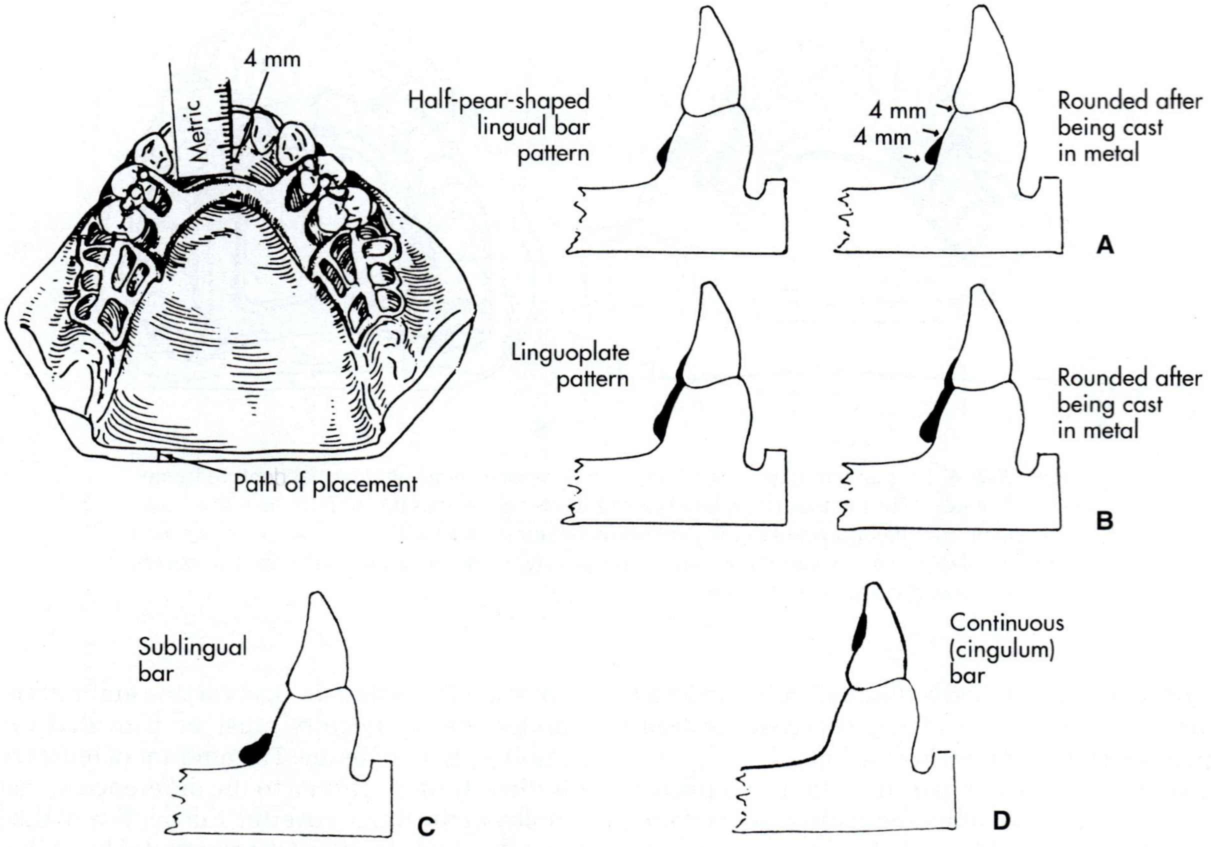

Figure 5-3 **A,** Lingual bar major connector should be located at least 4 mm inferior to gingival margins and more if possible. The vertical height of a finished lingual bar should be at least 4 mm for strength and rigidity. If less than 8 mm exists between gingival margins and movable floor of mouth, a linguoplate **(B)**, a sublingual bar **(C)**, or a continuous bar **(D)** is preferred as a major connector. Relief is provided for soft tissue under all portions of the mandibular major connector and any location where the framework crosses the marginal gingiva. The inferior border of mandibular major connectors should be gently rounded after being cast to eliminate a sharp edge.

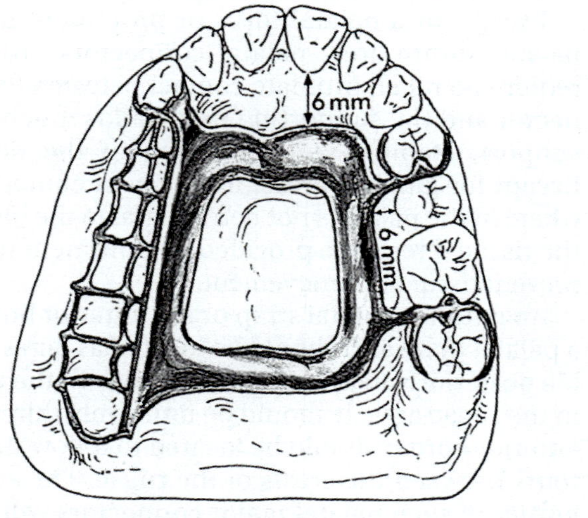

Figure 5-4 Palatal major connector should be located at least 6 mm away from gingival margins and parallel to their mean curvature. All adjoining minor connectors should cross gingival tissues abruptly and should join major connectors at nearly a right angle.

border must cross a ruga crest, it should be done abruptly, avoiding the crest as much as possible. The posterior limitation of a maxillary major connector should be just anterior to the vibrating line. A useful rule applied to major connectors and throughout partial denture design is to try to avoid adding any part of the denture framework to an already convex surface.

Characteristics of major connectors contributing to the maintenance of health of the oral environment and the well-being of the patient may be listed as shown in Box 5-1.

Mandibular Major Connectors

Six types of mandibular major connectors are:

1. Lingual bar (Figure 5-5, *A*)
2. Linguoplate (Figure 5-5, *B*)
3. Sublingual bar (Figure 5-5, *C*)
4. Lingual bar with cingulum bar (continuous bar) (Figure 5-5, *D*)

BOX 5-1 Characteristics of Major Connectors Contributing to Health and Well-Being

1. Made from an alloy compatible with oral tissue
2. Is rigid and provides cross-arch stability through the principle of broad distribution of stress
3. Does not interfere with and is not irritating to the tongue
4. Does not substantially alter the natural contour of the lingual surface of the mandibular alveolar ridge or of the palatal vault
5. Does not impinge on oral tissue when the restoration is placed, removed, or rotates in function
6. Covers no more tissue than is absolutely necessary
7. Does not contribute to the retention or trapping of food particles
8. Has support from other elements of the framework to minimize rotation tendencies in function
9. Contributes to the support of the prosthesis

5. Cingulum bar (continuous bar) (Figure 5-5, *E*)
6. Labial bar (Figure 5-5, *F*)

The lingual bar and linguoplate are by far the most common major connectors used in mandibular removable partial dentures.

Lingual Bar

The basic form of a mandibular major connector is a half-pear shape, located above moving tissue but as far below the gingival tissue as possible. It is usually made of reinforced, 6-gauge, half-pear-shaped wax or a similar plastic pattern (Figure 5-6).

The major connector must be contoured so that it does not present sharp margins to the tongue and cause irritation or annoyance by an angular form. The superior border of a lingual bar connector should be tapered toward the gingival tissue superiorly, with its greatest bulk at the inferior border, resulting in a contour that is a half-pear shape. Lingual bar patterns, both wax and plastic, are made in this conventional

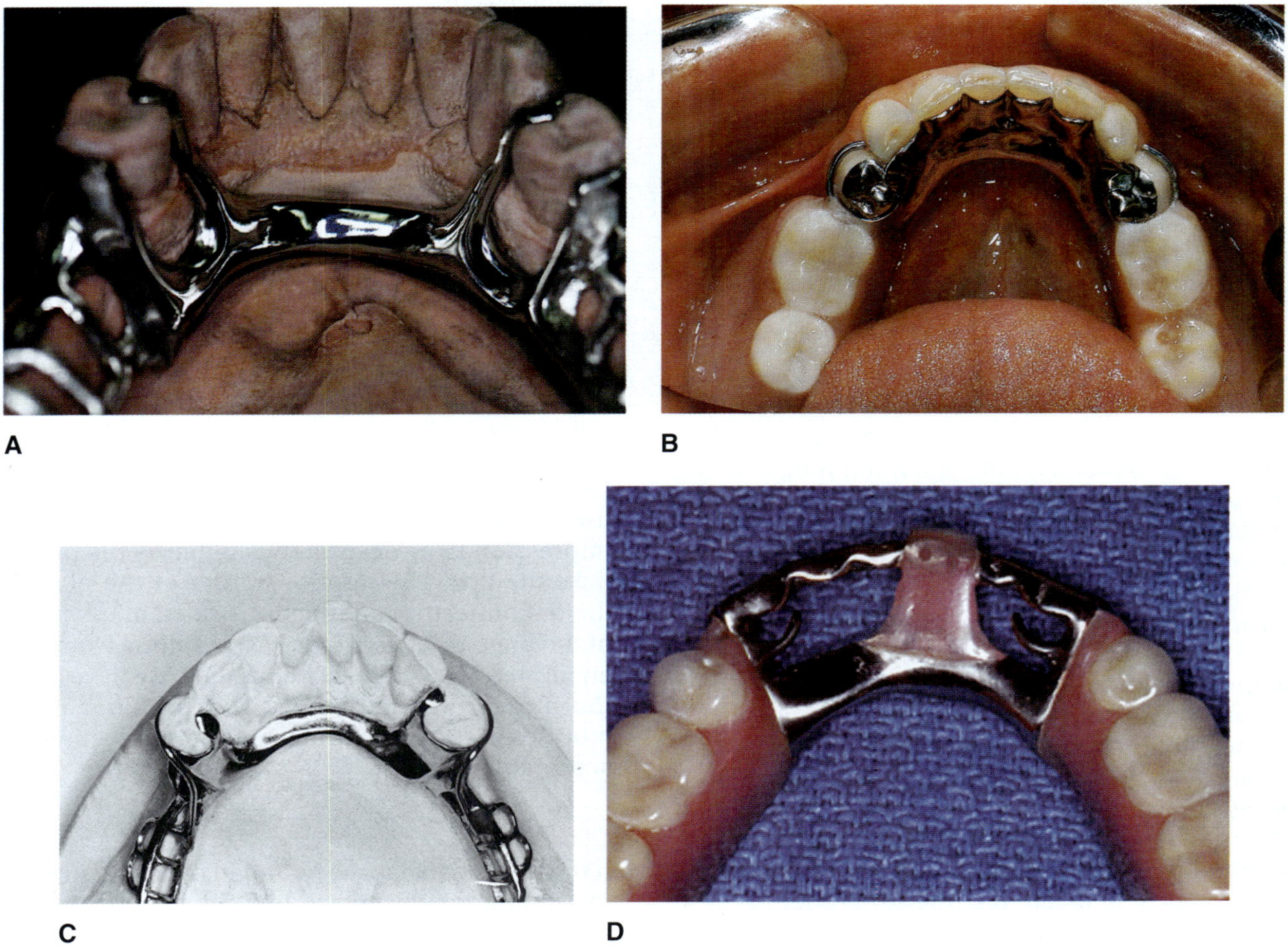

Figure 5-5 Mandibular major connectors. **A,** Lingual bar. **B,** Linguoplate. **C,** Sublingual bar. **D,** Lingual bar with continuous bar (cingulum bar).

Continued

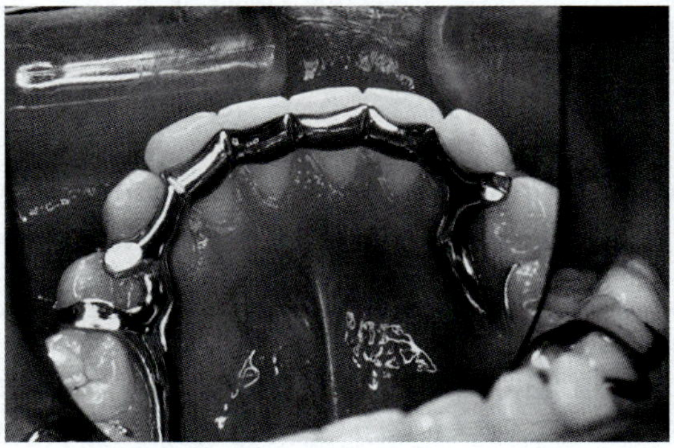

E

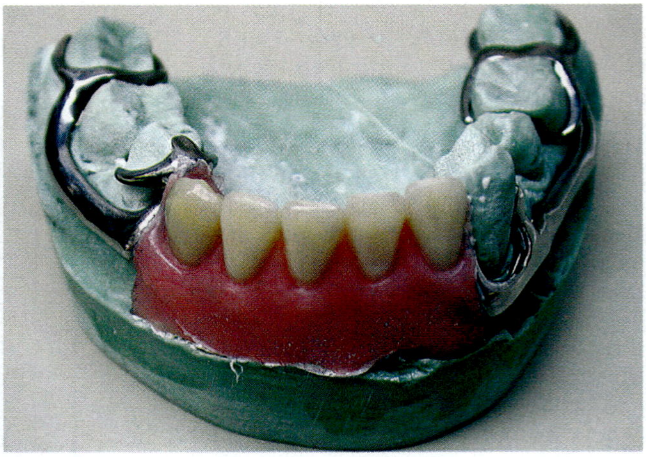

F

Figure 5-5 Cont'd **E,** Cingulum bar. **F,** Labial bar.

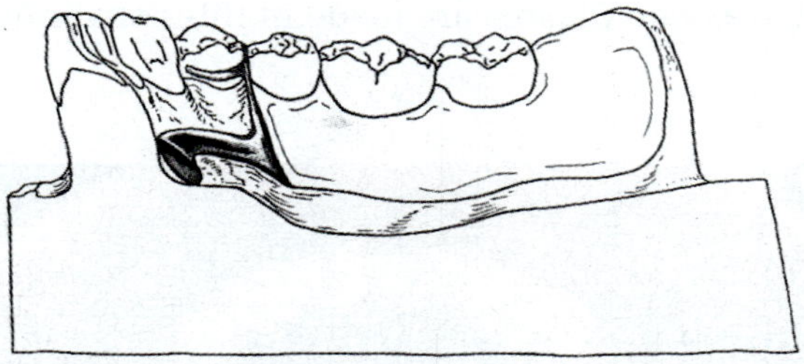

Figure 5-6 Sagittal section showing half-pear shape of lingual bar. A taper of superior border of the bar to the soft tissues above will minimize interference with tongue and will be more acceptable to the patient than would a dissimilar contour. Tissue relief is necessary to protect the soft tissue of the floor of the mouth.

shape. However, the inferior border of the lingual bar should be slightly rounded when the framework is polished. A rounded border will not impinge on the lingual tissue when the denture bases rotate inferiorly under occlusal loads. Frequently, additional bulk is necessary to provide rigidity, particularly when the bar is long or when a less rigid alloy is used. This is accomplished by underlying the ready-made form with a sheet of 24-gauge casting wax rather than altering the original half-pear shape.

The inferior border of a lingual mandibular major connector must be located so that it does not impinge on the tissue in the floor of the mouth because it changes elevations during the normal activities of mastication, swallowing, speaking, licking the lips, and so forth. Yet, at the same time it seems logical to locate the inferior border of these connectors as far inferiorly as possible to avoid interference with the resting tongue and trapping of food substances when they are introduced into the mouth. Additionally the more inferiorly a lingual bar can be located, the farther the superior border of the bar can be placed from the lingual gingival crevices of adjacent teeth, thereby avoiding impingement on the gingival tissue.

There are at least two clinically acceptable methods to determine the relative height of the floor of the mouth to locate the inferior border of a lingual mandibular major connector. The first method is to measure the height of the floor of the mouth in relation to the lingual gingival margins of adjacent teeth with a periodontal probe (Figure 5-7). During these measurements, the tip of the patient's tongue should be just lightly touching the vermilion border of the upper lip. Recording of these measurements permits their transfer to both diagnostic and master casts, thus ensuring a rather advantageous location of the inferior border of the major connector. The second method is to use an individualized impression tray having its lingual borders 3 mm short of the elevated floor of the mouth and then to use an impression material that will permit the impression to be accurately molded as the patient licks the lips. The inferior border of the planned major connector can then be located at the height of the lingual sulcus of the cast resulting from such an impression. Of the two methods, we have found the measuring of the height of the floor of the mouth to be less variable and more clinically acceptable.

Linguoplate

If the rectangular space bounded by the lingual bar, the anterior tooth contacts and cingula, and the bordering minor connectors is filled in, a linguoplate results (Figure 5-8).

A linguoplate should be made as thin as is technically feasible and should be contoured to follow

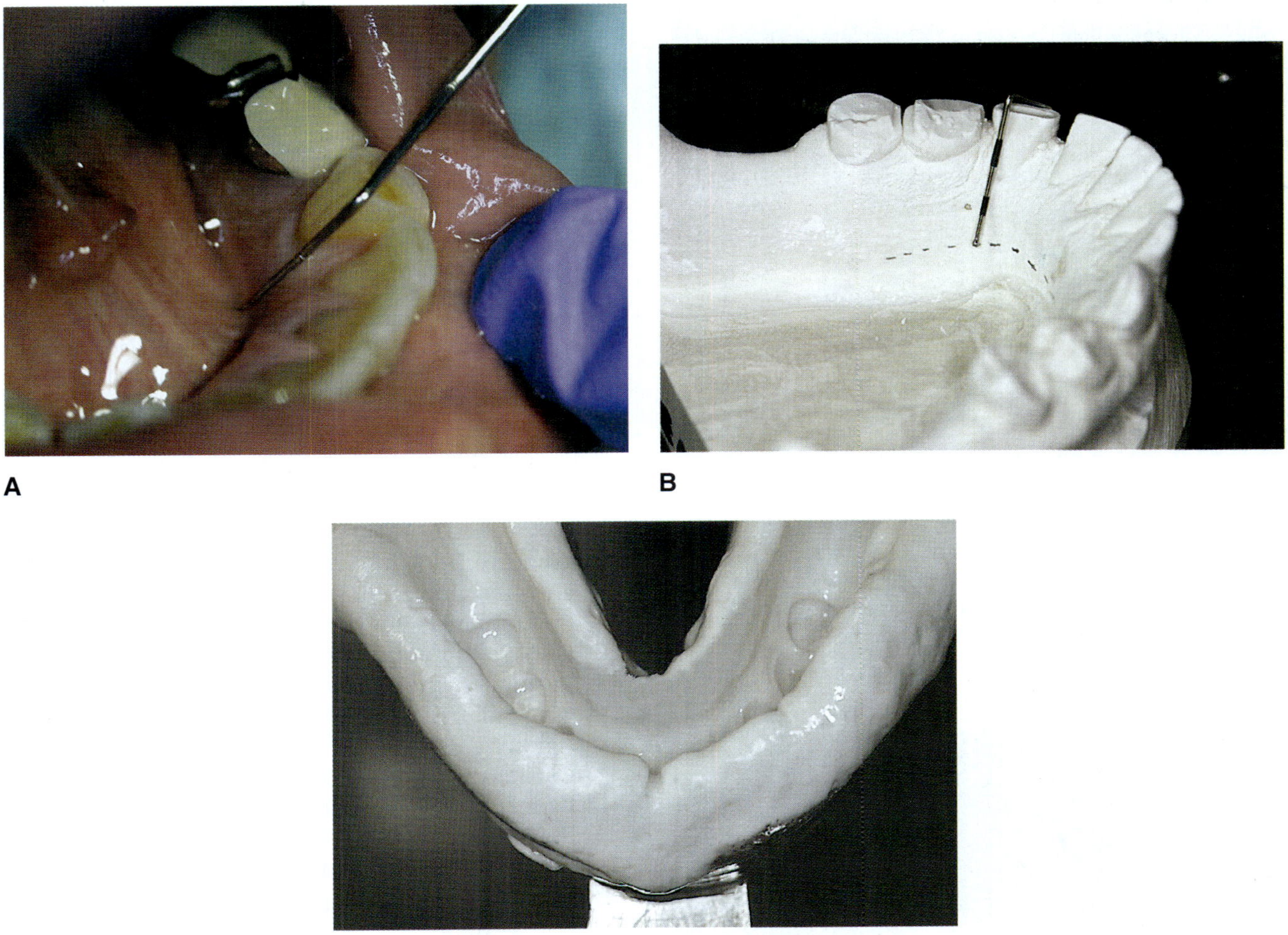

A B C

Figure 5-7 **A,** Height of floor of mouth (tongue elevated) in relation to lingual gingival sulci measured with a periodontal probe. **B,** Recorded measurements are transferred to diagnostic cast and then to master cast after mouth preparations are completed. Line connecting marks indicates location of inferior border of major connector. If periodontal surgery is performed, line on the cast can be related to incisal edges of teeth and the measurements recorded for subsequent use. **C,** Impression made with functional movement of the tongue to demonstrate maximum shortening of the floor of the mouth. This allows visualization of the anatomic feature that establishes the inferior extent of a major connector. If a stock tray causes impingement on this functional position, an individualized or custom tray may be used for the same purpose.

the contours of the teeth and the embrasures (Figure 5-9). The patient should be aware of as little added bulk and altered contours as possible. The upper border should follow the natural curvature of the supracingular surfaces of the teeth and should not be located above the middle third of the lingual surface except to cover interproximal spaces to the contact points. The half-pear shape of a lingual bar should still form the inferior border providing the greatest bulk and rigidity. All gingival crevices and deep embrasures must be blocked out parallel to the path of placement to avoid gingival irritation and any wedging effect between the teeth. In many instances the judicious recontouring of lingual proximal surfaces of overlapped anterior teeth permits a closer adaptation of the linguoplate major connector, eliminating otherwise deep interproximal embrasures to be covered (Figure 5-10).

The linguoplate does not in itself serve as an indirect retainer. When indirect retention is required, definite rests must be provided for this purpose. Both the linguoplate and the cingulum bar should ideally have a terminal rest at each end regardless of the need for indirect retention. However, when indirect retainers are necessary, these rests may also serve as terminal rests for the linguoplate or continuous bar.

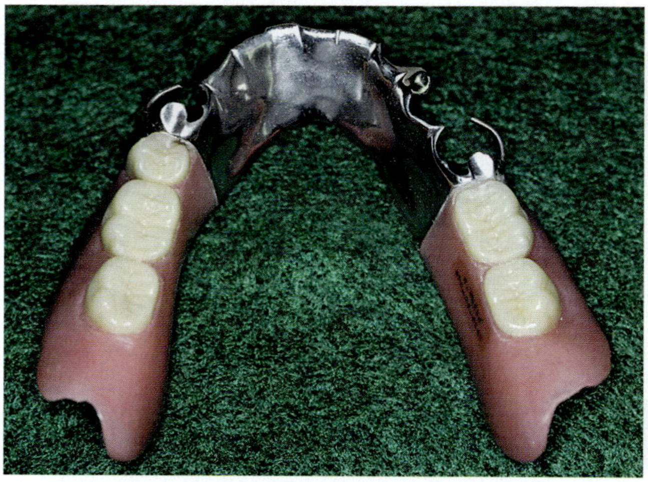

Figure 5-8 View of mandibular Class I design with contoured linguoplate. Linguoplate is made as thin as possible and should follow the lingual contours of the teeth contacted. Doing so will often result in a scalloped superior margin. In this example, the straight superior margin can be bulky at the cingulum region, causing tongue discomfort.

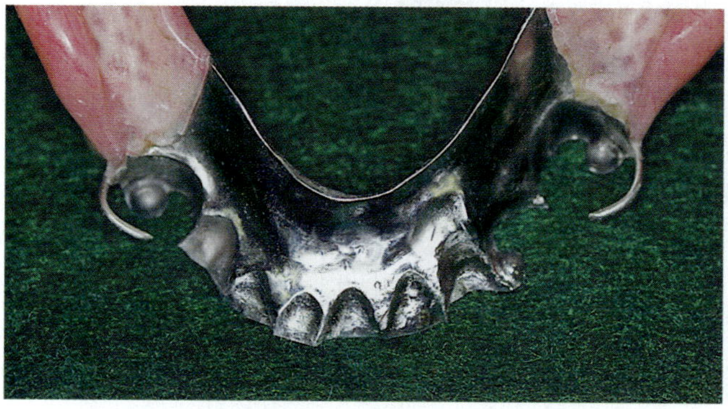

Figure 5-9 Apron of linguoplate (tissue side) is closely adapted to teeth extending into nonundercut interproximal embrasures, resulting in scalloped form. When well adapted, this form will benefit from some anterior teeth acting together to help resist horizontal rotational tendencies of the prosthesis, especially if the posterior ridge form does not resist such movement.

Since no component part of a removable partial denture should be added arbitrarily, each component should be added to serve a definite purpose. The indications for the use of a linguoplate may be listed as follows:

1. When the lingual frenum is high or the space available for a lingual bar is limited. In either instance the superior border of a lingual bar would have to be placed too close to the gingival tissue. Irritation could be avoided only by generous relief, which might be annoying to the tongue and create an undesirable food trap. Where a clinical measurement from the free gingival margins to the slightly elevated floor of the mouth is less than 8 mm, a linguoplate is indicated in lieu of a lingual bar. The use of a linguoplate permits the inferior border to be placed more superiorly without tongue and gingival irritation and without compromise of rigidity.
2. In Class I situations in which the residual ridges have undergone excessive vertical resorption. Flat residual ridges offer little resistance to the horizontal rotational tendencies of a denture. The bracing effect provided by the remaining teeth must be depended upon to resist such rotation. A correctly designed linguoplate will engage the remaining teeth to help resist horizontal rotations.
3. For stabilizing periodontally weakened teeth, splinting with a linguoplate can be of some value when used with definite rests on sound adjacent teeth. As described below, a cingulum bar may be used to accomplish the same purpose, because it actually represents the superior border of a linguoplate without the gingival apron. The cingulum bar accomplishes stabilization along with the other advantages of a linguoplate. However, it is frequently more objectionable to the patient's tongue and is certainly more of a food trap than is the contoured apron of a linguoplate.
4. When the future replacement of one or more incisor teeth will be facilitated by the addition of retention loops to an existing linguoplate. Mandibular incisors that are periodontally weak may thus be retained, with provisions for possible loss and future additions.

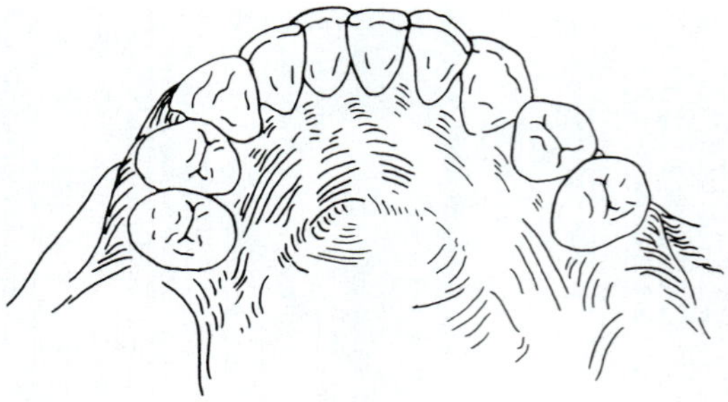

Figure 5-10 If linguoplate major connector was indicated for this patient with overlapped anterior teeth, judicious recontouring of lingual proximal surfaces of right lateral, right central, and left lateral incisors would eliminate excessive undercuts and permit closer adaptation of lingual apron of major connector.

The same reasons for use of a linguoplate anteriorly apply to its use elsewhere in the mandibular arch. If a lingual bar alone is to be used anteriorly, there is no reason for adding an apron elsewhere. However, when auxiliary splinting is used for stabilization of

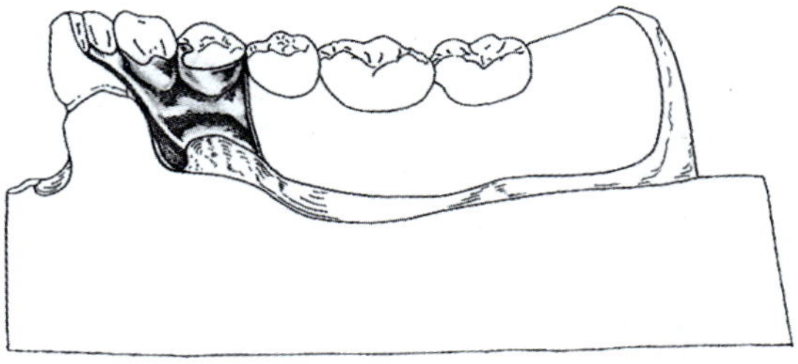

Figure 5-11 Sagittal section through linguoplate demonstrating basic half-pear-shaped inferior border with metallic apron extending superiorly. Extension of linguoplate to height of contour on premolar was accomplished to enclose a rather large triangular interproximal space inferior to contact point between canine and premolar. Such spaces may often be bridged to eliminate obvious food traps. Relief is provided for soft tissue under all portions of the mandibular major connector and any location where the framework crosses the marginal gingiva.

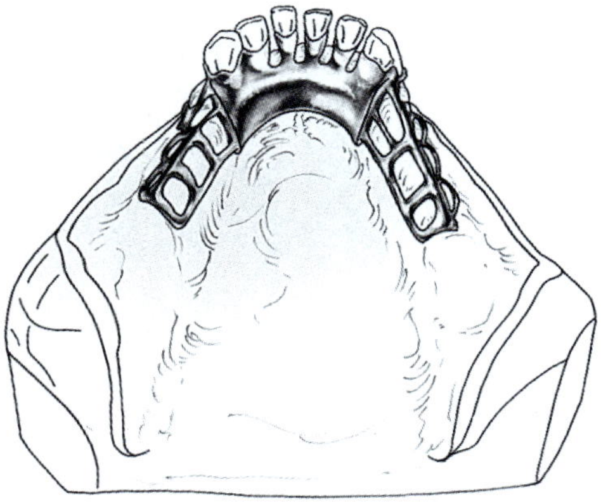

Figure 5-12 Interrupted linguoplate in presence of interproximal spaces.

the remaining teeth or for horizontal stabilizing of the prosthesis, or for both, small rectangular spaces sometimes remain. Tissue response to such small spaces is better when bridged with an apron than when it is left open. Generally the apron is used to avoid gingival irritation or entrapment of food debris or to cover generously relieved areas that would be irritating to the tongue (Figure 5-11).

Sometimes a dentist is faced with a clinical situation wherein a linguoplate is indicated as the major connector of choice even though the anterior teeth are quite spaced and the patient strenuously objects to metal showing through the spaces. The linguoplate can then be constructed so that the metal will not appreciably show through the spaced anterior teeth (Figure 5-12). Rigidity of the major connector is not greatly altered. However, such a design may be as much of a food trap as the continuous bar type of major connector.

Design of Mandibular Major Connectors

The following systematic approach to designing a mandibular lingual bar and linguoplate major connectors can be readily used with the diagnostic casts after considering the diagnostic data and relating them to the basic principles of major connector design:

Step 1: Outline the basal seat areas on the diagnostic cast (Figure 5-13, *A*)

Step 2: Outline the inferior border of the major connector (Figure 5-13, *B*)

Step 3: Outline the superior border of the major connector (Figure 5-13, *C*)

Step 4: Connect the basal seat area to the inferior and superior borders of the major connector, and add minor connectors to retain the acrylic resin denture base material (Figure 5-13, *D*)

Sublingual Bar

A modification of the lingual bar that has been demonstrated to be useful when the height of the floor of the mouth does not allow placement of the superior border of the bar at least 4 mm below the free gingival margin is the sublingual bar. The bar shape remains essentially the same as that of a lingual bar, but placement is inferior and posterior to the usual placement of a lingual bar, lying over and parallel to the anterior floor of the mouth. It is generally accepted that a sublingual bar can be used in lieu of a lingual plate if the lingual frenum does not interfere or in the presence of an anterior lingual undercut that would require considerable blockout for a conventional lingual bar. Contraindications include interfering lingual tori, high attachment of a lingual frenum, and interference with elevation of the floor of the mouth during functional movements.

Cingulum Bar (Continuous Bar)

When a linguoplate is the major connector of choice, but the axial alignment of the anterior teeth is such that excessive blockout of interproximal undercuts must be made, a cingulum bar may be considered. A cingulum bar located on or slightly above the cingula of the anterior teeth may be added to the lingual bar or can be used independently (Figure 5-14). Additionally, when wide diastemata exist between the lower anterior teeth, a continuous bar retainer may be more esthetically acceptable than a linguoplate.

Labial Bar

Fortunately there are few situations in which extreme lingual inclination of the remaining lower premolar and incisor teeth prevents the use of

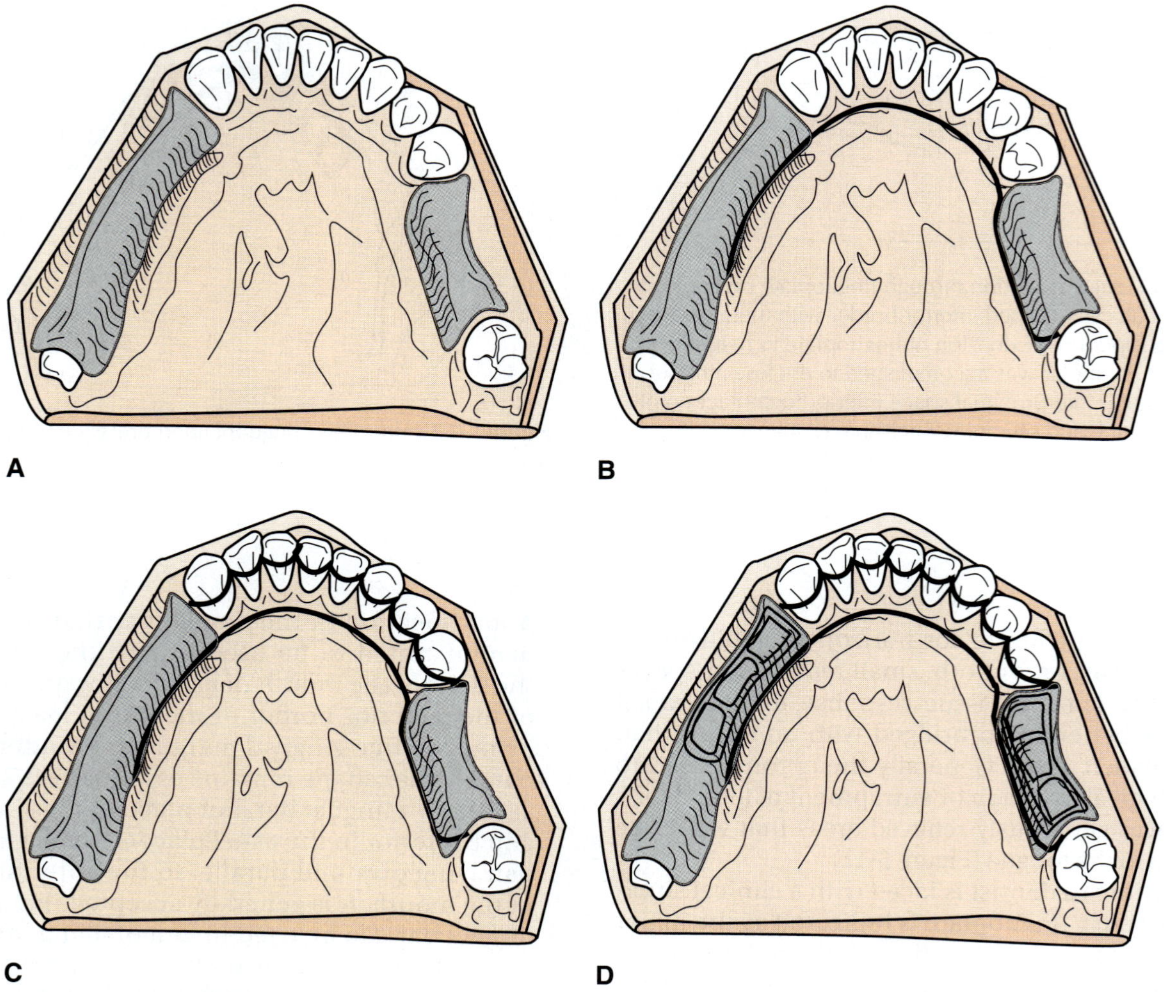

Figure 5-13 Sequence of design considerations for a mandibular major connector. **A,** Diagnostic cast with basal seat areas outlined. **B,** Inferior border of major connector is outlined. Location of inferior border was determined as suggested in Figure 5-7 and extends to the mesial of the mandibular right molar. **C,** Superior border of major connector is outlined. Limited space for lingual bar requires use of linguoplate major connector. Linguoplate requires that rest seats be used on canines and first premolar for positive support. **D,** Rest seat areas on posterior teeth are outlined, and minor connectors for retention of resin denture bases are sketched.

a lingual bar major connector. By conservative mouth preparations in the form of recontouring and by blockout, a lingual major connector can almost always be used. Lingually inclined teeth may sometimes have to be reshaped by means of crowns. Although the use of a labial major connector may be necessary in rare instances, it should be avoided by resorting to necessary mouth preparations rather than by accepting a condition that is otherwise correctable (Figure 5-15). The same applies to the use of a labial bar when a mandibular torus interferes with the placement of a lingual bar. Unless surgery is definitely contraindicated, interfering mandibular tori should be removed so that the use of a labial bar connector may be avoided.

A modification to the linguoplate is the hinged continuous labial bar. This concept is incorporated in the Swing-Lock* design, which consists of a labial or buccal bar that is connected to the major connector by a hinge on one end and a latch at the other end (Figure 5-16).

*Idea Development Co., Dallas, Texas.

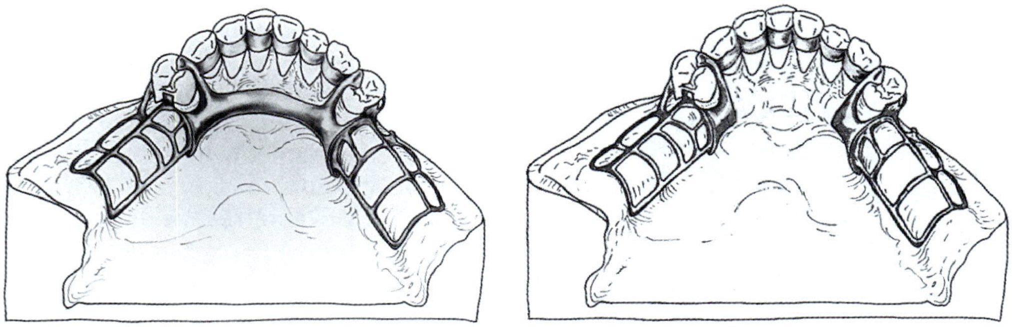

A B

Figure 5-14 **A,** Lingual bar and cingulum bar (continuous bar) major connector. Upper portion of this major connector is located on cingula of anterior teeth. Requirement of positive support by rest seats, at least as far anteriorly as the canines, is critical. Note that superior border of lingual bar portion is often placed objectionably close to gingival margins if sufficient bulk for rigidity is to be obtained. This type of major connector easily traps food and is often more objectionable to patients than a linguoplate. **B,** Cingulum bar (continuous bar) major connector. Although this design may reduce the possibility of food entrapment, it may not provide adequate rigidity.

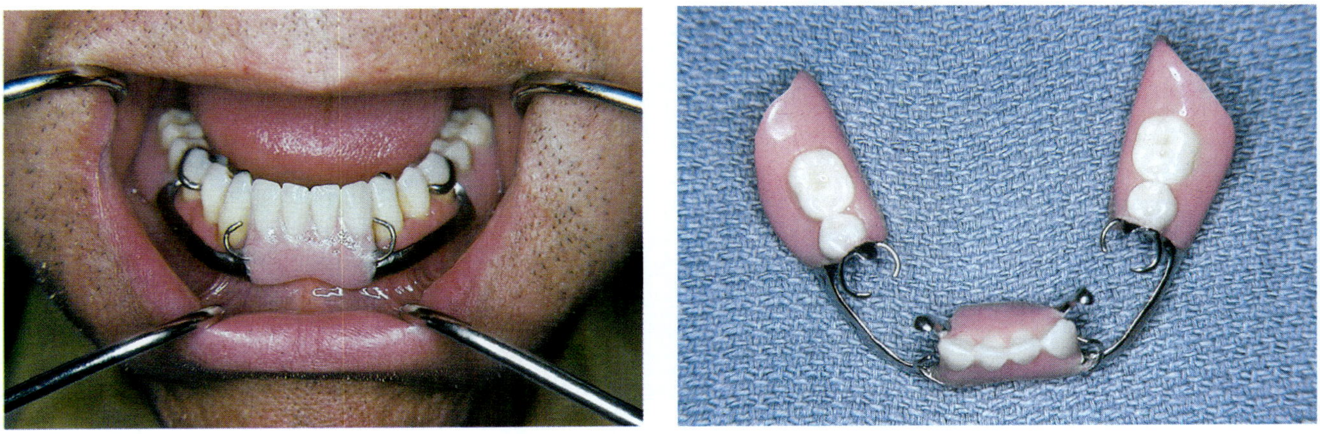

A B

Figure 5-15 **A,** Lingual inclination of patient's canines and premolars precludes use of lingual bar. **B,** Labial bar major connector was used in treatment. Retention was obtained on terminal abutments. Support and stabilization were gained by using rests, minor connectors arising from labial bar, and well-fitting denture bases.

Support is provided by multiple rests on the remaining natural teeth. Stabilization and reciprocation are provided by a linguoplate contacting the remaining teeth and are supplemented by the labial bar with its retentive struts. Retention is provided by a bar type of retentive clasp arms projecting from the labial or buccal bar and contacting the infrabulge areas on the labial surfaces of the teeth.

Use of the Swing-Lock concept would seem primarily indicated when the following conditions are present:

1. Missing key abutments. By using all the remaining teeth for retention and stability, the absence of a key abutment (such as a canine) may not present as serious a treatment problem with this concept as with more conventional designs (Figure 5-17).
2. Unfavorable tooth contours. When existing tooth contours (uncorrectable by recontouring with appropriate restorations) or excessive labial inclinations of anterior teeth prevent conventional clasp designs, the basic principles

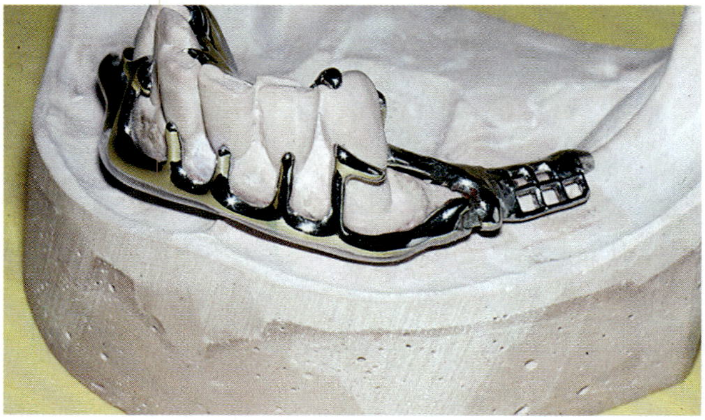

Figure 5-16 The hinge for this continuous labial bar connector is located buccal and distal to the remaining dentition (area of tooth #21). The latching mechanism is opposite to the hinge, adjacent to tooth #28. In this location it will be housed within the buccal flange of the denture.

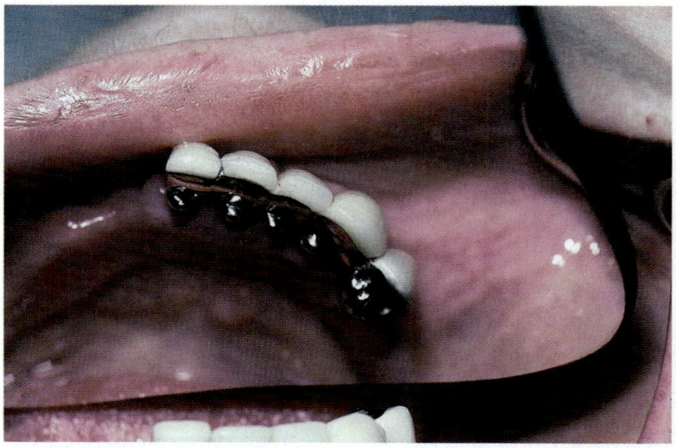

Figure 5-17 Absence of mandibular canine requires that all remaining anterior teeth be used for stabilization and retention of replacement restoration. Swing-Lock concept can be used to ensure group function of these remaining mandibular teeth.

of removable partial design may be better implemented with the Swing-Lock concept.

3. Unfavorable soft tissue contours. Extensive soft tissue undercuts may prevent proper location of component parts of a conventional removable partial denture or an overdenture (see. The hinged continuous labial bar concept may provide an adjunctive modality to accommodate such unfavorable soft tissue contours.
4. Teeth with questionable prognoses. The possibility of losing a key abutment tooth with a guarded prognosis seriously affects the stability and retention of a conventional prosthesis. Because all of the remaining teeth function as abutments in the Swing-Lock denture, the loss of a tooth would seemingly not compromise retention and stability to such a degree. The hinged labial bar type of restoration can be used satisfactorily for certain clinically compromised situations. As is true with any type of removable restoration, good oral hygiene, maintenance, regular recall, and close attention to details of design are paramount to successful implementation of this treatment concept.

Obvious contraindications to the use of this hinged labial bar concept are apparent. The most obvious is poor oral hygiene or lack of motivation for plaque control by the patient. Other contraindications are the presence of a shallow buccal or labial vestibule or a high frenal attachment. Any of these factors would prevent the proper placement of components of the Swing-Lock partial denture.

Maxillary Major Connectors

Six basic types of maxillary major connectors are considered:

1. Single palatal strap (Figure 5-18, *A*)
2. Combination anterior and posterior palatal strap-type connector (Figure 5-18, *B*)
3. Palatal plate-type connector (Figure 5-18, *C*)
4. U-shaped palatal connector (Figure 5-18, *D*)
5. Single palatal bar (Figure 5-18, *E*)
6. Anterior-posterior palatal bars (Figure 5-18, *F*)

Whenever it is necessary for the palatal connector to make contact with the teeth for reasons of support, definite tooth support must be provided. This is best accomplished by establishing definite rest seats on the predetermined abutment teeth. These should be located far enough above the gingival attachment to provide for bridging the gingival crevice with block-out. At the same time, they should be low enough on the tooth to avoid unfavorable leverage and low enough on the maxillary incisors and canine teeth to avoid incisal interference of the opposing dentition.

Major connector components resting on unprepared inclined tooth surfaces can lead to slippage of the denture or to orthodontic movement of the tooth, or to both. In either situation, settling into gingival tissue is inevitable. In the absence of the required vertical support provided by rests, the health of the surrounding tissue is usually impaired. Similarly, interproximal projections of the major connector that rest on the gingival third of the tooth and on gingival tissue that are structurally unable to render support may be traumatized. To prevent these sequelae, either support the major connector by definite rests on the teeth, provide adequate gingival

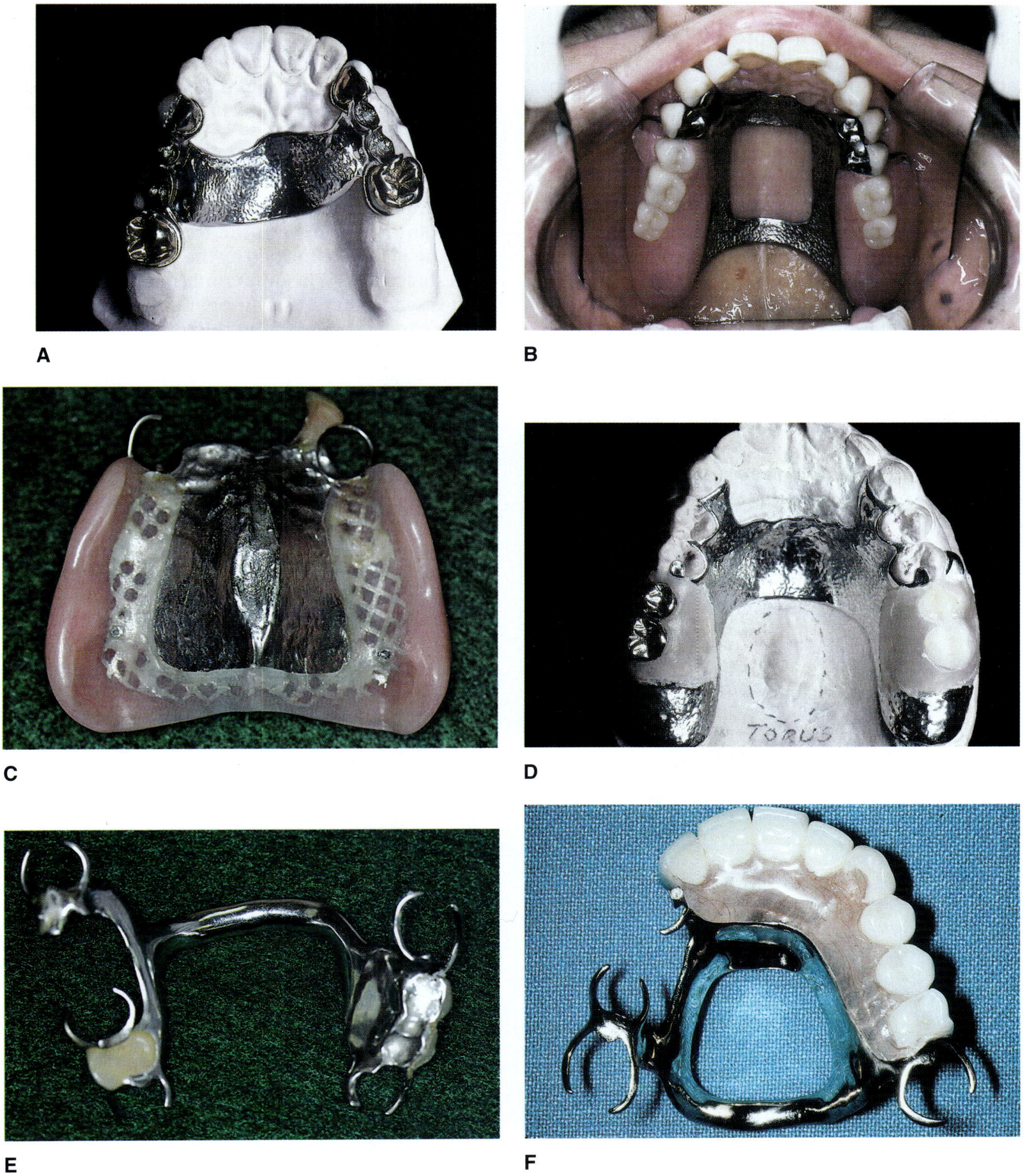

Figure 5-18 Maxillary major connectors: **A,** Single palatal strap. **B,** Anterior-posterior palatal strap. **C,** Palatal plate. **D,** U-shaped. **E,** Single palatal bar. **F,** Anterior-posterior palatal bars.

relief, and/or locate the connector far enough away from the gingival margin to avoid any possible restriction of blood supply and entrapment of food debris. All gingival crossings should be abrupt and at right angles to the major connector. Creating a sharp, angular form on any portion of a palatal connector should be avoided, and all borders should be tapered toward the tissue.

Single Palatal Strap

Bilateral tooth-supported prostheses, even those with short edentulous spaces, are effectively connected with a single, broad palatal strap connector, particularly when the edentulous areas are located posteriorly (Figure 5-19). Such a connector can be made rigid without objectionable bulk and interference with the tongue provided the cast framework material is distributed in three planes. Suitable rigidity, without excessive bulk, may be obtained for a single palatal strap by the laboratory technician casting a 22-gauge matte plastic pattern.

For reasons of torque and leverage, a single palatal strap major connector should not be used to connect anterior replacements with distal extension bases. To be rigid enough to resist torque and to provide adequate vertical support and horizontal stabilization, a single palatal strap would have to be objectionably bulky. When placed anteriorly, this bulk would become even more objectionable to the patient, because it could interfere with speech.

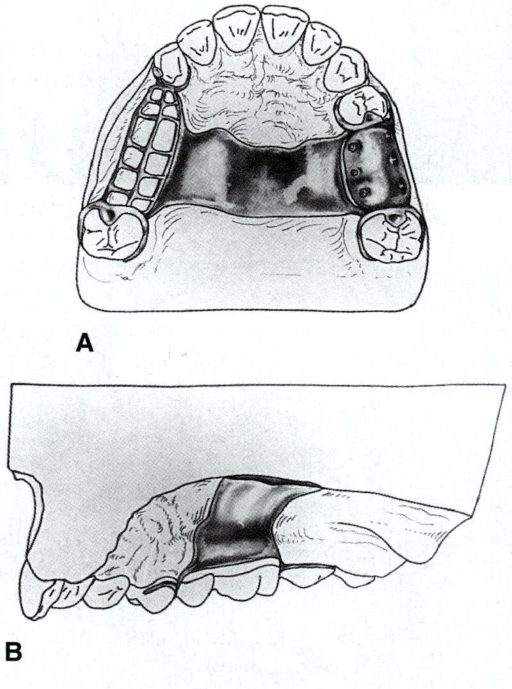

Figure 5-19 **A,** This single palatal strap-type major connector is better suited for the restoration of short span tooth-supported bilateral edentulous areas. It may also be used in tooth-supported unilateral edentulous situations with provision for cross-arch attachment by either extracoronal retainers or internal attachments. Width of palatal strap should be confined within the boundaries of supporting rests. **B,** Sagittal section. Midportion of major connector demonstrates slight elevation to provide rigidity. Such thickness of major connector does not appreciably alter palatal contours.

Combination Anterior and Posterior Palatal Strap-type Connector

Structurally, this is a rigid palatal major connector. The anterior and posterior palatal strap combination may be used in almost any maxillary partial denture design (Figure 5-20).

A posterior palatal strap should be flat and a minimum of 8 mm wide. Posterior palatal connectors should be located as far posteriorly as possible to avoid interference with the tongue but anterior to the line of flexure formed by the junction of the hard and soft palates. The only condition preventing their use is when there is an inoperable maxillary torus that extends posteriorly to the soft palate. In this situation, a broad, U-shaped major connector may be used as described elsewhere in this chapter.

The strength of this major connector design lies in the fact that the anterior and posterior components are joined together by longitudinal connectors on either side, forming a square or rectangular frame. Each component braces the others against possible torque and flexure. Flexure is practically nonexistent in such a design.

The anterior connector may be extended anteriorly to support anterior tooth replacements. In this form, a U-shaped connector is made rigid because of the added horizontal strap posteriorly. If a maxillary torus exists, it may be encircled by this type of major strap-type connector without sacrificing rigidity.

The combination anterior-posterior connector design may be used with any Kennedy class of partially edentulous arch. It is used most frequently in Classes II and IV, whereas the single wide palatal

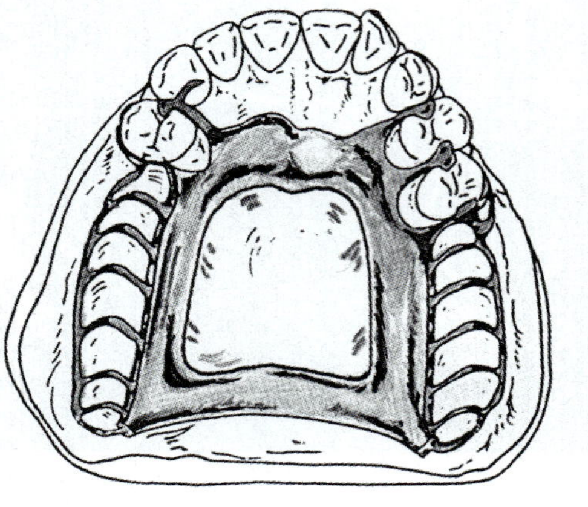

Figure 5-20 Anterior-posterior palatal strap-type major connector. Anterior component is a flat strap located as far posteriorly as possible to avoid rugae coverage and tongue interference. Anterior border of this strap should be located just posterior to a rugae crest or in the valley between two crests. Posterior strap is thin, a minimum of 8 mm wide, and is located as far posteriorly as possible, yet entirely on hard palate. It should be located at right angles to midline rather than diagonally.

strap is more frequently used in Class III situations. The palatal plate-type or complete coverage connector, described in this chapter, is used most frequently in Class I situations for reasons to be explained subsequently. All maxillary major connectors should cross the midline at a right angle rather than on a diagonal. It has been suggested that the tongue will accept symmetrically placed components far more readily than those placed without regard for symmetry.

Palatal Plate-type Connector

For the lack of better terminology, the words *palatal plate* are used to designate any thin, broad, contoured palatal coverage used as a maxillary major connector and covering one half or more of the hard palate (Figure 5-21). Anatomic replica palatal castings have uniform thickness and strength by reason of their corrugated contours. Through the use of electrolytic polishing, uniformity of thickness can be maintained, and the anatomical contours of the palate are faithfully reproduced in the finished denture.

The anatomic replica palatal major connector has several potential advantages:

1. It permits the making of a uniformly thin metal plate that reproduces faithfully the anatomic contours of the patient's own palate. Its uniform thinness and the thermal conductivity of the metal are designed to make the palatal plate more readily acceptable to the tongue and underlying tissue.
2. The corrugation in the anatomic replica adds strength to the casting; thus a thinner casting with adequate rigidity can be made.
3. Surface irregularities are intentional rather than accidental; therefore electrolytic polishing is all that is needed. The original uniform thickness of the plastic pattern is thus maintained.
4. By virtue of intimate contact, interfacial surface tension between metal and tissue provides the prosthesis with greater retention. Retention must be adequate to resist the pull of sticky foods, the action of moving border tissue against the denture, the forces of gravity, and the more violent forces of coughing and sneezing. These are all resisted to some extent by the retention of the base itself, which is proportional to the total area of denture base contact to the supporting tissue. The required amount of both direct and indirect retention will depend on the amount of retention provided by the denture base.

The palatal plate may be used in any one of three ways. It may be used as a plate of varying width that covers the area between two or more edentulous areas, as a complete or partial cast plate that extends posteriorly to the junction of the hard and soft palates (Figures 5-22 and 5-23), or in the form of an anterior palatal connector with a provision for extending an acrylic resin denture base posteriorly (Figure 5-24).

The palatal plate should be located anterior to the posterior palatal seal area. The maxillary complete denture's typical posterior palatal seal is not necessary

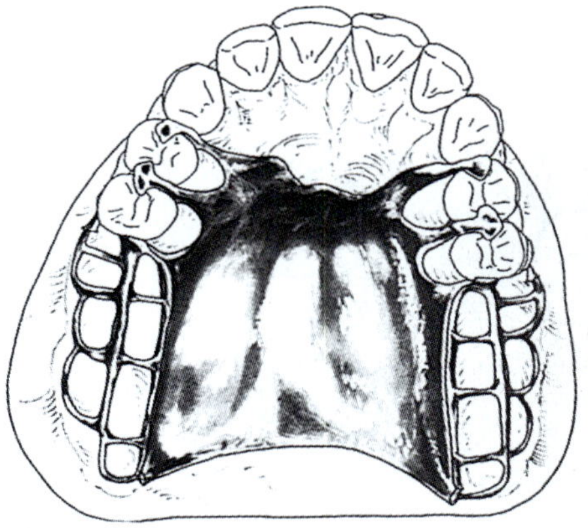

Figure 5-21 Palatal major connector covering two thirds of palate. Anterior border follows valleys between rugae and does not extend anterior to indirect retainers on first premolars. Posterior border is located at junction of hard and soft palates but does not extend onto soft palate. In bilateral distal extension situation illustrated, indirect retainers are a must to aid in resisting horizontal rotation of the restoration. Note that provisions have been made for a butt-type joint joining the denture bases and framework as denture base on each side passes through pterygomaxillary notch.

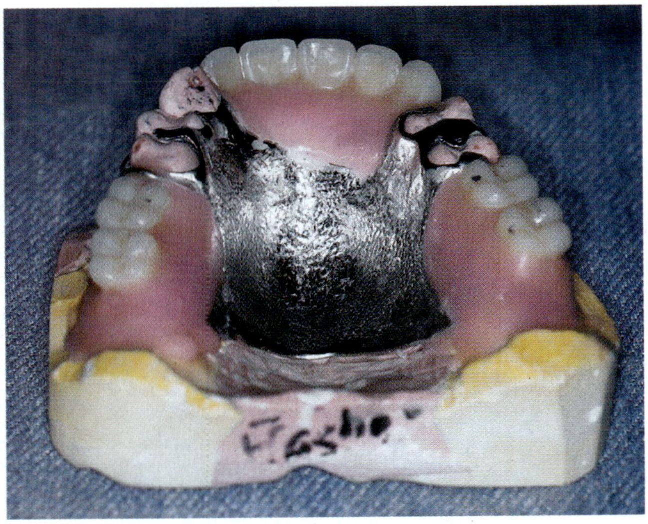

Figure 5-22 Palatal plate major connector for a Class I, modification 1, removable partial denture. Posterior border lies on immovable hard palate and crosses the midline at a right angle. Total contact provides excellent auxiliary retention without objectionable bulk.

with a maxillary partial denture's palatal plate because of the accuracy and stability of the cast metal.

When the last remaining abutment tooth on either side of a Class I arch is the canine or first premolar tooth, complete palatal coverage is strongly advised, especially when the residual ridges have undergone excessive vertical resorption. This may be accomplished in one of two ways. One method is to use a complete cast plate that extends to the junction of the hard and soft palates (see Figure 5-23). The other method is to use a cast major connector anteriorly, with retention posteriorly, for the attachment of an acrylic-resin denture base that extends posteriorly to the anatomic landmarks previously described (see Figure 5-24).

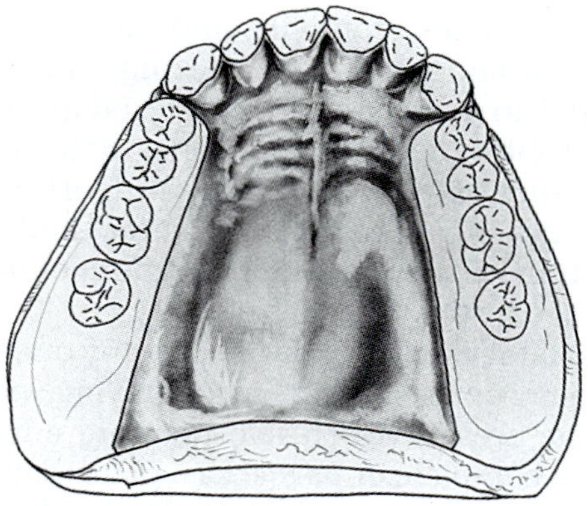

Figure 5-23 Complete coverage palatal major connector. Posterior border terminates at junction of hard and soft palates. Anterior portion, in the form of palatal linguoplate, is supported by positive lingual rest seats on canines. Location of finishing lines is most important in this type of major connector. Anteroposteriorly, they should be parallel to a line along the center of the ridge crest and located just lingual to an imaginary line contacting lingual surfaces of missing natural teeth. Alteration of natural palatal contour should be anticipated with its attendant detrimental effect on speech if these contours are not followed.

Despite increased cost, the advantages of a cast palate make it preferable to an acrylic-resin palate. However, the latter method may be used satisfactorily when relining is anticipated or cost is a factor. The complete palatal plate is not a connector that has received universal use. It has, however, become accepted as a satisfactory palatal connector for many maxillary partial dentures. In all circumstances, the portion contacting the teeth must have positive support from adequate rest seats. The dentist should be familiar with its use and, at the same time, with its limitations so that it may be used intelligently and to the fullest advantage.

Design of Maxillary Major Connectors

In 1953 Blatterfein described a systematic approach to designing maxillary major connectors. His method involves five basic steps and is certainly applicable to most maxillary removable partial denture situations. Using a diagnostic cast and knowledge of the relative displaceability of the palatal tissue, including that covering the median palatal raphe, he recommends the following basic steps:

Step 1: Outline of primary bearing areas. The primary bearing areas are those that will be covered by the denture base(s) (Figure 5-25, *A* and *B*).

Step 2: Outline of nonbearing areas. The nonbearing areas are the lingual gingival tissue within 5 to 6 mm of the remaining teeth, hard areas of the medial palatal raphe (including tori),

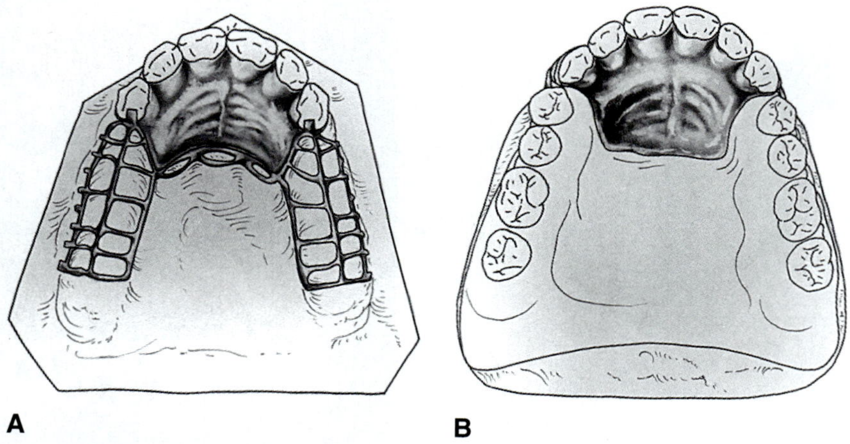

Figure 5-24 **A,** Maxillary major connector in the form of palatal linguoplate with provision for attaching full-coverage resin denture base. **B,** Completed removable partial denture with resin base. Palatal linguoplate is supported by rests occupying lingual rest seats prepared in cast restorations on canines. This type of removable partial denture is particularly applicable where (1) residual ridges have undergone extreme vertical resorption and (2) terminal abutments have suffered some bone loss and splinting cannot be accomplished.

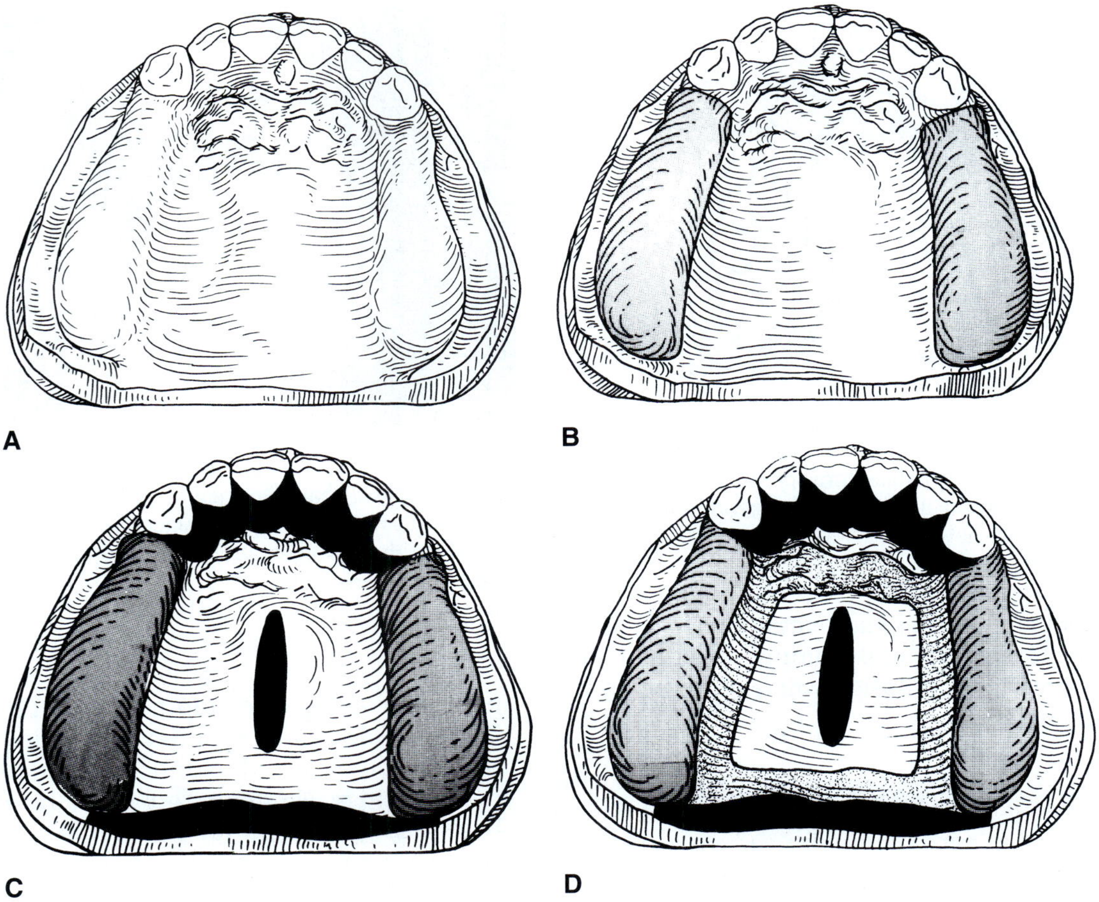

Figure 5-25 **A,** Diagnostic cast of partially edentulous maxillary arch. **B,** The palatal extent of the denture base areas are located 2 mm from the palatal surface of the posterior teeth. **C,** Nonbearing areas outlined in black, which include lingual soft tissue within 5 to 6 mm of teeth, an unyielding median palatal raphe area, and soft palate. The space bounded by bearing and nonbearing area outlines is available for placement of major connector. **D,** Major connector selected will be rigid and noninterfering with tongue and will cover a minimum of the palate.

and palatal tissue posterior to the vibrating line (Figure 5-25, *C*).

Step 3: Outline of connector areas. Steps 1 and 2, when completed, provide an outline or designate areas that are available to place components of major connectors (Figure 5-25, *C*).

Step 4: Selection of connector type. Selection of the type of connector(s) is based on four factors: mouth comfort, rigidity, location of denture bases, and indirect retention. Connectors should be of minimum bulk and should be positioned so that interference with the tongue during speech and mastication is not encountered. Connectors must have a maximum of rigidity to distribute stress bilaterally. The double-strap type of major connector provides the maximum rigidity without bulk and total tissue coverage. In many instances the choice of a strap type of major connector is limited by the location of the edentulous ridge areas. When edentulous areas are located anteriorly, the use of only a posterior strap is not recommended. By the same token, when only posterior edentulous areas are present, the use of only an anterior strap is not recommended. The need for indirect retention influences the outline of the major connector. Provision must be made in the major connector so that indirect retainers may be attached.

Step 5: Unification. After selection of the type of major connector based on the considerations in Step 4, the denture base areas and connectors are joined (Figure 5-25, *D*).

The indications for the use of complete palatal coverage have been previously discussed in this

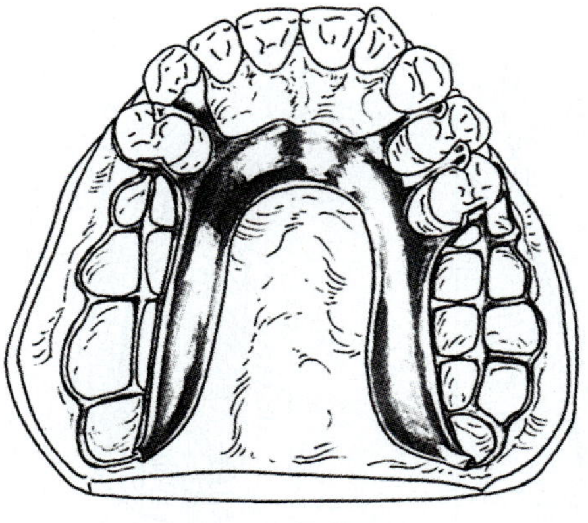

Figure 5-26 U-shaped palatal connector is probably the least rigid type of maxillary major connector and should be used only when large inoperable palatal torus prevents use of palatal coverage or combination anterior-posterior palatal strap-type designed framework.

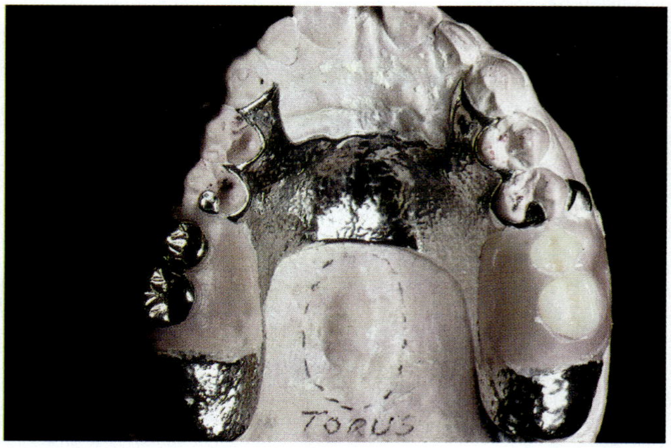

Figure 5-27 Removable partial denture design that uses an objectionable U-shaped palatal major connector. Such a connector lacks necessary rigidity, places bulk where it is most objectionable to patient, and impinges on gingival tissue lingual to remaining teeth.

chapter. Although there are many variations in palatal major connectors, a thorough comprehension of all factors influencing their design will lead to the best design for each patient.

U-shaped Palatal Connector

From both the patient's standpoint and a mechanical standpoint, the U-shaped palatal connector is the least desirable of maxillary major connectors. It should never be used arbitrarily. When a large inoperable palatal torus exists, and occasionally when several anterior teeth are to be replaced, the U-shaped palatal connector may have to be used (Figure 5-26). In most instances, however, other designs will serve more effectively.

The following are the principal objections to use of the U-shaped connector:

1. Its lack of rigidity (compared with other designs) can allow lateral flexure under occlusal forces, which may induce torque or direct lateral force to abutment teeth.
2. The design fails to provide good support characteristics and may permit impingement of underlying tissue when subjected to occlusal loading.
3. Bulk to enhance rigidity results in increased thickness in areas that are a hindrance to the tongue.

Many maxillary partial dentures have failed for no other reason than the flexibility of a U-shaped major connector (Figure 5-27). To be rigid, the U-shaped palatal connector must have bulk where the tongue needs the most freedom, which is the rugae area. Without sufficient bulk, the U-shaped design leads to increased flexibility and movement at the open ends. In distal extension partial dentures, when tooth support posterior to the edentulous area is nonexistent, movement is particularly noticeable and is traumatic to the residual ridge. No matter how well the extension base is supported or how harmonious the occlusion, without a rigid major connector the residual ridge suffers.

The wider the coverage of a U-shaped major connector, the more it resembles a palatal plate–type connector with its several advantages. But when used as a narrow U design, the necessary rigidity is usually lacking. A U-shaped connector may be made more rigid by providing multiple tooth support through definite rests. A common error in the design of a U-shaped connector, however, is its proximity to, or actual contact with, gingival tissue. The principle that the borders of major connectors should either be supported by rests in prepared rest seats or be located well away from gingival tissue has been stated previously. The majority of U-shaped connectors fail to do either, with resulting gingival irritation and periodontal damage to the tissue adjacent to the remaining teeth.

Single Palatal Bar

To differentiate between a palatal bar and a palatal strap, a palatal connector component of less than 8 mm in width is referred to as a bar in this textbook. The single palatal bar is perhaps the most widely used and yet the least logical of all palatal major connectors. It is difficult to say whether the bar or the U-shaped palatal connector is the more objectionable of palatal connectors.

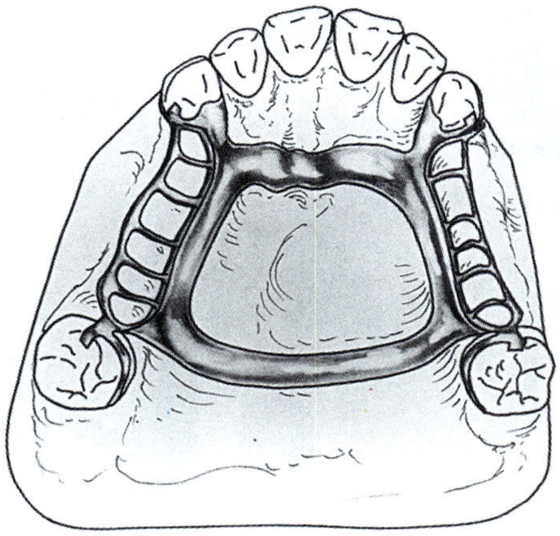

Figure 5-28 Combination anterior-posterior palatal bar. To be sufficiently rigid to provide required support and stability, these major connectors must be excessively bulky. Due to its bulk and location the anterior bar often interferes with the tongue.

For a single palatal bar to have the necessary rigidity for cross-arch distribution of stress, it must have concentrated bulk, which, unfortunately, is all too often ignored. For a single palatal bar to be effective, it must be rigid enough to provide support and cross-arch stabilization and must be centrally located between the halves of the denture. Mechanically, this practice may be sound enough. However, from the standpoint of patient comfort and alteration of palatal contours, it is highly objectionable.

A partial denture made with a single palatal bar is often either too thin and flexible or too bulky and objectionable to the patient's tongue. The decision to use a single palatal bar instead of a strap should be based on the size of the denture-bearing areas that are connected and on whether a single connector located between them would be rigid without objectionable bulk.

Combination Anterior and Posterior Palatal Bar-type Connectors

Structurally, this combination of major connectors exhibits many of the same disadvantages as the single palatal bar (Figure 5-28). To be sufficiently rigid and to provide the needed support and stability, these connectors could be too bulky and could interfere with tongue function.

Beading of the Maxillary Cast

Beading is a term used to denote the scribing of a shallow groove on the maxillary master cast outlining the palatal major connector exclusive of rugae areas (Figure 5-29). The purposes of beading are as follows:

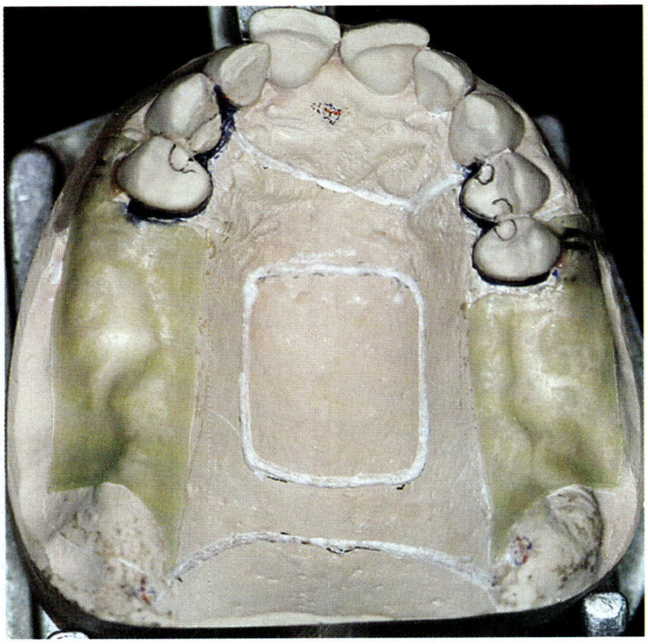

Figure 5-29 Framework design on master cast before preparation for duplication in refractory investment. Shallow groove (0.5 mm) has been scribed on outline of anterior and posterior borders of the major connector. Anterior outline follows valleys of rugae. Beading is readily accomplished with cleoid carver. Slightly rounded groove is preferred to V-shaped groove.

1. To transfer the major connector design to the investment cast (Figure 5-30, *A* and *B*)
2. To provide a visible finishing line for the casting (Figure 5-31)
3. To ensure intimate tissue contact of the major connector with selected palatal tissue

Beading is readily accomplished by using an appropriate instrument, such as a cleoid carver. Care must be exercised to create a groove not in excess of 0.5 mm in width or depth (Figures 5-32, *A* and *B*).

MINOR CONNECTORS

Minor connectors are those components that serve as the connecting link between the major connector or base of a removable partial denture and the other components of the prosthesis, such as the clasp assembly, indirect retainers, occlusal rests, or cingulum rests. In many instances a minor connector may be continuous with some other part of the denture. For example, an occlusal rest at one end of a linguoplate is actually the terminus of a minor connector, even though that minor connector is continuous with the linguoplate. Similarly the portion of a partial denture framework that supports the clasp and the occlusal rest is a minor connector, which joins the major connector with the clasp proper.

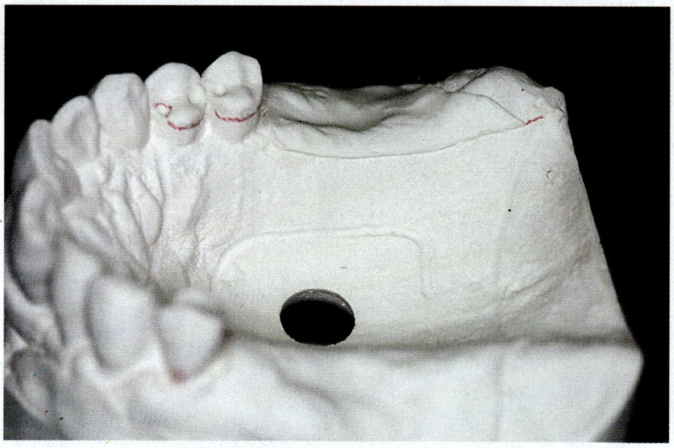

A

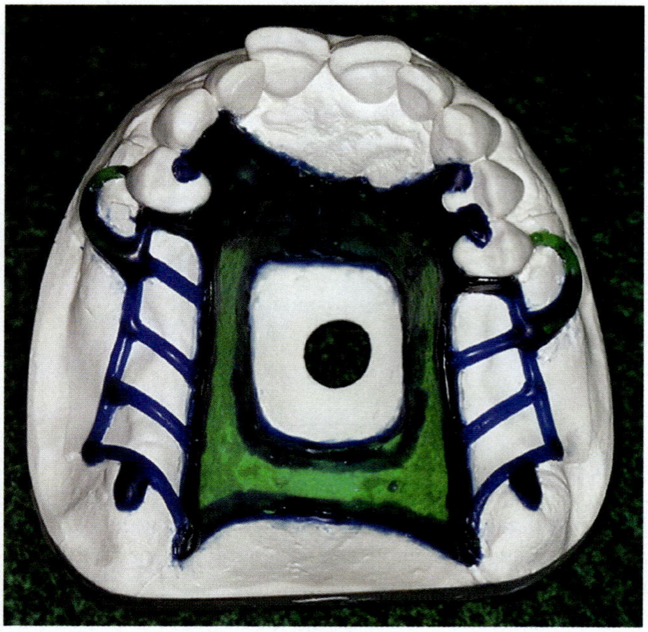

B

Figure 5-30 **A,** Refractory cast. Note definitive outline of major connector indicated by beading lines that were transferred in duplicating the master cast. **B,** Wax pattern for major connector is accurately executed by following the beading lines. Major connector is confined to previously scribed beading.

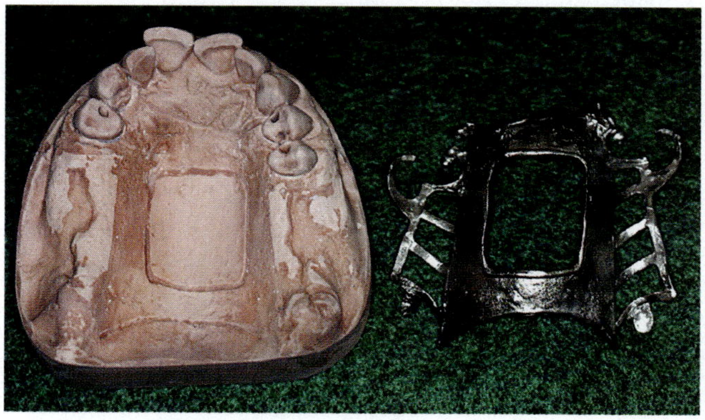

Figure 5-31 Cast and framework showing metal margin produced by the 0.5 mm beading line scribed on the cast. Such a margin is easily finished in the lab and provides intimate tissue contact, preventing food from easily dislodging the prosthesis. Care should be exercised in adapting such a beaded margin to non-compressible tissue, such as the median palatal raphe.

Those portions of a removable partial denture framework that retain the denture bases are also minor connectors.

Functions

In addition to joining denture parts, the minor connector serves two other purposes.

1. To transfer functional stress to the abutment teeth. This is a prosthesis-to-abutment function of the minor connector. Occlusal forces applied to the artificial teeth are transmitted through the base to the underlying ridge tissue if that base is primarily tissue supported. Occlusal forces applied to the artificial teeth are also transferred to abutment teeth through occlusal rests. The minor connectors arising from a rigid major connector make possible this transfer of functional stress throughout the dental arch.
2. To transfer the effect of the retainers, rests, and stabilizing components throughout the prosthesis. This is an abutment-to-prosthesis function of the minor connector. Thus forces applied on one portion of the denture may be resisted by other components placed elsewhere in the arch for that purpose. A stabilizing component on one side of the arch may be placed to resist horizontal forces originating on the opposite side. This is possible only because of the transferring effect of the minor connector, which supports that stabilizing component, and the rigidity of the major connector.

Form and Location

Like the major connector, the minor connector must have sufficient bulk to be rigid; otherwise the transfer of functional stresses to the supporting teeth and tissue will not be effective. At the same time, the bulk of the minor connector should not be objectionable.

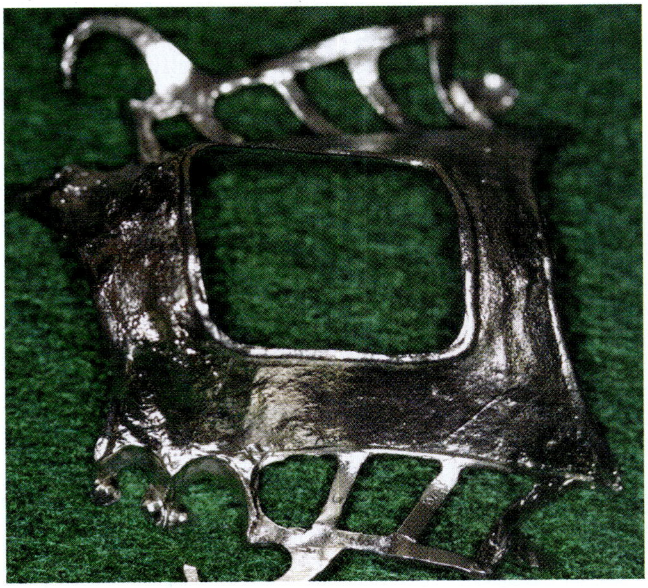

A

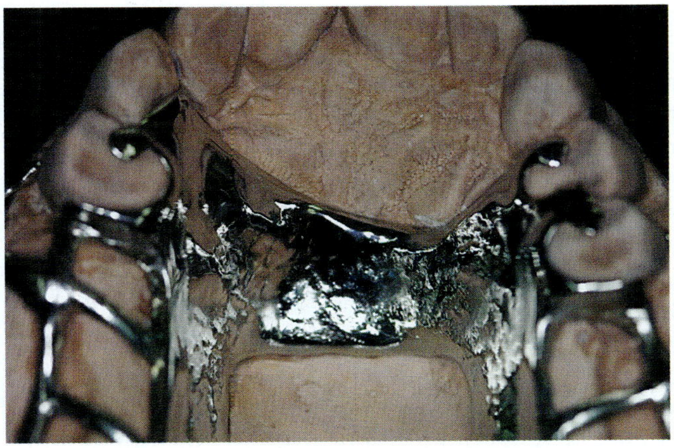

B

Figure 5-32 A, Tissue side of casting. Note slightly elevated ridges outlining anterior, posterior, and mid-palatal opening region of this anterior-posterior palatal strap major connector. B, Casting finished to demarcated outline and seated on the master cast showing intimate adaptation.

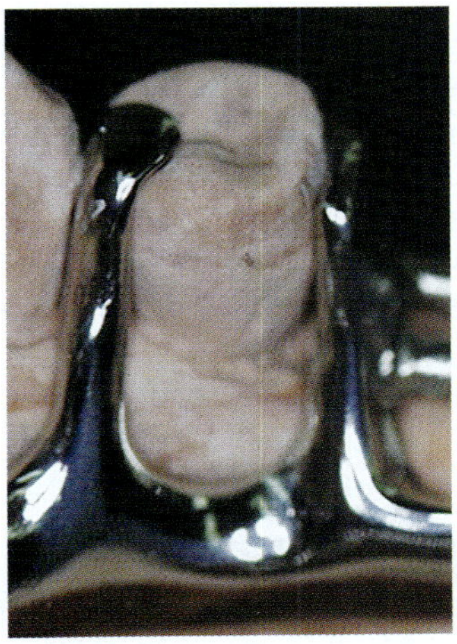

Figure 5-33 In an embrasure space, the minor connector is tapered to the tooth to avoid bulk and to accommodate the tongue.

A minor connector contacting the axial surface of an abutment should not be located on a convex surface. Instead it should be located in an embrasure (Figure 5-33) where it will be least noticeable to the tongue. It should conform to the interdental embrasure, passing vertically from the major connector so that the gingival crossing is abrupt and covers as little of the gingival tissue as possible. It should be thickest toward the lingual surface, tapering toward the contact area (Figure 5-34).

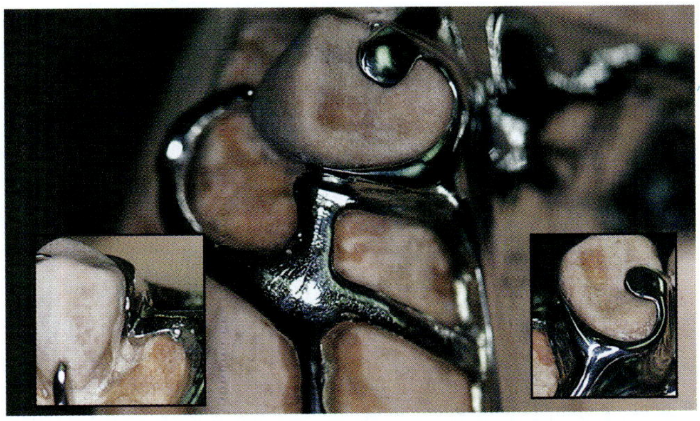

Figure 5-34 Minor connector that contacts the guiding plane is part of a clasp assembly. It can be separate from the other parts, or, as in this case, it can be connected to the lingual stabilizing portion of the clasp assembly. The proximal plate minor connector contact is about one half of the distance between tips of adjacent buccal and lingual cusps of the abutment tooth, and it extends gingivally, contacting an area of the abutment from the marginal ridge to two thirds the length of the enamel crown. Viewed from above, it is triangular, the apex of the triangle being buccally located and the base of the triangle being located lingually. Less interference with arrangement of adjacent artificial tooth is encountered with minor connectors so shaped.

The deepest part of the interdental embrasure should have been blocked out to avoid interference during placement and removal, and to avoid any wedging effect on the contacted teeth.

A modification of the conventional removable partial denture minor connector has been proposed. The application was suggested to be limited to the maxillary arch only, with the minor connector located in the center of the lingual surface of the maxillary abutment tooth.

It is suggested that this modification reduces the amount of gingival tissue coverage, provides enhanced guidance for the partial denture during insertion and removal, and increases stabilization against horizontal and rotational forces. However, because of its location, such a design variation could encroach on the tongue space and create a greater potential space for food entrapment. The proposed variation should be used with careful application.

When a minor connector contacts tooth surfaces on either side of the embrasure in which it lies, it should be tapered to the teeth. This avoids sharp angles, which could hinder tongue movement, and eliminates spaces that could trap food (Figure 5-35).

It is a minor connector that contacts the guiding plane surfaces of the abutment teeth, whether as a connected part of a direct retainer assembly or as a separate entity (see Figure 5-34). Here the minor connector must be wide enough to use the guiding plane to the fullest advantage. When it gives rise to a clasp arm, the connector should be tapered to the tooth below the origin of the clasp. If no clasp arm is formed (as when a bar clasp arm originates elsewhere), the connector should be tapered to a knife-edge the full length of its buccal aspect.

When an artificial tooth will be placed against a proximal minor connector, the minor connector's greatest bulk should be toward the lingual aspect of the abutment tooth. This way sufficient bulk is ensured with the least interference to placement of the artificial tooth. Ideally the artificial tooth should contact the abutment tooth with only a thin layer of metal intervening buccally. Lingually the bulk of the minor connector should lie in the interdental embrasure, the same as between two natural teeth.

As stated previously, those portions of a denture framework by which acrylic resin denture bases are attached are minor connectors. This type of minor connector should be so designed that it will be completely embedded within the denture base.

The junctions of these mandibular minor connectors with the major connectors should be strong butt-type joints but without appreciable bulk (see Figure 5-35). Angles formed at the junctions of the connectors should not be greater than 90 degrees, thus ensuring the most advantageous and strongest mechanical connection between the acrylic resin denture base and the major connector.

An open latticework or ladder type of design is preferable and is conveniently made by using preformed 12-gauge half-round and 18-gauge round wax strips. The minor connector for the mandibular distal extension base should extend posteriorly about two thirds the length of the edentulous ridge and have elements on both the lingual and buccal surfaces. Such an arrangement will not only add strength to the denture base but also may minimize distortion of the cured base from its inherent strains caused by processing. The minor connector must be planned with care so that it will not interfere with the arrangement of artificial teeth (Figure 5-36).

A means to attach acrylic resin individualized trays to the mandibular framework when a corrected impression is planned must be arranged when the framework pattern is being developed.

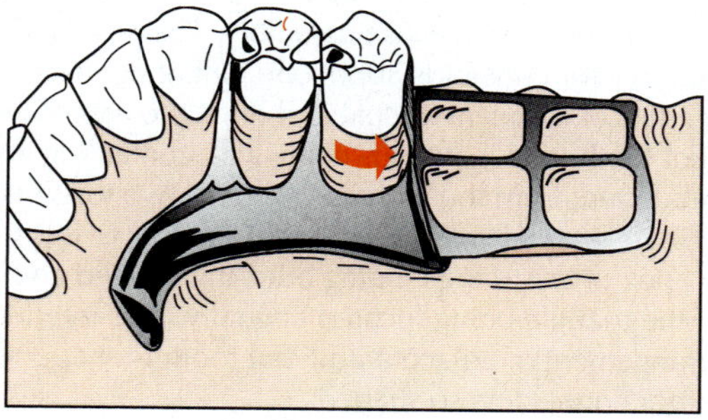

Figure 5-35 Finishing line at junction of ladderlike minor connector and major connector blends smoothly into minor connector contacting distal guiding plane on second premolar. Framework is *feathered* toward tissue anterior to finishing line to avoid as much bulk in this area as possible without compromising the strength of the butt-type joint.

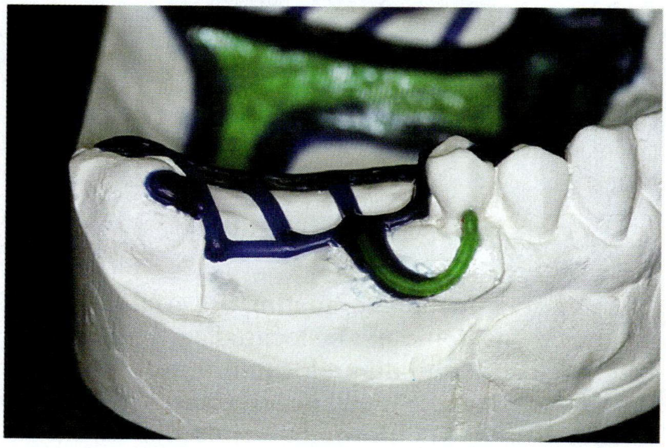

Figure 5-36 Minor connector for attaching the resin denture base should be designed so that denture tooth placement is not compromised. The minor connector design should not include a main lattice strut at the ridge crest or in a desired tooth location.

Three nailhead minor connectors fabricated as part of the denture base minor connector serve this purpose well. Unless some similar arrangement is made, the resin trays may become detached or loosened during impression-making procedures. Minor connectors for maxillary distal extension denture bases should extend the entire length of the residual ridge and should be of a ladderlike and loop design (Figure 5-37).

Tissue Stops

Tissue stops are integral parts of minor connectors designed for retention of acrylic resin bases. They provide stability to the framework during the stages of transfer and processing. They are particularly useful in preventing distortion of the framework during acrylic resin processing procedures. Tissue stops can engage buccal and lingual slopes of the residual ridge for stability (Figure 5-38).

Altered cast impression procedures often necessitate that tissue stops be augmented subsequent to the development of the altered cast. This can be readily accomplished with the addition of autopolymerizing acrylic resin (Figure 5-39).

Another integral part of the minor connector designed to retain the acrylic resin denture base is similar to a tissue stop but serves a different purpose. It is located distal to the terminal abutment and is a continuation of the minor connector contacting the guiding plane. Its purpose is to establish a definitive finishing index tissue stop for the acrylic resin base after processing (Figure 5-40).

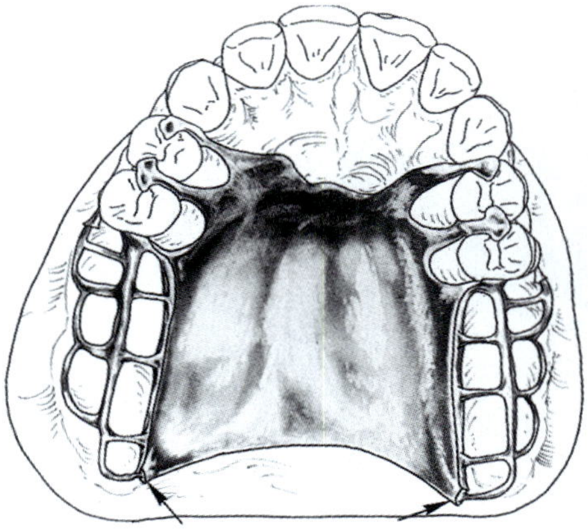

Figure 5-37 Extension of finishing line to area of pterygomaxillary notch provides butt-type joint for attachment of border portion of resin base through pterygomaxillary notch *(arrows)*.

FINISHING LINES

The finishing line junction with the major connector should take the form of an angle not greater than 90°, therefore being somewhat undercut (Figure 5-41). Of course the medial extent of the minor connector depends on the lateral extent of the major palatal connector. Too little attention is given to this finishing line location in many instances. If the finishing line is located too far medially, the natural contour of the palate will

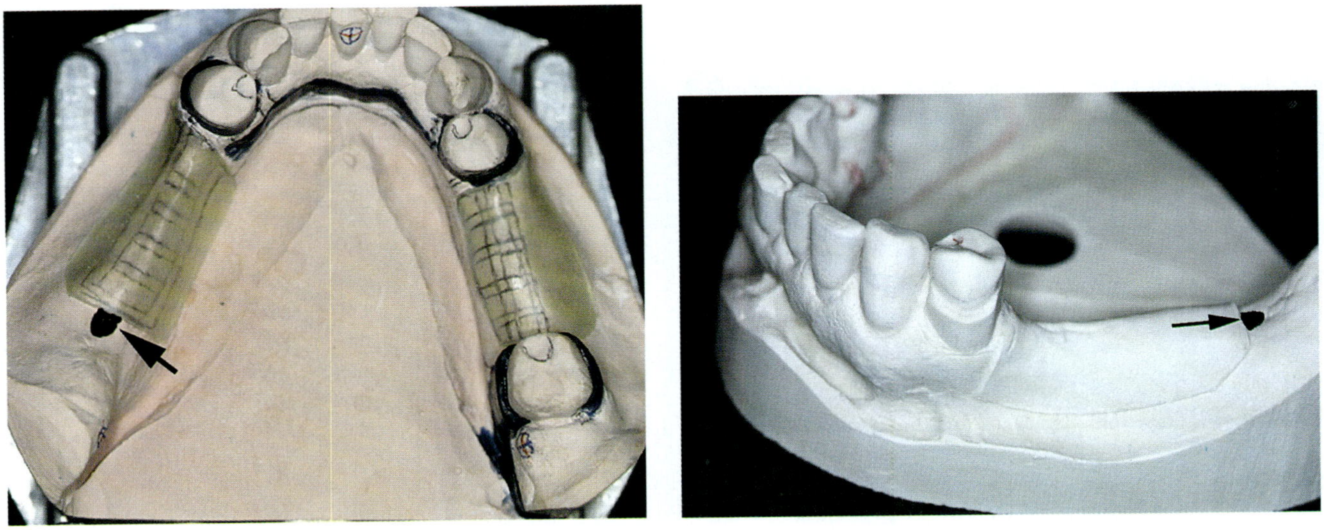

A

B

Figure 5-38 **A,** *Arrow* points to location of tissue stop. **B,** Master cast partially prepared for duplication in refractory investment. Posterior to relief wax, at the distal of the residual ridge *(arrow)*, a tissue stop will be waxed.

Continued

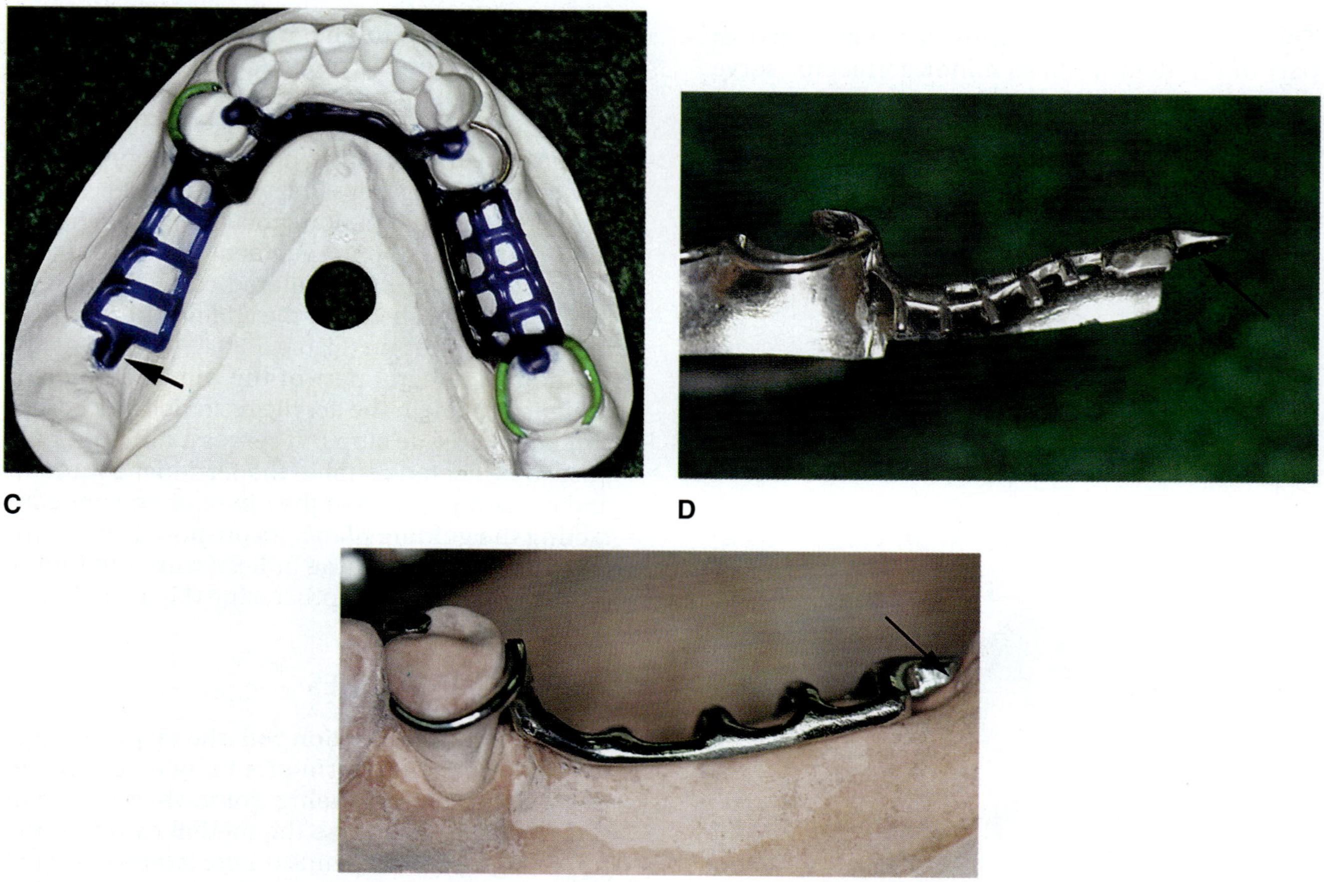

C D E

Figure 5-38 Cont'd **C,** Wax tissue stop placed distal to relief *(arrow)*. After casting this will result in tissue stop contact of the framework. **D,** Tissue stop seen from labial. **E,** Framework on cast showing tissue contact posterior to minor connector with planned relief. *Arrow* points to created tissue stop.

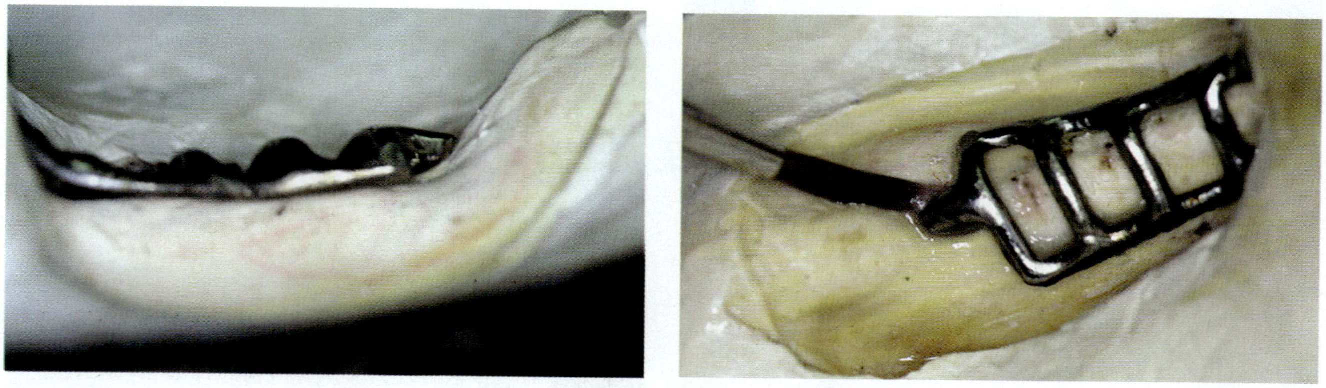

A B

Figure 5-39 **A,** Lower half of flask in which distal extension denture was invested. Note that terminal portion of minor connector (original tissue stop) is elevated from residual ridge. Framework was developed on cast, with residual ridge recorded in its anatomic form. Residual ridge was later recorded in its functional form by a corrected impression, thus the elevated tissue stop. **B,** Autopolymerizing resin is painted on between tissue stop and ridge to maintain position of minor connector during packing and processing procedures for a resin denture base.

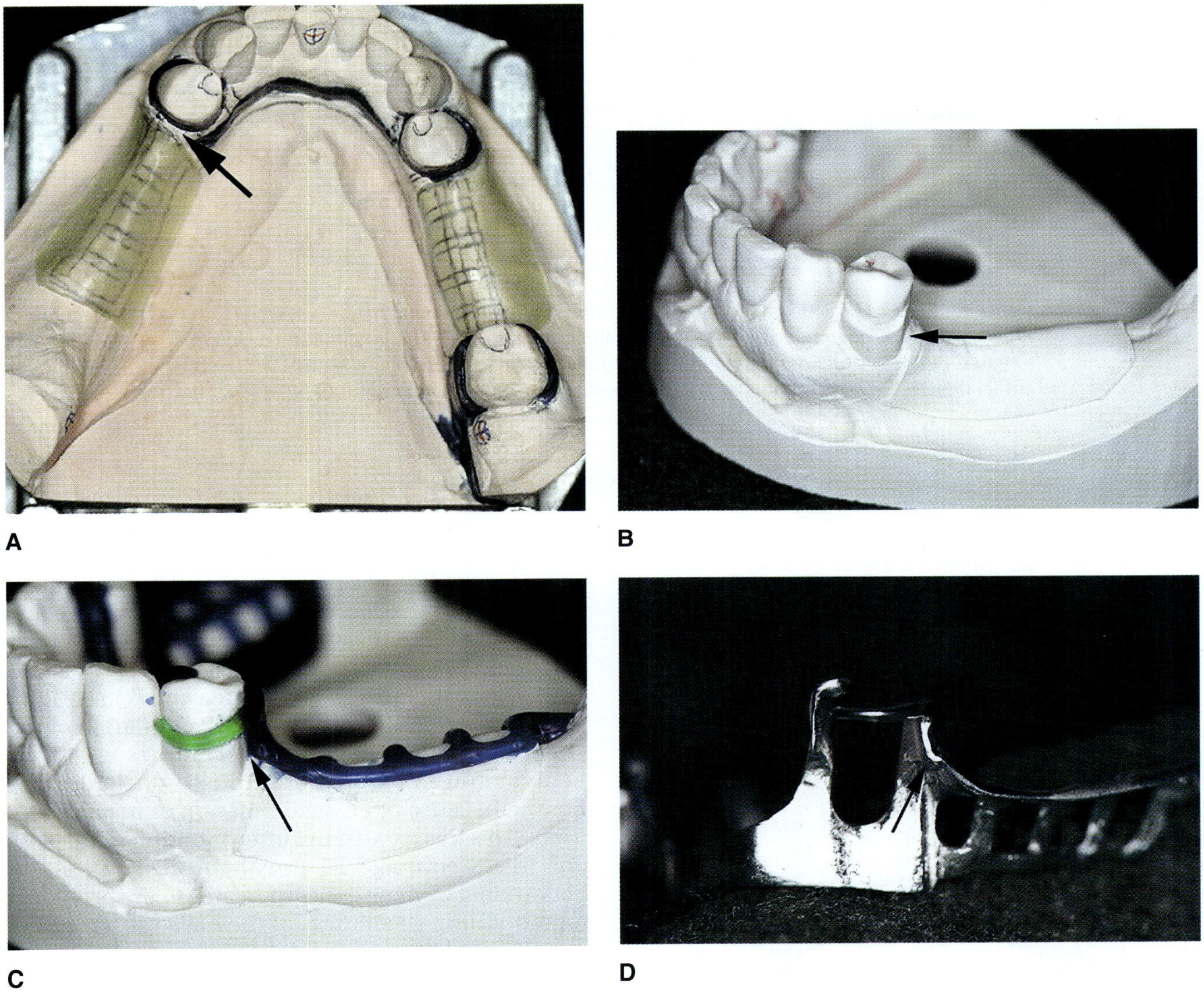

Figure 5-40 Finishing index tissue stop. **A,** Designed to facilitate finishing of the denture base resin at the region of the terminal abutment. Note space at anterior region of wax relief. Framework will be waxed to fill this space and provide positive tissue contact. **B,** Refractory cast showing space distal to abutment. **C,** Wax pattern filling space for future tissue index contact. **D,** Framework index tissue stop anterior to relief beneath the minor connector of the distal extension base and posterior to the primary abutment.

be altered by the thickness of the junction and the acrylic resin supporting the artificial teeth (Figure 5-42). If, on the other hand, the finishing line is located too far buccally, it will be most difficult to create a natural contour of the acrylic resin on the lingual surface of the artificial teeth. The location of the finishing line at the junction of the major and minor connector should be based on restoring the natural palatal shape, taking into consideration the location of the replacement teeth.

Equal consideration must be given to the junction of minor connectors and bar-type direct retainer arms. These junctions are 90° butt-type joints and should follow the guidelines for base contour and clasp length.

REACTION OF TISSUE TO METALLIC COVERAGE

The reaction of tissue to coverage by the metallic components of a removable partial denture has been the subject of significant controversy, particularly in regions of marginal gingiva and broad areas of tissue contact. These tissue reactions can result

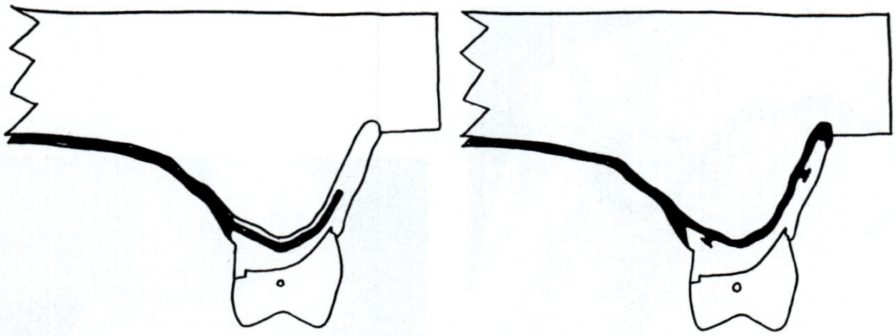

Figure 5-41 Frontal sections through lingual finishing lines of palatal major connectors. *Right image* is through full cast metal base major connector; *left image* is through resin denture base. In both situations, location of finishing lines minimizes bulk of resin attaching the artificial teeth. Palatal contours are restored, enhancing speech and contributing to a natural feeling for the patient.

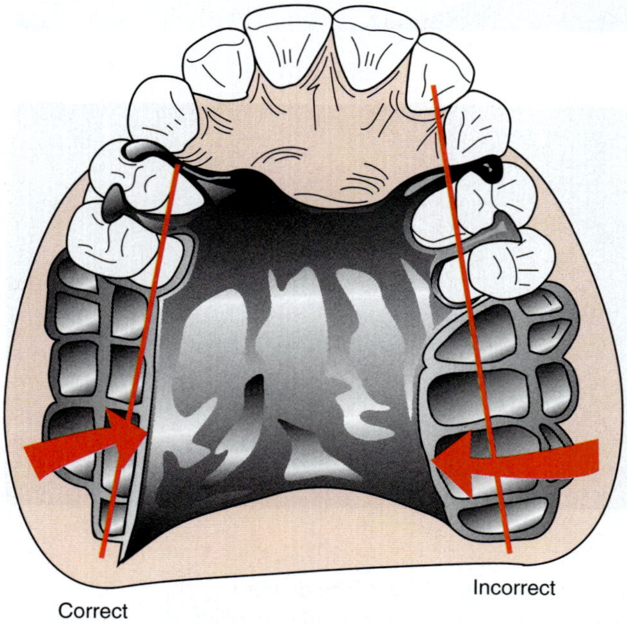

Figure 5-42 Junction of major connector and minor connector at palatal finishing lines should be located 2 mm medial from an imaginary line that would contact lingual surfaces of missing posterior teeth. Finish line on right is too far toward midline of palate. Natural contours of palate will be altered.

from pressure from lack of support, lack of adequate hygiene measures, and prolonged contact through continual use of a prosthesis.

Pressure occurs at regions where relief over gingival crossings and other areas of contact with tissue that are incapable of supporting the prosthesis is inadequate. Impingement will likewise occur if the denture settles because of loss of tooth and/or tissue support. This may be caused by failure of the rest areas as a result of improper design, caries involvement, fracture of the rest itself, or intrusion of abutment teeth under occlusal loading. It is important to maintain adequate relief and support from both teeth and tissue. Settling of the denture because of loss of tissue support may also produce pressure elsewhere in the arch, such as beneath major connectors. Settling of a prosthesis must be prevented or corrected if it has occurred. Excessive pressure must be avoided whenever oral tissue must be covered or crossed by elements of the partial denture.

Lack of adequate hygiene measures can result in tissue reactions because of an accumulation of food debris and bacteria. Coverage of oral tissue with partial dentures that are not kept clean irritates those tissue because of an accumulation of irritating factors. This has led to a misinterpretation of the effect of tissue coverage by prosthetic restorations. An additional hygiene concern relates to the problem of maintaining cleanliness of the tissue surface of the prosthesis.

The first two causes of untoward tissue reaction can be accentuated the longer a prosthesis is worn. It is apparent that mucous membranes cannot tolerate this constant contact with a prosthesis without resulting in inflammation and breakdown of the epithelial barrier. Some patients become so accustomed to wearing a removable restoration that they neglect to remove it often enough to give the tissue any respite from constant contact. This is frequently true when anterior teeth are replaced by the partial denture and the individual does not allow the prosthesis to be out of the mouth at any time except in the privacy of the bathroom during toothbrushing. Living tissue should not be covered all the time or changes in those tissue will occur. Partial dentures should be removed for several hours each day so that the effects of tissue contact can subside and the tissue can return to a normal state.

Clinical experience with the use of linguoplates and complete metallic palatal coverage has shown conclusively that when factors of pressure, cleanliness, and time are controlled, tissue coverage is not in itself detrimental to the health of oral tissue.

MAJOR CONNECTORS IN REVIEW

MANDIBULAR LINGUAL BAR

Indications for Use The lingual bar should be used for mandibular removable partial dentures where sufficient space exists between the slightly elevated alveolar lingual sulcus and the lingual gingival tissue.

Characteristics and Location (1) Half-pear shaped with bulkiest portion inferiorly located. (2) Superior border tapered to soft tissue. (3) Superior border located at least 4 mm inferior to gingival margins and more if possible. (4) Inferior border located at the ascertained height of the alveolar lingual sulcus when the patient's tongue is slightly elevated.

Blockout and Relief of Master Cast (1) All tissue undercuts parallel to path of placement. (2) An additional thickness of 32-gauge sheet wax when the lingual surface of the alveolar ridge is either undercut or parallel to the path of placement (see Figures 11-24 and 11-25). (3) No relief is necessary when the lingual surface of the alveolar ridge slopes inferiorly and posteriorly. (4) One thickness of baseplate wax over basal seat areas (to elevate minor connectors for attaching acrylic resin denture bases).

Waxing Specifications (1) Six-gauge, half-pear-shaped wax form reinforced by 22- to 24-gauge sheet wax or similar plastic pattern adapted to the design width. (2) Long bar requires more bulk than short bar; however, cross-sectional shape is unchanged.

Finishing Lines Butt-type joint(s) with minor connector(s) for retention of denture base(s).

MANDIBULAR LINGUOPLATE

Indications for Use (1) Where the alveolar lingual sulcus so closely approximates the lingual gingival crevices that adequate width for a rigid lingual bar does not exist. (2) In those instances in which the residual ridges in Class I arch have undergone such vertical resorption that they will offer only minimal resistance to horizontal rotations of the denture through its bases. (3) For using periodontally weakened teeth in group function to furnish support to the prosthesis and to help resist horizontal (off-vertical) rotation of the distal extension type of denture. (4) When the future replacement of one or more incisor teeth will be facilitated by the addition of retention loops to an existing linguoplate.

Characteristics and Location (1) Half-pear shaped with bulkiest portion inferiorly located. (2) Thin metal apron extending superiorly to contact cingula of anterior teeth and lingual surfaces of involved posterior teeth at their height of contour. (3) Apron extended interproximally to the height of contact points, i.e., closing interproximal spaces. (4) Scalloped contour of apron as dictated by interproximal blockout. (5) Superior border finished to continuous plane with contacted teeth. (6) Inferior border at the ascertained height of the alveolar lingual sulcus when the patient's tongue is slightly elevated.

Blockout and Relief of Master Cast (1) All involved undercuts of contacted teeth parallel to the path of placement. (2) All involved gingival crevices. (3) Lingual surface of alveolar ridge and basal seat areas the same as for a lingual bar.

Waxing Specifications (1) Inferior border—6-gauge, half-pear-shaped wax form reinforced with 24-gauge sheet wax or similar plastic pattern. (2) Apron—24-gauge sheet wax.

Finishing Lines Butt-type joint(s) with minor connector(s) for retention of denture base(s).

MANDIBULAR SUBLINGUAL BAR

Indications for Use (1) The sublingual bar should be used for mandibular removable partial dentures where the height of the floor of the mouth in relation to the free gingival margins will be less than 6 mm. It may also be indicated whenever it is desirable to keep the free gingival margins of the remaining anterior teeth exposed and there is inadequate depth of the floor of the mouth to place a lingual bar.

Contraindications for Use Remaining natural anterior teeth severely tilted toward the lingual.

Characteristics and Location The sublingual bar is essentially the same half-pear shape as a lingual bar except that the bulkiest portion is located to the lingual and the tapered portion is toward the labial. The superior border of the bar should be at least 3 mm from the free gingival margin of the teeth. The inferior border is located at the height of the alveolar lingual sulcus when the patient's tongue is slightly elevated. This necessitates a functional impression of the lingual vestibule to accurately register the height of the vestibule.

Blockout and Relief of Master Cast (1) All tissue undercuts parallel to path of placement. (2) An additional thickness of 32-gauge sheet wax when the lingual surface of the alveolar ridge is either undercut or parallel to the path of placement. (3) One thickness of baseplate wax over basal seat areas (to elevate minor connectors for attaching acrylic resin denture bases).

Waxing Specifications (1) Six-gauge, half-pear-shaped wax form reinforced by 22- to 24-gauge sheet wax or similar plastic pattern adapted to design width. (2) Long bar bulkier than short bar; however, cross-sectional shape unchanged.

Finishing Lines Butt-type joint(s) with minor connector(s) for retention of denture base(s).

MANDIBULAR LINGUAL BAR WITH CONTINUOUS BAR (CINGULUM BAR)

Indications for Use (1) When a linguoplate is otherwise indicated but the axial alignment of anterior teeth is such that excessive blockout of interproximal undercuts would be required. (2) When wide diastemata exist between mandibular anterior teeth and a linguoplate would objectionably display metal in a frontal view.

Characteristics and Location (1) Conventionally shaped and located same as lingual bar major connector component when possible. (2) Thin, narrow (3 mm) metal strap located on cingula of anterior teeth, scalloped to follow interproximal embrasures with inferior and superior borders tapered to tooth surfaces. (3) Originates bilaterally from incisal, lingual, or occlusal rests of adjacent principal abutments.

Blockout and Relief of Master Cast (1) Lingual surface of alveolar ridge and basal seat areas same as for lingual bar. (2) No relief for continuous bar except blockout of interproximal spaces parallel to path of placement.

Waxing Specifications (1) Lingual bar major connector component waxed and shaped same as lingual bar. (2) Continuous bar pattern formed by adapting two strips (3 mm wide) of 28-gauge sheet wax, one at a time, over the cingula and into interproximal embrasures.

Finishing Lines Butt-type joint(s) with minor connector(s) for retention of denture base(s).

MANDIBULAR CONTINUOUS BAR (CINGULUM BAR)

Indications for Use When a lingual plate or sublingual bar is otherwise indicated but the axial alignment of the anterior teeth is such that the excessive blockout of interproximal undercuts would be required.

Contraindications for Use (1) Anterior teeth severely tilted to the lingual. (2) When wide diastemata exist between the mandibular anterior teeth and the cingulum bar would objectionably display metal in a frontal view.

Characteristics and Location (1) Thin, narrow (3 mm) metal strap located on cingula of anterior teeth, scalloped to follow interproximal embrasures with inferior and superior borders tapered to tooth surfaces. (2) Originates bilaterally from incisal, lingual, or occlusal rests of adjacent principal abutments.

Blockout and Relief of Master Cast No relief for cingulum bar except blockout of interproximal spaces parallel to the path of placement.

Waxing Specifications Cingulum bar pattern formed by adapting two strips (3 mm wide) of 28-gauge sheet wax, one at a time, over the cingula and into interproximal embrasures.

Finishing Lines Butt-type joint(s) with minor connector(s) for retention of denture base(s).

MANDIBULAR LABIAL BAR

Indications for Use (1) When lingual inclinations of remaining mandibular premolar and incisor teeth cannot be corrected, preventing the placement of a conventional lingual bar connector. (2) When severe lingual tori cannot be removed and prevent the use of a lingual bar or lingual plate major connector. (3) When severe and abrupt lingual tissue undercuts make it impractical to use a lingual bar or lingual plate major connector.

Characteristics and Location (1) Half-pear shaped with bulkiest portion inferiorly located on the labial and buccal aspects of the mandible. (2) Superior border tapered to soft tissue. (3) Superior border located at least 4 mm inferior to labial and buccal gingival margins and more if possible. (4) Inferior border located in the labial-buccal vestibule at the juncture of attached (immobile) and unattached (mobile) mucosa.

Blockout and Relief of Master Cast (1) All tissue undercuts parallel to path of placement, plus an additional thickness of 32-gauge sheet wax when the labial surface is either undercut or parallel to the path of placement. (2) No relief necessary when the labial surface of the alveolar ridge slopes inferiorly to the labial or buccal. (3) Basal seat areas same as for lingual bar major connector.

Waxing Specifications (1) Six-gauge, half-pear-shaped wax form reinforced with 22- to 24-gauge sheet wax or similar plastic pattern. (2) Long bar necessitates more bulk than short bar; however, cross-sectional shape unchanged. (3) Minor connectors joined with occlusal or other superior components by a labial or buccal approach. (4) Minor connectors for base attachment joined by a labial or buccal approach.

Finishing Lines Butt-type joint(s) with minor connector(s) for retention of denture base(s).

SINGLE PALATAL STRAP-TYPE MAJOR CONNECTOR

Indications for Use Bilateral edentulous spaces of short span in a tooth-supported restoration.

Characteristics and Location (1) Anatomic replica form. (2) Anterior border follows the valleys between rugae as nearly as possible at right angles to median suture line. (3) Posterior border at right angle to median suture line. (4) Strap should be 8 mm wide or approximately as wide as the combined width of a maxillary premolar and first molar. (5) Confined within an area bounded by the four principal rests.

Blockout and Relief of Master Cast (1) Usually none required except slight relief of elevated medial palatal raphe or any exostosis crossed by the connector. (2) One thickness of baseplate wax over basal seat areas (to elevate minor connectors for attaching acrylic resin denture bases).

Beading (See Figures 5-39 to 5-42.)

Waxing Specifications (1) Anatomic replica pattern equivalent to 22- to 24-gauge wax, depending on arch width.

Finishing Lines (1) Undercut and slightly elevated. (2) No farther than 2 mm medial from an imaginary line contacting lingual surfaces of principal abutments and teeth to be replaced. (3) Follow curvature of arch.

SINGLE BROAD PALATAL MAJOR CONNECTOR

Indications for Use (1) Class I partially edentulous arches with residual ridges that have undergone little vertical resorption and will lend excellent support. (2) V- or U-shaped palates. (3) Strong abutments (single or made so by splinting). (4) More teeth in arch than six remaining anterior teeth. (5) Direct retention not a problem. (6) No interfering tori.

Characteristics and Location (1) Anatomic replica form. (2) Anterior border following valleys of rugae as near right angle to median suture line as possible and not extending anterior to occlusal rests or indirect retainers. (3) Posterior border located at junction of hard and soft palate but not extended onto soft palate; at right angle to the median suture line; extended to pterygomaxillary notches.

Blockout and Relief of Master Cast (1) Usually none required except relief of elevated median palatal raphe or any small exostoses covered by the connector. (2) One thickness of baseplate wax over basal seat areas (to elevate minor connectors for attaching acrylic resin denture bases).

Beading (See Figures 5-39 to 5-42.)

Waxing Specifications Anatomic replica pattern equivalent to 24-gauge sheet wax thickness.

Finishing Lines (1) Provision for butt-type joint at pterygomaxillary notches. (2) Undercut and slightly elevated. (3) No farther than 2 mm medial from an imaginary line contacting the lingual surfaces of the missing natural teeth. (4) Following curvature of arch.

ANTERIOR-POSTERIOR STRAP-TYPE MAJOR CONNECTOR

Indications for Use (1) Class I and II arches in which excellent abutment and residual ridge support exists, and direct retention can be made adequate without the need for indirect retention. (2) Long edentulous spans in Class II, modification 1 arches. (3) Class IV arches in which anterior teeth must be replaced with a removable partial denture. (4) Inoperable palatal tori that do not extend posteriorly to the junction of the hard and soft palates.

Characteristics and Location (1) Parallelogram shaped and open in center portion. (2) Relatively broad (8 to 10 mm) anterior and posterior palatal straps. (3) Lateral palatal straps (7 to 9 mm) narrow and parallel to curve of arch; minimum of 6 mm from gingival crevices of remaining teeth. (4) Anterior palatal strap: anterior border not placed farther anteriorly than anterior rests and never closer than 6 mm to lingual gingival crevices; follows the valleys of the rugae at right angles to the median palatal suture. Posterior border, if in rugae area, follows valleys of rugae at right angles to the median palatal suture. (5) Posterior palatal connector: posterior border located at junction of hard and soft palates and at right angles to median palatal suture and extended to hamular notch area(s) on distal extension side(s). (6) Anatomic replica or matte surface.

Blockout and Relief of Master Cast (1) Usually none required except slight relief of elevated median palatal raphe where anterior or posterior straps cross the palate. (2) One thickness of baseplate wax over basal seat areas (to elevate minor connectors for attaching acrylic resin denture bases).

Beading (See Figures 5-39 to 5-42.)

Waxing Specifications (1) Anatomic replica patterns or matte surface forms of 22-gauge thickness. (2) Posterior palatal component—A strap of 22-gauge thickness, 8 to 10 mm wide (a half-oval form of approximately 6-gauge thickness and width) may also be used.

Finishing Lines Same as for single broad palatal major connector.

COMPLETE PALATAL COVERAGE MAJOR CONNECTOR

Indications for Use (1) In most situations in which only some or all anterior teeth remain. (2) Class II arch with a large posterior modification space and some missing anterior teeth. (3) Class I arch with one to four premolars and some or all anterior teeth remaining, and abutment support is poor and cannot otherwise be enhanced; residual ridges have undergone extreme vertical resorption; direct retention is difficult to obtain. (4) In the absence of a pedunculated torus.

Characteristics and Location (1) Anatomic replica form for full palatal metal casting supported anteriorly by positive rest seats. (2) Palatal linguoplate supported anteriorly and designed for the attachment of acrylic resin extension posteriorly. (3) Contacts all or almost all of the teeth remaining in the arch. (4) Posterior border: terminates at the junction of the hard and soft palates; extended to hamular notch area(s) on distal extension side(s); at a right angle to median suture line.

Blockout and Relief of Master Cast (1) Usually none required except relief of elevated median palatal raphe or any small palatal exostosis. (2) One thickness of baseplate wax over basal seat areas (to elevate minor connectors for attaching acrylic resin denture bases).

Beading (See Figures 5-39 to 5-42.)

Waxing Specifications (1) Anatomic replica pattern equivalent to 22- to 24-gauge sheet wax thickness. (2) Acrylic resin extension from linguoplate the same as for a complete denture.

Finishing Lines As illustrated here and previously discussed.

U-SHAPED PALATAL MAJOR CONNECTOR

This connector should be used only in those situations in which inoperable tori extend to the posterior limit of the hard palate.

The U-shaped palatal major connector is the least favorable design of all palatal major connectors, because it lacks the rigidity of other types of connectors. Where it must be used, indirect retainers must support any portion of the connector extending anteriorly from the principal occlusal rests. Anterior border areas of this type of connector must be kept at least 6 mm away from adjacent teeth. If for any reason the anterior border must contact the remaining teeth, the connector must again be supported by rests placed in properly prepared rest seats. It should never be supported even temporarily by inclined lingual surfaces of anterior teeth.

Waxing specifications, finishing lines, etc., are the same as for full palatal castings or other previously discussed similar major connectors.

SELF-ASSESSMENT AIDS

1. A Class I removable partial denture should have seven components. Name the components.
2. Define the term *major connector* in your own words.
3. Several desirable characteristics of major connectors are listed in the first few pages of Chapter 5. What are five of these characteristics?
4. What purposes are served by rigid major connectors as contrasted with flexible connectors?
5. Major connectors should be located in a favorable relation to moving tissue, gingival tissue, and areas of bony and tissue prominences. What difficulties would the patient encounter if the preceding guidelines are not carried out?
6. Name and draw the cross-sectional form of the basic mandibular major connector.
7. Margins of major connectors adjacent to gingival tissue should be located far enough from the tissue to avoid possible impingement when the denture rotates from functional and parafunctional forces. The superior border of a lingual bar should be located at least ______ mm from gingival crevices.
8. The inferior border of a lingual bar is located as far inferiorly as possible without encroaching on the movable tissue in the alveolar lingual sulcus. Describe two methods by which the location of the inferior border can be accurately determined.
9. Sufficient relief must be provided beneath a major connector to avoid impingement and/or displacement of soft tissue resulting in an inflammatory response. What is meant by the word *relief*? Rationalize planned relief for a lingual bar and give quantitative rules of thumb that depend on the contour of the anterior, lingual alveolar ridge.

10. Discuss those clinical observations that indicate the choice of a lingual bar as a major connector.
11. What is the form of a mandibular linguoplate major connector?
12. Give four clinical observations that indicate use of a linguoplate rather than a lingual bar as a major connector.
13. Draw a sagittal section through a cast that shows the basic form of a linguoplate.
14. What is the difference in determining the location of the inferior borders for lingual bars and linguoplates?
15. Describe the superior extent of the apron portion of a linguoplate in relation to the lingual surfaces of teeth contacted by the major connector.
16. What are the indications for use of a lingual bar-, continuous bar-type of major connector?
17. Interpret in your own words the rationale of this statement made by McCracken: "No component of a partial denture should be added arbitrarily or conventionally. Each component should be added for a good reason and to serve a definite purpose."
18. How may a linguoplate be modified to avoid an over display of metal when used on an arch in which wide diastemata exist between anterior teeth?
19. The dentist alone is responsible for the design of the restoration, which is based on both biological and mechanical principles. Give the dimensional specifications of the wax patterns of mandibular major connectors.
20. At what point in treating the partially edentulous patient must the choice of maxillary and mandibular major connectors be made? Explain.
21. There are basically four types of maxillary major connectors. Name and describe them.
22. What objections are associated with the use of the single palatal bar-type major connector?
23. Which type of palatal major connector is probably the most rigid and at the same time covers the smallest amount of soft tissue?
24. In what situations would one be most likely to use a single palatal strap-type major connector?
25. There are definite rules of thumb for the location of the anterior and posterior borders of all palatal major connectors. Describe the relationship of the borders to rugae, junction of hard and soft palates, gingival crevices, pterygomaxillary notches, and palatal tori.
26. Can adequate support be obtained by resting the palatal major connector on tooth inclines? Why?
27. Rationalize this statement: "Either support the connector by definite rests on the teeth contacted, bridging the gingivae with adequate relief, or locate the connector far enough away from the gingivae to avoid any possible restriction of blood supply and entrapment of food debris."
28. Why should all gingival crossings by components of a framework be abrupt and at right angles to the major connector and bridge the gingivae with adequate relief?
29. Describe a continuous bar mandibular major connector and list the indications for its use.
30. Describe a sublingual bar mandibular major connector and list the indications for its use.
31. What clinical and diagnostic observations would lead to the selection of an anterior-posterior palatal strap-type major connector?
32. Under what circumstances is full palatal coverage, by the major connector, indicated?
33. Describe a palatal linguoplate major connector and explain why such a design would be selected.
34. Describe the five steps outlined by Blatterfein for the design of palatal major connectors on a diagnostic cast of a Class I maxillary arch.
35. What is a minor connector?
36. What are the functions of minor connectors?
37. Should minor connectors be structurally rigid or flexible? Why?
38. Describe the shape of a minor connector contacting axial surfaces of adjacent abutments at interproximal areas.
39. Identify six of the eight minor connectors in this drawing.

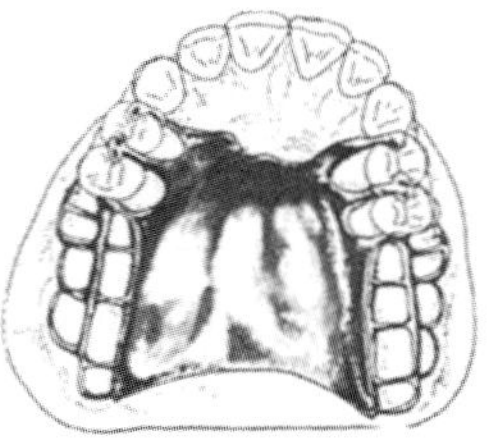

40. What modification in the design of a minor connector was suggested by Radford? What are the suggested advantages and the disadvantages of this variation in design? What is the limitation of this design?
41. Minor connectors used to attach acrylic resin denture bases to major connectors should be located on both buccal and lingual sides of the residual ridge. Why?
42. State rules of thumb for the form and length of minor connectors connecting acrylic resin denture bases to major connectors.
43. What advantages accrue to the restoration by having minor connectors for acrylic resin denture bases attached to the major connector in a butt-type joint?

44. Describe the best location for palatal finishing lines at the junction of major and minor connectors. How do you determine this optimum location on a cast? Why is it important that the natural contour of the palatal vault be restored with a removable restoration?
45. In addition to a more natural feeling contour, what other factors may be achieved by the use of anatomic replica patterns for palatal major connectors?
46. What are three ways to increase the bond strength between the minor connectors and the acrylic resin denture bases? How much is the bond strength increased?

6

RESTS AND REST SEATS

The capacity for teeth to resist functional forces and remain stable over time is provided through their sophisticated support mechanism. Studies have shown that displacement and recovery following loading is far better for natural teeth than for oral mucosa. Consequently, appropriate use of the teeth to help resist functional forces in removable prostheses is a critical strategy to control prosthesis movement and achieve functional stability.

Appropriate use of teeth requires consideration as to how best to engage a tooth for the supportive qualities they provide. Since the most effective resistance can be provided if the tooth is stressed along its long axis, the prosthesis framework should engage the tooth in a manner that encourages axial loading. The various forms of rests have as a main goal such a form for engaging natural teeth. It is important to realize that this goal can only be achieved through some form of tooth modification.

Vertical support must be provided for a removable partial denture. Any component of a partial denture on a tooth surface that provides vertical support is called a rest (Figure 6-1). Rests should always be located on properly prepared tooth surfaces. The prepared surface of an abutment to receive the rest is called the rest seat. Rests are designated by the surface of the tooth prepared to receive them (occlusal rest, lingual rest, and incisal rest). The topography of any rest should restore the topography of the tooth that existed before the rest seat was prepared.

The primary purpose of the rest is to provide vertical support for the partial denture. In doing so, it also does the following:

1. Maintains components in their planned positions
2. Maintains established occlusal relationships by preventing settling of the denture
3. Prevents impingement of soft tissue
4. Directs and distributes occlusal loads to abutment teeth

Thus rests serve to support the position of a partial denture and to resist movement toward the tissue. They serve to transmit vertical forces to the abutment teeth and to direct those forces along the long axes of the teeth. In this respect, tooth-supported removable partial denture rests function in a manner similar to fixed abutment retainers. It is obvious that for this degree of stability to exist, the rests must be rigid and must receive positive support from the abutment teeth.

In a removable partial denture that has one or more distal extension bases, the denture becomes increasingly tissue supported as the distance from the abutment increases. Closer to the abutment, however, more of the occlusal load is transmitted to the abutment tooth by means of the rest. The load is thereby distributed between the abutment and the supporting residual ridge tissue.

When rests prevent movement of the denture in an apical direction, the position of the retentive portion of clasp arms can be maintained in their designated

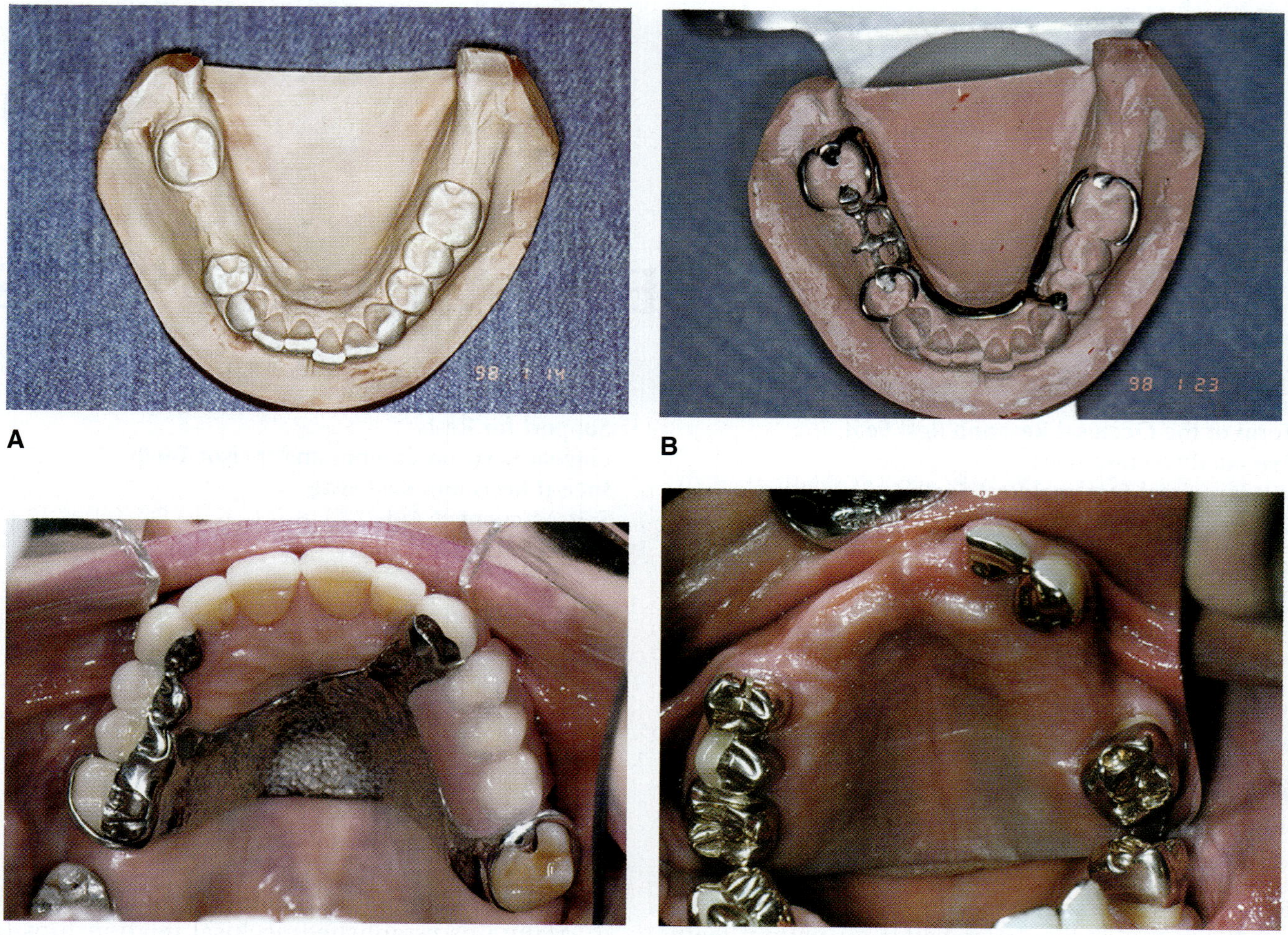

A B C D

Figure 6-1 **A,** Occlusal rest seats have been prepared on molar and premolar teeth to provide vertical support for the removable partial denture. **B,** Framework for tooth-supported removable partial denture. Rests on patient's right provide vertical support to the replacement dentition, while rests on patient's left provide cross-arch support and stabilization. **C,** Tooth support for this prosthesis is provided by rests occupying definite, prepared, rest seats on the canine and occlusal surfaces of selected posterior teeth. **D,** Kennedy Class III Mod I maxillary arch with rest seats prepared on the lingual surfaces of the canine and lateral incisor, and the occlusal surfaces of the premolar and molar.

relation to the tooth undercuts. Although passive when it is in its terminal position, the retentive portion of the clasp arm should remain in contact with the tooth, ready to resist a vertical dislodging force. Then, when a dislodging force is applied, the clasp arm should immediately become actively engaged to resist vertical displacement. If settling of the denture results in clasp arms that stand away from the tooth, some vertical displacement is possible before the retainer can become functional. The rest serves to prevent such settling and thereby helps to maintain the vertical stability of the partial denture.

FORM OF THE OCCLUSAL REST AND REST SEAT

1. The outline form of an occlusal rest seat should be a rounded triangular shape with the apex toward the center of the occlusal surface (Figure 6-2).
2. It should be as long as it is wide, and the base of the triangular shape (at the marginal ridge) should be at least 2.5 mm for both molars and premolars. Rest seats of smaller dimensions do not provide an adequate bulk of metal for rests, especially if the rest is contoured to restore the occlusal morphology of the abutment tooth.

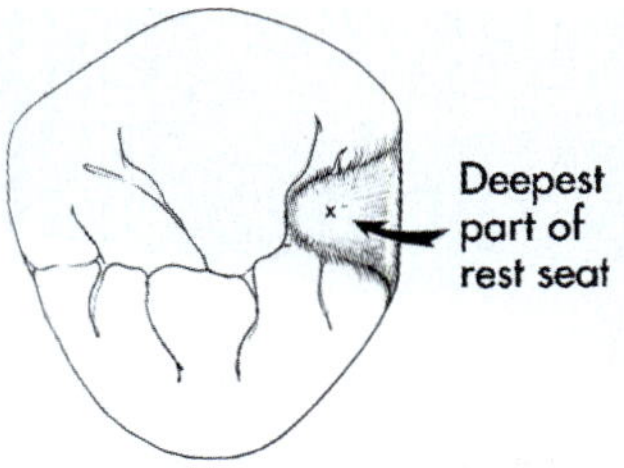

Figure 6-2 Deepest part of an occlusal rest preparation should be inside lowered marginal ridge at *X*. Marginal ridge is lowered to provide bulk and to accommodate the origin of the occlusal rest with the least occlusal interference.

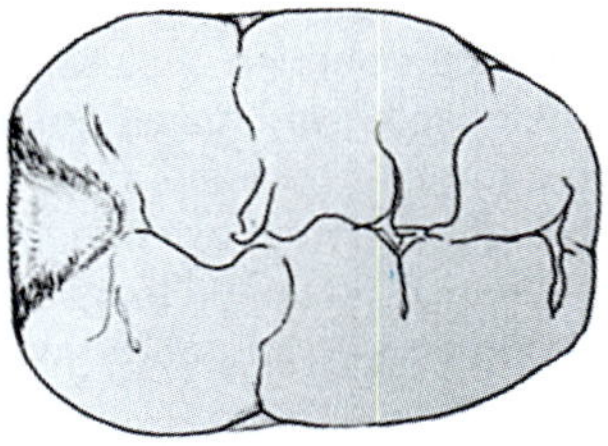

Figure 6-3 Occlusal rest seat preparation on molar. Preparation is rounded, and triangular concavity has smooth margins on occlusal surface and lowered, rounded marginal ridge.

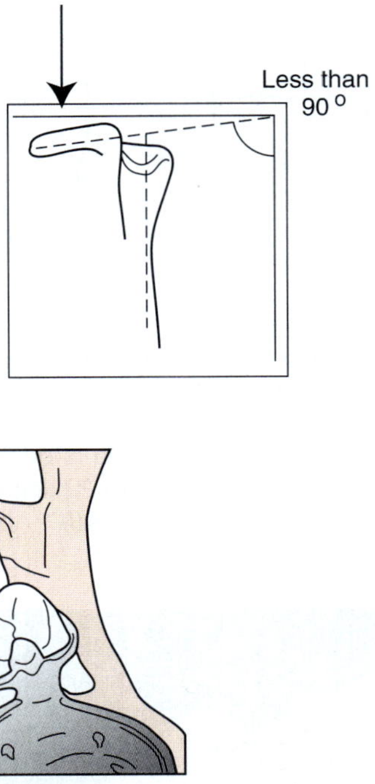

Figure 6-4 Occlusal rest should be spoon shaped and slightly inclined apically from marginal ridge. The rest should restore occlusal morphology of tooth that existed before preparation of rest seat.

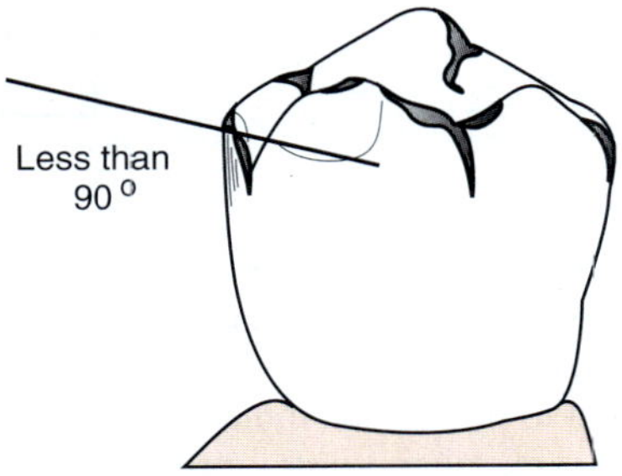

Figure 6-5 Floor of occlusal rest seat should be inclined apically from lowered marginal ridge. Any angle less than 90 degrees is acceptable as long as preparation of proximal surface and lowering and rounding of marginal ridge precede completion of rest seat itself.

3. The marginal ridge of the abutment tooth at the site of the rest seat must be lowered to permit a sufficient bulk of metal for strength and rigidity of the rest and the minor connector. This means that a reduction of the marginal ridge of approximately 1.5 mm is usually necessary.
4. The floor of the occlusal rest seat should be apical to the marginal ridge and the occlusal surface and should be concave, or spoon shaped (Figure 6-3). Caution should be exercised in preparing a rest seat to avoid creating sharp edges or line angles in the preparation.
5. The angle formed by the occlusal rest and the vertical minor connector from which it originates should be less than 90° (Figures 6-4 and 6-5). Only in this way can the occlusal forces be directed along the long axis of the abutment tooth. An angle greater than 90° fails to transmit occlusal forces along the supporting vertical axis of the abutment tooth. This also permits slippage of the prosthesis away from the abutment, which can result in orthodontic-like forces being applied to an inclined plane on the abutment, with possible tooth movement (Figure 6-6).

When an existing occlusal rest preparation is inclined apically toward the reduced marginal ridge and cannot be modified or deepened because of fear of perforation of the enamel or restoration, then a *secondary occlusal rest* must be employed to prevent slippage of the primary rest and orthodontic movement of the abutment tooth (Figure 6-7). Such a rest should pass over the lowered marginal ridge on the side of the tooth opposite the primary rest and should, if possible, be inclined slightly apically from the marginal ridge. However, two opposing occlusal rests on diverging tooth inclines will function to prevent unfavorable forces if all related connectors are sufficiently rigid. In any tooth-tissue-supported partial denture, the relation of the occlusal rest to the abutment should be that of a shallow ball-and-socket joint to prevent a possible transfer of horizontal stresses to the abutment tooth. The occlusal rest should provide only occlusal support. Stabilization against horizontal movement of the prosthesis must be provided by other components of the partial denture rather than by any locking effect

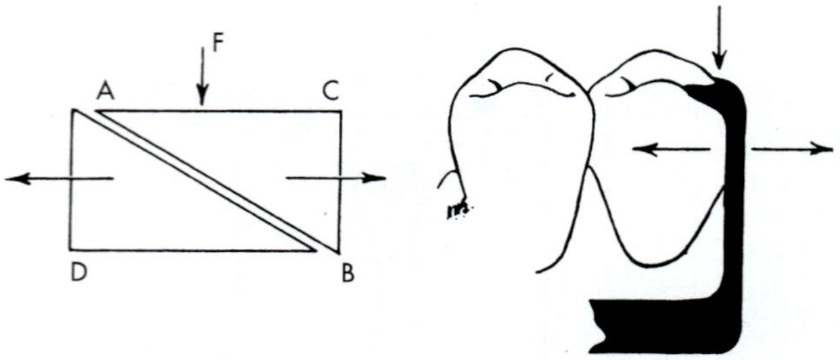

Figure 6-6 Result of force applied to an inclined plane when floor of occlusal rest preparation inclines apically toward marginal ridge of abutment tooth. *F,* Occlusal force applied to abutment tooth. *AB,* Relationship of occlusal rest to abutment tooth when angle is greater than 90 degrees. *ABC,* Removable partial denture framework. *ABD,* Abutment tooth.

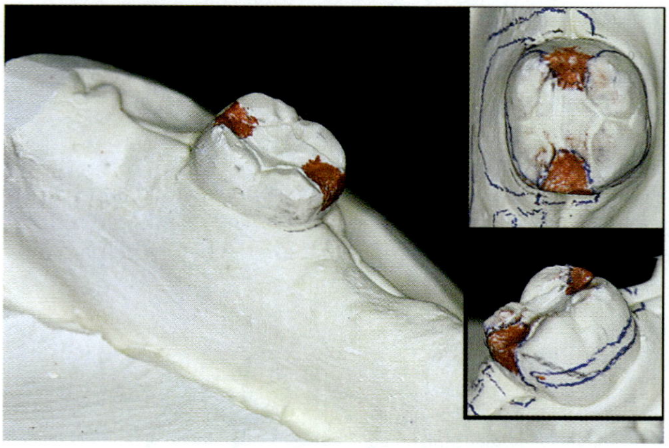

Figure 6-7 Diagnostic cast evaluation of mesially-tipped molar abutment. Anterior tilt of molar precludes preparation of acceptable rest seat on mesio-occlusal surface. Patient could not afford crown to improve axial alignment or orthodontic treatment to upright the molar. Occlusal rests will be used on mesio-occlusal and disto-occlusal surfaces to support restoration and direct forces over greatest root mass of abutment. Proposed ring clasp design is outlined.

of the occlusal rest, which will cause the application of leverages to the abutment tooth.

EXTENDED OCCLUSAL REST

In Kennedy Class II, modification 1, and Kennedy Class III situations in which the most posterior abutment is a mesially tipped molar, an extended occlusal rest should be designed and prepared to minimize further tipping of the abutment and to ensure that the forces are directed down the long axis of the abutment. This rest should extend more than one half the mesiodistal width of the tooth, be approximately one third the buccolingual width of the tooth, and allow for a minimum of 1-mm thickness of the metal, and the preparation should be rounded with no undercuts or sharp angles (Figure 6-8).

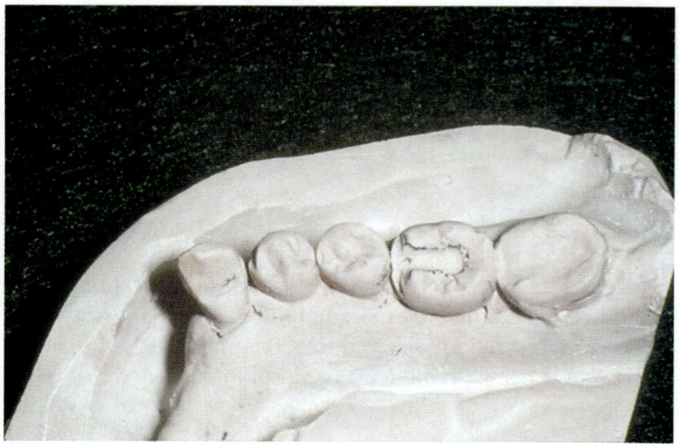

Figure 6-8 Cast showing extended occlusal rest on mandibular first molar, designed to ensure maximum bracing from the tooth. If placed on a mesially inclined molar next to a modification space (as in Figure 6-7) the extended rest would ensure that the forces are directed down the long axis of the abutment and therefore the distal-occlusal rest would not have been needed.

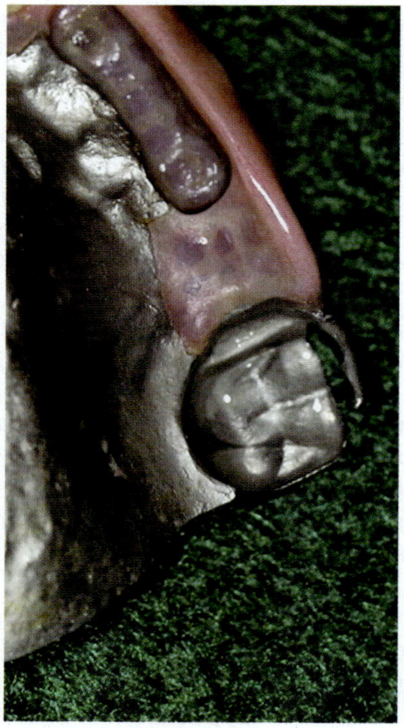

Figure 6-9 Intaglio surface of an onlay occlusal rest restoring contour and occlusion for this maxillary molar.

In situations in which the abutment is severely tilted, the extended occlusal rest may take the form of an onlay to restore the occlusal plane (Figure 6-9). The tooth preparation for this type of extended rest must include removing or restoring pits, fissures, and grooves; placing a 1- to 2-mm bevel on the buccal and lingual occlusal surfaces to allow the extended rest (onlay) to provide stabilization; allowing the rest

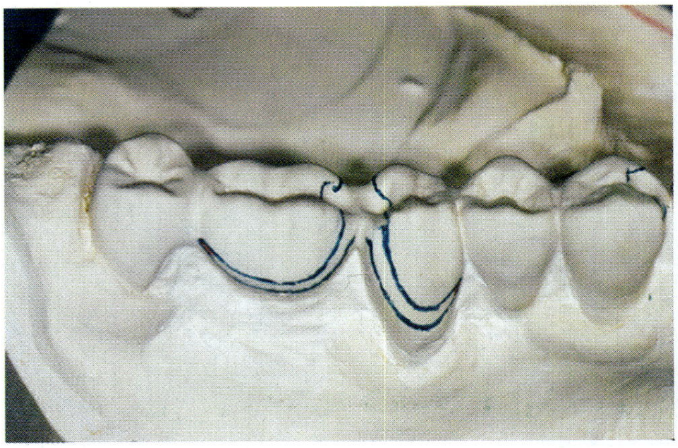

Figure 6-10 Drawing on cast showing the desired design of a direct retainer assembly on mandibular premolar and molar abutments that incorporates interproximal occlusal rests. The direct retainers on the distobuccal undercut of molar and mesiobuccal undercut of premolar are extended from the joined occlusal rests, which occupy specifically prepared adjoining rest seats.

to restore the contour and occlusion of the natural tooth; and ensuring the rest directs the forces down the long axis of the tooth. Tooth preparation must also include a 1- to 2-mm guiding plane on the mesial surface of the abutment.

INTERPROXIMAL OCCLUSAL REST SEATS

The design of a direct retainer assembly may require the use of interproximal occlusal rests (Figure 6-10). These rest seats are prepared as individual occlusal rest seats, with the exception that the preparations must be extended farther lingually than is ordinarily accomplished (Figure 6-11). Adjacent rests, rather than a single rest, are used to prevent interproximal wedging by the framework. Additionally the joined rests are designed to shunt food away from contact points.

In preparing such rest seats, care must be exercised to avoid reducing or eliminating contact points of abutment teeth. However, sufficient tooth structure must be removed to allow for adequate bulk of the component for strength and to permit the component to be so shaped that occlusion will not be altered. Therefore analysis of mounted diagnostic casts is mandatory to assess interocclusal contact areas where rests are to be placed. Sufficient space must be present or created to avoid interference with the placement of rests (Figure 6-12).

The lingual interproximal area requires only minor preparation. Creation of a vertical groove must be avoided to prevent a torquing effect on the abutments by the minor connector.

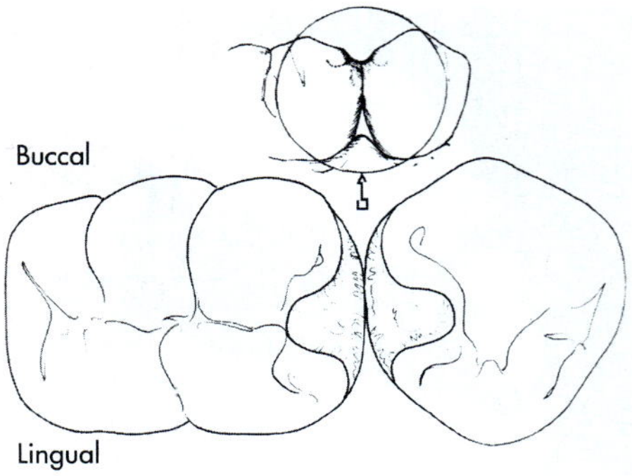

Figure 6-11 Rest seat preparations on premolar and molar fulfill requirements of properly prepared rest seats. Preparations are extended lingually to provide strength (through bulk) without overly filling interproximal space with minor connector. This type of preparation is challenging for natural tooth modification, and care must be exercised to avoid violation of contact points—yet marginal ridge of each abutment should be sufficiently lowered (1.5 mm).

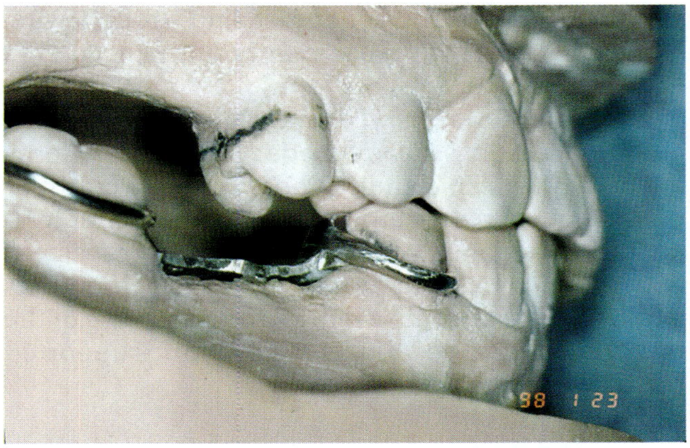

Figure 6-12 View of mounted casts with framework fully seated illustrates interocclusal space was made available by a properly prepared rest seat.

INTRACORONAL RESTS

A partial denture that is totally tooth supported by means of cast retainers on all abutment teeth may use intracoronal rests for both occlusal support and horizontal stabilization (Figure 6-13).

An intracoronal rest is not a retainer and should not be confused with an attachment. Occlusal support is derived from the floor of the rest seat. Horizontal stabilization is derived from the near-vertical walls of this type of rest seat. The form of the rest should be parallel to the path of placement, slightly tapered occlusally, and slightly dovetailed to prevent dislodgment proximally.

The main advantages of the internal rest are that it facilitates the elimination of a visible clasp arm buccally and permits the location of the rest seat in a more favorable position in relation to the *tipping axis* (horizontal) of the abutment. Retention is provided

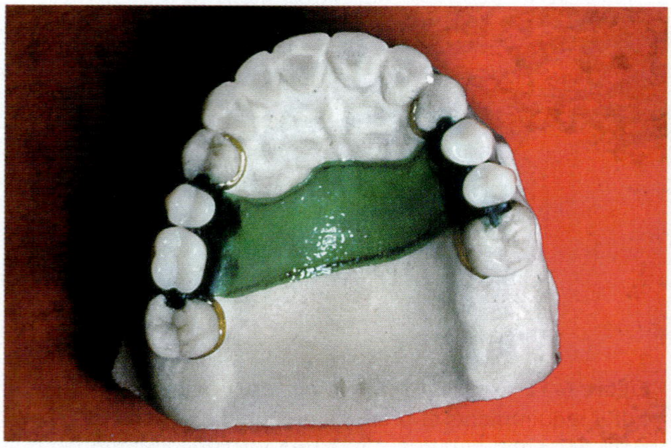

A

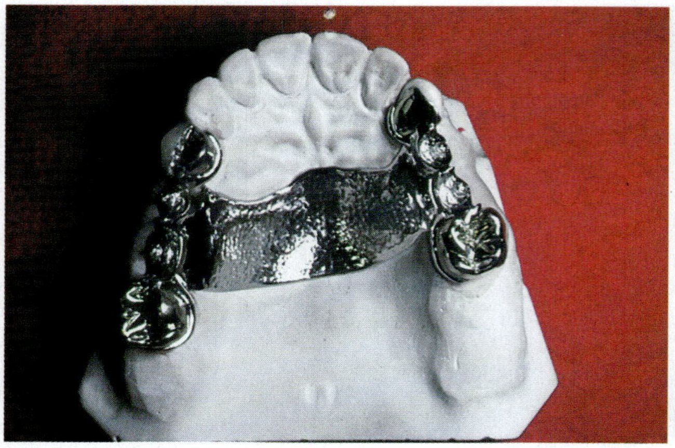

B

Figure 6-13 Maxillary tooth-supported removable partial denture utilizing internal occlusal rests. **A,** Wax pattern developed utilizing internal rests on canine, premolar, and molars. **B,** Maxillary framework on cast with the internal rests fitted within surveyed crowns.

by a lingual clasp arm, either cast or of wrought wire, lying in a natural or prepared infrabulge area on the abutment tooth.

Internal rests are carved in wax or spark eroded in abutment castings. Ready-made plastic rest patterns are readily available and can be waxed into crown or partial-veneer patterns, invested, and cast after having been positioned parallel to the path of placement with a dental cast surveyor. Further developments and techniques promise more widespread use of the internal occlusal rest but only for tooth-supported partial dentures.

SUPPORT FOR RESTS

Rests may be placed on sound enamel or on any restoration material that has been proven scientifically to resist fracture and distortion when subjected to applied forces.

Rests placed on sound enamel are not conducive to caries in a mouth with a low-caries index provided that good oral hygiene is maintained. Proximal tooth surfaces are much more vulnerable to caries attack than are the occlusal surfaces supporting an occlusal rest. The decision to use abutment coverage is usually based on needed mouth preparation, determined from the survey of diagnostic casts, to accommodate modifications of abutment teeth necessary to fabricate a removable partial denture (see Chapter 11). When precarious fissures are found in occlusal rest areas in teeth that are otherwise sound, they may be removed and appropriately restored without resorting to more extensive abutment protection. Although it cannot be denied that the best protection from caries for an abutment tooth is full coverage, it is imperative that such crowns be contoured properly to provide support, stabilization, and retention for the partial denture.

In deciding whether to use unprotected enamel surfaces for rests, future vulnerability of each tooth must be considered—for it is not easy to fabricate full crowns to accommodate rests and clasp arms after the partial denture has been made. In many instances sound enamel may be used safely for the support of occlusal rests. In such situations, the patient should be advised that future susceptibility to caries is not predictable and that much depends on oral hygiene and possible future changes in caries susceptibility. Although the decision to use unprotected abutments logically should be left up to the dentist, economic factors may influence the final decision. The patient should be informed of the risks involved and of his or her responsibility for maintaining good oral hygiene and for returning periodically for observation.

Rest seat preparations should be made in sound enamel. In most instances, preparation of proximal tooth surfaces is necessary to provide proximal guiding planes and to eliminate undesirable undercuts that rigid parts of the framework must pass over during placement and removal. The preparation of occlusal rest seats always must follow proximal preparation, never precede it. Only after the alteration of proximal tooth surfaces is completed may the location of the occlusal rest seat in relation to the marginal ridge be determined. When proximal preparation follows occlusal rest seat preparation, the inevitable consequence is that the marginal ridge is too low and too sharp, with the center of the floor of the rest seat too close to the marginal ridge. Therefore it is often impossible to correct the rest preparation without making it too deep, which causes irreparable damage to the tooth.

Occlusal rest seats in sound enamel may be prepared with burs and polishing points that leave the enamel surface as smooth as the original enamel

(Figure 6-14). The larger round bur is used first to lower the marginal ridge and to establish the outline form of the rest seat. The resulting occlusal rest seat is then complete except that the floor is not sufficiently concave. A slightly smaller round bur is then used to deepen the floor of the occlusal rest seat. At the same time, it forms the desired spoon shape inside the lowered marginal ridge. The preparation is smoothed by a polishing point of suitable size and shape.

When a small enamel defect is encountered in the preparation of an occlusal rest seat, it is usually best to ignore it until the rest preparation has been completed. Then, with small burs, prepare the remaining defect to receive a small restoration. This then may be finished flush with the floor of the rest preparation that was previously established.

A fluoride gel should be applied to abutment teeth following enamel recontouring. If the master cast will be fabricated from an irreversible hydrocolloid impression, application of the gel should be delayed until after impressions are made. This is because some fluoride gels and irreversible hydrocolloids may be incompatible.

Occlusal rest seat preparations in existing restorations are treated the same as those in sound enamel. Any proximal preparations must be done first, for if the occlusal rest seat is placed first and then the proximal surface is prepared, the outline form of the occlusal rest seat is sometimes irreparably altered.

The possibility that an existing restoration may be perforated in the process of preparing an ideal occlusal rest seat is always present. Although some compromise is permissible, the effectiveness of the occlusal rest seat should not be jeopardized for fear of perforating an existing restoration. The rest seat may be widened to compensate for shallowness, but the floor of the rest seat should still be slightly inclined apically from the marginal ridge. When this is not possible, a secondary occlusal rest should be used on the opposite side of the tooth to prevent slipping of the primary rest.

When perforation does occur, it may be repaired, but occasionally the making of a new restoration is unavoidable. In such a situation, the original preparation should be modified to accommodate the occlusal rest, thereby avoiding the risk of perforating the completed restoration or fabricating a restoration with an inadequate rest seat.

Occlusal rest seat location in new restorations should be known when the tooth is prepared so that sufficient clearance may be provided for the rest seat within the preparation. The final step in the preparation of the tooth should be to make sure such clearance exists and, if not, to make a depression to accommodate the depth of the rest (Figure 6-15).

Occlusal rest seats in crowns and inlays are generally made somewhat larger and deeper than those in enamel. Those made in abutment crowns for tooth-supported dentures may be made slightly deeper than those in abutments that support a distal extension base; thus they approach the effectiveness of boxlike internal rests.

Internal rest seats also should be created first in wax, either with suitable burs in a handpiece holder or by waxing around a lubricated mandrel, which is held in the surveyor. In either situation, the rest preparation must be finished on the casting with burs in a handpiece holder or with a precision drill press. Plastic and metal shoes that fit over a mandrel are also available for this purpose. Thus a smooth casting

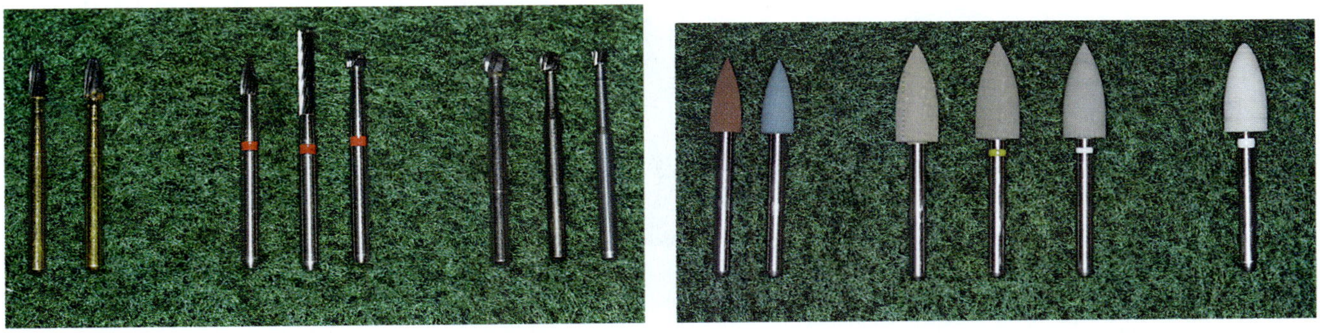

A B

Figure 6-14 Recontouring of axial surfaces and rest seat preparations in enamel may be readily accomplished by selected use of accessories. **A,** The three pear-shaped multi-fluted burs *(3 burs on left)* can be used for cingulum rests and rounding marginal ridges; the longer straight multi-fluted enamelplasty bur *(middle bur)* is ideal for height of contour adjustments and guide plane preparation; round multi-fluted or carbide burs *(3 burs right of middle)* are for occlusal rest preparation; and the inverted cone *(far right bur)* can be used for cingulum rests as well. **B,** Various abrasive rubber polishing points are necessary to assure a smooth surface finish following any enamelplasty procedure. Following the manufacturer's recommended sequence of abrasives should return the surface to smoothness comparable to the original condition. Diamonds are not recommended for this type of tooth reduction.

is ensured, and the need for finishing the inside of the internal rest with burs is eliminated. Sufficient clearance must be provided in the preparation of the abutment to accommodate the depth of the internal rest.

LINGUAL RESTS ON CANINES AND INCISOR TEETH

Analysis of mounted diagnostic casts is mandatory to assess incisal and lingual contact areas where rests are to be placed. Sufficient space must be present or created to avoid interference with placement of rests.

Although the preferred site for an external rest is the occlusal surface of a molar or a premolar, an anterior tooth may be the only abutment available for occlusal support of the denture. Also an anterior tooth occasionally must be used to support an indirect retainer or an auxiliary rest. A canine is much preferred over an incisor for this purpose. When a canine is not present, multiple rests that are spread over several incisor teeth are preferable to the use of a single incisor. Root form, root length, inclination of the tooth, and ratio of the length of the clinical crown to the alveolar support must be considered in determining the site and form of rests placed on incisors.

A lingual rest is preferable to an incisal rest, because it is placed nearer the horizontal axis of rotation (tipping axis) of the abutment and therefore will have less tendency to tip the tooth. In addition, lingual rests are more esthetically acceptable than are incisal rests.

If an anterior tooth is sound and the lingual slope is gradual rather than perpendicular, a lingual rest may sometimes be placed in an enamel seat at the cingulum or just incisally to the cingulum (Figure 6-16). This type of lingual rest is usually confined to maxillary canines that have a gradual lingual incline and a prominent cingulum. In a few instances, such a rest also may be placed on maxillary central incisors. The lingual slope of the mandibular canine is usually too steep for an adequate lingual rest seat to be placed in the enamel, and some other provision for rest support must be made. Lingual rest seat preparations in enamel are rarely satisfactory on mandibular anterior teeth because of a lack of thickness of enamel in which to prepare a seat of adequate form to be truly supportive.

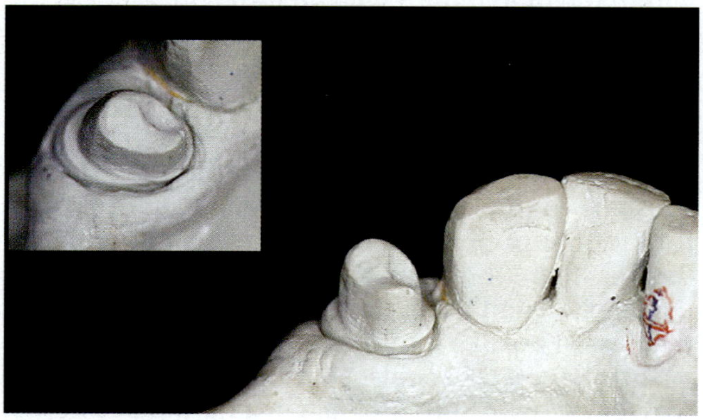

Figure 6-15 Preparation on mandibular premolar for surveyed crown incorporates space for mesio-occlusal rest seat. Adequate occlusal reduction was accomplished to accommodate the depth of the rest seat in the abutment crown. The modification for the rest seat is performed following the standard crown preparation.

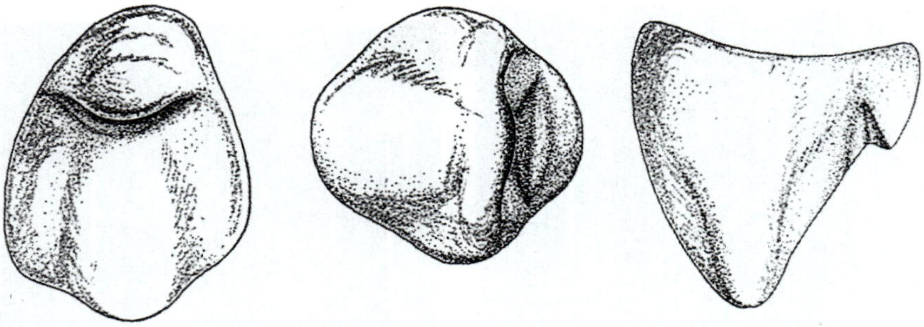

Figure 6-16 Three views of lingual rest seat prepared in enamel of maxillary canine. The rest seat, from lingual aspect, assumes form of a broad inverted V, maintaining natural contour sometimes seen in a maxillary canine cingulum. Inverted V notch form is self-centering for the rest and at the same time directs forces rather favorably in an apical direction. Looking at preparation from incisal view, it will be noted that rest seat preparation is broadest at most lingual aspect of canine. As preparation approaches proximal surfaces of tooth, it is less broad than at any other areas. Proximal view demonstrates correct taper of floor of rest seat. It also should be noted that borders of rest seat are slightly rounded to avoid line angles in its preparation. Mesiodistal length of preparation should be a minimum of 2.5 to 3 mm, labiolingual width about 2 mm, and incisal-apical depth a minimum of 1.5 mm. It is a risky preparation and should not be attempted on lower anterior teeth.

The preparation of an anterior tooth to receive a lingual rest may be accomplished in one of the two following ways:

1. A slightly rounded V is prepared on the lingual surface at the junction of the gingival and the middle one third of the tooth. The apex of the V is directed incisally. This preparation may be started by using an inverted, cone-shaped diamond stone and progressing to smaller, tapered stones with round ends to complete the preparation. All line angles must be eliminated, and the rest seat must be prepared within the enamel and must be highly polished. Shaped, abrasive rubber polishing points, followed by flour of pumice, produce an adequately smooth and polished rest seat. A predetermined path of placement for the denture must be kept in mind in preparing the rest seat. The lingual rest seat must not be prepared as though it was going to be approached from a direction perpendicular to the lingual slope. The floor of the rest seat should be toward the cingulum rather than the axial wall. Care must be taken not to create an enamel undercut, which interferes with placement of the denture (see Figure 6-16).
2. The most satisfactory lingual rest from the standpoint of support is one that is placed on a prepared rest seat in a cast restoration (Figure 6-17). This is done most effectively by planning and executing a rest seat in the wax pattern rather than by attempting to cut a rest in a cast restoration in the mouth. The contour of the framework may then restore the lingual form of the tooth.

By accentuating the cingulum in the wax pattern, the floor of the rest seat is readily carved to be the most apical portion of the preparation. A saddlelike shape, which provides a positive rest seat located favorably in relation to the long axis of the tooth, is formed. The framework of the denture is made to fill out the continuity of the lingual surface so that the tongue contacts a smooth surface without the patient being conscious of bulk or irregularities.

The lingual rest may be placed on the lingual surface of a cast veneer crown (Figure 6-18), a three-quarter crown, an inlay, a laminate veneer, a composite restoration, or an etched metal restoration. The latter displays less metal than the three-quarter crown, especially on the mandibular canine where the lingual rest that was placed on a cast restoration is frequently used, and it is a more conservative restoration. The three-quarter crown may be used if the labial surface of the tooth is sound and if the retentive contours are satisfactory. However, if the labial surface presents inadequate or excessive contours for placement of a retentive clasp arm, or if gingival decalcification or caries is present, a veneered complete coverage restoration should be used.

In some instances, ball type of rests may be used in prepared seats. Such rest seats may be cautiously prepared in tooth surfaces with overly sufficient enamel thickness or may be prepared in restorations placed in teeth where enamel thickness is inadequate. Conservative restorations (silver amalgam, pin inlays, composite resin, etc.) in anterior teeth may be better suited for ball type of rest seats than the less conservative inverted V type of rest seats.

There is some scientific evidence that demonstrates that individually cast chromium-cobalt alloy rest seat forms (attached to lingual surfaces of anterior teeth by use of composite resin cements with acid-etched tooth preparation), laminates, and composite resins have been successfully used as conservative approaches to forming rest seats on teeth with unacceptable lingual contours (Figure 6-19). Sapphire ceramic orthodontic brackets have also been bonded to the lingual surfaces of mandibular canines and shaped as rest seats. These have advantages over

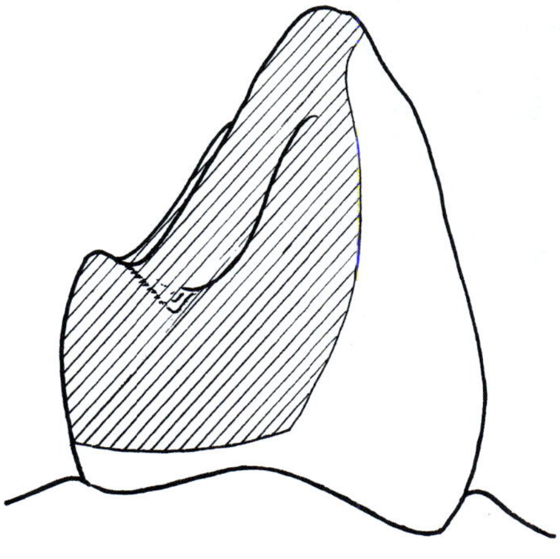

Figure 6-17 Rest seat preparation can be exaggerated for better support when it is prepared in cast restoration.

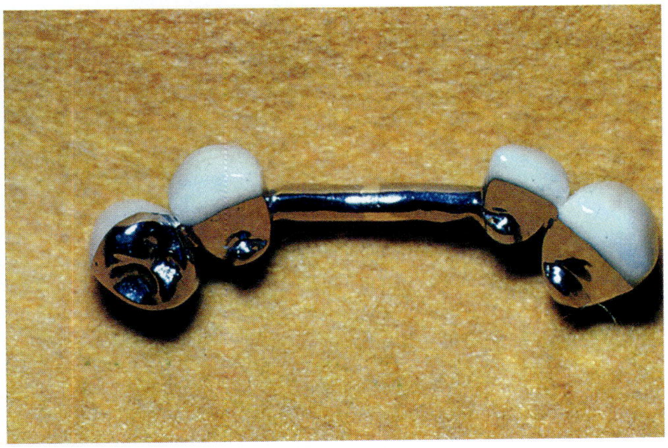

Figure 6-18 Positive vertical support for prosthesis is furnished by rest seats prepared in splinted metal ceramic crowns. The cingulum rest seats are optimally placed as near the horizontal axis of rotation as possible to minimize tipping forces.

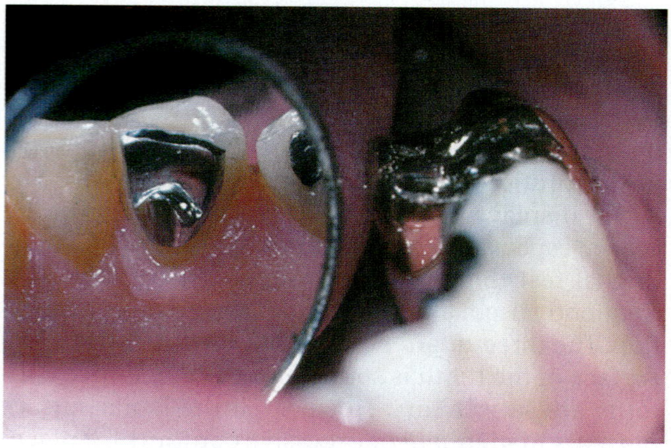

Figure 6-19 Chromium-cobalt lingual rest seat on mandibular canine retained by resin cement with acid-etched tooth preparation.

the metal acid-etched retained rest in that a laboratory step is avoided and increased bond strengths are achieved. The major disadvantage to using orthodontic brackets is that removal of the rest seat would necessitate that they be ground off with the potential of heat generation and possible pulpal damage.

INCISAL RESTS AND REST SEATS

Incisal rests are placed at the incisal angles of anterior teeth and on prepared rest seats. Although this is the least desirable placement of a rest seat for reasons previously mentioned, it may be used successfully for selected patients when the abutment is sound and when a cast restoration is not otherwise indicated. Therefore incisal rests generally are placed on enamel (Figure 6-20). Incisal rests are used predominantly as auxiliary rests or as indirect retainers.

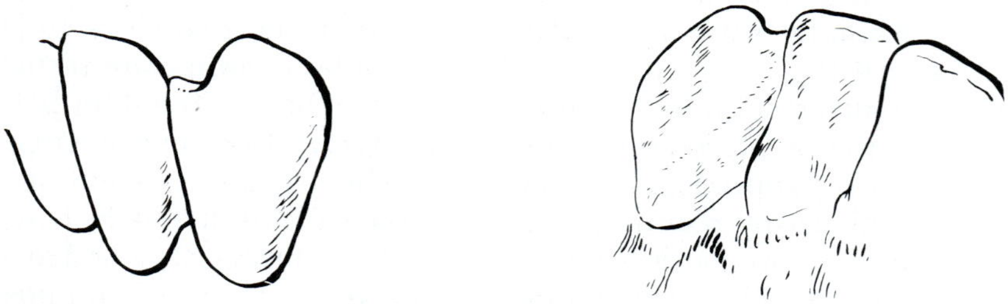

A

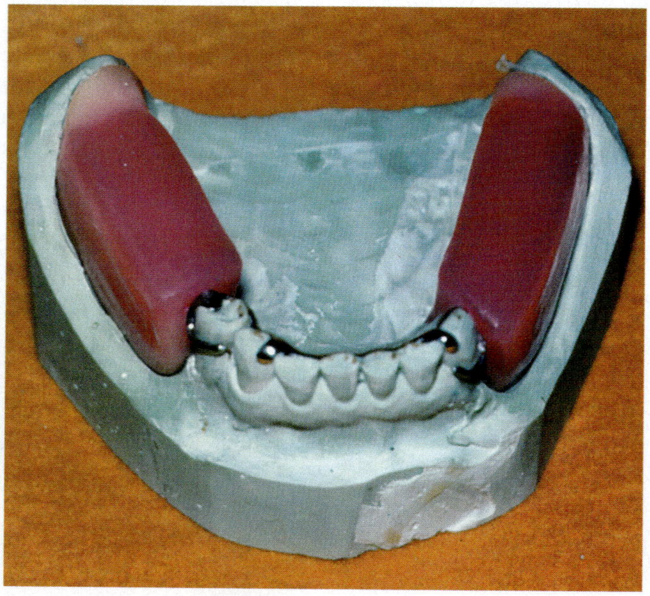

B

Figure 6-20 A, Incisal rest seat placed in mesial incisal edge of lower canine. Note that contact point is not involved in preparation of rest seat. B, Mesial incisal rests on the canines will furnish excellent vertical support and indirect retention for this prosthesis upon completion. Incisal rest on tooth #27 will also provide a third point of reference when establishing frame orientation during maintenance reline procedures.

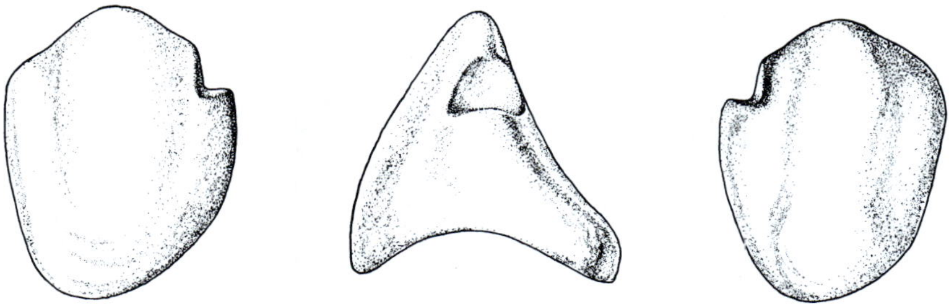

Figure 6-21 Three views of incisal rest seat preparation on mandibular canine adjacent to a modification space. Labial view demonstrates inclination of floor of rest seat, which allows forces to be directed along the long axis of tooth as nearly as possible. Note that floor of rest seat has been extended slightly onto labial aspect of tooth. As seen from a proximal view, proximal edge of rest seat is rounded rather than straight. Lingual view shows that all borders of rest seat are rounded to avoid sharp line angles. It is especially important to avoid a line angle at junction of axial wall of preparation and floor of rest seat. The rest that occupies such a preparation should be able to move slightly in a lateral direction to avoid torquing the abutment tooth.

Although the incisal rest may be used on a canine abutment in either arch, it is more applicable to the mandibular canine. This type of rest provides definite support with relatively little loss of tooth structure and little display of metal. Esthetically it is preferable to the three-quarter crown. The same criteria apply in deciding whether to use unprotected enamel for an occlusal rest on a molar or premolar. An incisal rest is more likely to lead to some orthodontic movement of the tooth because of unfavorable leverage factors than is a lingual rest.

An incisal rest seat is prepared in the form of a rounded notch at the incisal angle of a canine or on the incisal edge of an incisor, with the deepest portion of the preparation apical to the incisal edge (Figure 6-21). The notch should be beveled both labially and lingually, and the lingual enamel should be partly shaped to accommodate the rigid minor connector connecting the rest to the framework. An incisal rest seat should be approximately 2.5 mm wide and 1.5 mm deep so that the rest will be strong without having to exceed the natural contour of the incisal edge (Figure 6-22).

In the absence of other suitable placements for incisal rests and rest seats, incisal rests on multiple mandibular incisors may be considered (Figure 6-23). Use of such rests may be justified by the following factors:

1. They may take advantage of natural incisal faceting.
2. Tooth morphology does not permit other designs.
3. Such rests can restore defective or abraded tooth anatomy.
4. Incisal rests provide stabilization.
5. Full incisal rests may restore or provide anterior guidance.

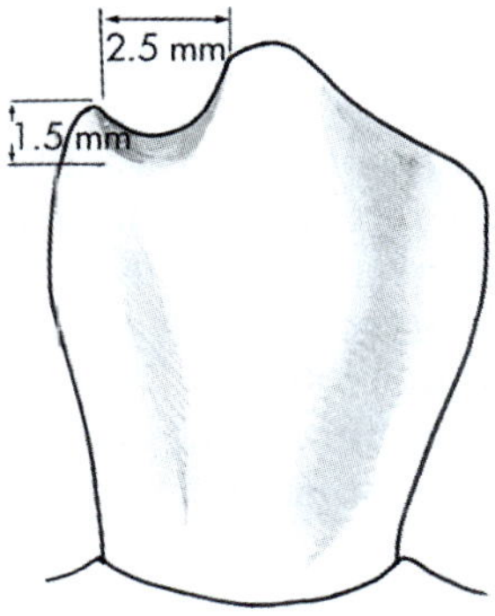

Figure 6-22 Dimensions given in illustration for incisal rest seat preparation will provide adequate strength of framework at junction of rest and minor connector. Rest seats of smaller dimension have proved unsatisfactory regardless of metal alloy from which framework is made.

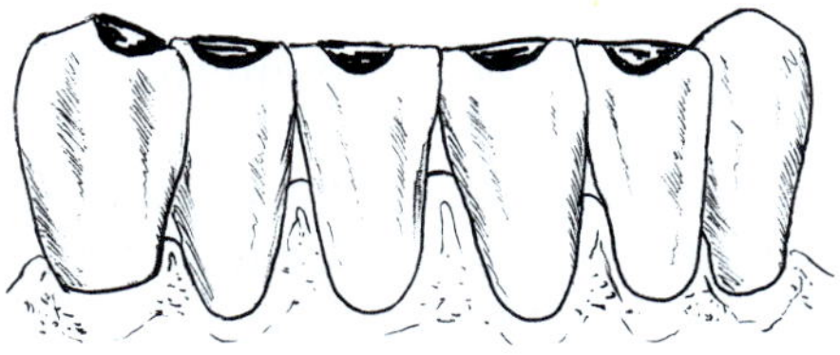

Figure 6-23 Labial view of configuration and location of incisal rests on mandibular incisors and right canine.

In the event that full incisal rests are considered, the patient should be thoroughly informed regarding their location, form, and esthetic impact.

It is, of course, essential that both the master cast and the casting be accurate if rests are to seat properly. The incisal rest should be over contoured slightly to allow for labial and incisal finishing to the adjoining enamel in much the same manner as a three-quarter crown or inlay margin is finished to enamel. In this way, minimal display of metal is possible without jeopardizing the effectiveness of the rest.

Care taken in selecting the type of rest seat to be used, in preparing it, and in fabricating the framework casting does much to ensure the success of any type of rest. The topography of any rest should be such that it restores the topography of the tooth existing before the rest seat is prepared.

SELF-ASSESSMENT AIDS

1. Define the word *rest* as a component of a removable partial denture.
2. What are the functions of a rest?
3. Rests are designated by the surface of the tooth that is prepared to receive the rest. Therefore rests are ______ rests, or ______ rests, or ______ rests.
4. Describe the form of an adequately prepared occlusal rest seat.
5. Where is the deepest portion of an occlusal rest seat located?
6. Draw a diagram of the approximate dimensions of an occlusal rest seat on a molar. A premolar.
7. Why should the angle formed by the rest and the vertical minor connector from which it originates be less than 90°?
8. Under what circumstances would one choose to prepare a secondary occlusal rest seat on the same tooth?
9. Describe the form of adjacent, interproximal occlusal rest seats.
10. What advantages are gained by using adjacent, interproximal occlusal rest seats rather than a single interproximal rest seat?
11. Describe an internal occlusal rest seat and relate the circumstances under which it may be used.
12. How does one fabricate an internal occlusal rest seat?
13. Rests may be placed on sound enamel, cast restorations, or silver amalgam alloy restorations. Which of the three structures is the least desirable for support of the rests? Why?
14. When preparing occlusal rest seats immediately adjacent to a proximal surface that has to be recontoured for optimum location of other components, which is accomplished first—rest seat preparation or recontouring of the axial surface of the abutment? Defend your answer.
15. What is the sequence of operations in preparing an occlusal rest seat in enamel? Name the cutting and polishing instruments used.
16. How do you handle a small enamel defect encountered in preparing a rest seat?
17. Suppose you expose dentin in preparing an occlusal rest seat in enamel—what then?
18. Describe the form of a lingual rest seat preparation.
19. Which unrestored teeth may sometimes have such a lingual contour that an acceptable lingual rest seat may be prepared in enamel?
20. Five morphologic or anatomic factors must be evaluated in determining whether an abutment can support a lingual rest. Enumerate these five factors.
21. Most often, unrestored canines and incisors should not be used for supports for lingual rests. Why?
22. For what reasons should a rounded, inverted V notch form be used for a lingual rest seat?
23. State the minimum dimensions for a lingual rest seat mesiodistally, labiolingually, and incisal-apically.
24. Give the sequence of use of rotary instruments in preparing a lingual rest seat in enamel.
25. The design of a framework is such that lingual rest seats must be placed on incisor teeth, yet dentin will knowingly be exposed in preparing acceptable rest seats. What are the options for providing adequate rest seats on the incisors?
26. The adequacy of a lingual rest seat is better accomplished with a cast restoration than a preparation confined to enamel. True or false?
27. Four conservative alternatives to forming rest seats on teeth with unacceptable lingual contours were described in the text. What are they and what are their advantages and disadvantages?
28. Describe the contour of an incisal rest seat preparation.
29. What are the minimum acceptable dimensions of an incisal rest seat?
30. Name and describe several indications for the use of incisal rests.
31. Which rest is the most unfavorable in relation to a possible tipping of the tooth? Which is the most favorable to avoid unfavorable leverage factors?
32. For what reasons must a rest restore the occlusal, lingual, or incisal morphology of the abutment tooth that existed before the rest seat preparation?

7

DIRECT RETAINERS

DIRECT RETAINER'S ROLE IN PROSTHESIS MOVEMENT CONTROL

Retention of a removable prosthesis is a unique concern when compared with other prostheses. When dealing with a crown or fixed partial denture, the use of preparation geometry (i.e., resistance and retention form) and a luting agent combine to fix the prosthesis to the tooth in a manner that resists all forces to which the teeth are subjected. As mentioned in Chapter 4, the direction of forces can be toward, across, or away from the tissue. In general, the forces acting to move prostheses toward and across the supporting teeth and/or tissue are the greatest in intensity. This is because they are most often forces of occlusion.

Forces acting to displace the prosthesis from the tissue can be gravity acting against a maxillary prosthesis, the action of adherent foods acting to displace a prosthesis on opening of the mouth in chewing, or functional forces acting across a fulcrum to unseat a prosthesis. The first two of these forces are seldom at the magnitude of functional forces and the latter is minimized through the use of adequate support. The component part applied to resist this movement away from the teeth and/or tissue provides retention for the prosthesis and is called the *direct retainer.* A direct retainer is any unit of a removable dental prosthesis that engages an abutment tooth to resist displacement of the prosthesis away from basal seat tissue. The direct retainer's ability to resist this movement is greatly influenced by the stability and support of the prosthesis provided by major and minor connectors, rests, and tissue bases. This relationship of the supportive and retentive components highlights the relative importance of these component parts. Though the forces working against a removable partial denture to move it away from the tissue are generally not as great as the functional forces causing stress toward the tissue, the removable partial denture must have retention appropriate to resist reasonable dislodging forces. Too often retention concerns are given greater importance than is appropriate, especially if such a focus detracts from more serious consideration of resistance of typical functional forces.

Sufficient retention is provided by two means. Primary retention for the removable partial denture is accomplished mechanically by placing retaining elements (direct retainers) on the abutment teeth. Secondary retention is provided by the intimate relationship of the minor connector contact with the guiding planes, denture bases, and major connectors (maxillary) with the underlying tissue. The latter is similar to the retention of a complete denture. It is proportionate to the accuracy of the impression registration, the accuracy of the fit of the denture bases, and the total involved area of contact.

TYPES OF DIRECT RETAINERS

Mechanical retention of removable partial dentures is accomplished by means of direct retainers of one type or another. Retention is accomplished by frictional means, by engaging a depression in the abutment tooth, or by engaging a tooth undercut lying cervically to its height of contour. There are two basic types of direct retainers, the intracoronal retainer and the extracoronal retainer. The extracoronal (clasp-type) retainer is the most commonly used retainer for removable partial dentures.

The intracoronal retainer is either cast or attached totally within the restored natural contours of an abutment tooth. It is typically composed of a prefabricated machined key and keyway, with opposing vertical parallel walls, which serve to limit movement and resist removal of the partial denture through frictional resistance (Figure 7-1). The intracoronal retainer is

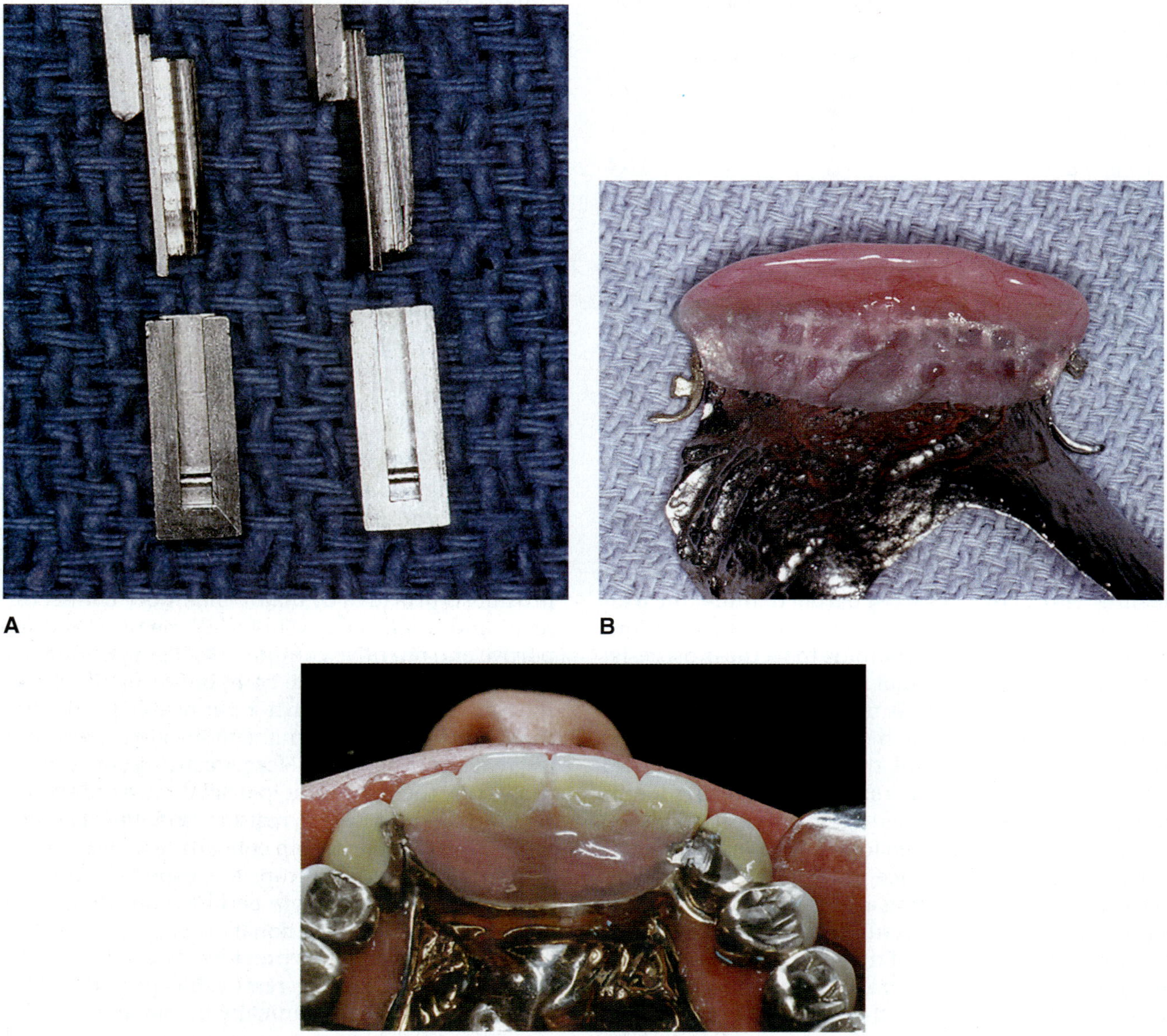

A B C

Figure 7-1 **A,** Intracoronal retainer consists of a key and keyway with extremely small tolerance. Keyways are contained within abutment crowns, and **B,** keys are attached to removable removable partial denture framework. **C,** Frictional resistance to removal and placement and limitation of movement serve to retain and stabilize prosthesis.

usually regarded as an **internal** or a precision attachment. The principle of the internal attachment was first formulated by Dr. Herman E.S. Chayes in 1906.

The other type of retainer is the extracoronal retainer, which uses mechanical resistance to displacement through components placed on or attached to the external surfaces of an abutment tooth (Figure 7-2). The extracoronal retainer comes in three principal forms. The clasp-type retainer (Figures 7-3 and 7-4), which is the most common form used, retains through a flexible clasp arm. The arm engages an external surface of an abutment tooth in an area cervical to the greatest convexity of the tooth, or it engages a depression prepared to receive the terminal tip of the arm. The other forms both involve manufactured attachments and include interlocking components such as the *Dalbo* (see Figure 7-2) or the use of a spring-loaded device that engages a tooth contour to resist occlusal displacement. A second type is a manufactured attachment, which uses flexible clips or rings that engage a rigid component that is cast or attached to the external surface of an abutment crown.

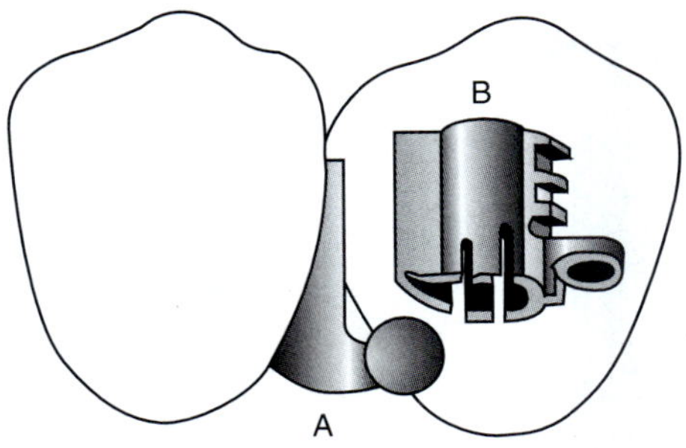

Figure 7-2 Dalbo extracoronal attachment. Components consist of *A*, L-shaped male portion that is attached to an abutment crown; *B*, female sleeve that is placed in artificial tooth adjacent to abutment, and coiled spring that fits into female portion. Design permits some vertical movement of denture under force through compression of coiled spring.

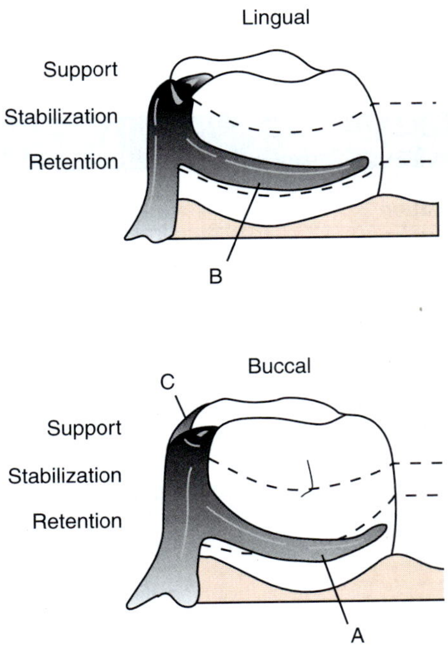

Figure 7-3 Extracoronal circumferential direct retainer. Assembly consists of *A*, buccal retentive arm; *B*, rigid lingual stabilizing (reciprocal) arm; and *C*, supporting occlusal rest. Terminal portion of retentive arm is flexible and engages measured undercut. Assembly remains passive until activated by placement or removal of restoration or when subjected to masticatory forces that tend to dislodge the denture base.

ANALYSIS OF TOOTH CONTOURS FOR RETENTIVE CLASPS

Although the extracoronal, or clasp-type, direct retainer is used more often than the internal attachment, it is commonly misused. It is hoped that a better understanding of the principles of clasp design will lead to a more intelligent use of this retainer. To best gain this understanding, it is vitally important to consider how tooth contour and removable partial denture components must interact (be related) to allow stable prosthetic function. Just as unaltered natural teeth are not appropriately contoured to receive fixed partial dentures without preparation, the teeth that are engaged by a removable partial denture must be contoured to support, stabilize, and retain the functioning prosthesis. Analysis and accomplishment of where tooth modification is required for optimum stability and retention are necessary for success of the prosthesis.

Critical areas of an abutment that provide for retention and stabilization (reciprocation) can only be identified with the use of a dental cast surveyor (Table 7-1). To enhance the understanding of direct retainers, an introduction of the dental cast surveyor is appropriate at this time. Surveying will be covered in detail in Chapter 11.

The cast surveyor (Figure 7-5) is a simple instrument essential to planning partial denture treatment. Its main working parts are the vertical arm and the adjustable table, which hold the cast in a fixed relation to the vertical arm. This relationship of the vertical arm to the cast represents the path of placement that the partial denture will ultimately take when inserted or removed from the mouth (Figure 7-6).

The adjustable table may be tilted in relation to the vertical arm of the surveyor until a path can be found that best satisfies all the involved factors (Figure 7-7). A cast in a horizontal relationship to the vertical arm represents a vertical path of placement; a cast in a tilted relationship represents a path of

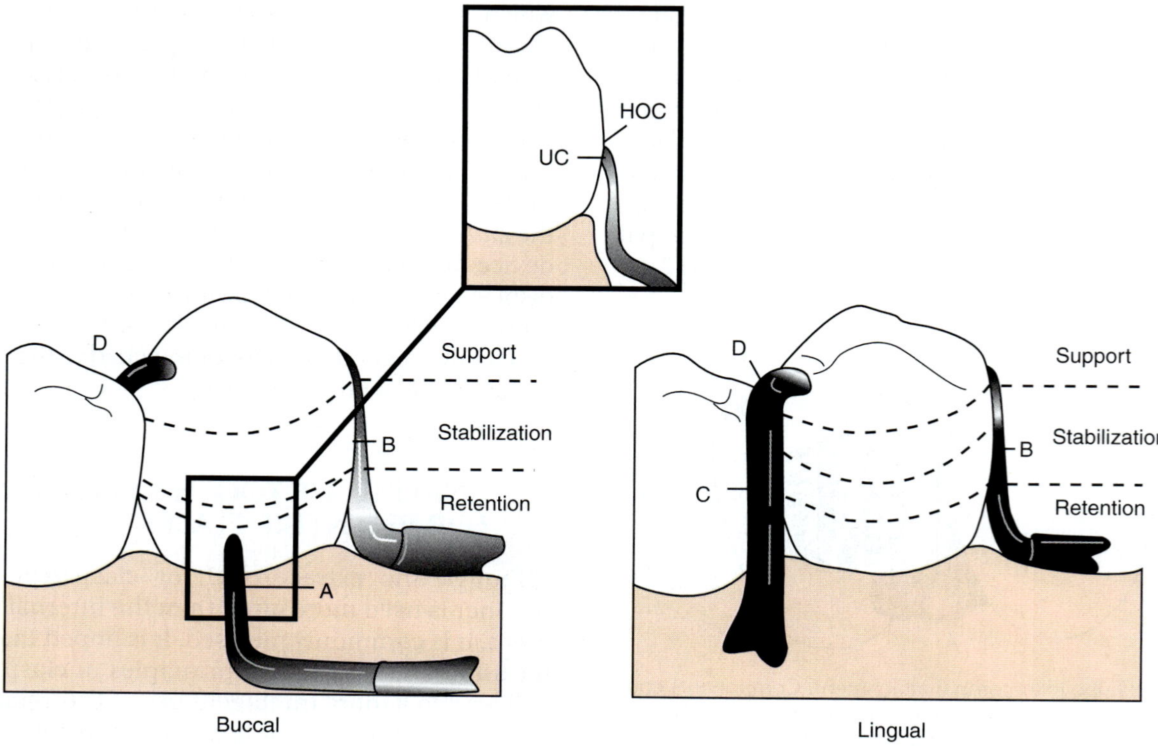

Figure 7-4 Extracoronal bar-type direct retainer. Assembly consists of *A*, buccal retentive arm engaging measured undercut (with slight occlusal extension for stabilization, see insert where *HOC* is height of contour and *UC* is undercut); *B*, stabilizing (reciprocal) elements; proximal plate minor connector on distal; *C*, lingually placed mesial minor connector for occlusal rest, which also serves as a stabilizing (reciprocal) component; and *D*, mesially placed supporting occlusal rest. Assembly remains passive until activated.

TABLE 7-1. Function and Position of Clasp Assembly Parts

Component Part	Function	Location
Rest	Support	Occlusal, lingual, incisal
Minor connector	Stabilization	Proximal surfaces extending from a prepared marginal ridge to the junction of the middle and gingival one third of abutment crown
Clasp arms	Stabilization (reciprocation)	Middle one third of crown
	Retention	Gingival one third of crown in measured undercut

placement toward the side of the cast that is on an upward slant. The vertical arm, when brought in contact with a tooth surface, identifies the location on the clinical crown where the greatest convexity exists. This line, called the *height of contour* (specific to the surveyor-defined path), is the boundary between (1) an occlusal or incisal region of the tooth that is freely accessible to a prosthesis, and (2) a gingival region of the tooth that can only be accessed if a portion of the prosthesis elastically deforms and recovers to contact the tooth. This surveyor-defined path and the subsequent tooth height of contour will indicate the areas available for retention and those available for support, and the existence of

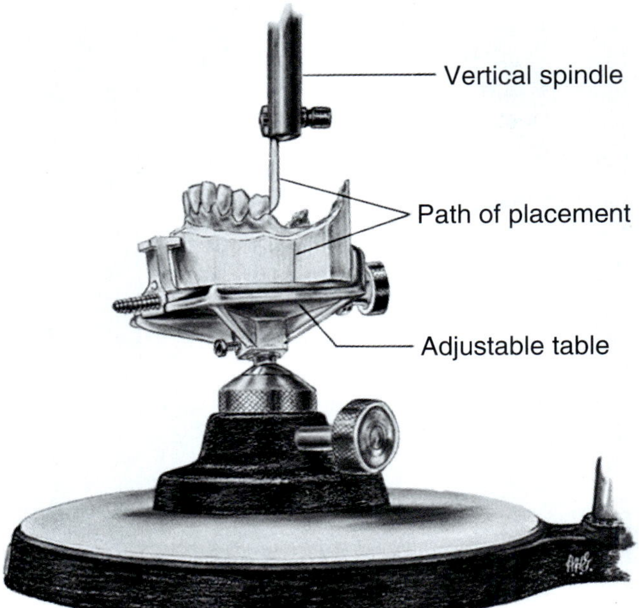

Figure 7-5 Essential parts of a dental surveyor (Ney Parallelometer), showing vertical spindle in relation to adjustable table.

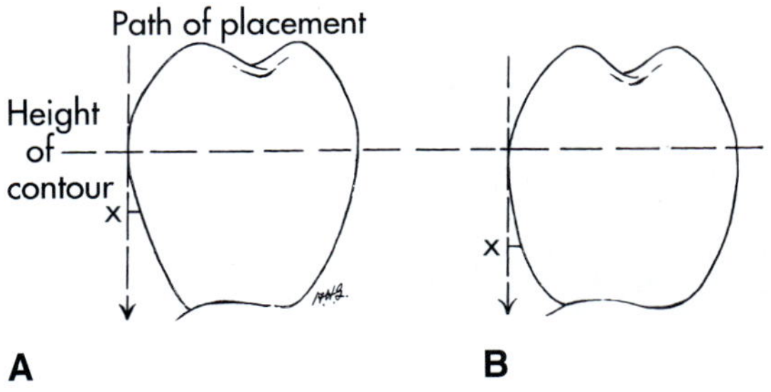

Figure 7-6 Angle of cervical convergence on two teeth presenting dissimilar contours. Greater angle of cervical convergence on tooth **A** necessitates placement of clasp terminus, *X*, nearer the height of contour than when lesser angle exists, as in **B**. It is apparent that uniform clasp retention depends on depth (amount) of tooth undercut rather than on distance below the height of contour at which clasp terminus is placed.

tooth and other tissue interference to the path of placement.

When the surveyor blade contacts a tooth on the cast at its greatest convexity, a triangle is formed. The apex of the triangle is at the point of contact of the surveyor blade with the tooth, and the base is the area of the cast representing the gingival tissue (see Figure 11-19). The apical angle is called the angle of cervical convergence (see Figure 7-6). This angle may be measured as described in Chapter 11, or it may be estimated by observing the triangle of light visible between the tooth and the surveyor blade. For this reason, a wide surveyor blade rather than a small cylindrical tool is used so it is easier to see the triangle of light. The importance of this angle lies in its relationship to the amount of retention.

AMOUNT OF RETENTION

Clasp retention is based on the resistance to deformation of the metal. For a clasp to be retentive, it must be placed in an undercut area of the tooth where it is forced to deform upon application of a vertical dislodging force (Figure 7-8). It is this resistance to deformation along an appropriately selected path that generates retention (Figure 7-9). Such resistance to deformation is dependent on several factors and is also proportionate to the flexibility of the clasp arm.

An interaction of a number of factors under the control of the clinician combines to produce retention. These include both tooth (planned and executed by the clinician) and prosthesis (to be planned by the dentist and executed by the laboratory technician) factors.

Tooth factors are the size of the angle of cervical convergence (depth of undercut) and how far the clasp terminal is placed into the angle of cervical convergence. Prosthesis factors include the flexibility of the clasp arm. Clasp flexibility is the product of clasp length (measured from its point of origin to its terminal end), clasp relative diameter (regardless of its cross-sectional form), clasp cross-sectional form or shape (whether it is round, half round, or some other form), and the material used in making the clasp. The retention characteristics of gold alloy, chrome alloy, titanium, or titanium alloy depend on whether it is in cast or wrought form.

Size of and Distance Into the Angle of Cervical Convergence

To be retentive, a tooth must have an angle of convergence cervical to the height of contour. When it is surveyed, any single tooth will have a height of contour or an area of greatest convexity. Areas of cervical convergence may not exist when the tooth is viewed in relation to a given path of placement. Also, certain areas of cervical convergence may not be usable for the placement of retentive clasps because of their proximity to gingival tissue.

This is best illustrated by mounting a spherical object, such as an egg, on the adjustable table of a dental surveyor (see Figure 7-7). The egg now represents the cast of a dental arch or, more correctly, one tooth of a dental arch. The egg is first placed perpendicular to the base of the surveyor and surveyed to determine the height of contour. The vertical arm of the surveyor represents the path of placement

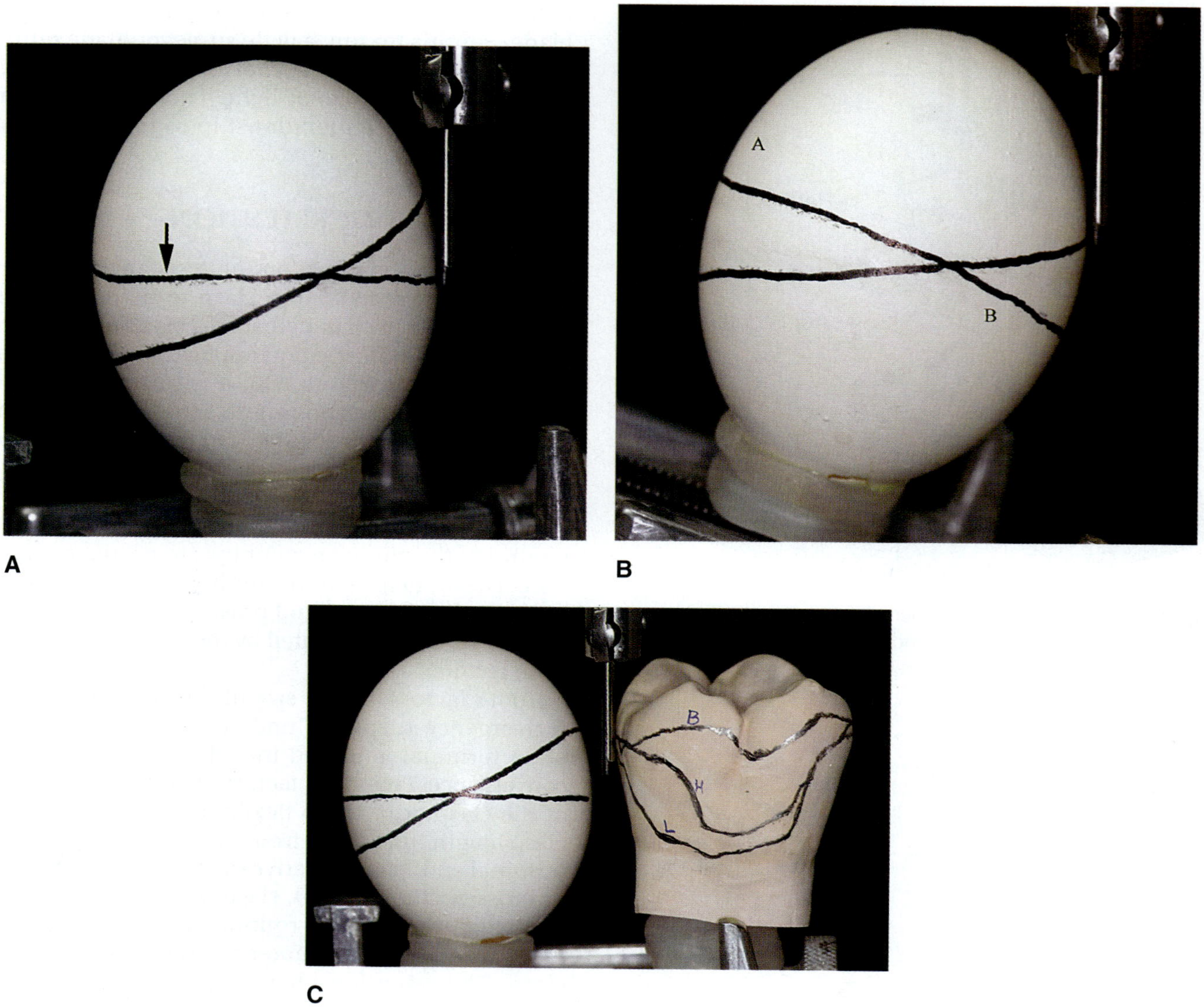

Figure 7-7 Relationship of height of contour, suprabulge, and infrabulge. **A,** When an egg is placed with its long axis parallel to the surveying tool, the height of contour is found at its greatest circumference, here designated by the *arrow*. In this example the second line is diagonal to the line outlining the height of contour and is either above the height of contour (right side of egg), referred to as the **suprabulge region**, or below the height of contour (left side of egg), referred to as the **infrabulge region**. **B,** If the long axis of the egg is reoriented so that the previous diagonal line is now at the greatest circumference, the original "height of contour line" no longer is at the greatest circumference. The line segment at *A* is in the suprabulge region and the line segment *B* is in the infrabulge region. Changing the orientation alters the relationship of surfaces relative to the greatest circumference and consequently alters supra- and infrabulge locations. **C,** Just as height of contour changes as orientation changes for the egg, when a tooth orientation changes the height of contour is altered. For this molar, the line *H* was produced with a horizontal orientation. When the tooth was inclined bucally, the height of contour moved to *B* relative to the horizontal location. Alternately, when the tooth was inclined lingually, the height of contour move to *L* relative to the horizontal location.

that a denture would take, and conversely its path of removal.

With a carbon marker, a circumferential line has been drawn on an egg at its greatest circumference, as shown by the arrow in Figure 7-7, *A*. This line, which Kennedy called the *height of contour*, is its greatest convexity. Cummer spoke of it as the guideline because it is used as a guide in the placement of retentive and nonretentive clasps. To this, DeVan added the terms *suprabulge*, denoting the

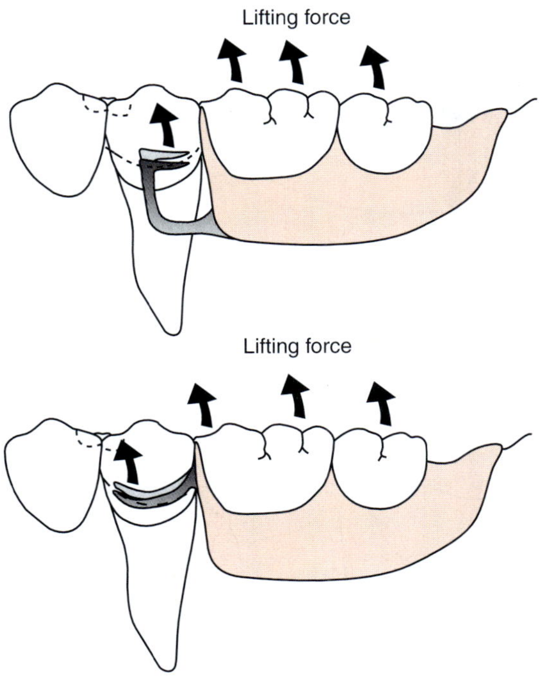

Figure 7-8 Retention is provided primarily by flexible portion of clasp assembly. Retentive terminals are ideally located in measured undercuts in gingival third of abutment crowns. When force acts to dislodge restoration in occlusal direction, retentive arm is forced to deform as it passes from undercut location over height of contour. Amount of retention provided by clasp arm is determined by its length, diameter, taper, cross-sectional form, contour, type of alloy, and location and depth of undercut engaged.

surfaces sloping superiorly, and *infrabulge*, denoting the surfaces sloping inferiorly.

Any areas cervical to the height of contour may be used for the placement of retentive clasp components, whereas areas occlusal to the height of contour may be used for the placement of nonretentive, stabilizing, or reciprocating components. Obviously, only flexible components may be placed gingivally to the height of contour because rigid elements would not flex over the height of contour or contact the tooth in the undercut area.

With the original height of contour marked on the egg, the egg is now tilted from the perpendicular to an angular relation with the base of the surveyor (see Figure 7-7, *B*). Its relation to the vertical arm of the surveyor has now been changed, just as a change in the position of a dental cast would bring about a different relationship with the surveyor. The vertical arm of the surveyor still represents the path of placement. However, its relation to the egg is totally different.

Again, the carbon marker is used to delineate the height of contour or the greatest convexity. It will be seen that areas that were formerly infrabulge are now suprabulge, and vice versa. A retentive clasp arm placed below the height of contour in the original position may now be either excessively retentive or totally nonretentive, whereas a nonretentive stabilizing or reciprocal arm that is located above the height of contour in the first position may now be located in an area of undercut. Figure 7-7, *C* illustrates this principle compared with a tooth example showing that changes in tilt can alter heights of contour significantly.

The location and depth of a tooth undercut available for retention are therefore only relative to the path of placement and removal of the partial denture. At the same time, nonretentive areas on which rigid components of the clasp may be placed exist only for a given path of placement (see Figure 7-8).

If conditions are found that are not favorable for the particular path of placement under consideration, a study should be conducted for a different path of placement. The cast is merely tilted in relation to the vertical arm until the most suitable path is found. The most suitable path of placement is generally considered to be the path of placement that will require the least amount of mouth preparation necessary to place the components of the partial denture in their ideal position on the tooth surfaces and in relation to the soft tissue. Then mouth preparations are planned with a definite path of placement in mind.

It is important to remember that tooth surfaces can be recontoured by selective grinding or the placement of restorations (mouth preparations) to achieve a more suitable path of placement. The path of placement also must take into consideration the presence of tissue undercuts that would interfere with the placement of major connectors, the location of vertical minor connectors, the origin of bar clasp arms, and the denture bases.

When the theory of clasp retention is applied to the abutment teeth in a dental arch during the surveying of the dental cast, each tooth may be considered individually and in relation to the other abutment teeth as far as the designs of retentive and stabilizing (reciprocating) components are concerned. This is necessary because the relationship of each tooth to the rest of the arch and to the design of the rest of the prosthesis has been considered previously in selecting or modifying the teeth to achieve the most suitable path of placement. Once this relationship of the cast to the surveyor has been established, the height of contour on each abutment tooth becomes fixed, and the clasp design for each must be considered separately.

A positive path of placement and removal is made possible by the contact of rigid parts of the denture framework with parallel tooth surfaces, which act as guiding planes. Because guiding planes control the

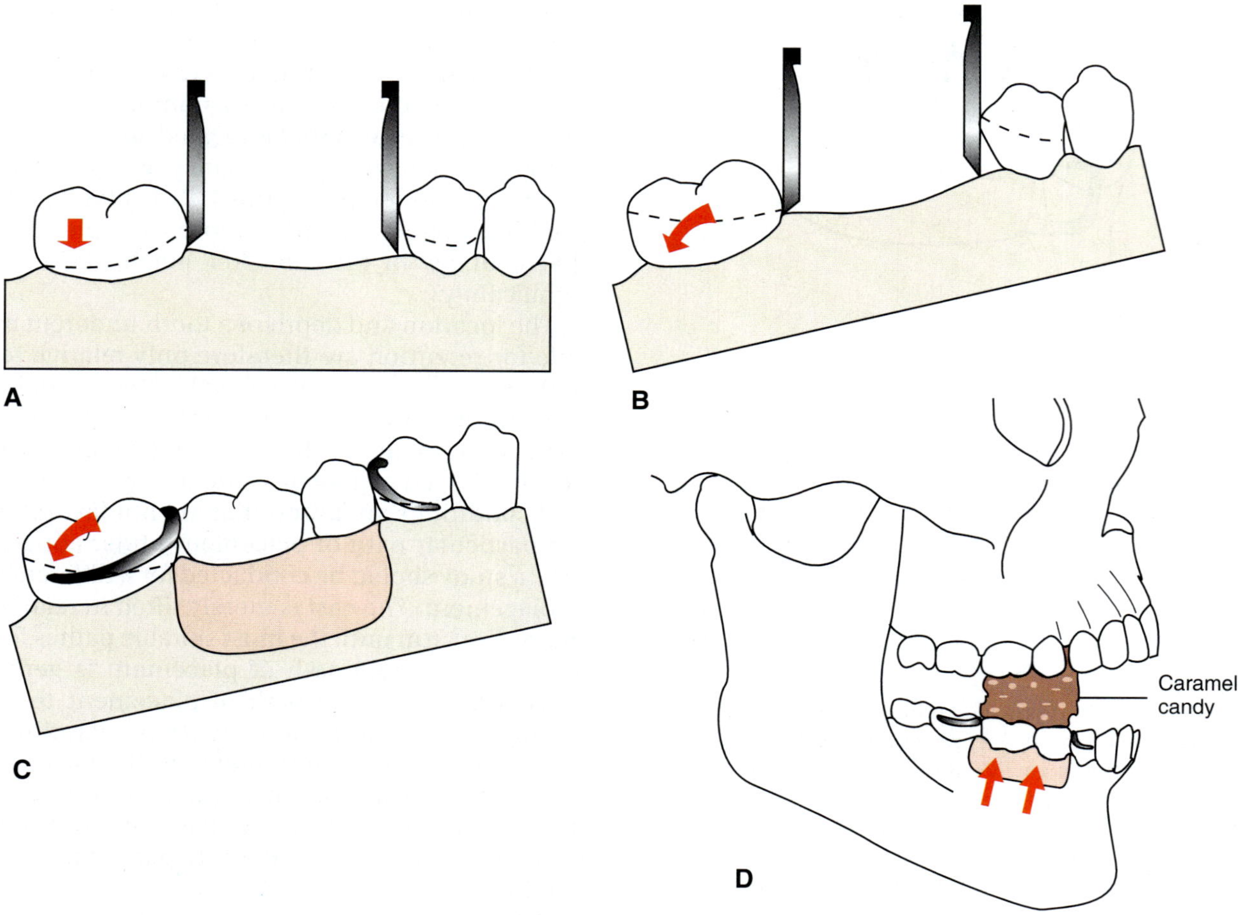

Figure 7-9 **A,** Retentive areas are not sufficient to resist reasonable dislodging forces when cast is surveyed at its most advantageous position (occlusal plane parallel to surveyor table) even though guide planes could be established with minor tooth modification. **B,** Tilting cast creates functionally ineffective tooth contours, which are present only in relation to surveying rod and do not exist when compared with most advantageous position (position in which restoration will be subject to dislodging forces in an occlusal direction). **C** and **D,** Clasps designed at tilt are ineffective without development of corresponding guide planes to resist displacement when restoration is subject to dislodging forces in occlusal direction.

path of placement and removal, they can also provide additional retention for the partial denture by limiting the possibilities that exist for its dislodgment. The more vertical walls (guiding planes) that are prepared parallel, the fewer the possibilities that exist for dislodgment. If some degree of parallelism does not exist during placement and removal, trauma to the teeth and supporting structures and strain on the denture parts are inevitable. This ultimately results in damage either to the teeth and their periodontal support or to the denture itself or both. Therefore without guiding planes, clasp retention will either be detrimental or practically nonexistent. If clasp retention is only frictional because of an active relationship of the clasp to the teeth, then orthodontic movement or damage to periodontal tissue, or both, will result. Instead a clasp should bear a passive relationship to the teeth except when a dislodging force is applied.

In addition to the degree of the angle of cervical convergence and the distance a clasp is placed into the angle of cervical convergence, the amount of retention generated by a clasp depends on its flexibility.

The amount of retention also depends on the flexibility of a clasp arm. This is a function of clasp length, diameter, cross-sectional form, and material.

Length of Clasp Arm

The longer the clasp arm the more flexible it will be, all other factors being equal. The length of a circum-

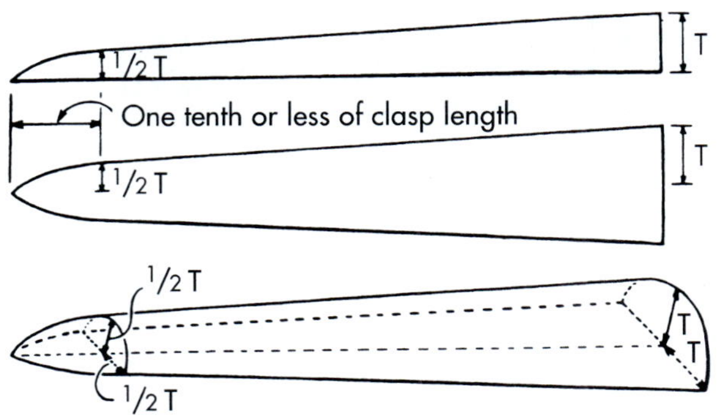

Figure 7-10 Retentive cast clasp arm should be tapered uniformly from its point of attachment at clasp body to its tip. Dimensions at tip are about half those at point of attachment. Clasp arm so tapered is approximately twice as flexible as one without any taper. *T* is clasp thickness. *(Courtesy J.F. Jelenko & Company, New York, NY.)*

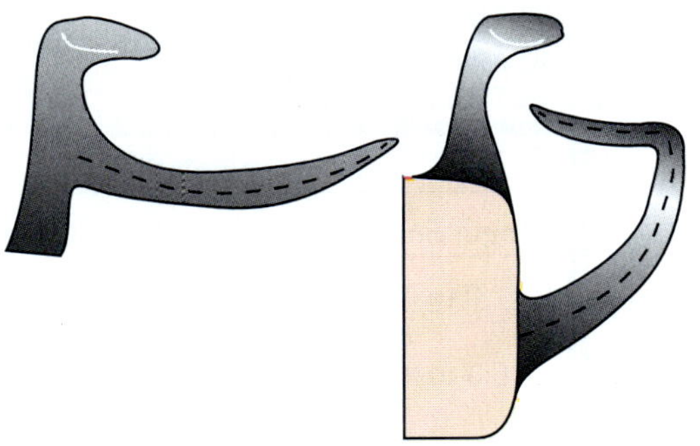

Figure 7-11 Length of tapered cast retentive clasp arm is measured along center portion of arm until it either joins clasp body (circumferential) or becomes part of denture base or is embedded in the base (bar-type clasp).

ferential clasp arm is measured from the point at which a uniform taper begins. Tooth modification providing increased length to a suprabulge retentive clasp by allowing the retentive tip to approach the undercut from a gingival direction optimizes clasp retention (see Figure 7-3). The retentive circumferential clasp arm should be tapered uniformly from its point of origin through the full length of the clasp arm (Figure 7-10).

The length of a bar clasp arm also is measured from the point at which a uniform taper begins. Generally the taper of a bar clasp arm should begin at its point of origin from a metal base or at the point at which it emerges from a resin base (Figure 7-11). Although a bar clasp arm will usually be longer than a circumferential clasp arm, its flexibility will be less because its half-round form lies in several planes, which prevents its flexibility from being proportionate to its total length. Tables 7-2 and 7-3 give an approximate depth of undercut that may be used for the cast gold and chromium-cobalt retentive clasp arms of circumferential and bar-type clasps. Based on a proportional limit of 60,000 psi and on the assumption that the clasp arm is properly tapered, the clasp arm should be able to flex repeatedly within the limits stated without hardening or rupturing because of fatigue. It has been estimated that alternate stress applications of the fatigue type are placed on a retainer arm during mastication and other force-producing functions about 300,000 times a year.

Diameter of Clasp Arm

The greater the average diameter of a clasp arm the less flexible it will be, all other factors being equal. If its taper is absolutely uniform, the average diameter will be at a point midway between its origin and its terminal end. If its taper is not uniform, a point of flexure—and therefore a point of weakness—will exist, which will then be the determining factor in its flexibility regardless of the average diameter of its entire length.

Cross-sectional Form of the Clasp Arm

Flexibility may exist in any form, but it is limited to only one direction in the case of the half-round form. The only universally flexible form is the round form, which is practically impossible to obtain by casting and polishing.

Because most cast clasps are essentially half round in form, they may flex away from the tooth, but edgewise flexing (and edgewise adjustment) is limited. For this reason, cast retentive clasp arms are more acceptable in tooth-supported partial dentures in which they are called on to flex only during placement and removal of the prosthesis. A retentive clasp arm on an abutment adjacent to a distal extension base not only must flex during placement and removal but also must be capable of flexing during functional movement of the distal extension base. It must either have universal flexibility to avoid transmission of tipping stresses to the abutment tooth or be capable of disengaging the undercut when vertical forces directed against the denture are toward the residual ridge. A round clasp is the only circumferential clasp form that may be safely used to engage a tooth undercut on the side of an abutment tooth away from the distal extension base. The location of the undercut is perhaps the single most important factor in selecting a clasp for use with distal extension partial dentures.

Material Used for the Clasp Arm

Although all cast alloys used in partial denture construction possess flexibility, their flexibility is

TABLE 7-2. Permissible Flexibilities of Retentive Cast Circumferential and Bar-type Clasp Arms of Type IV Gold Alloys*

Circumferential		Bar-type	
Length (inches)	Flexibility (inches)	Length (inches)	Flexibility (inches)
0 to 0.3	0.01	0 to 0.7	0.01
0.3 to 0.6	0.02	0.7 to 0.9	0.02
0.6 to 0.8	0.03	0.9 to 1.0	0.03

*Based on the approximate dimensions of Jelenko *preformed* plastic patterns, JF Jelenko, New York.

TABLE 7-3. Permissible Flexibilities of Retentive Cast Circumferential and Bar-type Clasp Arms for Chromium-Cobalt Alloys*

Circumferential		Bar-type	
Length (inches)	Flexibility (inches)	Length (inches)	Flexibility (inches)
0 to 0.3	0.004	0 to 0.7	0.004
0.3 to 0.6	0.008	0.7 to 0.9	0.008
0.6 to 0.8	0.012	0.9 to 1.0	0.012

*Based on the approximate dimensions of Jelenko *preformed* plastic patterns, JF Jelenko, New York.

proportionate to their bulk. If this were not true, other components of the partial denture could not have the necessary rigidity. A disadvantage of a cast gold partial denture is that its bulk must be increased to obtain the needed rigidity at the expense of added weight and increased cost. It cannot be denied that greater rigidity with less bulk is possible through the use of chromium-cobalt alloys.

Although cast gold alloys may have greater resiliency than do cast chromium-cobalt alloys, the fact remains that the structural nature of the cast clasp does not approach the flexibility and adjustable nature of the wrought-wire clasp. Having been formed by being drawn into a wire, the wrought-wire clasp arm has toughness exceeding that of a cast clasp arm. The tensile strength of a wrought structure is at least 25% greater than that of the cast alloy from which it was made. It may therefore be used in smaller diameters to provide greater flexibility without fatigue and ultimate fracture.

Relative Uniformity of Retention

Having reviewed the factors inherent to a determination of the amount of retention from individual clasps, it is important to consider coordination of relative retention between various clasps in a single prosthesis.

The size of the angle of convergence will determine how far a given clasp arm should be placed into that angle. Disregarding—for the time being—variations in clasp flexibility, relative uniformity of retention will depend on the location of the retentive part of the clasp arm, not in relation to the height of contour, but in relation to the angle of cervical convergence.

The retention on all principal abutments should be as equal as possible. Although esthetic placement of clasp arms is desirable, it may not be possible to place all clasp arms in the same occlusocervical relationship because of variations in tooth contours. However, retentive surfaces may be made similar by altering tooth contours or by using cast restorations with similar contours.

Retentive clasp arms must be located so that they lie in the same approximate degree of undercut on each abutment tooth. In Figure 7-6, this is at point **X** on both teeth—*A* and *B*—despite the variation in the distance below the height of contour. Should both clasp arms be placed equidistant below the height of contour, the higher location on tooth *B* would have too little retention, whereas the lower location on tooth *A* would be too retentive.

The measurement of the degree of undercut by mechanical means using a surveyor is important. However, undercut identification is only one factor that is important to consider in providing appropriate retention for a removable partial denture.

Stabilizing-reciprocal Cast Clasp Arm

When the direct retainer comes into contact with the tooth, the framework must be stabilized against horizontal movement for the required clasp deformation to occur. This stabilization is derived from either cross-arch framework contacts or a stabilizing or reciprocal clasp in the same clasp assembly. To provide true reciprocation, the reciprocal clasp must be in contact during the entire period of retentive clasp deformation. This is best provided with lingual-palatal, guide-plane surfaces.

A stabilizing (reciprocal) clasp arm should be rigid. Therefore it is shaped somewhat differently than is the cast retentive clasp arm, which must be flexible. Its average diameter must be greater than the average diameter of the opposing retentive arm to increase desired rigidity. A cast retentive arm is tapered in two dimensions, as illustrated in Figure 7-10, whereas a reciprocal arm should be tapered in one dimension only, as shown in Figure 7-12. Achieving such a form for the arm requires freehand waxing of patterns.

CRITERIA FOR SELECTING A GIVEN CLASP DESIGN

In selecting a particular clasp design for a given situation, its function and limitations must be carefully evaluated. Extracoronal direct retainers, as part of the clasp assembly, should be considered as a component of a removable partial denture framework. They should be designed and located to perform the specific functions of support, stabilization, reciprocation, and retention. It does not matter whether the direct retainer-clasp assembly components are physically attached to each other, or originate from major and minor connectors of the framework (Figure 7-13). If attention is directed to the separate function of each component of the direct retainer-clasp assembly, then selection of a direct retainer is simplified.

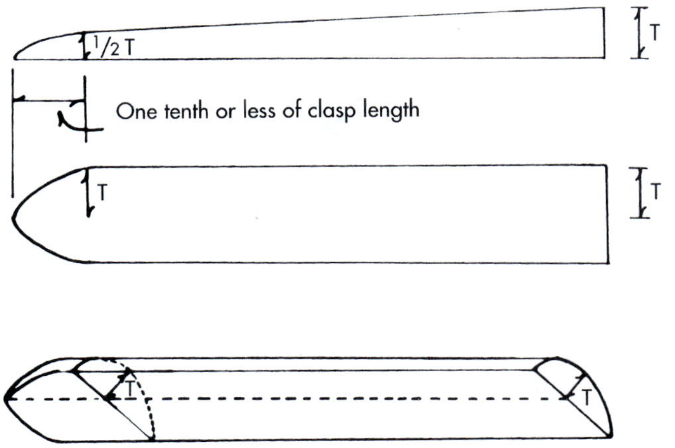

Figure 7-12 Reciprocal arm of direct retainer assembly should be rigid. Arm tapered both lengthwise and widthwise is more flexible than arm of the same dimensions tapered only lengthwise. *T* is clasp thickness.

Although there are some rather complex designs for clasp arms, they may all be classified into one of two basic categories. One is the circumferential clasp arm, which approaches the retentive undercut from an occlusal direction. The other is the bar clasp arm, which approaches the retentive undercut from a cervical direction. A clasp assembly may be a combination of cast circumferential and bar clasp arms, and/or wrought-wire retentive arms in one of several possible combinations as illustrated in buccal and lingual views in Figure 7-14.

A clasp assembly should consist of four component parts. First, there should be one or more minor connectors from which the clasp components originate. Second, there should be a principal rest designed to direct stress along the long axis of the tooth. Third, there should be a retentive arm engaging a tooth undercut. For most clasps, the retentive region is only at its terminus. Fourth, there should be a nonretentive arm (or other component) on the opposite side of the tooth for stabilization and reciprocation against horizontal movement of the prosthesis (rigidity of this clasp arm is essential to its purpose).

No confusion should exist between the choice of clasp arm and the purpose for which it is used. Either type of cast clasp arm (bar or circumferential) may be made tapered and retentive, or nontapered (rigid) and nonretentive. The choice depends on whether it is used for retention, stabilization, or reciprocation. An auxiliary occlusal rest, such as in the RPI concept, may be used rather than a reciprocal clasp arm to satisfy the need for encirclement provided it is located in a way to accomplish the same purpose (Figure 7-15; see also Figure 7-4). The addition of a lingual apron to a cast reciprocal clasp arm alters neither its primary purpose nor the need for proper location to accomplish that purpose.

BASIC PRINCIPLES OF CLASP DESIGN

The clasp assembly serves a similar function for a removable partial denture that a retainer crown serves for a fixed partial denture. Both must encircle

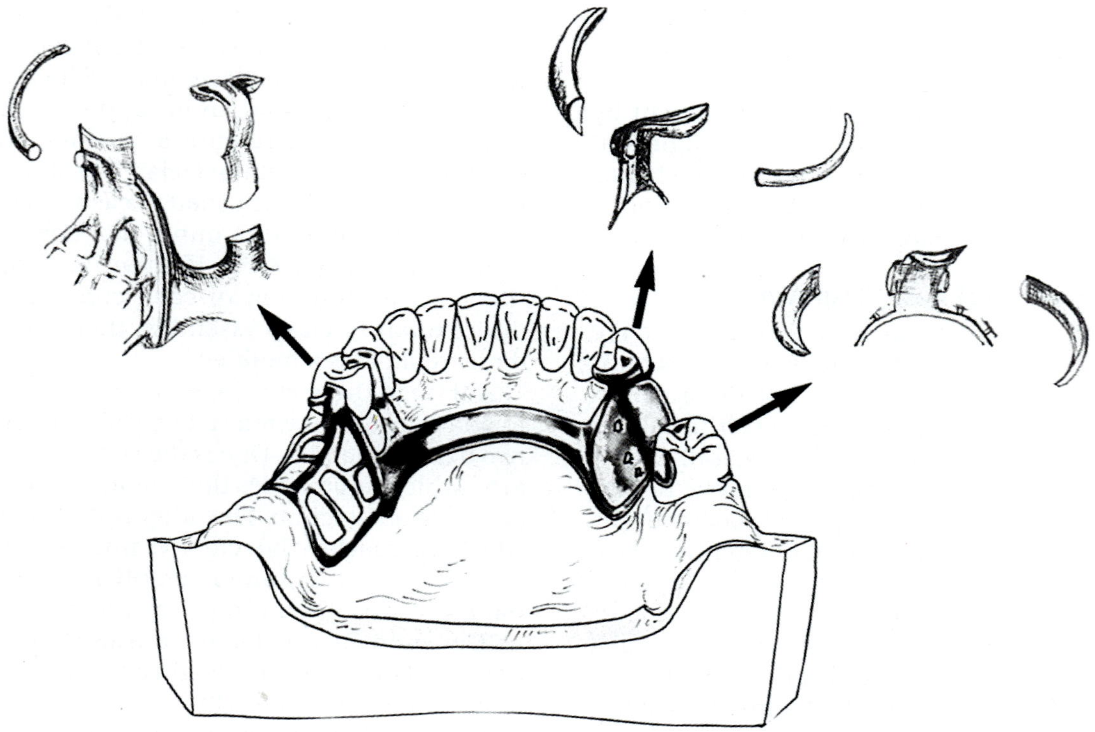

Figure 7-13 Choice and definitive location of each component of direct retainer assembly must be based on preserving health of periodontal attachment in spite of rotational tendencies of distal extension denture. Knowledge of characteristics of each component of collective assemblies for a particular arch and rationalized rotational tendencies of denture simplifies design of removable restorations.

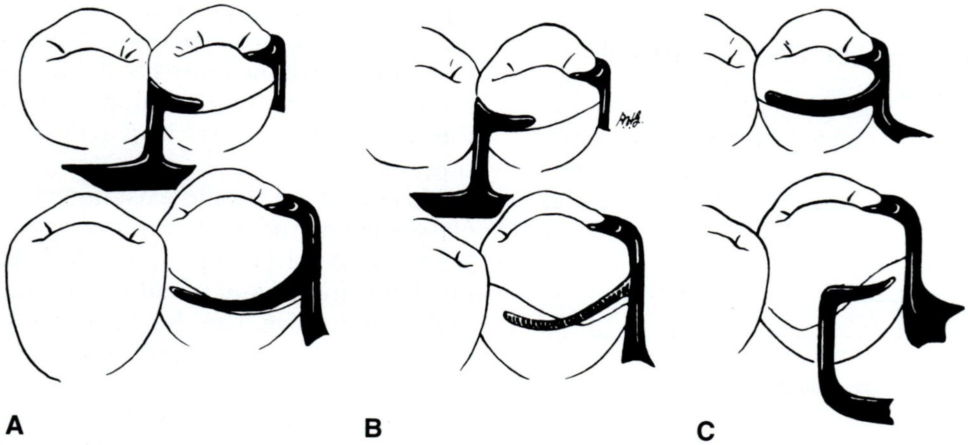

Figure 7-14 Clasp assembly *(with mirror views)*, including rest, may be combination of circumferential and bar clasp arms in one of several possible combinations. These mirror views are for abutments bounding a modification space. **A,** Cast circumferential retentive clasp arm with nonretentive bar clasp arm on opposite side for stabilization and reciprocation. **B,** Tapered wrought-wire circumferential retentive clasp arm with nonretentive bar clasp arm on opposite side for stabilization and reciprocation. **C,** Retentive bar clasp arm with nonretentive cast circumferential clasp arm on opposite side for stabilization and reciprocation.

the prepared tooth in a manner that prevents movement of the tooth separate from the retainer. To borrow from a fixed prosthodontic term, *limiting the freedom of displacement* refers to the effect of one cylindrical surface (the framework encircling the tooth) on another cylindrical surface (the tooth). It implies that the curve that defines the framework is properly shaped if it prevents move-

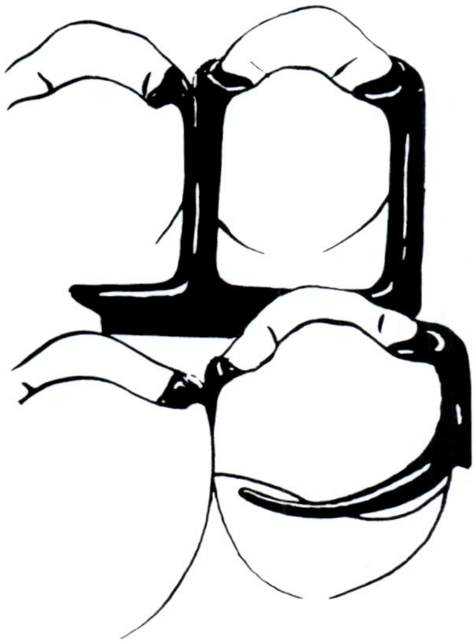

Figure 7-15 Auxiliary occlusal rest (*mirror view*) may be used rather than reciprocal clasp arm without violating any principle of clasp design. Its greatest disadvantages are that second rest seat must be prepared and that enclosed tissue space at the gingival margin can result in a food trap. Auxiliary occlusal rest is also sometimes used to prevent slippage when principal occlusal rest seat cannot be inclined apically from marginal ridge. Minor connectors used to close interproximal space most often require rests on adjacent teeth to avoid wedging effect when force is placed on denture.

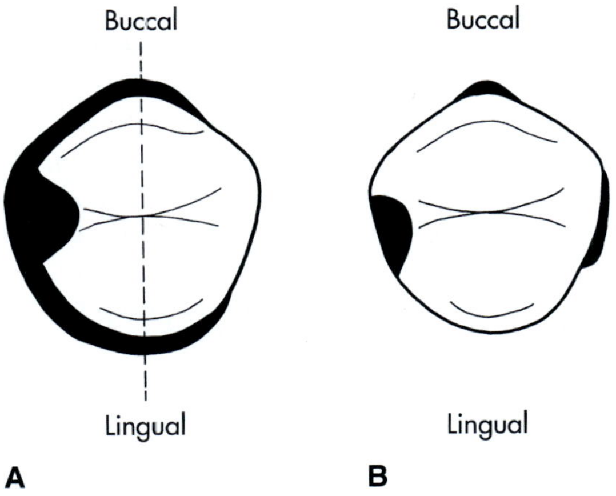

Figure 7-16 **A,** Line drawn through illustration represents 180 degrees of greatest circumference of abutment from occlusal rest. Unless portions of lingual reciprocal arm and retentive buccal arm are extended beyond the line, clasp would not accomplish its intended purpose. If respective arms of retainer were not extended beyond the line, abutment tooth could be forced away from retainer by torquing action of clasp or removable partial denture could move away from abutment. **B,** Bar-type clasp assembly engagement of more than 180 degrees of circumference of abutment is realized by minor connector for occlusal rest, minor connector contacting guiding plane on distal proximal surface, and retentive bar arm.

ment at right angles to the tooth axis. This basic principle of clasp design offers a two-way benefit. First, it ensures the stability of the tooth position because of the restraint from encirclement, and second, it ensures stability of the clasp assembly because of the controlled position of the clasp in three dimensions.

Therefore the basic principle of clasp design referred to as the *principle of encirclement* means that more than 180 degrees in the greatest circumference of the tooth, passing from diverging axial surfaces to converging axial surfaces, must be engaged by the clasp assembly (Figure 7-16). The engagement can be in the form of continuous contact, such as in a circumferential clasp, or discontinuous contact, such as in the use of a bar clasp. Both provide tooth contact in at least three areas encircling the tooth: the occlusal rest area, the retentive clasp terminal area, and the reciprocal clasp terminal area.

In addition to encirclement, other basic principles of clasp design are as follows:

1. The occlusal rest must be designed to prevent the movement of the clasp arms toward the cervical.
2. Each retentive terminal should be opposed by a reciprocal component capable of resisting any transient pressures exerted by the retentive arm during placement and removal. Stabilizing and reciprocal components must be rigidly connected bilaterally (cross-arch) to realize reciprocation of the retentive elements (Figure 7-17).

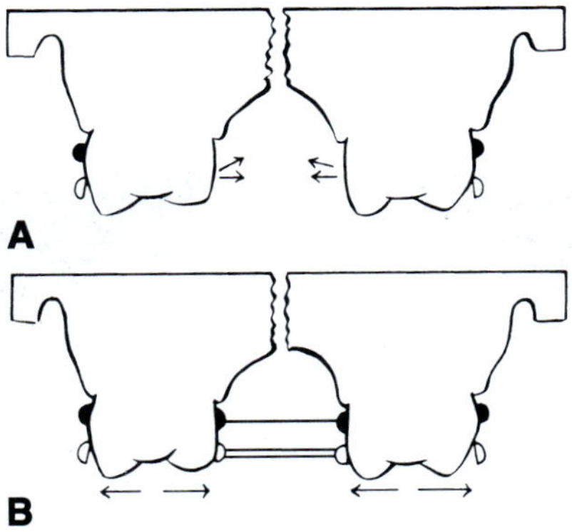

Figure 7-17 **A,** Flexing action of retentive clasp arm initiates medially directed pressure on abutment teeth as its retentive tip springs over height of contour. **B,** Reciprocation to medially directed pressure is counteracted either by rigid lingually placed clasp arms contacting abutments simultaneously with buccal arms or by rigid stabilizing components of framework contacting lingual guiding planes when buccal arms begin to flex.

3. Clasp retainers on abutment teeth adjacent to distal extension bases should be designed so that they will avoid direct transmission of tipping and rotational forces to the abutment. In effect, they must act as stress-breakers either by their design or by their construction. This is accomplished through proper location of the retentive terminal relative to the rest or by use of a more flexible clasp arm in relation to the anticipated rotation of the denture under functional forces.
4. Unless guiding planes will positively control the path of removal and stabilize abutments against rotational movements, retentive clasps should be bilaterally opposed, i.e., buccal retention on one side of the arch should be opposed by buccal retention on the other, or lingual on one side opposed by lingual on the other. In Class II situations, the third abutment may have either buccal or lingual retention. In Class III situations, retention may be either bilaterally or diametrically opposed (Figure 7-18).
5. The path of escapement for each retentive clasp terminal must be other than parallel to the path of removal for the prosthesis to require clasp engagement with the resistance to deformation that is retention (see Figure 7-8).
6. The amount of retention should always be the minimum necessary to resist reasonable dislodging forces.
7. Reciprocal elements of the clasp assembly should be located at the junction of the gingival and middle thirds of the crowns of abutment teeth. The terminal end of the retentive arm is optimally placed in the gingival third of the crown (Figures 7-19 through 7-21). These locations permit better resistance to horizontal and torquing forces because of a reduction in the effort arm as described in Chapter 4.

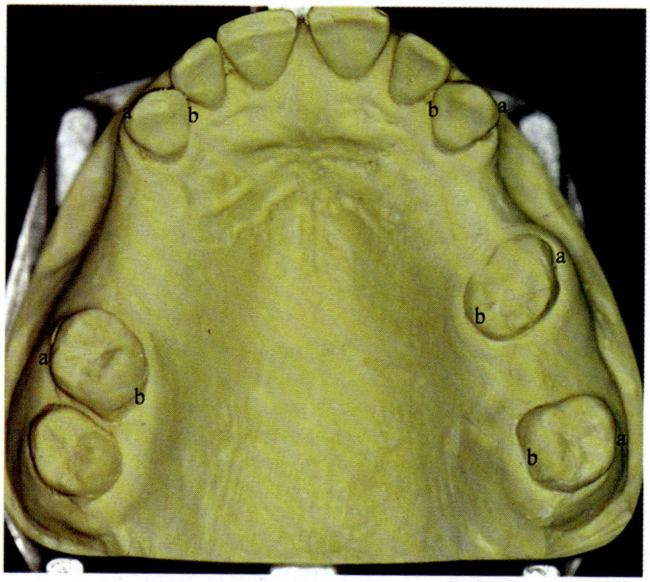

Figure 7-18 Retentive clasps should be bilaterally opposed. This means using bilateral buccal or bilateral lingual undercuts as shown on this Class III, modification 2, arch where the retention may be either *(a)* bilaterally buccal or *(b)* bilaterally lingual.

Reciprocal Arm Functions

As mentioned earlier, reciprocal arms are intended to resist tooth movements in response to the retainer arm deforming as it engages a tooth height of contour. The opposing clasp arm reciprocates the effect of this deformation as it prevents tooth movement. For this to occur, the reciprocal arm must be in contact during the time of retainer arm deformation. Unless the abutment tooth has been specifically contoured, the reciprocal clasp arm will not come into contact with the tooth until the denture is fully seated and the retentive clasp arm has again become passive. When this happens, a momentary tipping force is applied to the abutment teeth during each placement and removal. This may not be a damaging force—because it is transient—so long as the force does not exceed the normal elasticity of the periodontal attachments. True reciprocation during placement and removal is possible only through the use of crown surfaces made parallel to the path of placement. The use of cast restorations permits the parallel surfaces to be contacted by the reciprocal arm in such a manner that true reciprocation is made possible. This is discussed in Chapter 14.

Reciprocal arms also can have additional functions. The reciprocal clasp arm should be located so that the denture is stabilized against horizontal movement. Stabilization is possible only through

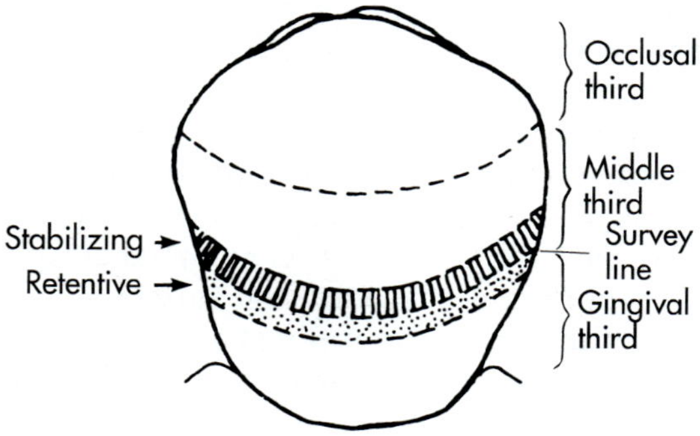

Figure 7-19 Simple mechanical laws demonstrate that the nearer stabilizing-reciprocal and retentive elements of direct retainer assemblies are located to horizontal axis of rotation of abutment, the less likely that physiologic tolerance of periodontal ligament will be exceeded. Horizontal axis of rotation of abutment tooth is located somewhere in its root.

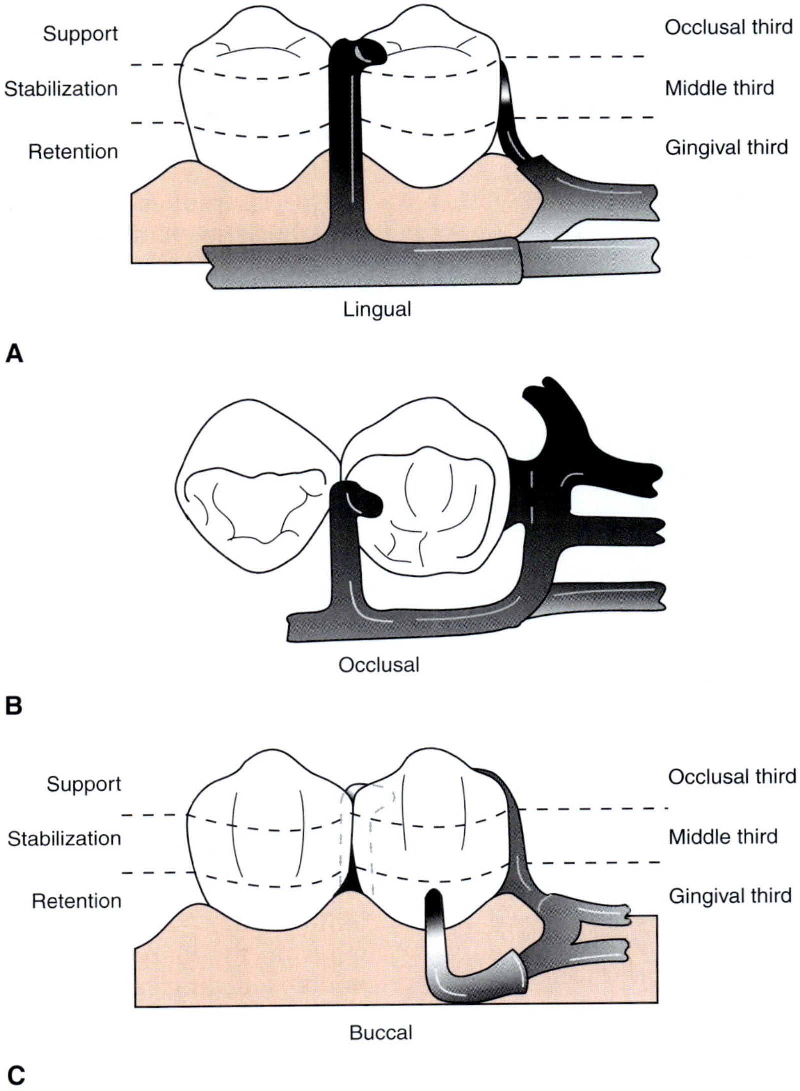

Figure 7-20 Bar-type clasp on mandibular premolar. **A,** Support is provided by occlusal rest. **B,** Stabilization is provided by occlusal rest and mesial and distal minor connectors. **C,** Retention is provided by buccal I-bar. Reciprocation is obtained through location of minor connectors. Engagement of more than 180 degrees of circumference of the abutment is accomplished by proper location of components contacting axial surfaces. (Minor connector supports occlusal rest, proximal plate minor connector, and buccal I-bar.)

the use of rigid clasp arms, rigid minor connectors, and a rigid major connector. Horizontal forces applied on one side of the dental arch are resisted by the stabilizing components on the opposite side providing cross-arch stability. Obviously the greater the number of such components, within reason, the greater will be the distribution of horizontal stresses.

The reciprocal clasp arm also may act to a minor degree as an indirect retainer. This is only true when it rests on a suprabulge surface of an abutment tooth lying anterior to the fulcrum line (see Figure 8-8). Lifting of a distal extension base away from the tissue is thus resisted by a rigid arm, which is not easily displaced cervically. The effectiveness of such an indirect retainer is limited by its proximity to the fulcrum line, which gives it a relatively poor leverage advantage, and by the fact that slippage along tooth inclines is always possible. The latter may be prevented by the use of a ledge on a cast restoration; however, enamel surfaces are not ordinarily so prepared.

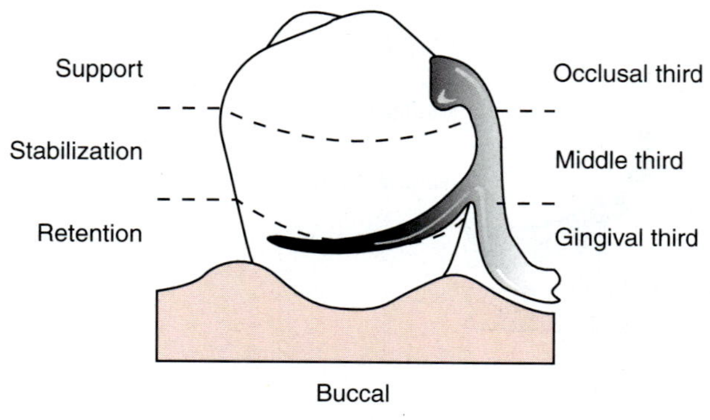

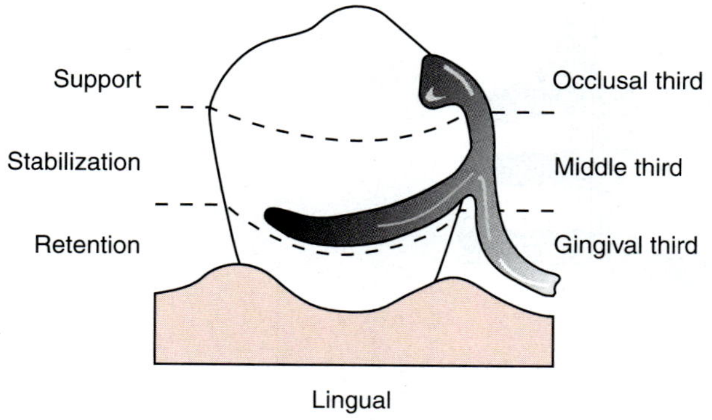

Figure 7-21 Circumferential clasp on mandibular premolar. Support is provided by occlusal rest; stabilization is provided by occlusal rest, proximal minor connector, lingual clasp arm, and rigid portion of buccal retentive clasp arm occlusal to height of contour; retention is realized by retentive terminal of buccal clasp arm; reciprocation is provided by nonflexible lingual clasp arm. Assembly engages more than 180 degrees of abutment tooth's circumference.

TYPES OF CLASP ASSEMBLIES

A wide variety of clasp assemblies are available for clinicians to use. The variety exists largely because of the imagination of clinicians and technicians providing prostheses when tooth modification was not or could not be provided. To simplify clasp designs and to improve functional predictability of prostheses, today's clinician must realize the need for tooth modification.

Some clasp assemblies are designed to accommodate prosthesis functional movement (as mentioned in the basic principles above) and others do not incorporate such design features. While it has been demonstrated by Kapur and others that adverse outcomes are not always associated with the use of rigid clasp assemblies in distal extension classifications, the following clasp assemblies will be described as clasps designed to accommodate distal extension functional movement and clasps designed without movement accommodation. The clinician should not interpret these categories as mutually exclusive since most any clasp assembly can be used to retain a well-supported and maintained prosthesis.

Clasps Designed to Accommodate Functional Movement

RPI, RPA, and Bar Clasp

Clasp assemblies that accommodate functional prosthesis movement are designed to address the concern of a Class I lever. The concern is that the distal extension acts as a long "effort arm" across the distal rest "fulcrum" to cause the clasp tip "resistance arm" to engage the tooth undercut. This results in a harmful tipping or torquing of the tooth and is greater with stiff clasps and more denture base movement. Two strategies are adopted to either change the fulcrum location and subsequently the "resistance arm" engaging effect (mesial rest concept clasp assemblies), or to minimize the effect of the lever by use of a flexible arm (wrought-wire retentive arm).

Mesial rest concept clasps are proposed to accomplish movement accommodation by changing the fulcrum location. This concept includes the RPI and RPA clasps. The RPI is a current concept of bar clasp design, and refers to the rest, proximal plate, and I-bar component parts of the clasp assembly. Basically, this clasp assembly consists of a mesioocclusal rest with the minor connector placed into the mesiolingual embrasure, but not contacting the adjacent tooth (Figure 7-22, *A*). A distal guiding plane, extending from the marginal ridge to the junction of the middle and gingival thirds of the abutment tooth, is prepared to receive a proximal plate (Figure 7-22, *B*). The buccolingual width of the guiding plane is determined by the proximal contour of the tooth (Figure 7-22, *A* and *C*). The proximal plate, in conjunction with the minor connector supporting the rest, provides the stabilizing and reciprocal aspects of the clasp assembly. The I-bar should be located in the gingival third of the buccal or labial surface of the abutment in a 0.01-inch undercut (Figure 7-22, *D*). The whole arm of the I-bar should be tapered to its terminus, with no more than 2 mm of its tip contacting the abutment. The retentive tip contacts the tooth from the undercut to the height of contour (Figure 7-22, *E*). This area of contact along with the rest and proximal plate contact provides stabilization through encirclement (see Figure 7-22, *C*). The horizontal portion of the approach arm must be located at least 4 mm from the gingival margin and even farther if possible.

There are three basic approaches to the application of the RPI system. The location of the rest, the design of the minor connector (proximal plate) as it relates to the guiding plane, and the location of the retentive arm are factors that influence how this clasp system functions. Variations in these factors

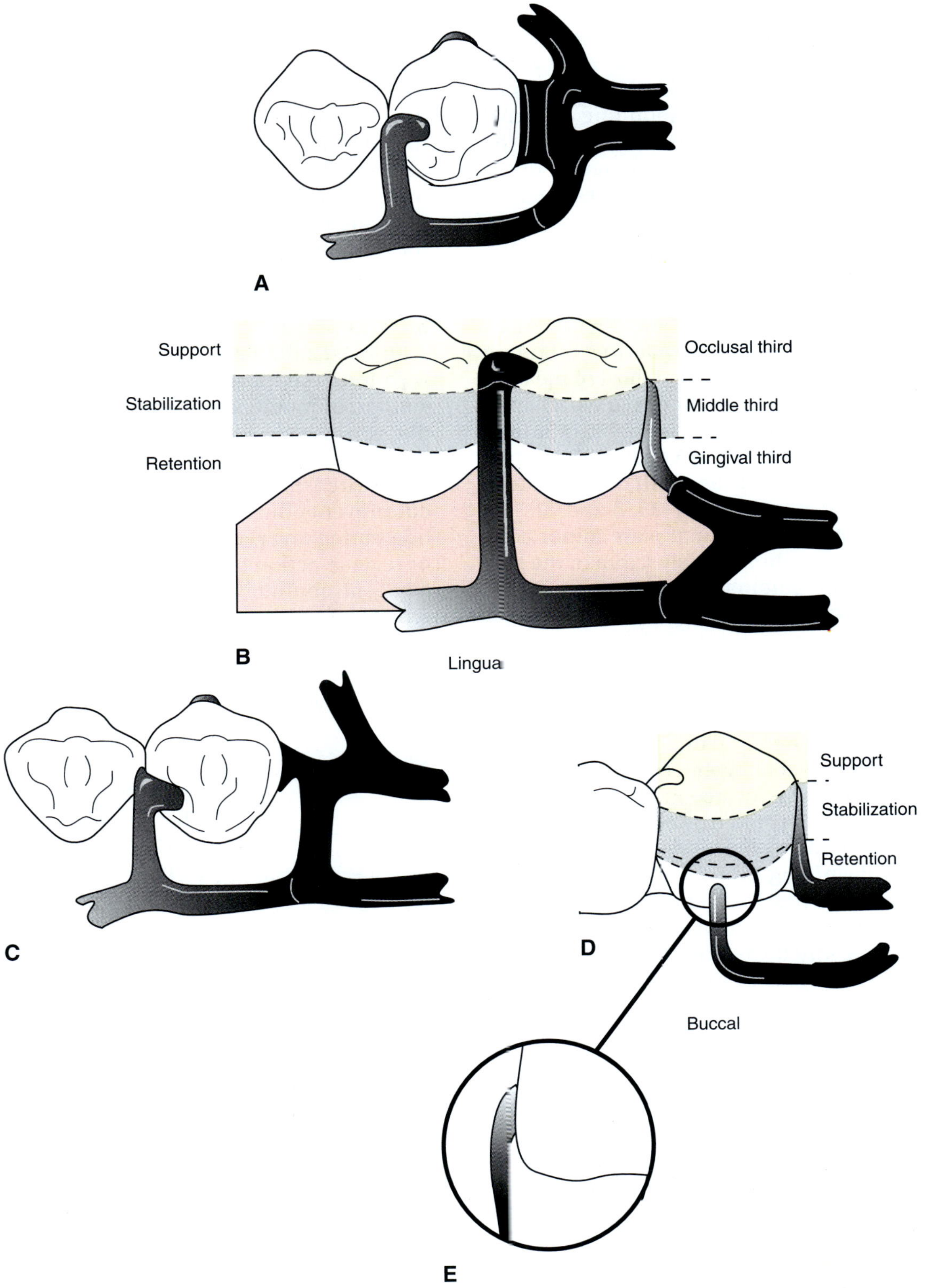

Figure 7-22 Bar-type clasp assembly. **A,** Occlusal view. Component parts (proximal plate minor connector, rest with minor connector, and retentive arm) tripod abutment to prevent its migration. **B,** Proximal plate minor connector extends just far enough lingually so that together with mesial minor connector lingual migration of abutment is prevented. **C,** On narrow or tapered abutments (mandibular first premolars), proximal plate should be designed to be as narrow as possible but still sufficiently wide to prevent lingual migration. **D,** I-bar retainer located at greatest prominence of tooth in gingival third. **E,** Mesial view of I-bar illustrating the retentive tip relationship to the undercut and a region superior toward the height of contour, which serves a stabilization function in encirclement.

provide the basis for the differences among these approaches. All advocate the use of a rest located mesially on the primary abutment tooth adjacent to the extension base area. One approach recommends that the guiding plane and corresponding proximal plate minor connector extend the entire length of the proximal tooth surface, with physiological tissue relief to eliminate impingement of the free gingival margin (Figure 7-23). A second approach suggests that the guiding plane and corresponding proximal plate minor connector extend from the marginal ridge to the junction of the middle and gingival thirds of the proximal tooth surface (Figure 7-24). Both approaches recommend that the retaining clasp arm be located in the gingival third of the buccal or labial surface of the abutment in a 0.01-inch undercut. Placement of the retaining clasp arm is generally in an undercut located at the greatest mesiodistal prominence of the tooth or adjacent to the extension base area (Figure 7-25, *A* and *B*). The third approach favors a proximal plate minor connector that contacts approximately 1 mm of the gingival portion of the guiding plane (Figure 7-26, *A*) and a retentive clasp arm located in a 0.01-inch undercut in the gingival third of the tooth at the greatest prominence or to the mesial away from the edentulous area (see Figure 7-25, *C*). If the abutment teeth demonstrate contraindications for a bar-type clasp (i.e., exaggerated buccal or lingual tilts, severe tissue undercut, or a shallow buccal vestibule) and the desirable undercut is located in the gingival third of the tooth away from the extension base area, a modification should be considered for the RPI system (the RPA clasp) (Figure 7-26, *B*). Application of each approach is predicated on the distribution of load to be applied to the tooth and edentulous ridge.

The bar clasp, which gave rise to the RPI, is discussed here because of this association. It may not be configured to allow functional movement but can be. The term *bar clasp* is generally preferred over the less descriptive term *Roach clasp arm.* Reduced to its simplest term, the *bar clasp arm* arises from the denture framework or a metal base and approaches the retentive undercut from a gingival direction (see Figure 7-22). The bar clasp arm has been classified by the shape of the retentive terminal. Thus it has been identified as a T, modified T, I, or Y. The form the terminal takes is of little significance as long as it is mechanically and functionally effective, covers as little tooth surface as possible, and displays as little metal as possible.

In most situations the bar clasp arm can be used with tooth-supported partial dentures, with tooth-supported modification areas, or when an undercut that can be logically approached with a bar clasp arm lies on the side of an abutment tooth adjacent to a distal extension base (Figure 7-27). If a tissue undercut prevents the use of a bar clasp arm, a mesially originating ring clasp, a cast, or a wrought-wire clasp or reverse-action clasp may be used. Preparation of adjacent abutments (natural teeth) to receive any type of interproximal direct retainer, traversing from lingual to buccal surfaces, is most difficult to ade-

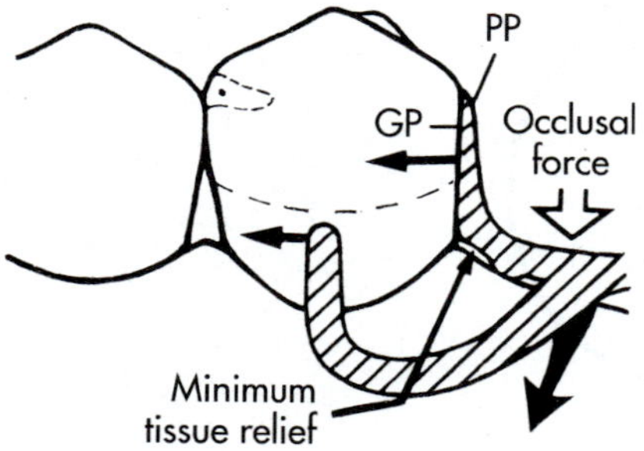

Figure 7-23 Bar clasp assembly in which guiding plane *(GP)* and corresponding proximal plate *(PP)* extend entire length of proximal tooth surface. Physiologic relief is required to prevent impingement of gingival tissues during function. Extending proximal plate to contact greater surface area of guide plane directs functional forces in horizontal direction, thus tooth (teeth) are loaded more than edentulous ridge.

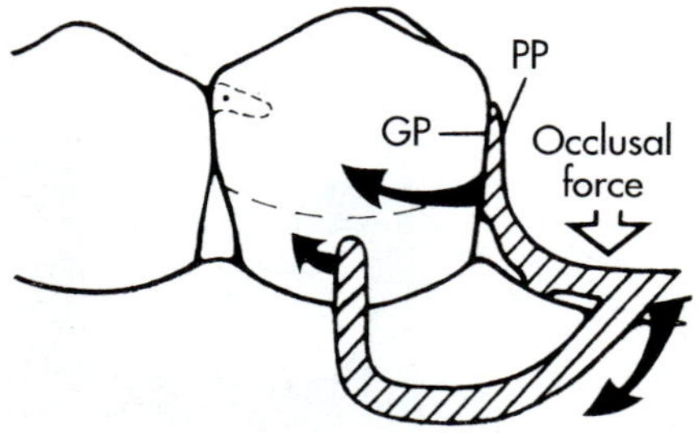

Figure 7-24 Bar clasp assembly in which guiding plane *(GP)* and corresponding proximal plate *(PP)* extend from marginal ridge to junction of middle and gingival thirds of proximal tooth surface. This decrease (compared with Figure 7-23) in amount of surface area contact of proximal plate on guiding plane more evenly distributes functional force between tooth and edentulous ridge.

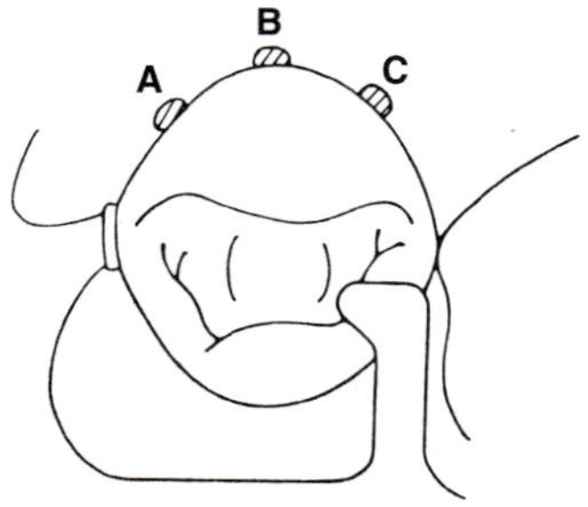

Figure 7-25 Occlusal view of RPI bar clasp assembly. Placement of I-bar in 0.01-inch undercut: **A,** on distobuccal surface; **B,** at greatest mesiodistal prominence; and **C,** on mesiobuccal surface.

quately accomplish. Inevitably the relative size of the occlusal table is increased, contributing to undesirable and additional functional loading.

The specific indications for using a bar clasp arm are (1) when a small degree of undercut (0.01 inch) exists in the cervical third of the abutment tooth, which may be approached from a gingival direction; (2) on abutment teeth for tooth-supported partial dentures or tooth-supported modification areas (Figure 7-28); (3) in distal extension base situations;

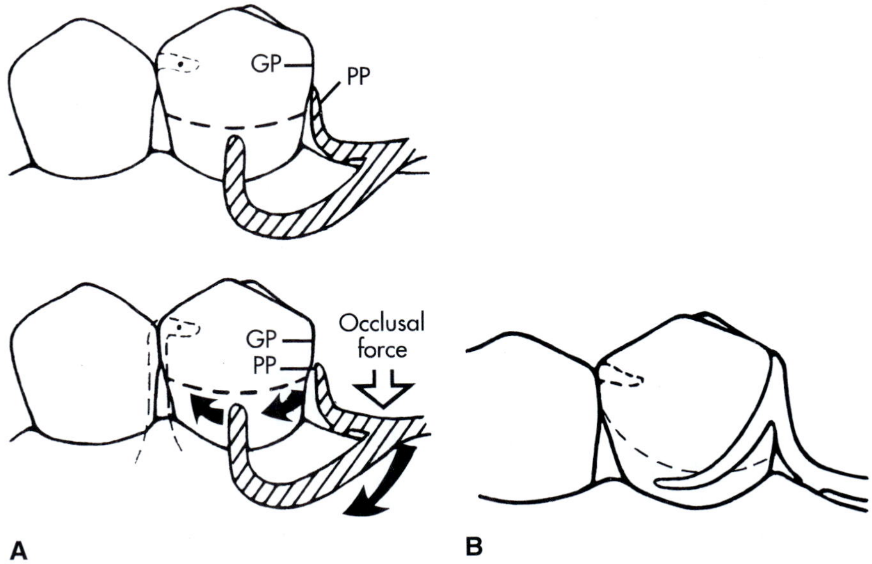

Figure 7-26 **A,** Bar clasp assembly in which proximal plate *(PP)* contacts approximately 1 mm of gingival portion of guiding plane *(GP)*. During function, proximal plate and I-bar clasp arm are designed to move in mesiogingival direction, disengaging tooth. Lack of sustained contact between proximal plate and guiding plane distributes more functional force to edentulous ridge. Asterisk (*) indicates center of rotation. **B,** Modification of RPI system (RPA clasp) is indicated when bar-type clasp is contraindicated and desirable undercut is located in gingival third of tooth away from extension base area.

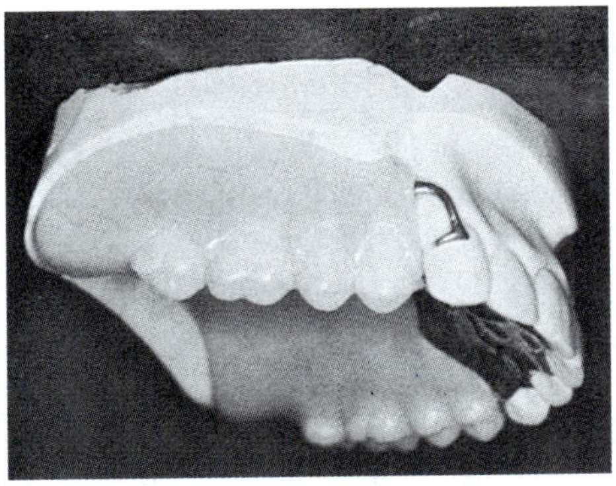

Figure 7-27 Bar clasp arm properly used on terminal abutment. Combination of rest, proximal plate, and bar clasp contacting the abutment tooth provides more than 180 degrees encirclement. Uniform taper to the bar ensures proper flexibility and internal stress distribution. Taper can originate from minor connector junction or at a finishing line indicating the anterior extent of the denture base. Encirclement does not require that retentive tip modification (in the form of a T) be provided, and such a modification adds little to the clasp assembly.

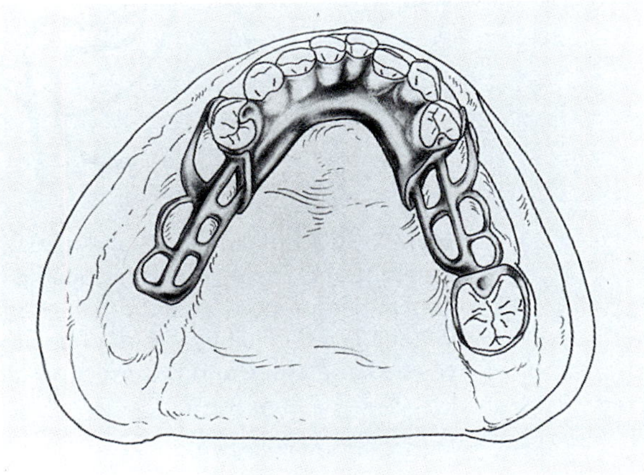

Figure 7-28 Bar retainer is used on anterior abutment of modification space, and its terminus engages distobuccal undercut. Denture is designed to rotate around terminal abutments when force is directed toward basal seat on left. Such rotation would impart force on right premolar directed superiorly and anteriorly. However, this direction of force is resisted in great part by mesial contact with canine. Direct retainer on right premolar engaging mesiobuccal undercut would tend to force tooth superiorly and posteriorly.

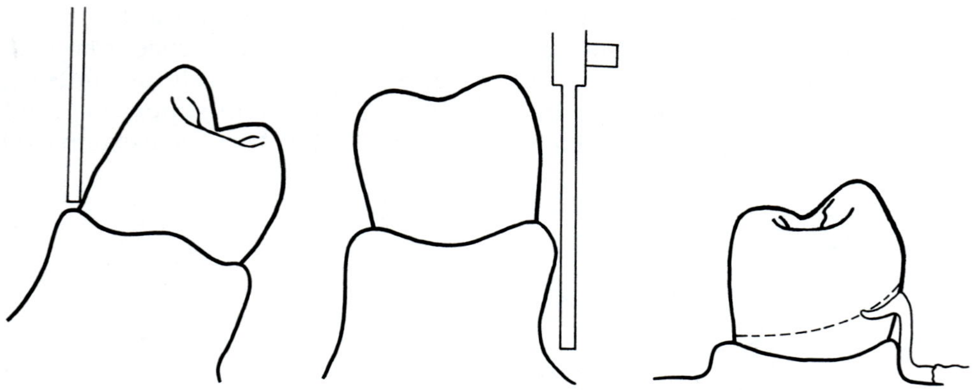

Figure 7-29 Contraindications for selection of bar-type clasps. **A,** Severe buccal or lingual tilts of abutment teeth. **B,** Severe tissue undercuts. **C,** Shallow buccal or labial vestibules.

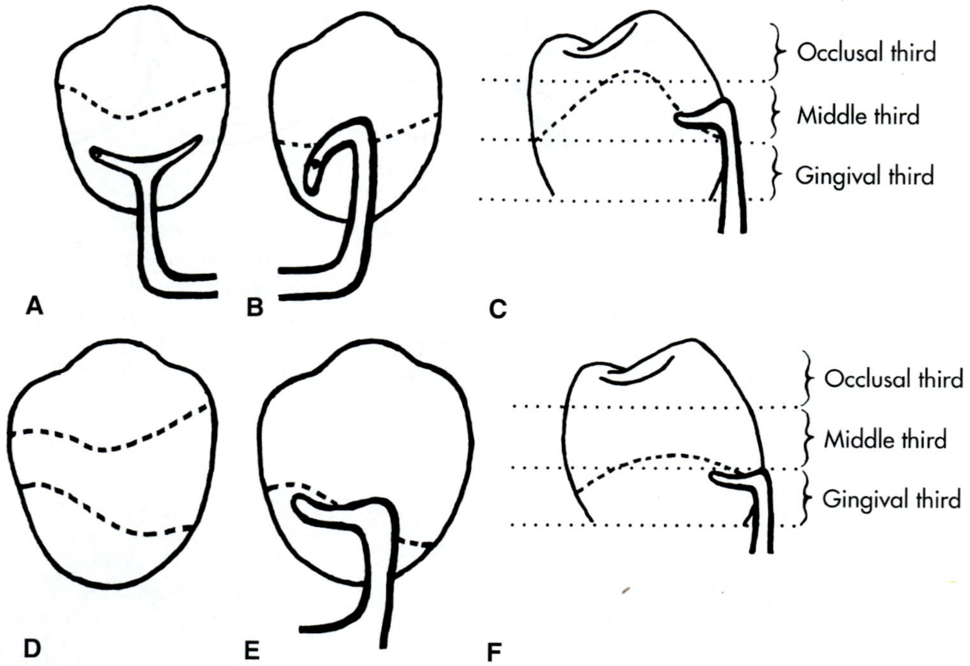

Figure 7-30 Common errors and recommended corrections in design of bar-type clasp assemblies. **A,** Survey line is unsuitable for bar clasp (too high). **B,** Retentive portion of bar clasp arm improperly contoured to resist dislodging force in occlusal direction. **C,** Retentive tip not located in gingival third of abutment. **D,** Contour of abutment correctly altered to receive bar clasp. **E** and **F,** Correct position of bar clasp assembly.

and (4) in situations in which esthetic considerations must be accommodated and a cast clasp is indicated. Thus use of the bar clasp arm is contraindicated when a deep cervical undercut exists or when a severe tooth and/or tissue undercut exists, either of which must be bridged by excessive blockout. When severe tooth and tissue undercuts exist, a bar clasp arm usually is an annoyance to the tongue and cheek and also traps food debris. Other limiting factors in the selection of a bar clasp assembly include a shallow vestibule or an excessive buccal or lingual tilt of the abutment tooth (Figure 7-29). Some common errors in the design of bar-type clasps are illustrated in Figure 7-30.

The bar clasp arm is not a particularly flexible clasp arm because of the effects of its half-round form and its several planes of origin. Although the cast circumferential clasp arm can be made more flexible than the bar clasp arm, the combination clasp is preferred for use on terminal abutments when torque and tipping are possible, because of engaging an undercut away from the distal extension base. Situations often exist, however, in which a bar clasp arm may be used to advantage without jeopardizing a terminal abutment. A bar clasp arm swinging distally into the undercut may be a logical choice, since movement of the clasp on the abutment as the distal extension base moves tissueward is minimized by the distal location of the clasp terminal.

There are several other types of bar clasps, one of which is the infrabulge clasp. It is designed so that the bar arm arises from the border of the denture base, either as an extension of a cast base or attached to the border of a resin base (Figure 7-31). It is made more flexible than the usual bar clasp arm in that the portion of the cast base that gives rise to the clasp arm is separated from the clasp arm itself, either by a saw cut or by being cast against a separating shim of matrix metal, which is later removed with acid. It may be made more flexible through the use of wrought wire, which is attached to a metal base by soldering or is embedded in the border of a resin base.

Some of the advantages attributed to the infrabulge clasp are (1) its interproximal location, which may be used to esthetic advantage; (2) increased retention without tipping action on the abutment; and (3) less chance of accidental distortion resulting from its proximity to the denture border. The wearer should be meticulous in the care of a denture so made, not only for reasons of oral hygiene but also to prevent cariogenic debris from being held against tooth surfaces.

The T and Y clasp arms are the most frequently misused. It is unlikely that the full area of a T or Y terminal is ever necessary for adequate clasp retention. Although the larger area of contact would provide greater frictional resistance, this is not true clasp retention, and only that portion engaging an undercut area should be considered retentive. Only one terminal of such a clasp arm should be placed in an undercut area (Figure 7-32). The remainder of the clasp arm may be superfluous unless it is needed as part of the clasp assembly to encircle the abutment tooth by more than 180° at its greatest circumference. If the bar clasp arm is made to be flexible for retentive purposes, any portion of the clasp above the height of contour will provide only limited stabilization, because it is also part of the

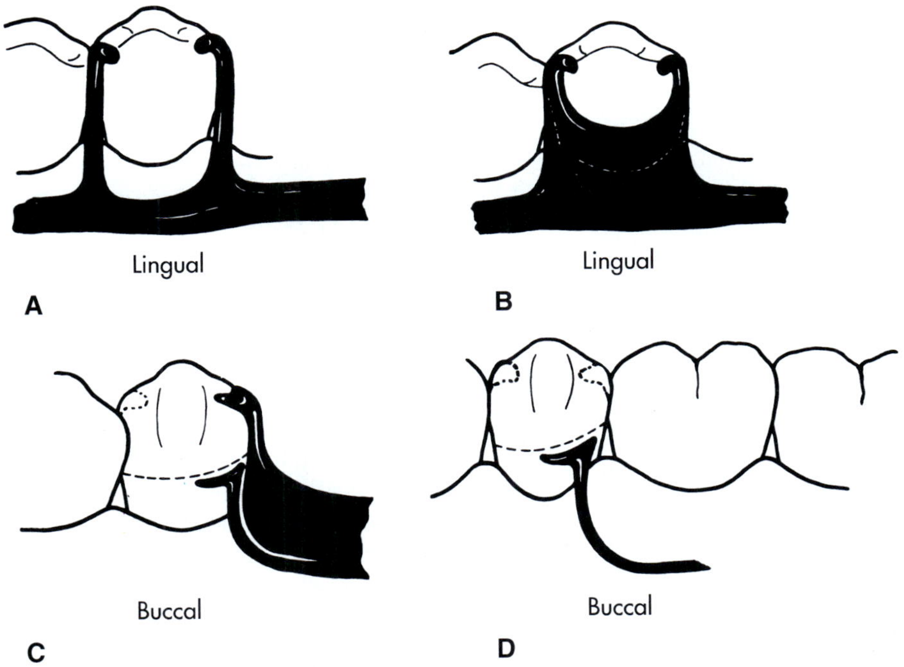

Figure 7-31 Infrabulge clasp designed by M.M. DeVan *(mirror view)*. **A** and **B,** Lingual aspect may be open or plated. DeVan recommended that two occlusal rests be used on each abutment. **C,** Clasp arm arises from border of metal base and is separated by saw cut or by having been cast against a metal shim, which is later removed. Wrought-wire retentive arm may be soldered to metal base to accomplish same purpose. **D,** Clasp arm is attached to buccal flange of resin denture base with autopolymerizing resin. This is usually a wrought-wire arm.

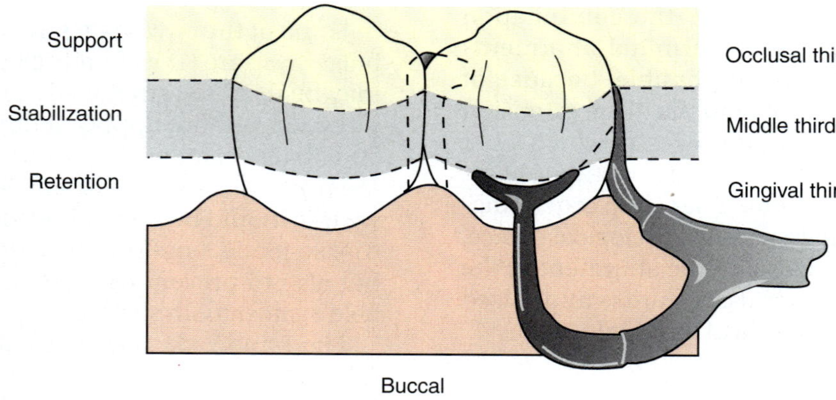

Figure 7-32 Only one terminal of retentive arm engages undercut in gingival third of abutment. Suprabulge portion of retentive clasp arm provides only limited stabilization and may be eliminated.

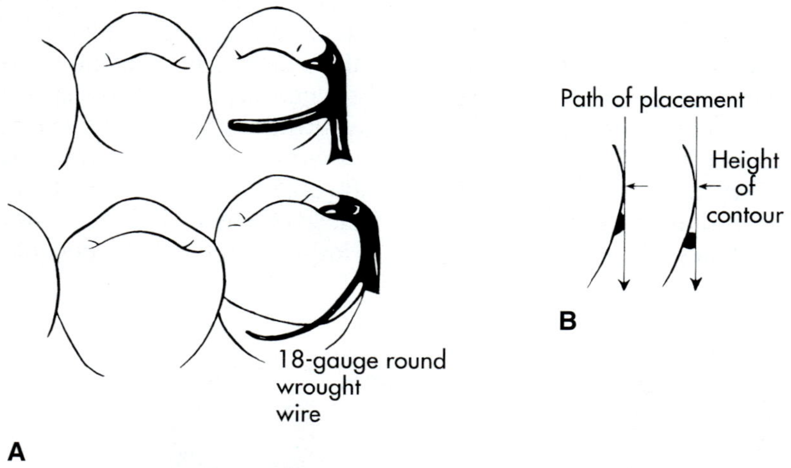

Figure 7-33 **A,** Combination clasp consists of cast reciprocal arm and tapered, round wrought-wire retentive clasp arm. The latter is either cast to, or soldered to, a cast framework. This design is recommended for anterior abutment of posterior modification space in Class II partially edentulous arch, where only a mesiobuccal undercut exists, to minimize the effects of first-class lever system. **B,** In addition to advantages of flexibility, adjustability, and appearance, wrought-wire retentive arm makes only line contact with abutment tooth, rather than broader contact of cast clasp.

flexible arm. Therefore in many instances this suprabulge portion of a T or Y clasp arm may be removed, and the retentive terminal of the bar clasp should be designed to be biologically and mechanically sound rather than to conform to any alphabetical configuration.

Combination Clasp

Another strategy to reduce the effect of the Class I lever in distal extension situations is to use a flexible component in the "resistance arm," which is the strategy employed in the combination clasp. The combination clasp consists of a wrought-wire retentive clasp arm and a cast reciprocal clasp arm (Figure 7-33). Although the latter may be in the form of a bar clasp arm, it is usually a circumferential arm. The retentive arm is almost always circumferential, but it also may be used in the manner of a bar, originating gingivally from the denture base.

The advantages of the combination clasp lie in the flexibility, the adjustability, and the appearance of the wrought-wire retentive arm. It is used when maximum flexibility is desirable, such as on an abutment tooth adjacent to a distal extension base or on a weak abutment when a bar-type direct retainer is contraindicated. It may be used for its adjustability when precise retentive requirements are unpredictable and later adjustment to increase or decrease retention may be necessary. A third justification for its use is its esthetic advantage over cast clasps. Wrought in structure, it may be used in smaller diameters than a cast clasp, with less danger of fracture. Because it is round, light is reflected in such a manner that the display of metal is less noticeable than with the broader surfaces of a cast clasp.

The most common use of the combination clasp is on an abutment tooth adjacent to a distal extension base where only a mesial undercut exists on the abutment or where a large tissue undercut contraindicates a bar-type retainer (Figure 7-34). When a distal undercut exists that may be approached with a properly designed bar clasp arm or with a ring clasp (despite its several disadvantages), a cast clasp can be located so that it will not cause abutment tipping as the distal extension base moves tissueward. When the undercut is on the side of the abutment away from the extension base, the tapered wrought-wire retentive arm offers greater flexibility than does the cast clasp arm and therefore better dissipates functional stresses. For this reason the combination clasp is preferred (Figure 7-34, *D*).

The combination clasp has several disadvantages: (1) it involves extra steps in fabrication, particularly when high-fusing chromium alloys are used; (2) it may be distorted by careless handling on the part of the patient; (3) because it is bent by hand, it may be less accurately adapted to the tooth and therefore provide less stabilization in the suprabulge portion, and (4) it may distort with function and not engage the tooth. The disadvantages of the wrought-wire clasp are offset by its several advantages, which are (1) its flexibility; (2) its adjustability; (3) its esthetic advantage over other retentive circumferential clasp arms; (4) a minimum of tooth surface covered because of its line contact with the tooth, rather than having the surface contact of a cast clasp arm; and (5) a less likely occurrence of fatigue failures in service with the tapered wrought-wire retentive arm versus the cast, half-round retentive arm.

The disadvantages listed previously should not prevent its use regardless of the type of alloy being used for the cast framework. Technical problems are minimized by selecting the best wrought wire for this purpose and then either casting to it or soldering it to the cast framework. Selection of wrought wire, attachment of it to the framework, and subsequent laboratory procedures to maintain its optimum physical properties are presented in Chapter 12.

The patient may be taught to avoid distortion of the wrought wire by explaining that to remove the partial dentures, the fingernail should always be applied to its point of origin, where it is held rigid by the casting, rather than to the flexible terminal end. Often, lingual retention may be used rather than buccal retention, especially on a mandibular abutment, so that the patient never touches the wrought-wire arm during removal of the denture. Instead, removal may be accomplished by lifting against the cast reciprocal arm located on the buccal side of the tooth. This may negate the esthetic advantage of the wrought-wire

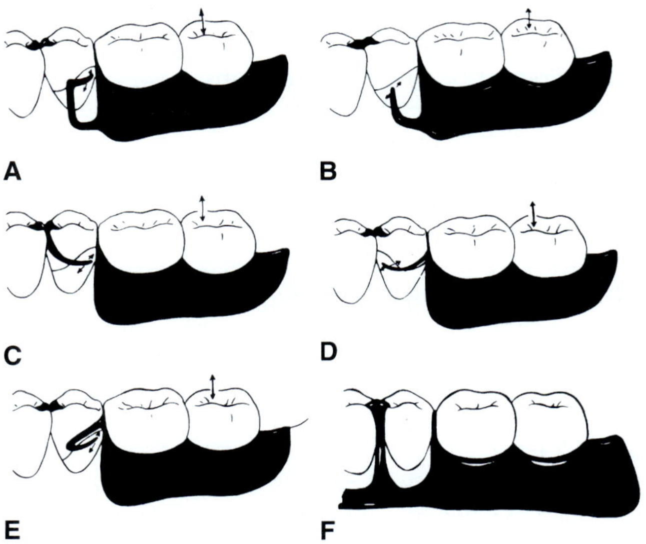

Figure 7-34 Five types of extracoronal direct retainer assemblies that may be used on abutments adjacent to distal extension base to avoid or minimize the effects of cantilever design. Arrows indicate general direction of movement of retentive tips of retainer arms when denture base rotates toward and away from edentulous ridge. **A,** Distobuccal undercut engaged by one-half T-type bar clasp. Portion of clasp arm on and above height of contour might afford some stabilization against horizontal rotation of denture base. **B,** I-bar placed in undercut at middle (anteroposteriorly) of buccal surface. This retainer contacts tooth only at its tip. Note that guiding plane on distal aspect of abutment is contacted by metal of denture framework and that mesial rest is used. **C,** Interproximal ring clasp engaging distobuccal undercut. Bar-type retainer cannot be used because of tissue undercuts inferior to buccal surface of abutment. **D,** Round, uniformly tapered 18-gauge wrought-wire circumferential retainer arm engaging mesiobuccal undercut. A wrought-wire arm, instead of a cast arm, should be used in this situation because of ability of wrought wire to flex omnidirectionally. Cast half-round retainer arm would not flex edgewise, which could result in excessive stress on tooth when rotation of denture base occurs. **E,** Hairpin clasp may be used when undercut lies cervical to origin of retainer arm. Both hairpin and interproximal ring clasps may be used to engage distobuccal undercut on terminal abutment of distal extension denture. However, distobuccal undercut on terminal abutment should be engaged by bar-type clasp in the absence of large buccal tissue undercut cervical to terminal abutment. Hairpin and interproximal ring clasps are least desirable of clasping situations illustrated here. **F,** Lingual view shows use of double occlusal rests, connected to lingual bar by minor connector in illustrated designs. This design eliminates need for lingual clasp arm, places fulcrum line anteriorly to make better use of residual ridge for support, and provides stabilization against horizontal rotation of denture base.

clasp arm, and esthetics should be given preference when the choice must be made between buccal and lingual retention. In most situations, however, retention must be used where it is possible and the clasp designed accordingly.

Clasps Designed Without Movement Accommodation

Circumferential Clasp

Although a thorough knowledge of the principles of clasp design should lead to a logical application of those principles, it is better that some of the more common clasp designs be considered individually. The circumferential clasp will be considered first as an all-cast clasp.

The circumferential clasp is usually the most logical clasp to use with all tooth-supported partial dentures because of its retentive and stabilizing ability (Figure 7-35). Only when the retentive undercut may be approached better with a bar clasp arm or when esthetics will be enhanced should the latter be used. The circumferential clasp arm does have the following disadvantages:

1. More tooth surface is covered than with a bar clasp arm because of its occlusal origin.
2. On some tooth surfaces, particularly the buccal surface of mandibular teeth and the lingual surfaces of maxillary teeth, its occlusal approach may increase the width of the occlusal surface of the tooth.
3. In the mandibular arch, more metal may be displayed than with the bar clasp arm.
4. As with all cast clasps, its half-round form prevents adjustment to increase or decrease retention. Adjustments in the retention afforded by a cast clasp arm should be made by moving a clasp terminal cervically into the angle of cervical convergence or occlusally into a lesser area of undercut. Tightening a clasp against the tooth or loosening it away from the tooth increases or decreases frictional resistance and does not affect the retentive potential of the clasp. True adjustment is, therefore, impossible with most cast clasps.

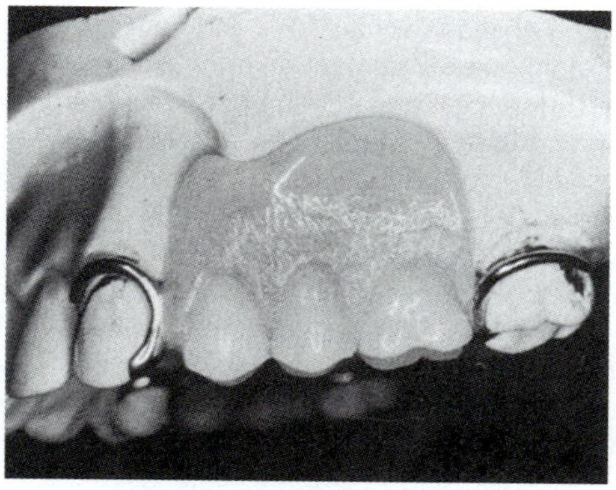

Figure 7-35 Cast circumferential retentive clasp arms properly designed. They originate on or occlusal to height of contour, which they then cross in their terminal third, and engage retentive undercuts progressively as their taper decreases and their flexibility increases.

Despite its disadvantages the cast circumferential clasp arm may be used effectively, and many of these disadvantages may be minimized by mouth preparation. Adequate mouth preparation will permit its point of origin to be placed far enough below the occlusal surface to avoid poor esthetics and increased tooth dimension (see Figure 7-35). Although some of the disadvantages listed imply that the bar-type clasp may be preferable, the circumferential clasp is actually superior to a bar clasp arm that is improperly used or poorly designed.

Experience has shown that faulty application and design too often negate the possible advantages of the bar clasp arm, whereas the circumferential clasp arm is not as easily misused.

The basic form of the circumferential clasp is a buccal and lingual arm originating from a common body (Figure 7-36). This clasp is used improperly when two retentive clasp arms originate from the body and occlusal rest areas and approach bilateral retentive areas on the side of the tooth away from the point of origin. The correct form of this clasp has only one retentive clasp arm, opposed by a nonretentive reciprocal arm on the opposite side. A common error is to use this clasp improperly by making both clasp terminals retentive. This not only is unnecessary but also disregards the need for reciprocation and bilateral stabilization. Other common errors in the design of circumferential clasps are illustrated in Figure 7-37.

Ring clasp. The circumferential type of clasp may be used in several forms. It appears as though many of these forms of the basic circumferential clasp design were developed to accommodate situations in which corrected tooth modifications could not be or were not accomplished by the dentist. One is the ring clasp, which encircles nearly all of a tooth from its point of origin (Figure 7-38). It is used when a proximal undercut cannot be approached by other means. For example, when a mesiolingual undercut on a lower molar abutment cannot be approached directly because of its proximity to the occlusal rest area and cannot be approached with a bar clasp arm because of lingual inclination of the tooth, the

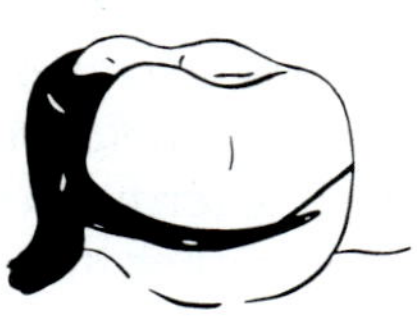

Figure 7-36 Cast circumferential retentive clasp arm.

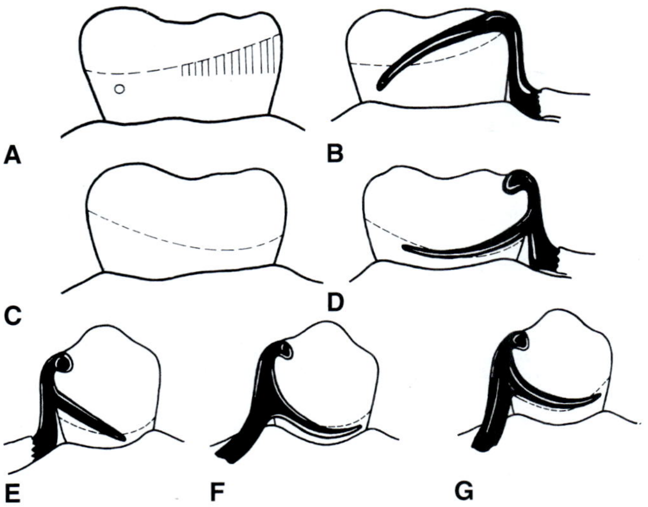

Figure 7-37 Some improper applications of circumferential clasp design and their recommended corrections. **A,** Tooth with undesirable height of contour in its occlusal third. **B,** Unsuitable contour and location of retentive clasp arm on unmodified abutment. **C,** More favorable height of contour achieved by modification of abutment. **D,** Retentive clasp arm properly designed and located on modified abutment. **E,** Unsuitable contour and location of retentive arm in relation to height of contour (straight arm configuration provides poor approach to retentive area and is less resistant to dislodging force). **F,** Terminal portion of retentive clasp arm located too close to gingival margin. **G,** Clasp arm that is properly designed and located.

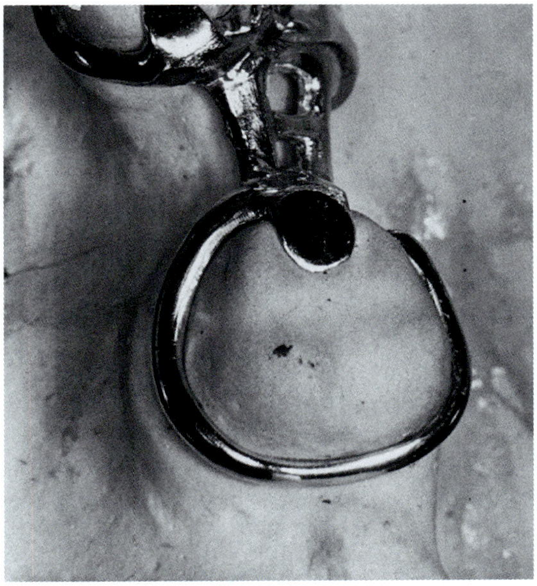

Figure 7-39 Improperly designed ring clasp lacking necessary support. Such a clasp lacks any reciprocating or stabilizing action because entire circumference of clasp is free to open and close. Supporting strut should always be added on nonretentive side of abutment tooth, which then becomes, in effect, a minor connector from which tapered and flexible retentive clasp arm originates.

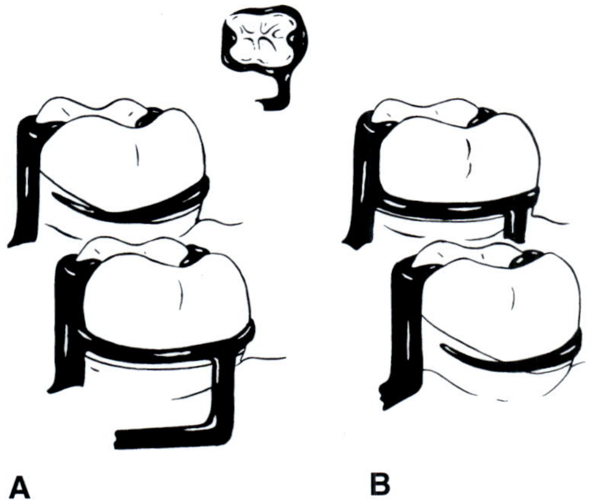

Figure 7-38 Ring clasp(s) encircling nearly all of tooth from its point of origin. **A,** Clasp originates on mesiobuccal surface and encircles tooth to engage mesiolingual undercut. **B,** Clasp originates on mesiolingual surface and encircles tooth to engage mesiobuccal undercut. In either example, supporting strut is used on nonretentive side (drawn both as direct view of near side of tooth and as mirror view of opposite side).

ring clasp encircling the tooth allows the undercut to be approached from the distal aspect of the tooth.

The clasp should never be used as an unsupported ring (Figure 7-39), because if it is free to open and close as a ring, it cannot provide either reciprocation or stabilization. Instead the ring-type clasp should always be used with a supporting strut on the nonretentive side, with or without an auxiliary occlusal rest on the opposite marginal ridge. The advantage of an auxiliary rest is that further movement of a mesially inclined tooth is prevented by the presence of a distal rest. In any event the supporting strut should be regarded as being a minor connector from which the flexible retentive arm originates. Reciprocation then comes from the rigid portion of the clasp lying between the supporting strut and the principal occlusal rest.

The ring-type clasp should be used on protected abutments whenever possible, because it covers such a large area of tooth surface. Esthetics need not be considered on such a posteriorly located tooth.

A ring-type clasp may be used in reverse on an abutment located anterior to a tooth-bounded edentulous space (Figure 7-40). Although potentially an effective clasp, this clasp covers an excessive amount of tooth surface and can be esthetically objectionable. The only justification for its use is when a distobuccal or distolingual undercut cannot be approached directly from the occlusal rest area and/or tissue undercuts prevent its approach from a gingival direction with a bar clasp arm.

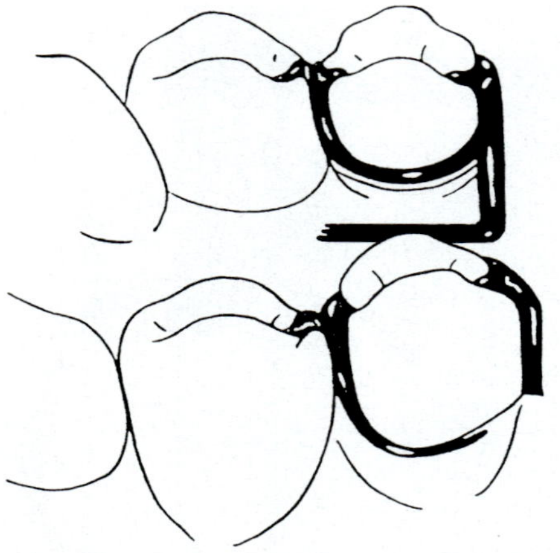

Figure 7-40 Ring clasp may be used in reverse on abutment located anterior to tooth-bound edentulous space.

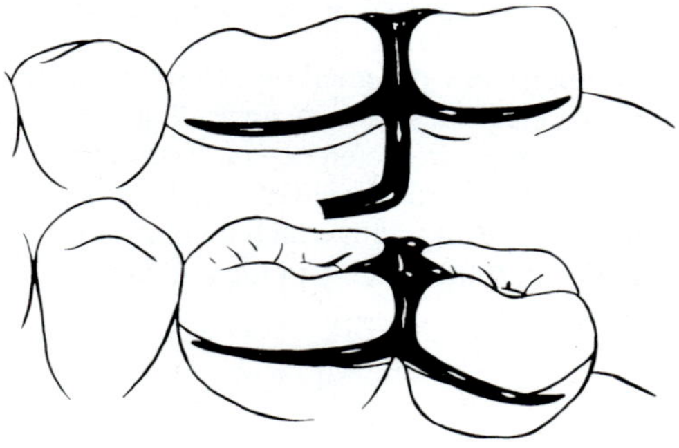

Figure 7-41 Embrasure clasp used where no edentulous space exists. Although in this drawing both retentive clasp arms are located on buccal surface and nonretentive arms on lingual surface, retention and reciprocation can be reversed on both teeth or on either tooth, depending on respective contours of the teeth. However, if second molar is sound and suitable stabilizing and retentive areas can be found, circumferential clasp originating on distal surface of abutment is preferable.

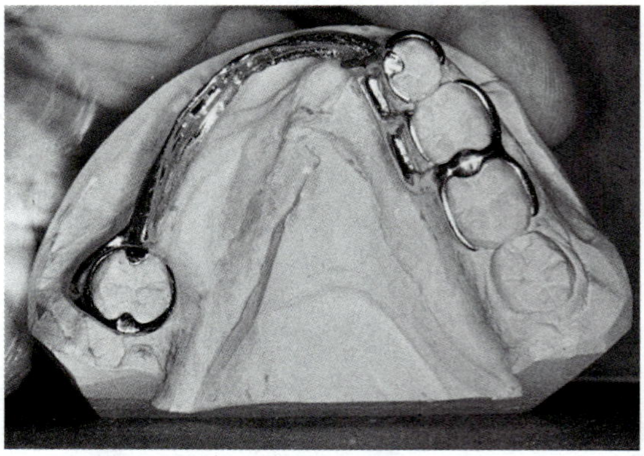

Figure 7-42 Multiple clasping in surgically mutilated mouth. On the right are embrasure clasp, bar clasp arm, and conventional circumferential clasp engaging lingual undercuts on three abutment teeth. On the left is well-designed ring clasp engaging lingual undercut, with supporting strut on buccal surface and auxiliary occlusal rest to prevent mesial tipping. Note rigid design of major connector.

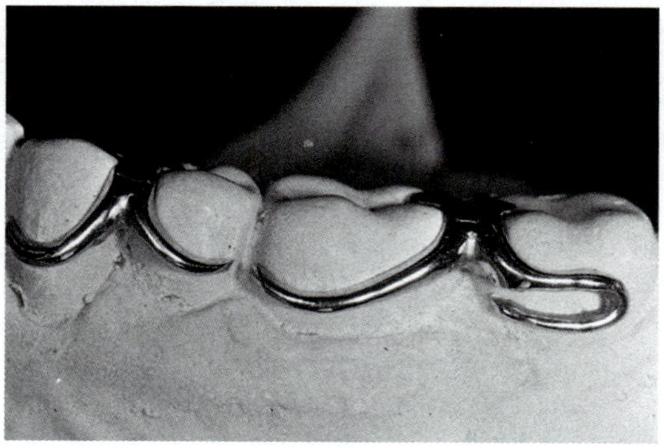

Figure 7-43 Embrasure and hairpin circumferential retentive clasp arms. The terminus of each engages suitable retentive undercut. Use of hairpin-type clasp on second molar is made necessary by the fact that the only available undercut lies directly below point of origin of clasp arm.

Embrasure clasp. In the fabrication of an unmodified Class II or Class III partial denture, there are no edentulous spaces on the opposite side of the arch to aid in clasping. Mechanically, this is a disadvantage. However, when the teeth are sound and retentive areas are available or when multiple restorations are justified, clasping can be accomplished by means of an embrasure clasp (Figures 7-41 and 7-42).

Sufficient space must be provided between the abutment teeth in their occlusal third to make room for the common body of the embrasure clasp (Figure 7-43), yet the contact area should not be eliminated entirely. Historically, this clasp assembly demonstrates a high percentage of fracture caused by inadequate tooth preparation in the contact area. Because vulnerable areas of the teeth are involved, abutment protection with inlays or crowns is recommended. The decision to use unprotected abutments must be made at the time of oral examination and should be based on the patient's age, caries index, and oral hygiene, as well as on whether existing tooth contours are favorable or can be made favorable by tooth modification. Preparation of adjacent, contacting, uncrowned abutments to receive any type of embrasure clasp of adequate interproximal bulk is difficult, especially when opposed by natural teeth.

The embrasure clasp always should be used with double occlusal rests, even when definite proximal shoulders can be established (Figure 7-44). This is done to avoid interproximal wedging by the prosthesis, which could cause separation of the abutment teeth and result in food impaction and clasp displacement. In addition to providing support, occlusal rests also serve to shunt food away from contact

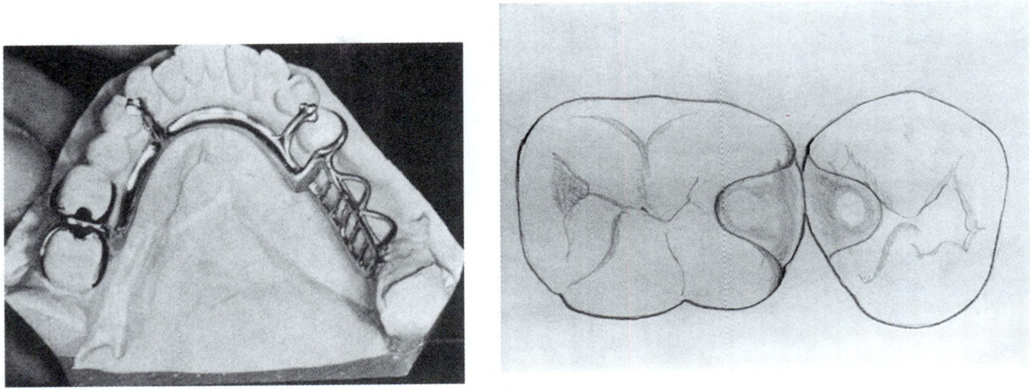

A B

Figure 7-44 **A,** Example of use of embrasure clasp for a Class II partially edentulous arch. Embrasure clasp on two left molar abutments was used in the absence of posterior modification space. **B,** Occlusal and proximal surfaces of adjacent molar and premolar prepared for embrasure clasp. Note that rest seat preparations are extended both buccally and lingually to accommodate retentive and reciprocal clasp arms. *Adequate preparation confined to enamel can rarely be accomplished for such a clasp, especially when clasped teeth are opposed by natural teeth.*

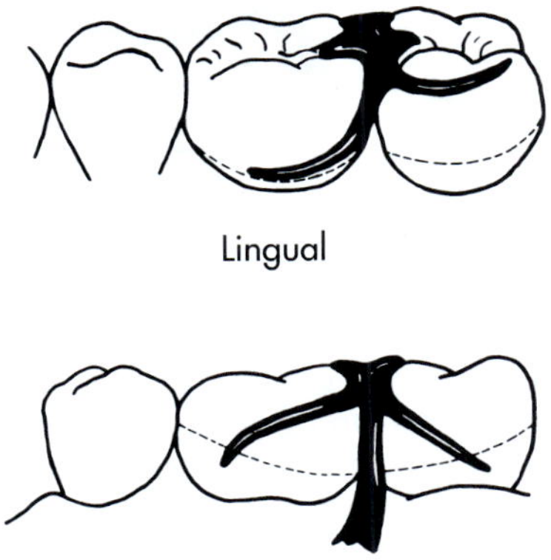

Figure 7-45 Improper application of embrasure clasp design *(mirror view).* Failure to locate retentive and reciprocating-stabilizing arms in most advantageous positions (proper third of crowns) is quite evident.

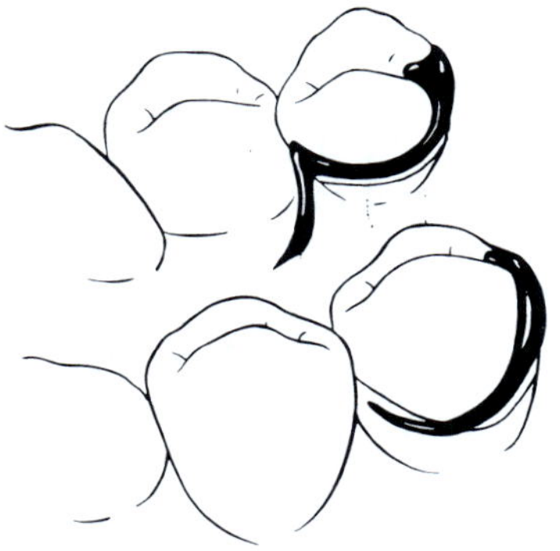

Figure 7-46 Back-action circumferential clasp used on premolar abutment anterior to edentulous space.

areas. For this reason, occlusal rests should always be used whenever food impaction is possible.

Embrasure clasps should have two retentive clasp arms and two reciprocal clasp arms, either bilaterally or diagonally opposed. An auxiliary occlusal rest or a bar clasp arm can be substituted for a circumferential reciprocal arm as long as definite reciprocation and stabilization result. A lingually placed retentive bar clasp arm may be substituted if a rigid circumferential clasp arm is placed on the buccal surface for reciprocation, provided lingual retention is used on the opposite side of the arch. Common errors in the design of embrasure-type clasps are illustrated in Figure 7-45.

Other less commonly used modifications of the cast circumferential clasp are the multiple clasp, the half-and-half clasp, and the reverse-action clasp.

Back-action clasp. The back-action clasp is a modification of the ring clasp, which has all of the same disadvantages and no apparent advantages (Figure 7-46). It is difficult to justify its use. The undercut can usually be approached just as well using a conventional circumferential clasp, with less tooth coverage and less display of metal. With the circumferential clasp, the proximal tooth surface can be used as a guiding plane as it should be, and the occlusal rest can have the rigid support it requires. An occlusal rest always should be attached to some rigid minor connector and should never be supported by a clasp arm alone. If

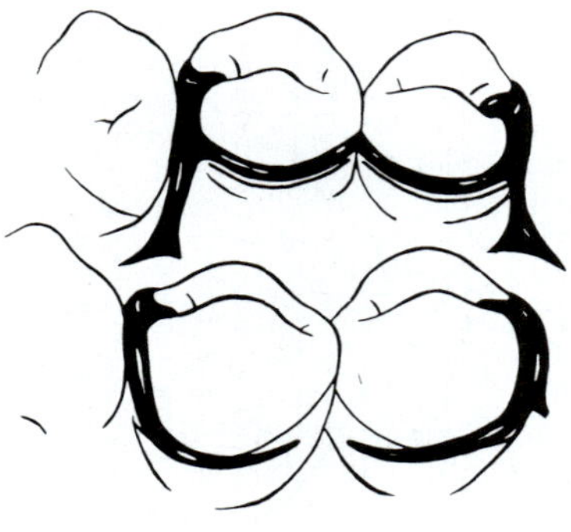

Figure 7-47 Multiple clasp is actually two opposing circumferential clasps joined at terminal end of two reciprocal arms *(mirror* view*)*.

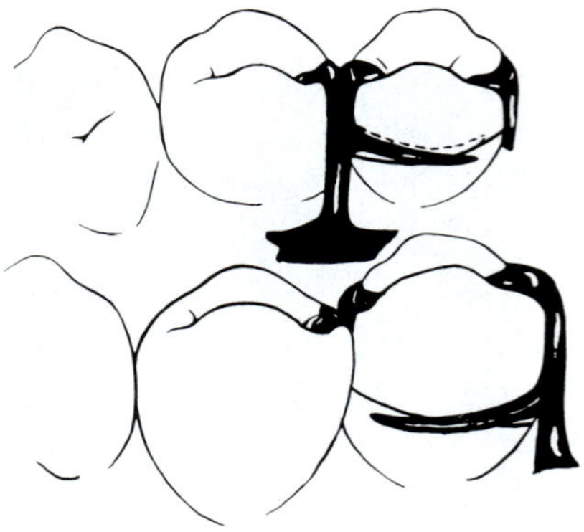

Figure 7-48 Half-and-half clasp consists of one circumferential retentive arm arising from distal aspect and a second circumferential arm arising from mesial aspect on the opposite side, with or without secondary occlusal rest. Broken line illustrates nonretentive reciprocal clasp arm used without secondary occlusal rest *(mirror* view*)*.

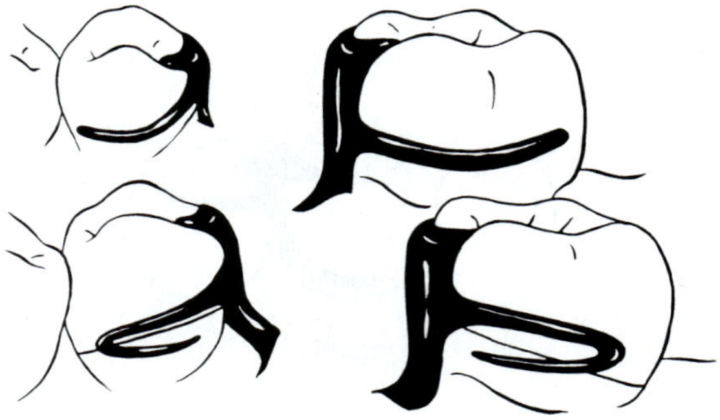

Figure 7-49 Reverse-action, or hairpin, clasp arm may be used on abutments of tooth-supported dentures when proximal undercut lies below point of origin of clasp *(mirror view)*. It may be esthetically objectionable and covers considerable tooth surface. It should be used only when a bar-type retentive arm is contraindicated because of a tissue undercut, tilted tooth, or shallow vestibule.

the occlusal rest is part of a flexible assembly, it cannot function adequately as an occlusal rest.

Multiple clasp. The multiple clasp is simply two opposing circumferential clasps joined at the terminal end of the two reciprocal arms (Figure 7-47). It is used when additional retention and stabilization are needed, usually on tooth-supported partial dentures. It may be used for multiple clasping in instances in which the partial denture replaces an entire half of the dental arch. It may be used rather than an embrasure clasp when the only available retentive areas are adjacent to each other. Its disadvantage is that two embrasure approaches are necessary rather than a single common embrasure for both clasps.

Half-and-half clasp. The half-and-half clasp consists of a circumferential retentive arm arising from one direction and a reciprocal arm arising from another (Figure 7-48). The second arm must arise from a second minor connector, and this arm is used with or without an auxiliary occlusal rest. Reciprocation arising from a second minor connector can usually be accomplished with a short bar or with an auxiliary occlusal rest, thereby avoiding so much tooth coverage. There is little justification for the use of the half-and-half clasp in bilateral extension base partial dentures. Its design was originally intended to provide dual retention, a principle that should be applied only to unilateral partial denture design.

Reverse-action clasp. The reverse-action, or hairpin, clasp arm is designed to permit engaging a proximal undercut from an occlusal approach (Figure 7-49). Other methods of accomplishing the same result are with a ring clasp originating on the opposite side of the tooth or with a bar clasp arm originating from a gingival direction. However, when a proximal undercut must be used on a posterior abutment and when tissue undercuts, tilted teeth, or high tissue attachments prevent the use of a bar clasp arm, the reverse-action clasp may be used successfully. Although the ring clasp may be preferable, lingual undercuts may prevent the placement of a supporting strut without tongue interference. In this limited situation, the hairpin clasp arm serves adequately, despite its several disadvantages. The clasp covers considerable tooth surface and may trap debris; its occlusal origin may increase the functional load on the tooth, and its flexibility is limited. Esthetics usually need not be considered when the clasp is used on a posterior abutment, but the hairpin clasp arm does have the additional disadvantage of displaying too much metal for use on an anterior abutment.

Properly designed, the reverse-action clasp should make a hairpin turn to engage an undercut below the point of origin (see Figure 7-49). The upper part of the arm of this clasp should be considered a minor connector, giving rise to the tapered lower part of the arm. Therefore only the lower part of the arm should be flexible. With the retentive portion beginning beyond the turn, only the lower part of the arm should flex over the height of contour to engage a retentive undercut. The bend that connects the upper and lower parts of the arm should be rounded to prevent stress accumulation and fracture of the arm at the bend. The clasp should be designed and fabricated with this in mind.

These are the various types of cast circumferential clasps. As mentioned previously, they may be used in combination with bar clasp arms as long as differentiation is made between retention and reciprocation by their form and location. Circumferential and bar clasp arms may be made either flexible (retentive) or rigid (reciprocal) in any combination as long as each retentive clasp arm is opposed by a rigid reciprocal component.

The use of many of the less desirable clasp forms can be avoided by changing the crown forms of the abutments by tooth modification within the enamel or with restorations. In fabricating abutment coverage, tooth contours should be established that will permit the use of the most desirable clasp forms rather than a form that makes it necessary to use a less desirable clasp design. This is best accomplished by first altering the crown contour of abutment teeth not designated for restoration to meet the requirements of guiding planes and survey line location. This is followed by the prescribed crown preparations. Before tooth reduction for the prescribed crown preparations, the requirements of guiding planes and survey line location should be met.

OTHER TYPES OF RETAINERS

Lingual Retention in Conjunction With Internal Rests

The internal rest is covered in Chapter 6. It is emphasized that the internal rest is not used as a retainer, but that its near-vertical walls provide for reciprocation against a lingually placed retentive clasp arm. For this reason, visible clasp arms may be eliminated, thus avoiding one of the principal objections to the extracoronal retainer.

Such a retentive clasp arm, terminating in an existing or prepared infrabulge area on the abutment tooth, may be of any acceptable design. It is usually a circumferential arm arising from the body of the denture framework at the rest area. It should be wrought, because the advantages of adjustability and flexibility make the wrought clasp arm preferable. It may be cast with gold or a low-fusing, chromium-cobalt alloy, or it may be assembled by being soldered to one of the higher-fusing, chromium-cobalt alloys. In any event, future adjustment or repair is facilitated.

The use of lingual extracoronal retention avoids much of the cost of the internal attachment yet disposes of a visible clasp arm when esthetics must be considered. Often it is employed with a tooth-supported partial denture only on the anterior abutments, and when esthetics is not a consideration, the posterior abutments are clasped in the conventional manner.

One of the dentist's prime considerations in clasp selection is the control of stress transferred to the abutment teeth when the patient exerts an occluding force on the artificial teeth. The location and design of rests, the clasp arms, and the position of minor connectors as they relate to guiding planes are key factors in controlling transfer of stress to abutments. Errors in the design of a clasp assembly can result in uncontrolled stress to abutment teeth and their supporting tissues. Some common errors and their corrections are illustrated in Figures 7-50 and 7-51.

The choice of clasp designs should be based on biological and mechanical principles. The dentist responsible for the treatment being rendered must be able to justify the clasp design

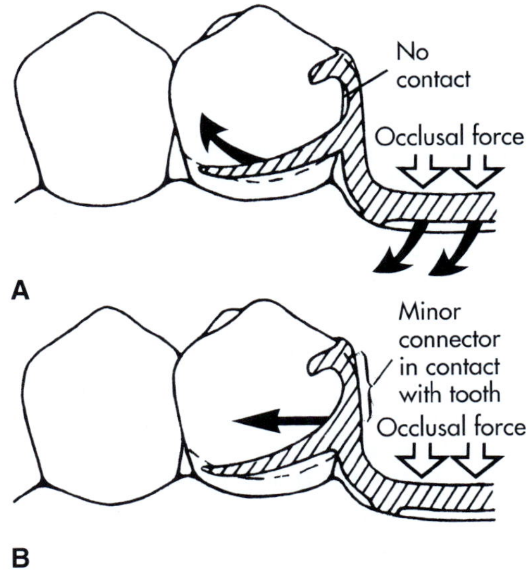

Figure 7-50 **A,** Minor connector supporting distal rest does not contact prepared guiding plane, resulting in uncontrolled stress to abutment tooth. **B,** Minor connector contacts prepared guiding plane and directs stresses around arch through proximal contacts.

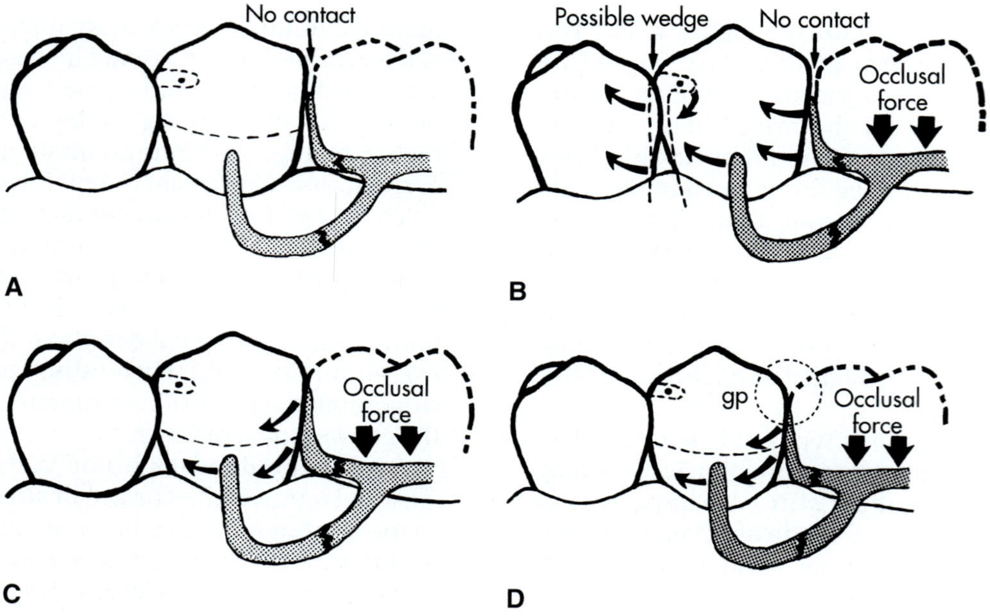

Figure 7-51 **A,** Clasp assembly designed so that vertical occlusal force results in proximal plate moving cervically and out of contact with guiding plane as illustrated in **B**. This lack of contact may contribute to possible wedging effect. **C,** Extending contact of proximal plate on prepared guiding plane or, as in **D,** eliminating space between artificial tooth and guiding plane *(gp)* will help direct stresses around arch through proximal contacts.

used for each abutment tooth in keeping with these principles.

INTERNAL ATTACHMENTS

As mentioned earlier in the chapter, the principle of the internal attachment was first formulated by Dr. Herman E.S. Chayes in 1906. One such attachment manufactured commercially still carries his name. Although it may be fabricated by the dental technician as a cast dovetail fitting into a counterpart receptacle in the abutment crown, the alloys used in manufactured attachments and the precision with which they are constructed make the ready-made attachment preferable to any of this type that can be fabricated in the dental laboratory. Much credit is due the manufacturers of metals used in dentistry for the continued improvements in the design of internal attachments.

The internal attachment has two major advantages over the extracoronal attachment: elimination of visible retentive and support components, and better vertical support through a rest seat located more favorably in relation to the horizontal axis of the abutment tooth. For these reasons, the internal attachment may be preferable in selected situations. It provides horizontal stabilization similar to that of an internal rest. However, additional extracoronal stabilization is usually desirable. It has been claimed that stimulation to the underlying tissue is greater when internal attachments are used because of intermittent vertical massage. This is probably no more than is possible with extracoronal retainers of similar construction.

Some of the disadvantages of internal attachments are: (1) they require prepared abutments and castings; (2) they require somewhat complicated clinical and laboratory procedures; (3) they eventually wear, with progressive loss of frictional resistance to denture removal; (4) they are difficult to repair and replace; (5) they are effective in proportion to their length and are therefore least effective on short teeth; (6) they are difficult to place completely within the circumference of an abutment tooth because of the size of the pulp; and (7) they are considered more costly.

Because the principle of the internal attachment does not permit horizontal movement, all horizontal, tipping, and rotational movements of the prosthesis are transmitted directly to the abutment tooth. The internal attachment therefore should not be used in conjunction with extensive tissue-supported distal extension denture bases unless some form of stress-breaker is used between the movable base and the rigid attachment. Although stress-breakers may be used, they do have some disadvantages—which are discussed later—and their use adds to the cost of the partial denture.

Numerous other types of retainers for partial dentures have been devised that cannot be classified as being primarily of the intracoronal or extracoronal type. Neither can they be classified as relying primarily on frictional resistance or placement of an element in an undercut to prevent displacement of the denture. However, all of these use some type of locking device, located either intracoronally or extracoronally, for providing retention without visible clasp retention. Although the motivation behind the development of other types of retainers has usually been a desire to eliminate visible clasp retainers, the desire to minimize torque and tipping stresses on the abutment teeth has also been given consideration.

All of the retainers that are discussed herein have merit, and much credit is due to those who have developed specific devices and techniques for the retention of partial dentures. The use of patented retaining devices and other techniques falls in the same limited category as the internal attachment prosthesis and is for economic and technical reasons available to only a small percentage of those patients needing partial denture service.

Internal attachments of the locking or dovetail type unquestionably have many advantages over the clasp-type denture in tooth-supported situations. However, it is questionable whether the locking type of internal attachments is indicated for distal extension removable partial dentures, with or without stress-breakers and with or without splinted abutments, because of inherent excessive leverages most often associated with these attachments.

The nonlocking type of internal attachments, in conjunction with sound prosthodontic principles, can be advantageously used in many instances in Class I and Class II partially edentulous situations. However, unless the cross-arch axis of rotation is common to the bilaterally placed attachments, torque on the abutments may be experienced (Figure 7-52). Excellent textbooks devoted to the use of manufactured intracoronal and extracoronal retainer systems are available. For this reason, this text concerns itself primarily with the extracoronal type of direct retainer assemblies (clasps). Numerous well-designed internal attachments are available in the dental market that may be used in situations requiring special retention. Descriptive literature and technique manuals are available from the manufacturers.

Other conservative treatment of partially edentulous arches with removable partial dentures can be accomplished in a variety of ways. Treatment is still contingent on the location and condition of the remaining teeth and the contour and quality of the residual ridges. Basic principles and concepts of design relative to support and stability must be respected even though a variety of retaining devices can be incorporated. Examples of some of these retaining devices are illustrated in Figures 7-53 through 7-64.

Text continued on p. 115.

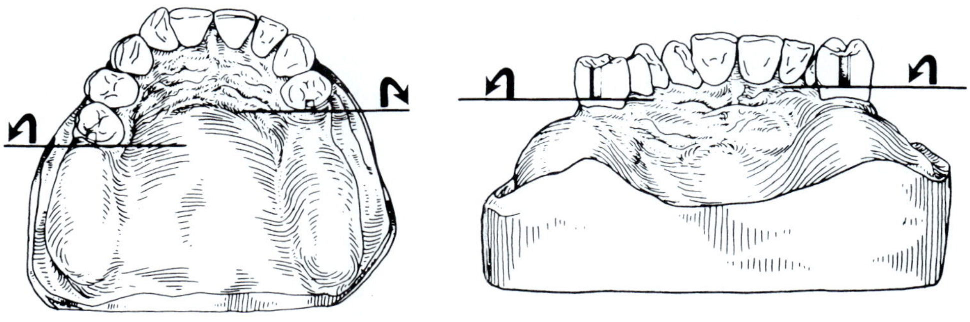

A B

Figure 7-52 **A,** Axes of rotation, although parallel, are not common because one axis is located anterior to other axis. **B,** When one nonlocking internal attachment is elevated farther from residual ridge than its cross-arch counterpart, the axes of rotation do not fall on a common line; thus some torquing of abutments should be anticipated. However, in many instances the effect produced by this situation will not exceed physiologic tolerance of supporting structures of abutments—all other torquing factors being equal.

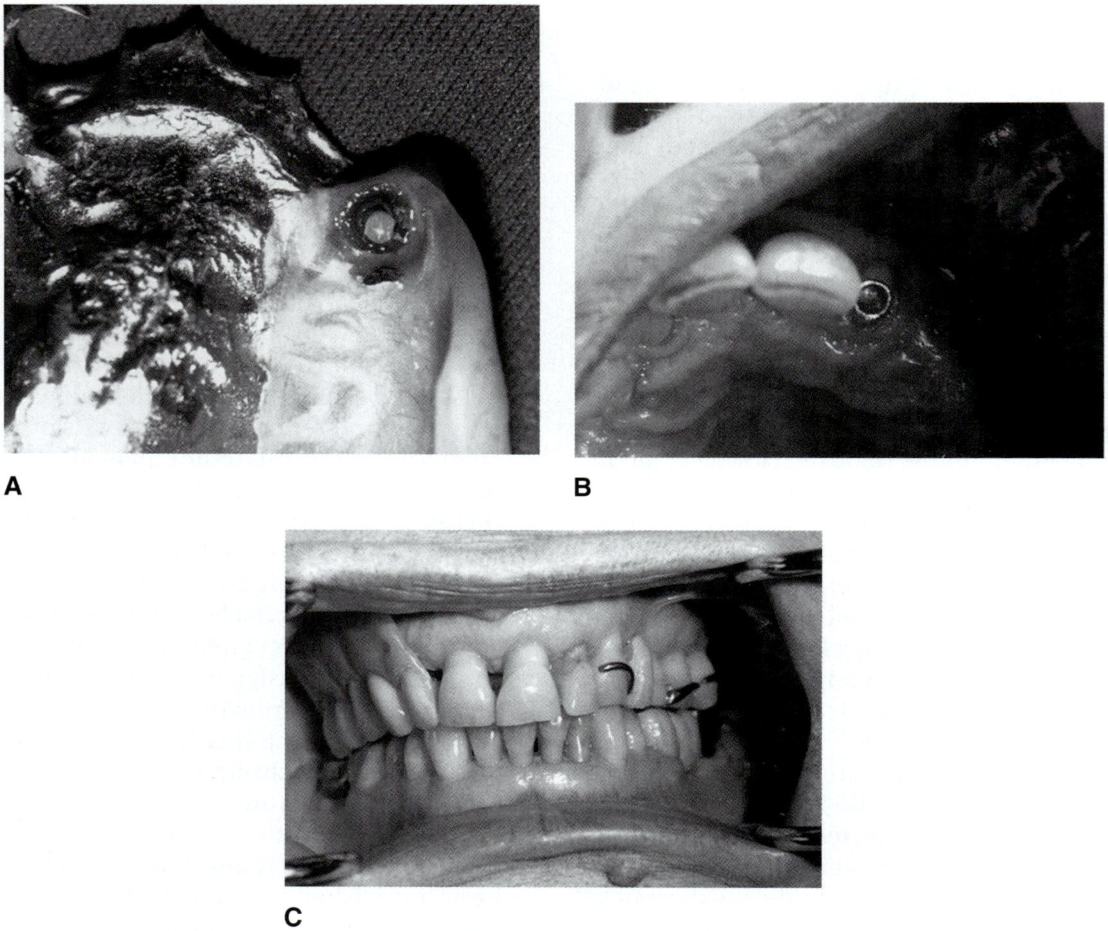

Figure 7-53 **A,** Intracoronal retaining device (Zest Anchor) consisting of nylon male post secured to denture base. **B,** Female insert cemented in dowel space of clinical root. **C,** Esthetic result.

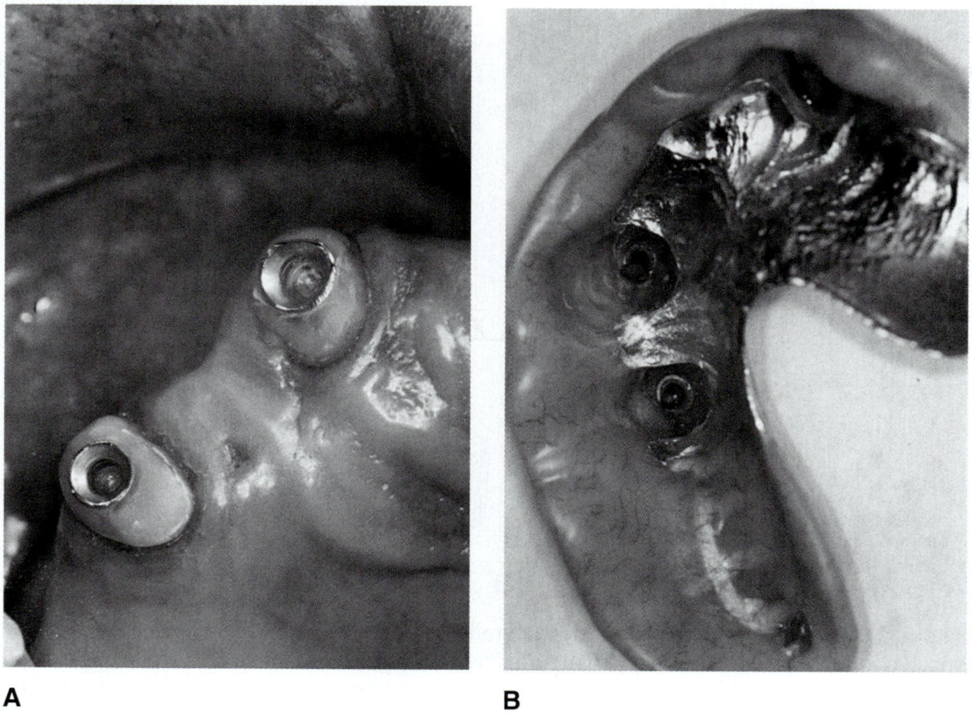

Figure 7-54 Intracoronal retaining device (Zagg attachment). **A,** Female retaining device secured in endodontically treated teeth. **B,** Nylon male post secured in denture base. *(Courtesy Dr. Walter Homayoon, Long Island, NY.)*

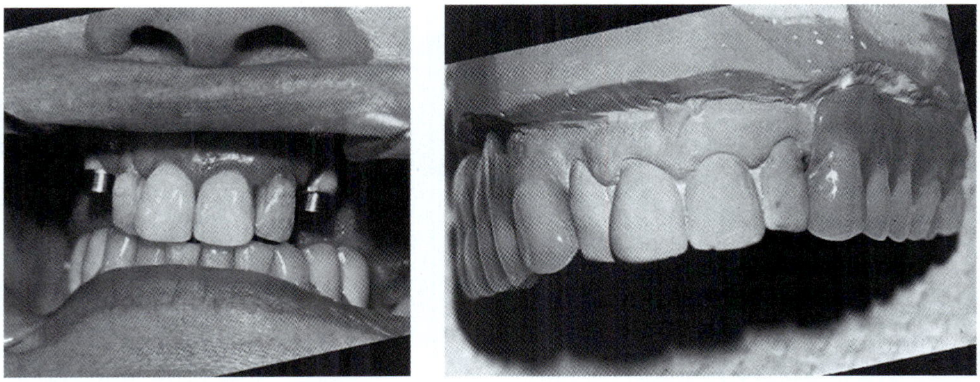

A B

Figure 7-55 Intracoronal magnets used for retention in partial denture applications. **A,** Magnets positioned on retained roots of canines. Keepers are cemented into endodontically treated roots, and magnets are processed into the denture base. **B,** Cast and prosthesis illustrating the esthetic advantage and simplicity of using magnets for retention. *(Courtesy Magnet-Dent Dental Ventures of America, Yorba Linda, Calif.)*

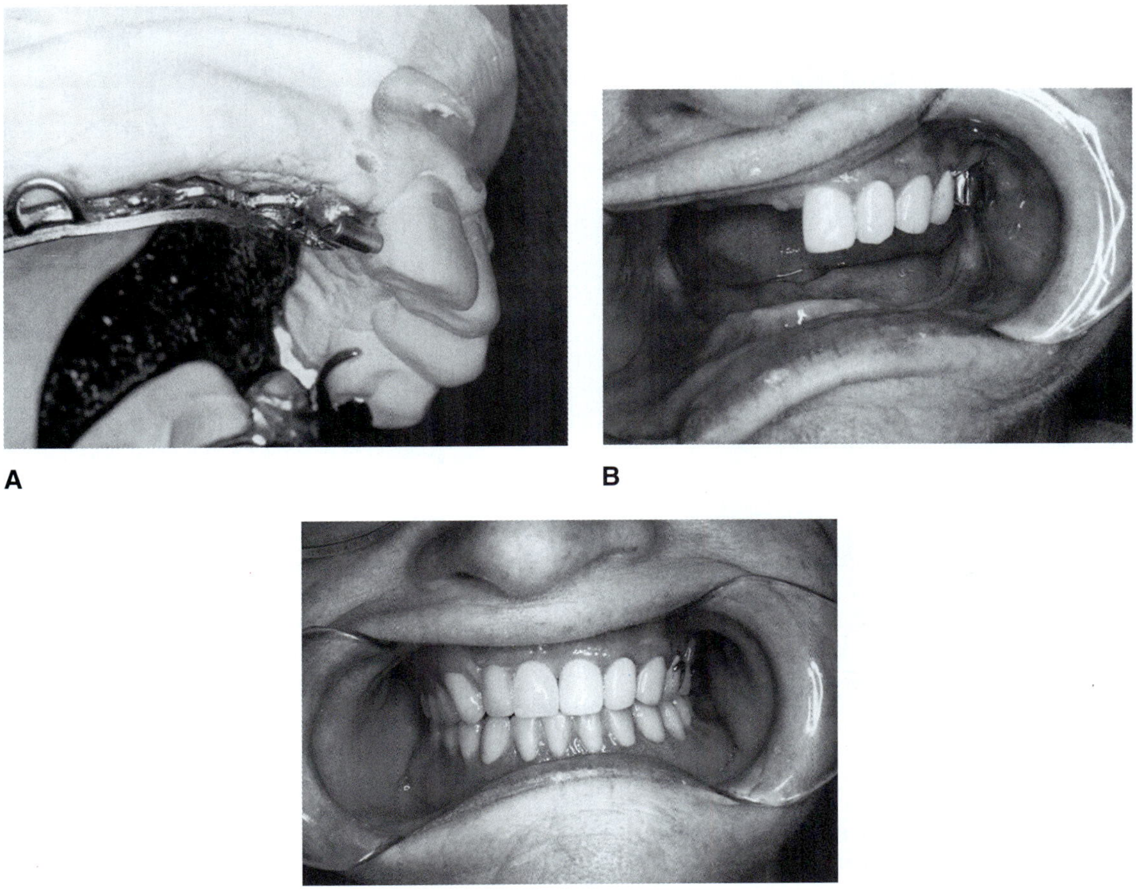

A B C

Figure 7-56 Extracoronal spring-loaded plunger retaining device (Hannes Anchor/IC plunger). Permits full range of motion. **A,** Male plunger fits into dimple or female recess in porcelain-fused-to-metal crown located below height of contour on proximal surface of left central incisor. **B** and **C,** Acceptable retention and esthetics achieved if sufficient space is available.

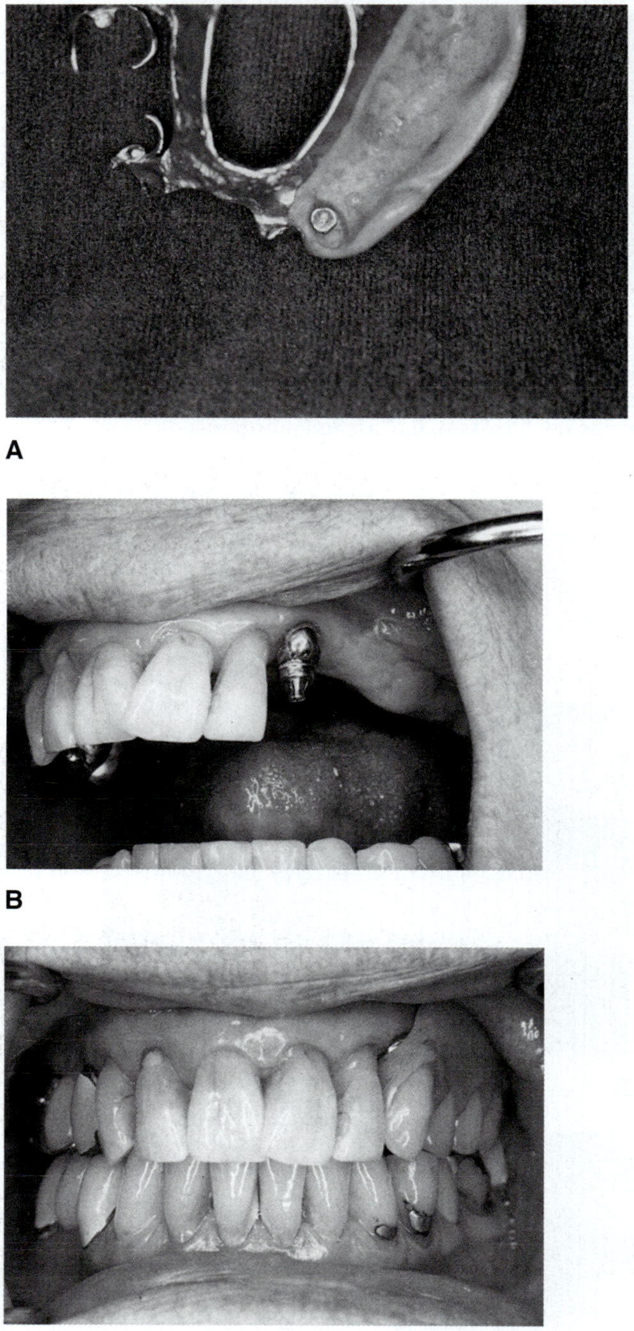

A

B

C

Figure 7-57 Intracoronal retaining device (Servo Anchor-SA/Ceka). **A,** Female retaining device secured in denture base (spacing ring provides for variable resiliency). **B,** Threaded male stud and base soldered or cast to post and coping. **C,** Acceptable retention and esthetics achieved if sufficient space available to accommodate retaining device.

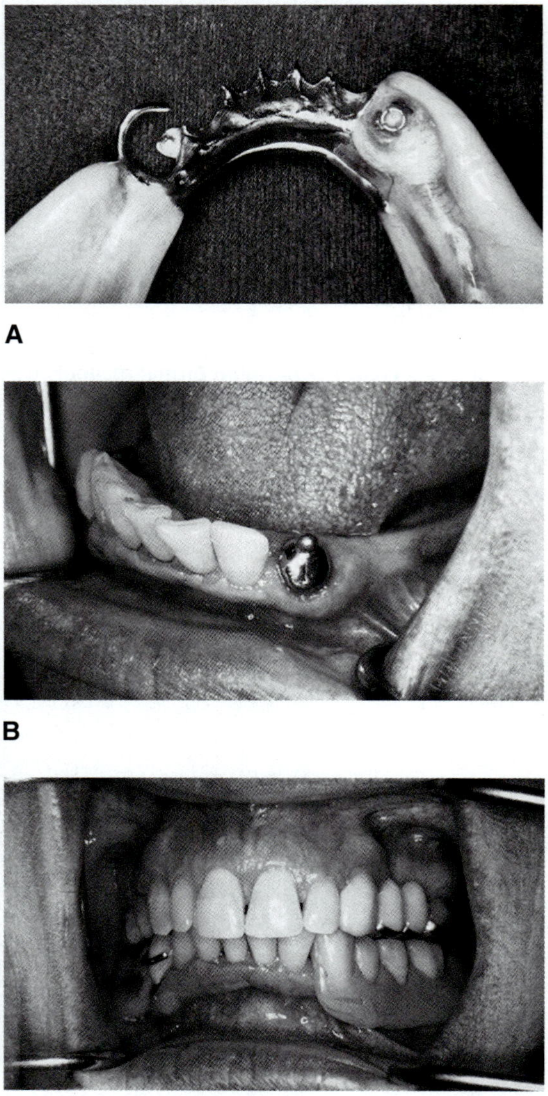

A

B

C

Figure 7-58 Intracoronal retaining device (Bona Ball). **A,** Female retaining device secured in denture base. **B,** Male stud cast or soldered to post and coping. **C,** Acceptable retention and esthetics if sufficient space available to accommodate retaining device.

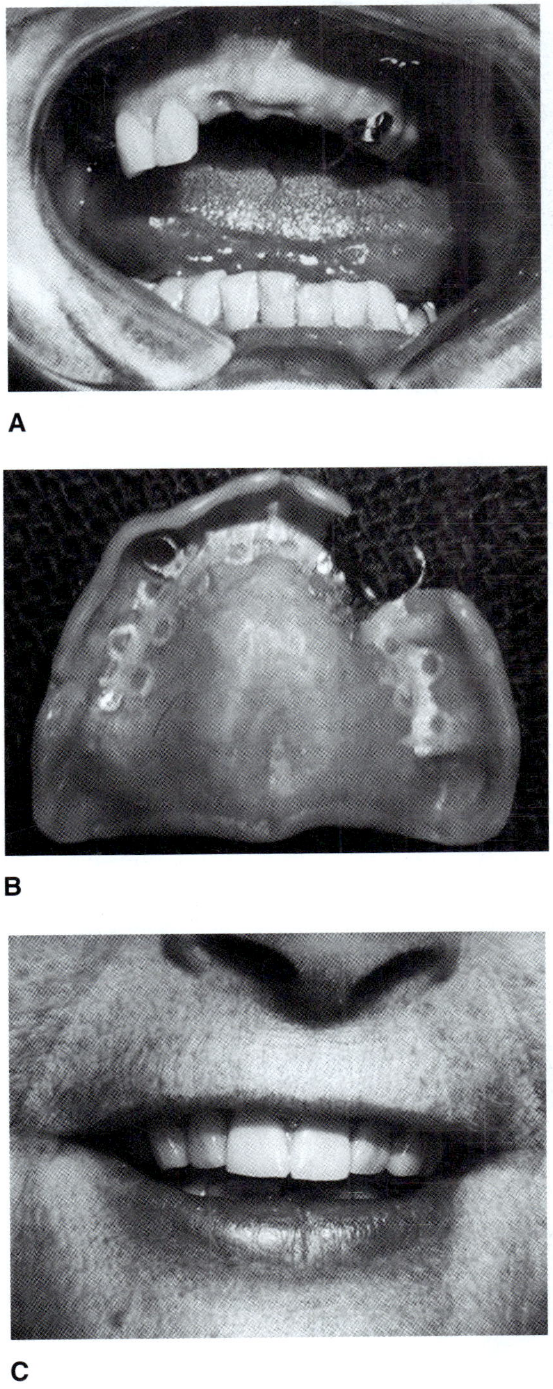

Figure 7-59 Intracoronal retaining device (Rotherman). **A,** Low-profile retaining device allows both hinge and vertical resiliency. Male stud cast or soldered to post and coping. **B,** Female retentive clip secured in denture base. Retention can be altered by compressing or spreading retention clips. **C,** Low profile provides acceptable esthetics. *(Courtesy Dr. Jerry Walker, Milwaukee, Wis.)*

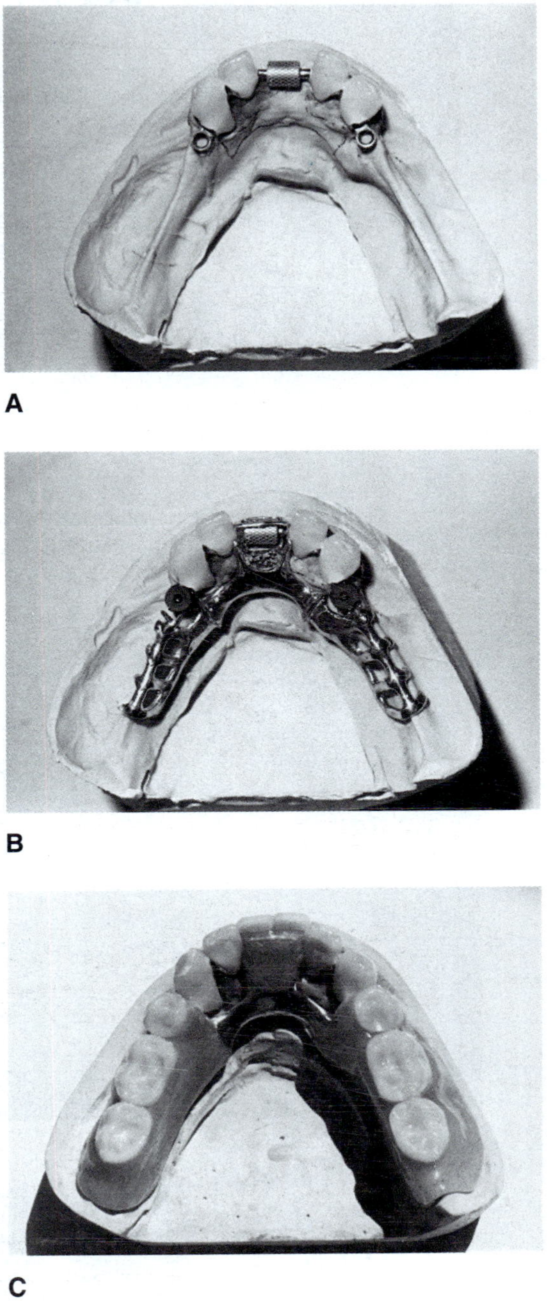

Figure 7-60 **A,** Cast with splinted crowns, Hader bar assembly, Hader bar clip, and two ERA receptors. **B,** Framework positioned on cast; ERA processing male components in place. **C,** Finished distal extension partial denture.

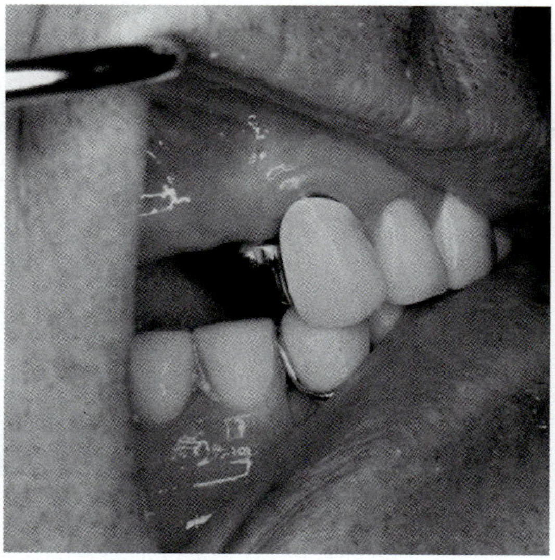

A

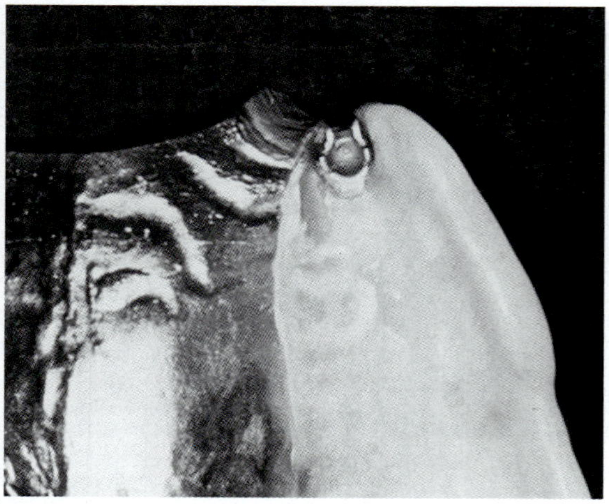

B

Figure 7-61 **A,** Dalbo extracoronal attachment with L-shaped male portion attached to abutment crown on maxillary right canine; **B,** female sleeve placed in artificial tooth adjacent to abutment.

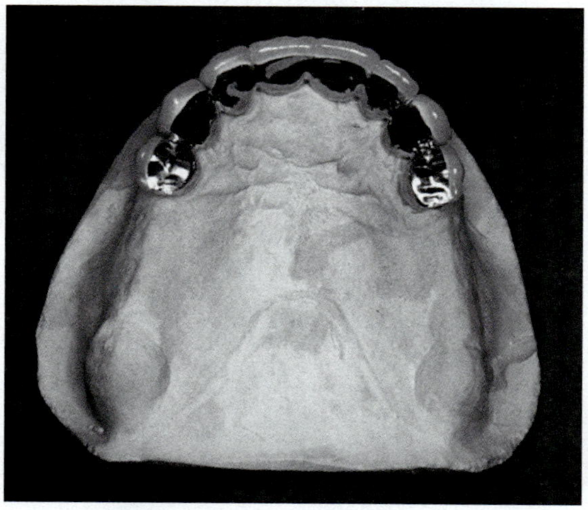

A

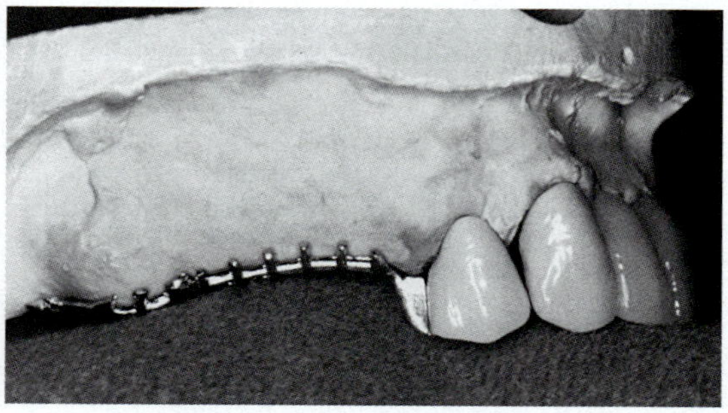

B

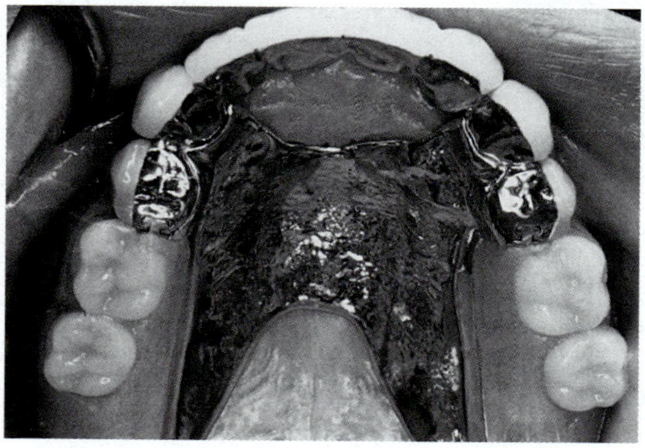

C

Figure 7-62 **A,** Sterngold GL internal attachments with female portions cast into distal proximal surfaces of splinted maxillary first premolars. **B,** Profile view of male portion attached to partial denture frame. **C,** Finished partial denture with male portion seated into female portions within primary abutments.

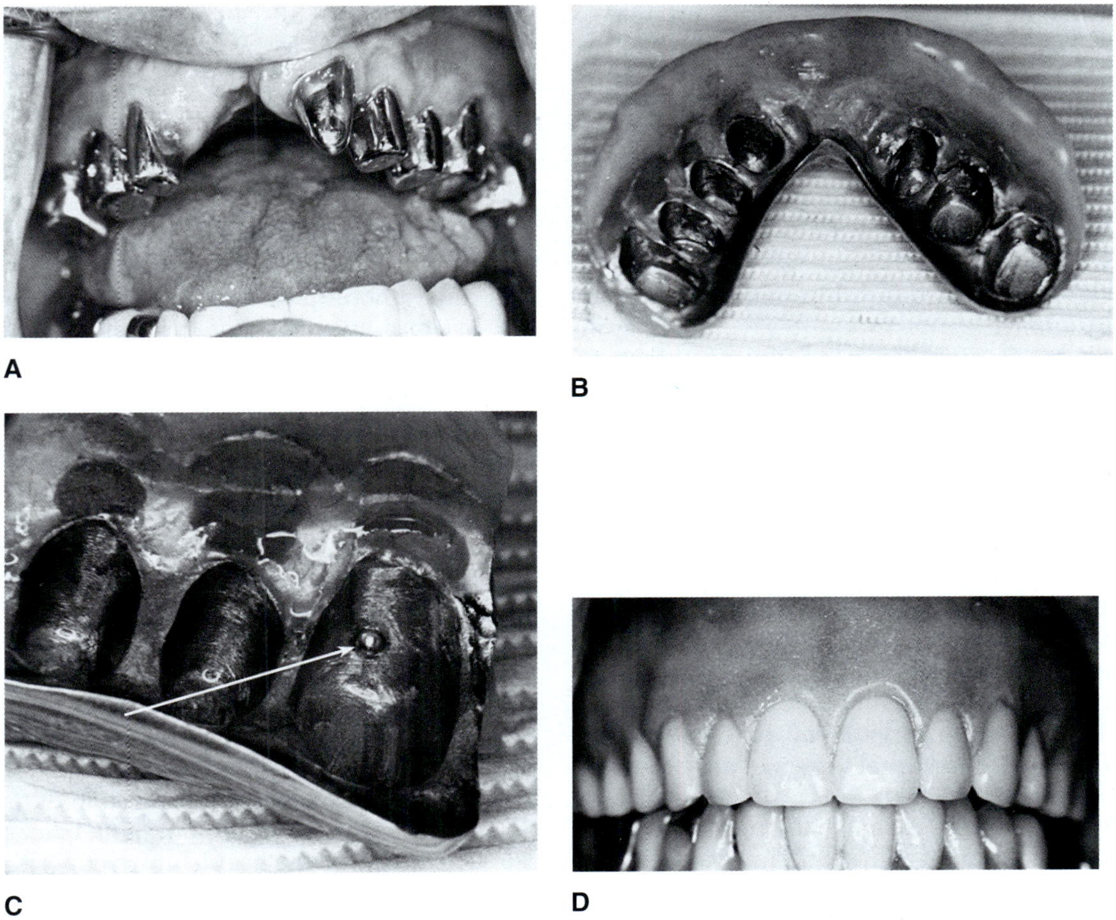

Figure 7-63 Long copings on prepared natural abutments can provide support and retention in compromised dentition. **A,** Patient is adult with repaired Class IV cleft with resultant cross-bite, Class III occlusion, and severe anterior occlusal deficit. **B,** Internal surface of prosthesis fabricated to restore the arch. **C,** View of the internal overdenture structure with an IC attachment (*arrow*) that engages a dimpled crown preparation. Several such copings are placed to enhance retention. **D,** Labial view of completed overdenture prosthesis.

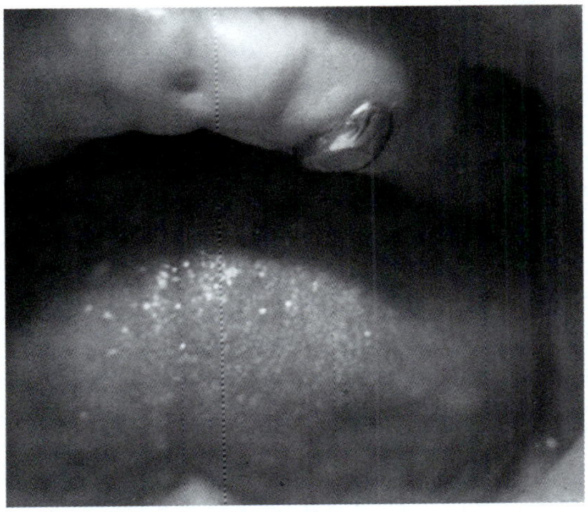

Figure 7-64 Low-profile coping contributes some additional retention but primarily provides improved support and stability.

SELF-ASSESSMENT AIDS

1. The framework of a removable partial denture must furnish **support, stabilization against horizontal (off vertical) movement, and mechanical retention**. How is mechanical retention accomplished?
2. What factor other than mechanical retention contributes to resistance of the denture to dislodging forces?
3. What is the function of a direct retainer (clasp)?
4. There are basically two types of direct retainers. Draw and label their component parts in their correct positions on an abutment tooth.
5. Describe the principles by which the extracoronal direct retainer and the intracoronal retainer provide retention for the removable partial denture.
6. What is meant by the *height of contour* of an abutment tooth?

7. Draw a diagram of an abutment tooth and illustrate the *angle of cervical convergence.*
8. A direct retainer is an assembly of the following three components that perform individual function: (1) support, by a rest; (2) stabilization-reciprocation, by a rigid clasp arm or other rigid component; and (3) a retentive element. Do these elements necessarily have to arise from a common source?
9. Flexibility is permitted for which component of a clasp assembly?
10. The amount of retention that a direct retainer is capable of generating depends on three factors. What are these factors?
11. The retentive arm of a direct retainer must be flexible to engage an undercut with its terminal portion. Flexibility of the arm is a product of four physical and composition factors. What are these important factors?
12. Retention on all principal abutments should be as equal as possible. To obtain this, which is the more important factor—the relation of the tip of the retentive arm to the height of contour or its depth in the angle of cervical convergence?
13. Describe the proportional tapers of a cast, half-round retentive arm.
14. Describe the taper of a cast, half-round stabilizing-reciprocal arm of a direct retainer assembly. For what reason must there be a difference in form between a retentive arm and a stabilizing-reciprocal arm?
15. Name the two basic types of retentive clasp arms.
16. A circumferential clasp arm approaches the retentive undercut from an occlusal direction. From which direction does a bar clasp arm approach the undercut?
17. A clasp assembly may be a combination of cast circumferential and bar clasp arms and/or wrought-wire retentive arms in one of several combinations. True or false?
18. A bar clasp arm is tapered in exactly the same way that a cast, half-round circumferential retentive clasp arm is tapered, differing only in configuration. Which arm is the more flexible if the two different arms are the same length? Why?
19. Permissible flexibilities of retentive cast circumferential and bar clasp arms based on length have been given in Tables 7-2 and 7-3. Can a 0.7-inch, bar-type arm be safely placed in the same depth of undercut as a 0.7-inch circumferential arm? Based on the information contained in Tables 7-2 and 7-3, explain the differences between permissible flexibilities of duplicate retentive clasp arms made from a type IV gold alloy and a chromium-cobalt alloy.
20. Cast clasp arms are essentially half round in form, permitting flexing in only one direction. Which direction is this?
21. Wrought wire, 18-gauge round, is often used as a circumferential clasp arm. Its round form will permit flexing in which directions?
22. We speak of a reciprocal clasp arm. Explain what is meant by reciprocation and describe the condition that must be met for true reciprocation to occur.
23. A basic principle of direct retainer (clasp) design is that the retentive and reciprocal arms must encompass more than 180° of the greatest circumference of the tooth, passing from diverging to converging axial surfaces. What would probably happen if a clasp failed to meet this criterion?
24. Simple mechanical laws (of levers) demonstrate that the closer a direct retainer assembly is located to the tipping axis of the tooth, the less likely that the periodontal ligament will be taxed from rotation tendencies of the denture. Draw the coronal portion of an abutment; divide the enamel crown into thirds; and locate support, retentive, stabilizing, and reciprocal components optimally.
25. Clasp retainers on abutment teeth adjacent to distal extension bases should be designed so that they will minimize direct transmission of tipping and rotational forces to the abutment. True or false?
26. The location of a usable undercut is perhaps the most important single factor in selecting a clasp for use with distal extension partial dentures. True or false?
27. There are many types and configurations of clasps. What factors are important to determine clasp retention and design?
28. Under what circumstances may circumferential embrasure clasps be used? What are some real disadvantages of this type of retainer?
29. Give the indications for the use of a cast circumferential direct retainer.
30. What observations would lead to the selection of a bar-type clasp?
31. What is a combination clasp and what are the indications for its use?
32. State three advantages of the combination clasp.
33. Name the essential parts of a dental surveyor.
34. There are six factors that determine the amount of retention a clasp is capable of generating. One of these is the type of metal from which it is made. Name the other five.
35. How does **tilting the cast** affect the selected areas available for clasp retention?
36. The provisions for support and retention are two of the six basic principles of design of an extracoronal retainer. What are the other four?
37. Draw four common errors in the design of a circumferential retainer. A bar-type retainer.

38. Would you agree that the single most important factor in selecting a type of direct retainer for a distal extension partial denture is the location of the undercut? Why? (Explain your answer.)
39. We know that guiding planes control the path of placement and removal of a removable partial denture. Can they also contribute to additional retention? If so, how?
40. Explain why it is necessary for retentive clasp arms to be bilaterally opposed in Class I partial dentures.
41. In Class III partial dentures should the retention be bilaterally or diametrically opposed? Explain.
42. Differentiate between three basic approaches to the application of the RPI retainer system.
43. How does the amount of contact of the minor connector proximal plate with the corresponding guiding plane in the RPI system influence the way stress is transferred to the abutment tooth and the residual ridge?

8

INDIRECT RETAINERS

As described in Chapter 4, partial denture movement can exist in three planes. Tooth-supported partial dentures effectively use teeth to control movement away from the tissue. Tooth-tissue supported partial dentures do not have this capability since one end of the prosthesis is free to move away from the tissue. This may occur because of the effects of gravity in the maxillary arch or adhesive foods in either arch. Attention to the details of design and location of partial denture component parts to control functional movement is the strategy used in partial denture design.

When the distal extension denture base is dislodged from its basal seat, it tends to rotate around the fulcrum lines. Theoretically, this movement away from the tissue can be resisted by the activation of the direct retainer, the stabilizing components of the clasp assembly, and the rigid components of the partial denture framework that are located on definite rests on the opposite side of the fulcrum line away from the distal extension base. These components are referred to as indirect retainers (Figures 8-1 and 8-2). The indirect retainer components should be placed as far as possible from the distal extension base, which provides the best leverage advantage against dislodgment (Figure 8-3).

For the sake of clarity in discussing the location and functions of indirect retainers, fulcrum lines should be considered the axis about which the denture will rotate when the bases move away from the residual ridge.

An indirect retainer consists of one or more rests and the supporting minor connectors (Figures 8-4 and 8-5). The proximal plates, adjacent to the edentulous areas, also provide indirect retention. Although it is customary to identify the entire assembly as the indirect retainer, it should be remembered that the rest is actually the indirect retainer united to the major connector by a minor connector. This is noted to avoid interpreting any contact with tooth inclines as being part of the indirect retainer. An indirect retainer should be placed as far from the distal extension base as possible in a prepared rest seat on a tooth capable of supporting its function.

Although the most effective location of an indirect retainer is commonly in the vicinity of an incisor tooth, that tooth may not be strong enough to support an indirect retainer and may have steep inclines that cannot be favorably altered to support a rest. In such a situation, the nearest canine tooth or the mesioocclusal surface of the first premolar may be the best location for the indirect retention, despite the fact that it is not as far removed from the fulcrum line. Whenever possible, two indirect retainers closer to the fulcrum line are then used to compensate for the compromise in distance.

FACTORS INFLUENCING EFFECTIVENESS OF INDIRECT RETAINERS

The following factors influence the effectiveness of an indirect retainer:

1. The principal occlusal rests on the primary abutment teeth must be reasonably held in their seats

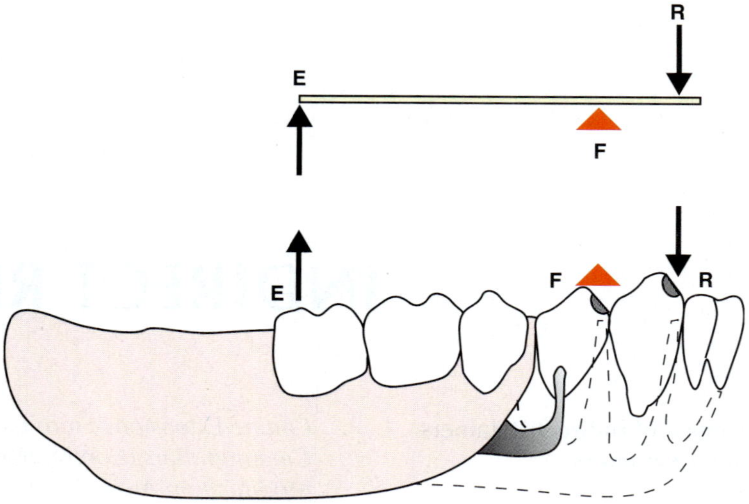

Figure 8-1 Mandibular distal extension removable partial denture showing distal extension base being lifted from the ridge, the clasp assembly being activated and engaged, with the indirect retainer providing stabilization against dislodgement. Lift of distal extension base is effectively controlled by the indirect retainer when the direct retainer and proximal plate act to maintain the clasp assembly in place during base movement away from the supporting tissue.

by the retentive arms of the direct retainers. If rests are held in their seats, rotation about an axis should occur, which activates the indirect retainers. If total displacement of the rests occurs, there would be no rotation about the fulcrum, and the indirect retainers would not be activated.

2. Distance from the fulcrum line. The following three areas must be considered:
   a. Length of the distal extension base
   b. Location of the fulcrum line
   c. How far beyond the fulcrum line the indirect retainer is placed
3. Rigidity of the connectors supporting the indirect retainer. All connectors must be rigid if the indirect retainer is to function as intended.
4. Effectiveness of the supporting tooth surface. The indirect retainer must be placed on a definite rest seat on which slippage or tooth movement will not occur. Tooth inclines and weak teeth should never be used to support indirect retainers.

AUXILIARY FUNCTIONS OF INDIRECT RETAINERS

In addition to effectively activating the direct retainer to prevent movement of a distal extension base away from the tissue, an indirect retainer may serve the following auxiliary functions:

1. It tends to reduce anteroposterior-tilting leverages on the principal abutments. This is particularly important when an isolated tooth is being used as an abutment, a situation that should be avoided whenever possible. Ordinarily, proximal contact with the adjacent tooth prevents such tilting of an abutment as the base lifts away from the tissue.
2. Contact of its minor connector with axial tooth surfaces aids in stabilization against horizontal movement of the denture. Such tooth surfaces, when made parallel to the path of placement, may also act as auxiliary guiding planes.
3. Anterior teeth supporting indirect retainers are stabilized against lingual movement.
4. It may act as an auxiliary rest to support a portion of the major connector facilitating stress distribution. For example, a lingual bar may be supported against settling into the tissue by the indirect retainer acting as an auxiliary rest. One must be able to differentiate between an auxiliary rest placed for support for a major connector, one placed for indirect retention, and one serving a dual purpose. Some auxiliary rests are added solely to provide rest support to a segment of the denture and should not be confused with indirect retention.
5. It may provide the first visual indications for the need to reline an extension base partial denture. Deficiencies in basal seat support are manifested by the dislodgment of indirect retainers from their prepared rest seats when the denture base is depressed and rotation occurs around the fulcrum.

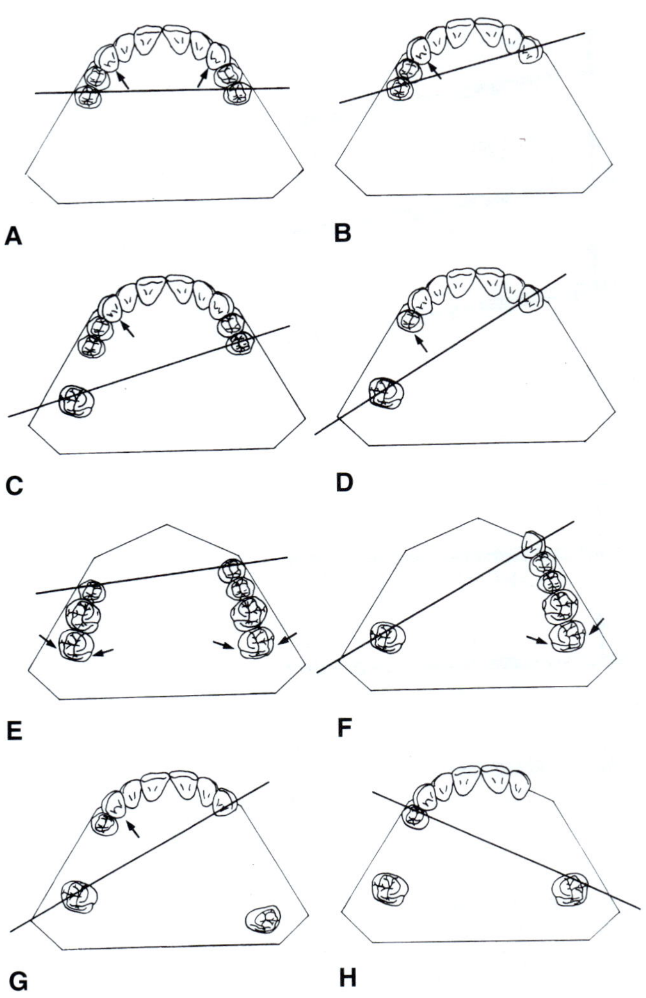

Figure 8-2 Fulcrum lines found in various types of partially edentulous arches, around which denture may rotate when bases are subjected to forces directed toward or away from residual ridge. Arrows indicate most advantageous position of indirect retainer(s). **A** and **B,** In Class I arch, fulcrum line passes through the most posterior abutments, provided some rigid component of framework is occlusal to abutment's heights of contour. **C,** In Class II arch, fulcrum line is diagonal, passing through abutment on distal extension side and the most posterior abutment on opposite side. **D,** If abutment tooth anterior to modification space lies far enough removed from fulcrum line, it may be used effectively for support of indirect retainer. **E** and **F,** In Class IV arch, fulcrum line passes through two abutments adjacent to single edentulous space. **G,** In Class III arch with posterior tooth on right side, which has a poor prognosis and will eventually be lost, fulcrum line is considered the same as though posterior tooth were not present. Thus its future loss may not necessitate altering original design of the removable partial denture framework. **H,** In Class III arch with nonsupporting anterior teeth, adjacent edentulous area is considered to be tissue-supported end, with diagonal fulcrum line passing through two principal abutments as in Class II arch.

These auxiliary functions derived from indirect retainers are important to consider, especially given the reported controversy as to the effectiveness of indirect retainers.

FORMS OF INDIRECT RETAINERS

The indirect retainer may be in one of several forms. All are effective in proportion to their support and the distance from the fulcrum line.

Auxiliary Occlusal Rest

The most commonly used indirect retainer is an auxiliary occlusal rest located on an occlusal surface and as far away from the distal extension base as possible. In a mandibular Class I arch, this location is usually on the mesial marginal ridge of the first premolar on each side of the arch (see Figure 8-4). The ideal position for the indirect retainer perpendicular to the fulcrum line would be in the vicinity of the central incisors, which are too weak and have lingual surfaces that are too perpendicular to support a rest. Bilateral rests on the first premolars are quite effective, even though they are located closer to the axis of rotation.

The same principle applies to any maxillary Class I partial denture when indirect retainers are used. Bilateral rests on the mesial marginal ridge of the first premolars are generally used in preference to rests on incisor teeth (see Figure 8-5). Not only are they effective without jeopardizing the weaker single-rooted teeth, but also interference with the tongue is far less when the minor connector can be placed in the embrasure between canine and premolar rather than anterior to the canine teeth.

Indirect retainers for Class II partial dentures are usually placed on the marginal ridge of the first premolar tooth on the opposite side of the arch from the distal extension base (Figure 8-6). Bilateral rests are seldom indicated except when an auxiliary occlusal rest is needed for support of the major connector or when the prognosis of the distal abutment is poor and provision is being considered for later conversion to a Class I partial denture.

Canine Rests

When the mesial marginal ridge of the first premolar is too close to the fulcrum line or when the teeth are overlapped so that the fulcrum line is not accessible, a rest may be used on the adjacent canine tooth. Such a rest may be made more effective by placing the minor connector in the embrasure anterior to the canine, either curving back onto a prepared lingual rest seat or extending to a mesioincisal rest. The same types of canine rests as those previously outlined, which are the lingual or incisal rests, may be used (see Chapter 6).

Canine Extensions From Occlusal Rests

Occasionally a finger extension from a premolar rest is placed on the prepared lingual slope of the adjacent canine tooth (Figure 8-7). Such an

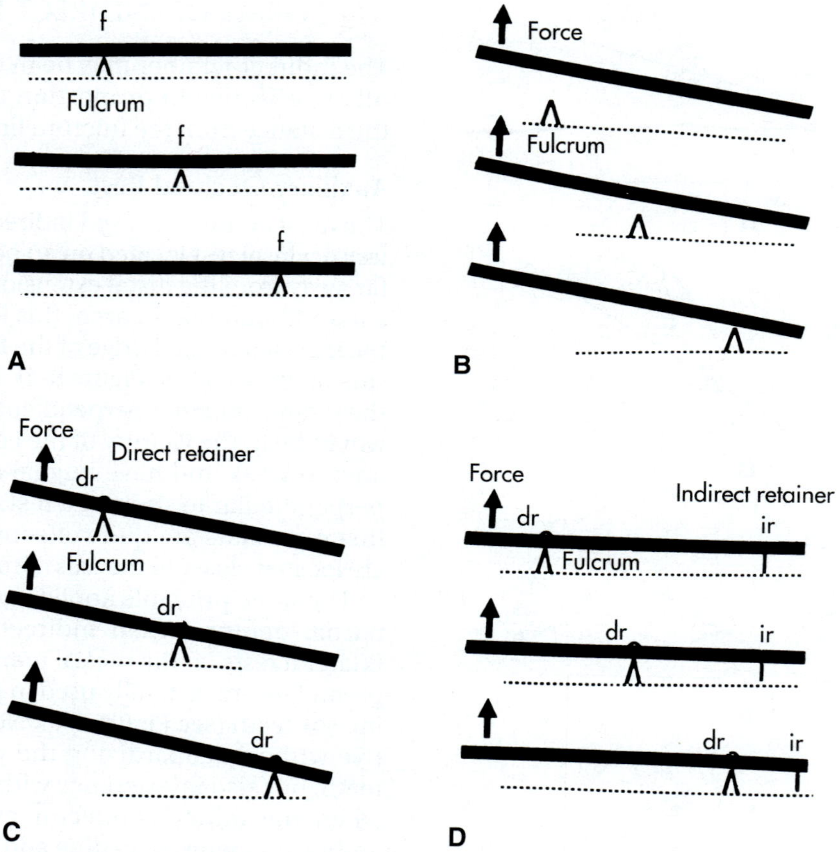

Figure 8-3 Indirect retainer principle. **A,** Beams are supported at various points. **B,** Lifting force will displace entire beam in absence of retainers. **C,** With direct retainers *(dr)* at fulcrum, lifting force will depress one end of beam and elevate other end. **D,** With both direct and indirect retainers *(ir)* functioning, lifting force will not displace beam. The farther the indirect retainer is from the fulcrum, the more efficiently it should control movement.

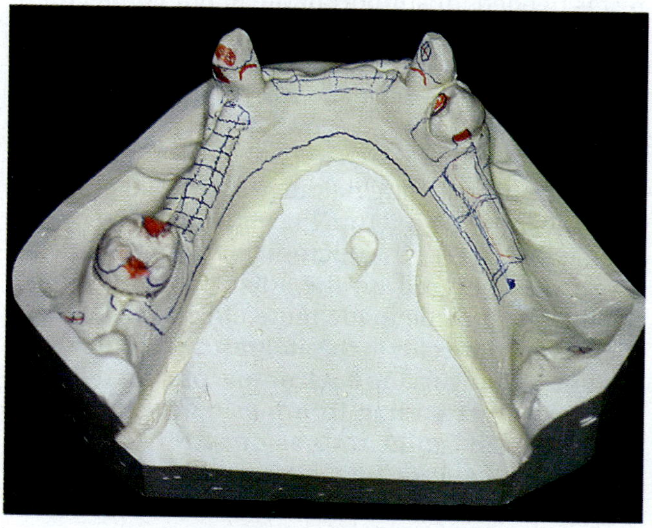

Figure 8-4 Planning location for indirect retainer for Class II Mod 2 removable partial denture. The greatest distance from axis of rotation around most distal rests *(fulcrum line)* would fall on tooth #22. Decision to use incisal rest or cingulum rest will depend on patients concern for esthetic impact of incisal rest versus having a crown (which could have a cingulum rest).

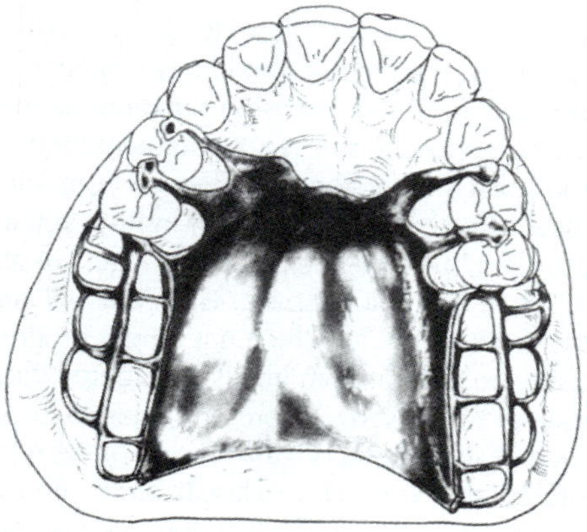

Figure 8-5 Example of indirect retention used in conjunction with palatal plate-type major connector. Indirect retainers are proximal plates on second premolars and occlusal rests located on first premolars. A secondary function of auxiliary occlusal rest assemblies is to prevent settling of anterior portion of major connector and to provide stabilization against horizontal rotation.

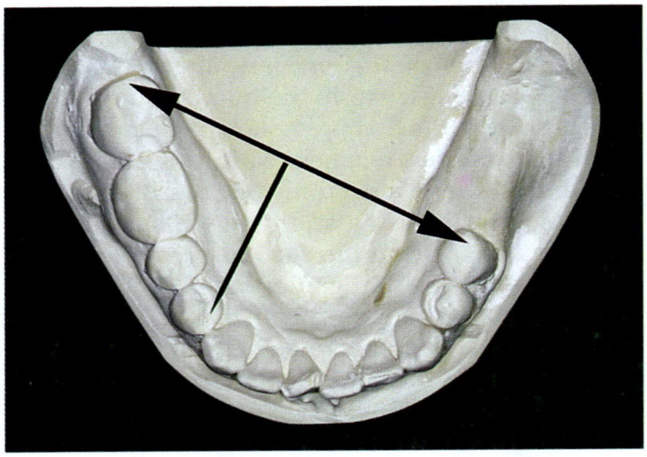

Figure 8-6 Mandibular Class II design showing best location for the indirect retainer on mesial-occlusal of first premolar #28. This location is at 90 degrees to the fulcrum line between primary rests, DO of #20 and DO of #31, and provides an efficient resistance to denture base lift.

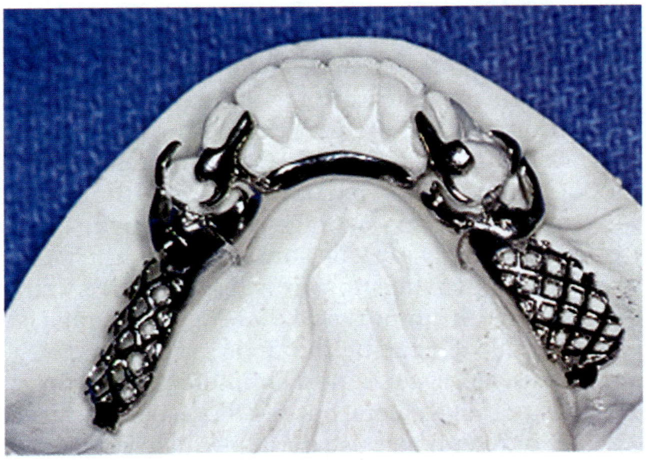

Figure 8-7 Mandibular Class I design using canine extensions from occlusal rests as indirect retainers. Canine extensions must be placed on prepared rest seats so that resistance will be directed as nearly as possible along long axes of canine abutments.

extension is used to effect indirect retention by increasing the distance of a resisting element from the fulcrum line. This method is particularly applicable when a first premolar must serve as a primary abutment. The distance anterior to the fulcrum line is only the distance between the mesioocclusal rest and the anterior terminal of the finger extension. In this instance, although the extension rests on a prepared surface, it is used in conjunction with a terminal rest on the mesial marginal ridge of the premolar tooth. Even when they are not used as indirect retainers, canine extensions, continuous bar retainers, and linguoplates should never be used without terminal rests because of the resultant forces effective when they are placed on inclined planes alone.

Cingulum Bars (Continuous Bars) and Linguoplates

Technically, cingulum bars (continuous bars) and linguoplates are not indirect retainers because they rest on unprepared lingual inclines of anterior teeth. The indirect retainers are actually the terminal rests at either end in the form of auxiliary occlusal rests or canine rests (see Chapter 5).

In Class I and Class II partial dentures, a cingulum bar or linguoplate may extend the effectiveness of the indirect retainer if it is used with a terminal rest at each end. In tooth-supported partial dentures, a cingulum bar or linguoplate is placed for other reasons but always with terminal rests (see Chapter 5).

In Class I and Class II partial dentures especially, a continuous bar retainer or the superior border of the linguoplate should never be placed above the middle third of the teeth so that orthodontic movement is prevented during the rotation of a distal extension denture. This guideline is not as important when the six anterior teeth are in nearly a straight line, but when the arch is narrow and tapering, a cingulum bar or linguoplate on anterior teeth extends well beyond the terminal rests—and orthodontic movement of those teeth is more likely. Although these are intended primarily to stabilize weak anterior teeth, they may have the opposite effect if not used with discretion.

Modification Areas

Occasionally the occlusal rest on a secondary abutment in a Class II partial denture may serve as an indirect retainer. This use will depend on how far from the fulcrum line the secondary abutment is located.

The primary abutments in a Class II, modification 1 partial denture are the abutment adjacent to the distal extension base and the most distal abutment on the tooth-supported side. The fulcrum line is a diagonal axis between the two terminal abutments (Figure 8-8).

The anterior abutment on the tooth-supported side is a secondary abutment, serving to support and retain one end of the tooth-supported segment and adding horizontal stabilization to the denture. If the modification space were not present, as in an unmodified Class II arch, auxiliary occlusal rests and stabilizing components in the

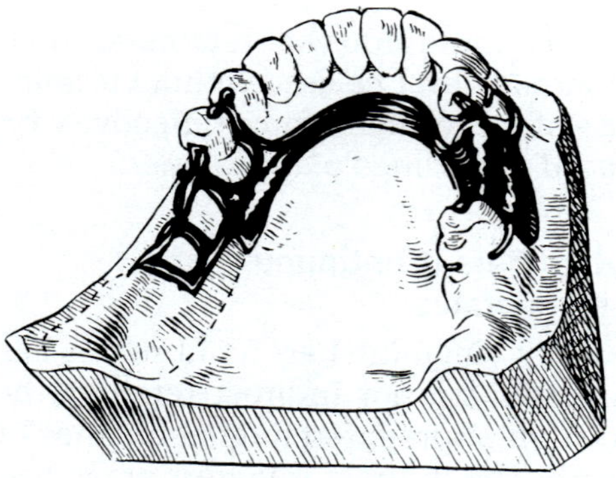

Figure 8-8 Class II, mod 1, removable partial denture framework. Fulcrum line, when denture base is displaced toward residual ridge, runs from left second premolar to right second molar. When forces tend to displace denture away from its basal seat, supportive element (distal occlusal rest) of direct retainer assembly on right first premolar serves as indirect retainer.

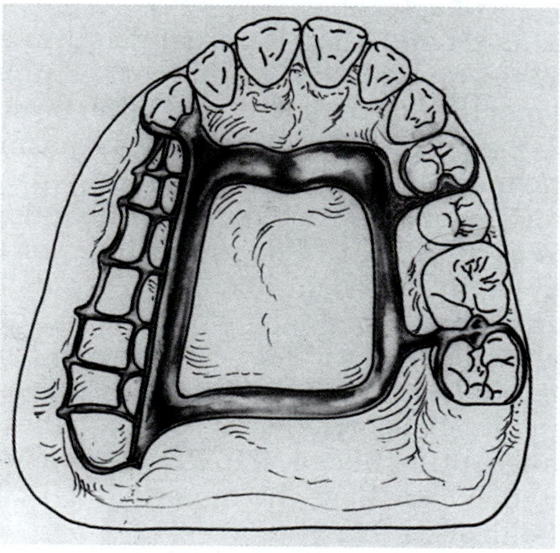

Figure 8-9 Class II maxillary removable partial denture framework design. Fulcrum line runs from patient's right canine to left second molar. Forces that tend to unseat denture from its basal seat will be resisted by activation of retentive elements on canine and molar, using supportive elements on left first premolar as indirect retainer.

same position would still be essential to the design of the denture (Figure 8-9). However, the presence of a modification space conveniently provides an abutment tooth for support, stabilization, and retention.

If the occlusal rest on the secondary abutment lies far enough from the fulcrum line, it may serve adequately as an indirect retainer. Its dual function then is tooth support for one end of the modification area and support for an indirect retainer. The most typical example is a distal occlusal rest on a first premolar when a second premolar and first molar are missing and the second molar serves as one of the primary abutments. The longest perpendicular to the fulcrum line falls in the vicinity of the first premolar, making the location of the indirect retainer nearly ideal.

On the other hand, if only one tooth, such as a first molar, is missing on the modification side, the occlusal rest on the second premolar abutment is too close to the fulcrum line to be effective. In such a situation, an auxiliary occlusal rest on the mesial marginal ridge of the first premolar is needed, both for indirect retention and for support for an otherwise unsupported major connector.

Support for a modification area extending anteriorly to a canine abutment is obtained by any one of the accepted canine rest forms, as previously outlined in Chapter 6. In this situation the canine tooth provides nearly ideal indirect retention and support for the major connector as well.

Rugae Support

Some clinicians consider coverage of the rugae area of the maxillary arch as a means of indirect retention because the rugae area is firm and usually well situated to provide indirect retention for a Class I removable partial denture. Although it is true that broad coverage over the rugae area can conceivably provide some support, the facts remain that tissue support is less effective than positive tooth support and that rugae coverage is undesirable if it can be avoided.

The use of rugae support for indirect retention is usually part of a palatal horseshoe design. Because posterior retention is usually inadequate in this situation, the requirements for indirect retention are probably greater than can be satisfied by this type of tissue support alone.

In the mandibular arch, retention from the distal extension base alone is usually inadequate to prevent lifting of the base away from the tissue. In the maxillary arch, where only anterior teeth remain, full palatal coverage is usually necessary. In fact, with any Class I maxillary removable partial denture extending distally from the first premolar teeth, except when a maxillary torus prevents its use, palatal coverage may be used to advantage. Although complete coverage may be in the form of a resin base, the added retention and reduced bulk of a cast metal palate make the latter preferable (see Chapter 5). However, in the absence of full palatal coverage, an indirect retainer should be used with other designs of major palatal connectors for the Class I removable partial denture.

SELF-ASSESSMENT AIDS

1. What elements prevent movement of the base(s) of a tooth-supported denture toward the basal seats?
2. Support of a distal extension removable partial denture is shared by abutment teeth and residual ridges. The quality of support furnished by the residual ridges is proportionate to at least three factors. Please name them.
3. Movement of a distal extension base away from basal seats will occur as a rotational movement or as ______.
4. What is the difference between fulcrum line and axis of rotation?
5. Identify the fulcrum line on a Class I arch; a Class II, modification 1; and a Class IV.
6. Define the term **indirect retainer**.
7. What components of a removable partial denture framework usually make an indirect retainer?
8. From the standpoint of leverage advantage, where should an indirect retainer be located?
9. An indirect retainer performs one major function and four auxiliary functions. State these five functions.
10. The effectiveness of an indirect retainer is influenced by four factors. What are they?
11. What are the probable sequelae of trying to use a continuous bar retainer or linguoplate to serve the purpose of an indirect retainer?
12. In a Class II, modification 1 arch—especially if the modification is a long edentulous space—what component may act as an indirect retainer?
13. Discuss the inadequacy of the use of coverage of rugae to act as support for indirect retention.
14. Each design of the extension base-type removable partial denture should include an indirect retainer or some component that will act as an indirect retainer. True or false?
15. Bilaterally placed indirect retainers contribute to stability of the Class I restoration to a greater extent than does a single indirect retainer. True or false?

9

DENTURE BASE CONSIDERATIONS

FUNCTIONS OF DENTURE BASES

The denture base supports the artificial teeth and consequently receives the functional forces from occlusion and transfers functional forces to supporting oral structures (Figure 9-1). This function is most critical for the distal extension prosthesis, as functional stability and comfort often relate directly to the ability for this transfer of forces to occur without undue movement.

Although its primary purpose is related to masticatory function, the denture base also may add to the cosmetic effect of the replacement, particularly when techniques are used for tinting and reproducing natural-looking contours. Most of the techniques for creating a natural appearance in complete denture bases are applicable equally to partial denture bases.

Still another function of the denture base is the stimulation of the underlying tissue of the residual ridge. Some vertical movement occurs with any denture base, even those supported entirely by abutment teeth, because of the physiological movement of those teeth under function. It is clearly evident that oral tissues placed under functional stress within their physiological tolerance maintain their form and tone better than similar tissues suffering from disuse. The term *disuse atrophy* is applicable to both periodontal tissue and the tissue of a residual ridge.

Tooth-supported Partial Denture Base

Denture bases differ in functional purpose and may differ in the material of which they are made. In a tooth-supported prosthesis, the denture base is primarily a span between two abutments supporting artificial teeth. Thus occlusal forces are transferred directly to the abutments through rests. Also, the denture base and the supplied teeth serve to prevent horizontal migration of all of the abutment teeth in the partially edentulous arch and vertical migration of teeth in the opposing arch.

When only posterior teeth are being replaced, esthetics is usually only a secondary consideration. On the other hand, when anterior teeth are replaced, esthetics may be of primary importance. Theoretically, the tooth-supported partial denture base that replaces anterior teeth must perform the following functions: (1) provide desirable esthetics; (2) support and retain the artificial teeth in such a way that they provide masticatory efficiency and assist in transferring occlusal forces directly to abutment teeth through rests; (3) prevent vertical and horizontal migration of remaining natural teeth; (4) eliminate

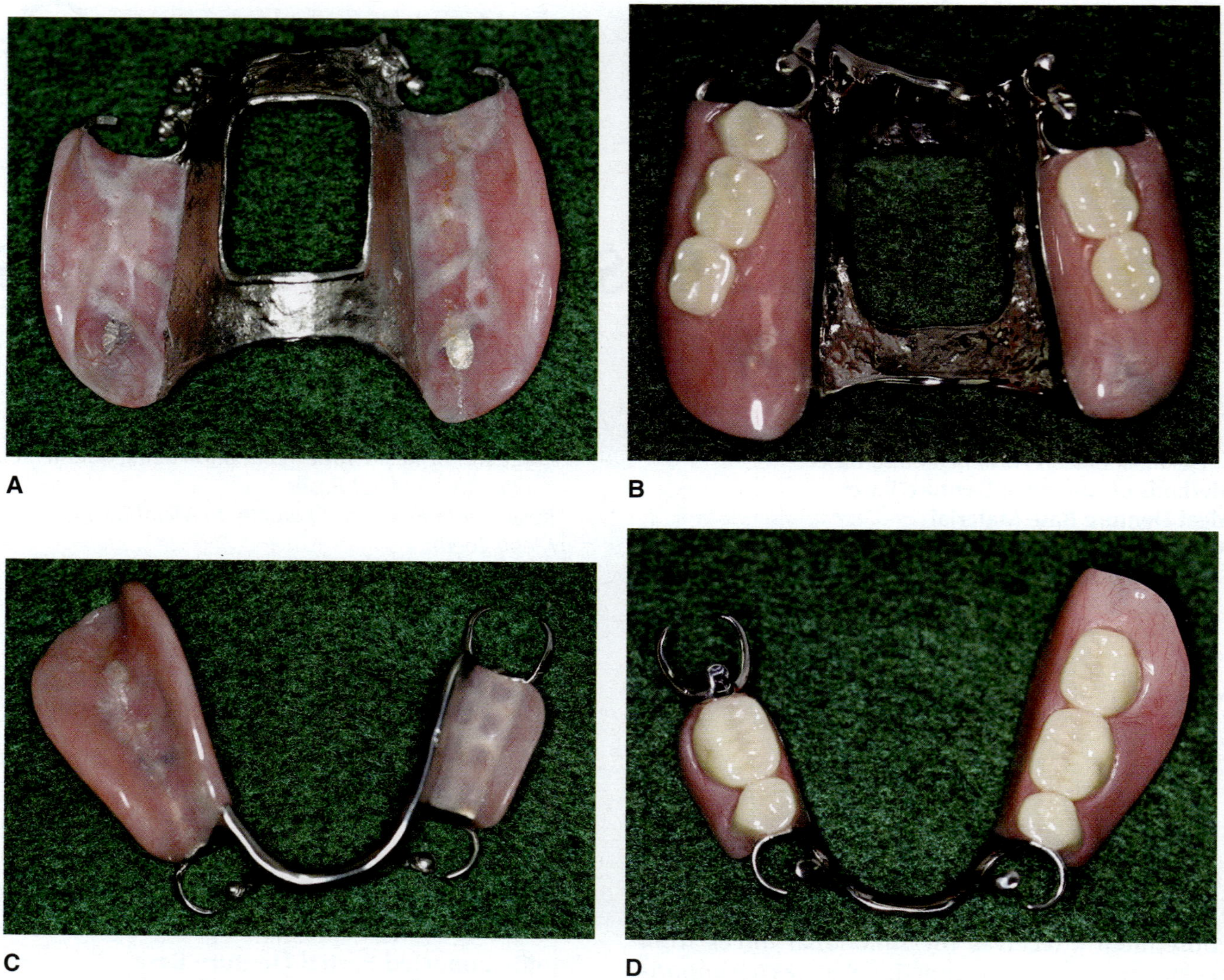

Figure 9-1 **A,** Class I maxillary distal extension removable partial denture showing tissue side (intaglio) of denture bases. **B,** Occlusal side of maxillary prosthesis, posterior artificial teeth are attached to bases. **C,** Class II Mod 1 mandibular distal extension removable partial denture showing intaglio of both extension and modification bases. **D,** Occlusal side of mandibular prosthesis, posterior artificial teeth are attached to bases. For both prostheses, the bases are extended within limits of physiologic activity of surrounding oral structures.

undesirable food traps (oral cleanliness); and (5) stimulate the underlying tissue.

Distal Extension Partial Denture Base

In a distal extension partial denture, the denture bases other than those in tooth-supported modifications must contribute to the support of the denture. Such support is critical to the goal of minimizing functional movement and improving prosthesis stability. Although the abutment teeth provide support for the distal extension base, as the distance from the abutment increases, the support from the underlying ridge tissue becomes increasingly important. Maximum support from the residual ridge may be obtained by using broad, accurate denture bases, which spread the occlusal load equitably over the entire area available for such support. The space available for a denture base is determined by the structures surrounding the space and by their movement during function. Maximum support for the denture base therefore can be accomplished only by using knowledge of the limiting anatomic structures and of the histological nature of the basal seat areas, accuracy of the impression, and accuracy of the denture base (Figure 9-2). The first two of these support features relate to the gross size and cellular characteristics of the residual ridge tissue. These are quite variable between patients, and consequently

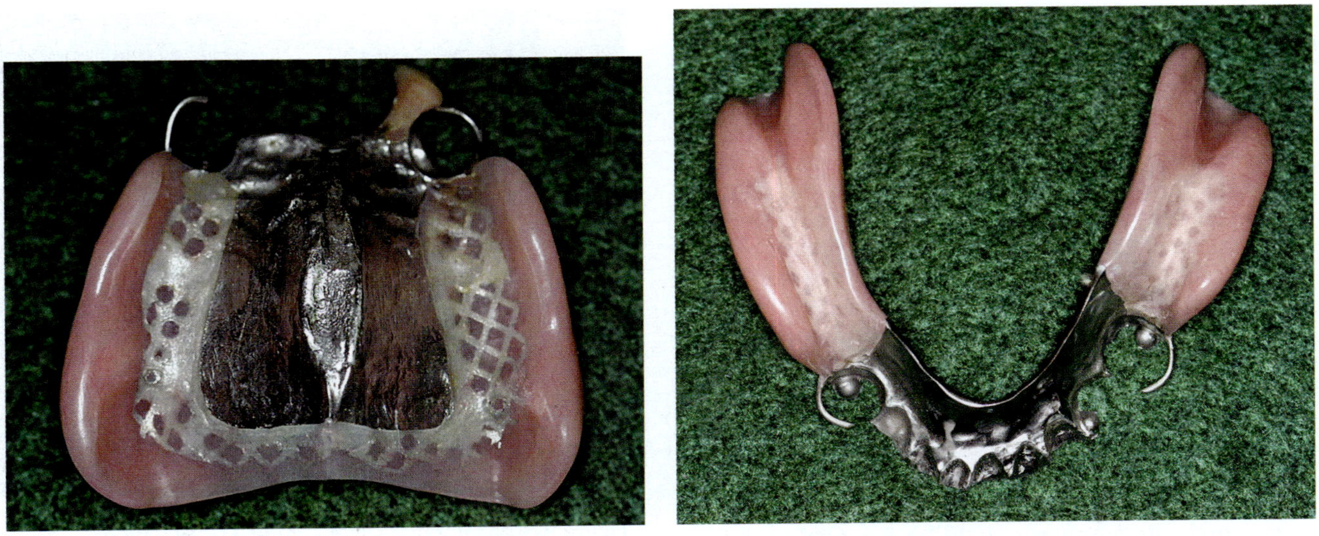

A B

Figure 9-2 Maxillary and mandibular distal extension removable partial dentures with resin denture bases. Bases are extended buccally within physiologic tolerance of border structures. **A,** Maxillary denture bases cover both the maxillary tuberosities, extend into the pterygomaxillary notches, and provide for adaptation along the posterior border, taking care not to extend beyond the soft palatal flexure. **B,** Mandibular bilateral distal extension removable partial denture bases cover the retromolar pads and extend into the retromylohyoid fossae. Impression procedure used established buccal shelves as primary stress-bearing areas of basal seats.

not all residual ridges can provide the same quality of support. Therefore the ability to control the functional displacement of the distal extension base is a determination that is unique for the individual patients.

The snowshoe principle, which suggests that broad coverage furnishes the best support with the least load per unit area, is the principle of choice for providing maximum support. Therefore support should be the primary consideration in selecting, designing, and fabricating a distal extension partial denture base. Of secondary importance (but to be considered nevertheless) are esthetics, stimulation of the underlying tissue, and oral cleanliness. Methods used to accomplish maximum support of the restoration through its base(s) are presented in Chapters 15 and 16.

In addition to their difference in functional purposes, denture bases vary in material of fabrication. This difference is directly related to their function because of the need for realignment of some dentures.

Because the tooth-supported base has an abutment tooth at each end on which a rest has been placed, future relining or rebasing may not be necessary to reestablish support. Relining is necessary only when tissue changes have occurred beneath the tooth-supported base to the point that poor esthetics or accumulation of debris result. For these reasons alone, tooth-supported bases made soon after extractions should be of a material that permits later relining. Such materials are the denture resins, the most common of which are copolymer and methyl methacrylate resins.

Primary retention for the removable partial denture is accomplished mechanically by placing retaining elements on the abutment teeth. *Secondary retention* is provided by the intimate relationship of denture bases and major connectors (maxillary) with the underlying tissue. The latter is similar to the retention of complete dentures and is proportionate to the accuracy of the impression registration, the accuracy of the fit of the denture bases, and the total area of contact involved.

Retention of denture bases has been described as the result of the following forces: (1) adhesion, which is the attraction of the saliva to the denture and tissue; (2) cohesion, which is the attraction of the molecules of the saliva for each other; (3) atmospheric pressure, which is dependent on a border seal and results in a partial vacuum beneath the denture base when a dislodging force is applied; (4) the physiological molding of the tissue around the polished surfaces of the denture; and (5) the effect of gravity on the mandibular denture.

Boucher, writing on the subject of complete denture impressions, described these forces as follows:

> Adhesion and cohesion are effective when there is perfect apposition of the impression surface of the denture to the mucous membrane surfaces. These forces lose their effectiveness if any horizontal displacement of the dentures breaks the continuity of this contact. Atmospheric pressure is effective primarily as a rescue force when extreme dislodging forces are applied to the denture. It depends on a perfect border seal to keep the pressure applied on only one side of the denture. The presence of air on the impression surface would neutralize the pressure of the air against the polished surface. Because each of these forces is directly proportional to the area covered by the dentures, the dentures should be extended to the limits of the supporting structures.
>
> The molding of the soft tissue around the polished surfaces of denture bases helps to perfect the border seal. Also, it forms a mechanical lock at certain locations on the dentures, provided these surfaces are properly prepared. This lock is developed automatically and without effort by the patient if the impression is made with an understanding of the anatomic possibilities.*

Few partial dentures are made without some mechanical retention. Retention from the denture bases may contribute significantly to the overall retention of the partial denture and therefore must not be discounted. Denture bases should be designed and fabricated so that they will contribute as much retention to the partial denture as possible. However, it is questionable whether atmospheric pressure plays as important a role in retention of removable partial dentures because a border seal cannot be obtained as readily as it can be with complete dentures. Therefore adhesion and cohesion gained by excellent apposition of the denture base and soft tissue of the basal seat play an important retentive role.

METHODS OF ATTACHING DENTURE BASES

Acrylic resin bases are attached to the partial denture framework by means of a minor connector designed so that a space exists between the framework and the underlying tissue of the residual ridge (Figure 9-3). Relief of at least a 20-gauge thickness over the basal seat areas of the master cast is used to create a raised platform on the investment cast on which the pattern for the retentive frame is formed (Figure 9-4). Thus after casting, the portion of the retentive framework to which the acrylic resin base will be attached will stand away from the tissue surface sufficiently to permit a flow of acrylic resin base material beneath its surface.

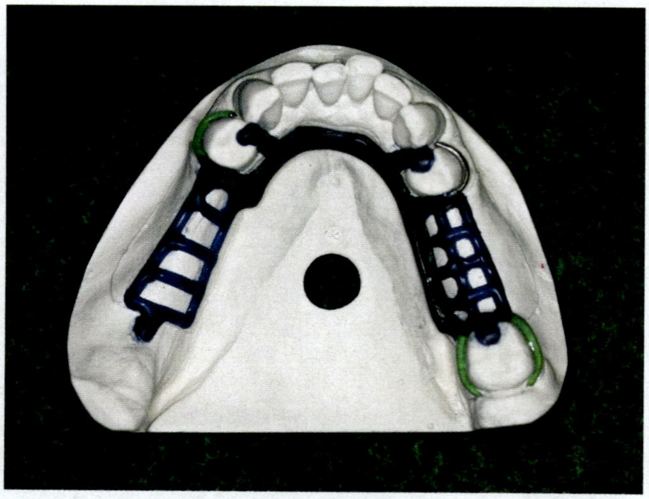

Figure 9-3 Mandibular Class II, mod 1, wax pattern developed on investment cast. Adequate provision is made for attaching resin base to major connector on edentulous side by way of ladderlike minor connector and butt-type joint. Similar minor connector design will be used for modification space. Note, relief space beneath minor connectors is established by relief wax placed on the original master cast and duplicated in this refractory cast. This allows processed resin to surround the minor connectors in creating the denture base.

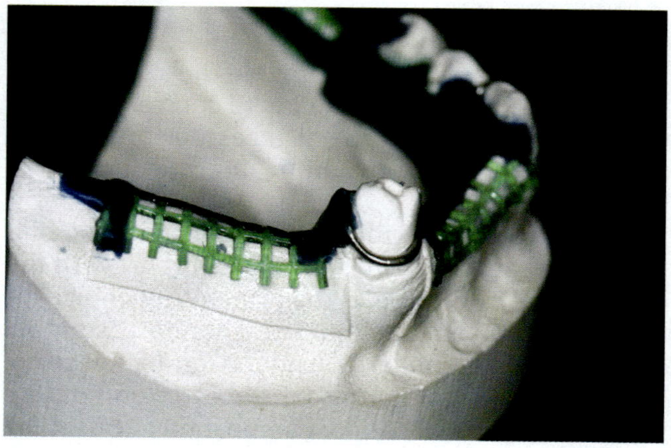

Figure 9-4 Unlike the minor connector designs in Figure 9-3, the designs used for this prosthesis are a plastic mesh pattern. Although such designs can be reinforced to be more rigid, the bulk of connector itself may contribute to weakening of resin base. A more open type of minor connector seems preferable.

*Paraphrased from Boucher CO: Complete denture impression based upon the anatomy of the mouth, J Am Dent Assoc 31:117-1181, 1994.

The retentive framework for the base should be embedded in the base material with sufficient thickness of resin (1.5 mm) to allow for relieving if this becomes necessary during the denture adjustment period or during relining procedures. Thickness is also necessary to prevent weakness and subsequent fracture of the acrylic resin base material surrounding the metal framework.

The use of plastic mesh patterns in forming the retentive framework is generally less satisfactory than a more open framework (see Figure 9-4). Less weakening of the resin by the embedded framework results from the use of the more open form. Pieces of 12- or 14-gauge half-round wax and 18-gauge round wax are used to form a ladderlike framework rather than the finer latticework of the mesh pattern. The precise design of the retentive framework, other than that it should be located both buccally and lingually, is not so important as its effective rigidity and strength when it is embedded in the acrylic resin base. It should also be free of interference with future adjustment, not interfere with the arrangement of artificial teeth, and be open enough to prevent weakening any portion of the attached acrylic resin. Designing the retentive framework for denture bases by having elements located buccally and lingually to the residual ridge not only will strengthen the acrylic resin base but also will minimize distortion of the base created by the release of inherent strains in the acrylic resin base during use or storage of the restoration (Figure 9-5).

Metal bases are usually cast as integral parts of the partial denture framework (Figure 9-6). Mandibular metal bases may also be assembled and attached to the framework with acrylic resin.

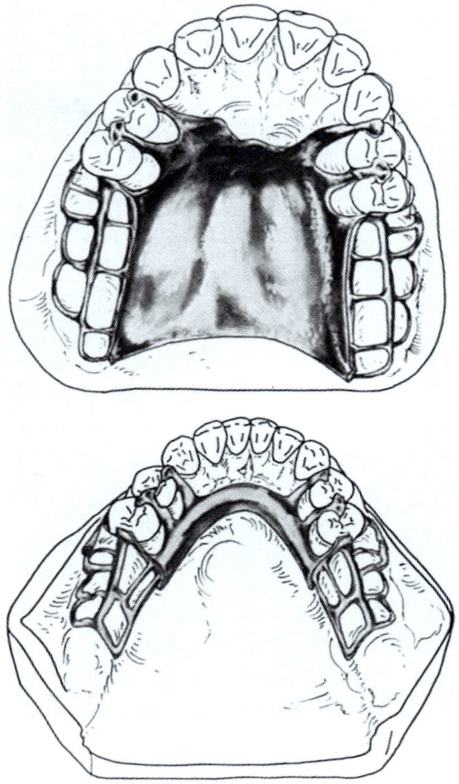

Figure 9-5 Note that minor connectors by which resin denture bases will be attached to framework are open, ladderlike configurations extending on both buccal and lingual surfaces. This not only provides excellent attachment of resin bases but also minimizes warping of bases resulting from the release of inherent strains in compression-molded resin.

IDEAL DENTURE BASE MATERIAL

The requirements for an ideal denture base are as follows:

1. Accuracy of adaptation to the tissue, with minimal volume change
2. Dense, nonirritating surface capable of receiving and maintaining a good finish
3. Thermal conductivity
4. Low specific gravity; lightweight in the mouth
5. Sufficient strength; resistance to fracture or distortion
6. Easily kept clean
7. Esthetic acceptability
8. Potential for future relining
9. Low initial cost

Such an ideal denture base material does not exist, nor is it likely to be developed in the near future. However, any denture base, whether of resin or metal and regardless of the method of fabrication, should come as close to this ideal as possible.

ADVANTAGES OF METAL BASES

Except for those edentulous ridges with recent extractions, metal can be used for tooth-supported bases and is thought to provide several advantages. Its principal disadvantages are that it is difficult to adjust and reline. A commonly stated advantage is that the stimulation it gives to the underlying tissue is so beneficial that it prevents some alveolar atrophy that would otherwise occur under a resin base and thereby would prolong the health of the tissue that it contacts. Some of the advantages of a metal base are discussed in the following sections.

Accuracy and Permanence of Form

Cast metal bases, whether of gold, chrome, or titanium alloys, not only may be cast more accurately than denture resins but also can maintain their accuracy of form without change in the mouth. Internal strains that may be released later to cause distortion are not present. Although some resins and some processing techniques are superior

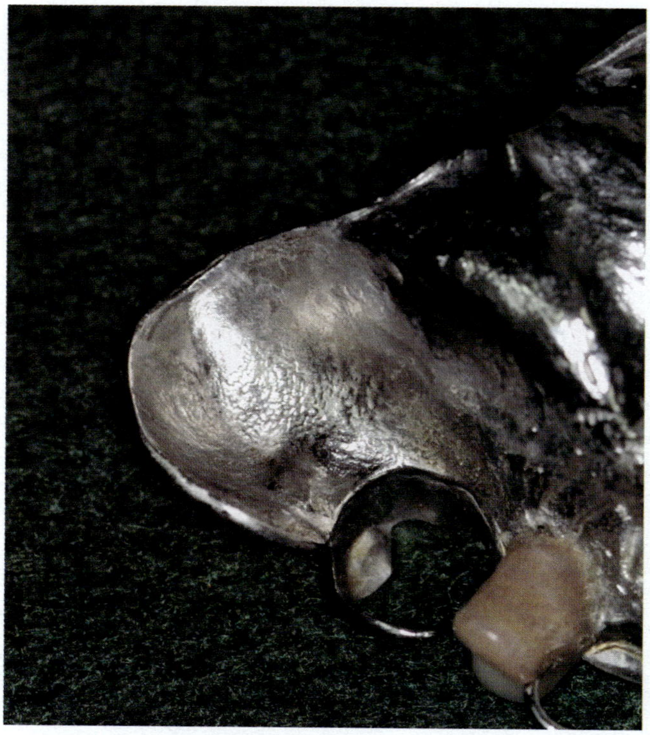

Figure 9-6 Cast distal extension base of maxillary removable partial denture. Cast bases are an integral part of the framework and not only provide support to the prosthetic dentition but reinforce framework rigidity.

to others in accuracy and permanence of form, modern cast alloys are generally superior in this respect. Evidence of this fact is that an additional posterior palatal seal may be eliminated entirely when a cast palate is used for a complete denture, as compared with the need for a definite post-dam when the palate is made of acrylic resin. Distortion of an acrylic resin base is manifest in the maxillary denture by a distortion away from the palate in the midline and toward the tuberosities on the buccal flanges. The greater the curvature of the tissue, the greater is this distortion. Similar distortions occur in a mandibular denture but are more difficult to detect. Accurate metal castings are not subject to distortion by the release of internal strains as are most denture resins.

Because of its accuracy, the metal base provides an intimacy of contact that contributes considerably to the retention of a denture prosthesis. Sometimes called interfacial surface tension, direct retention from a cast denture base is significant in proportion to the involved area. This has been previously mentioned as an important factor in both direct and direct-indirect retention of maxillary restorations. Such intimacy of contact is not possible with acrylic resin bases.

Permanence of form of the cast base is also ensured because of its resistance to abrasion from denture cleaning agents. Cleanliness of the denture base should be stressed; however, constant brushing of the tissue side of the acrylic resin denture base inevitably causes some loss of accuracy by abrasion. Intimacy of contact, which is never as great with an acrylic resin base compared with a metal base, is therefore jeopardized further by cleaning habits. The metal bases, particularly the harder chrome alloys, withstand repeated cleaning without significant changes in surface accuracy.

Comparative Tissue Response

Clinical observations have demonstrated that the inherent cleanliness of the cast metal base contributes to the health of oral tissue when compared with an acrylic resin base. Perhaps some of the reasons for this are the greater density and the bacteriostatic activity contributed by ionization and oxidation of the metal base. Acrylic resin bases tend to accumulate mucinous deposits containing food particles and calcareous deposits. Unfavorable tissue reaction to decomposing food particles, bacterial enzymes, and mechanical irritation from calculus results if the denture is not kept meticulously clean. Although calculus, which must be removed periodically, can precipitate on a cast metal base, other deposits do not accumulate as they do on an acrylic resin base. For this reason a metal base is naturally cleaner than an acrylic resin base.

Thermal Conductivity

Temperature changes are transmitted through the metal base to the underlying tissue, thereby helping to maintain the health of that tissue. Freedom of interchange of temperature between the tissue covered and the surrounding external influences (temperature of liquid, solid foods, and inspired air) contributes much to the patient's acceptance of a denture and may help prevent the feeling of the presence of a foreign body. Conversely, denture acrylic resins have insulating properties that prevent interchange of temperature between the inside and the outside of the denture base.

Weight and Bulk

Metal alloy may be cast much thinner than acrylic resin and still have adequate strength and rigidity. Cast gold must be given slightly more bulk to provide the same amount of rigidity but may still be made with less thickness than acrylic resin materials. Even less weight and bulk are possible when the denture bases are made of chrome or titanium alloys.

There are times, however, when both weight and thickness may be used to advantage in denture bases. In the mandibular arch, the weight of the denture may be an asset in regard to retention, and for this reason a cast gold base may be preferable. On the other hand, extreme loss of residual alveolar bone may make it necessary to add fullness to the denture base to restore normal facial contours and to fill out the buccal vestibule to prevent food from being trapped in the vestibule beneath the denture. In such situations an acrylic resin base may be preferable to the thinner metal base.

In the maxillary arch, an acrylic resin base may be preferable to the thinner metal base to provide fullness in the buccal flanges or to fill a maxillary buccal vestibule. Acrylic resin may also be preferred over the thinner metal base for esthetic reasons. In these instances the thinness of the metal base may be of no advantage, but in areas where the tongue and cheek need maximum room, thinness may be desirable.

Denture base contours for functional tongue and cheek contact can best be accomplished with acrylic resin. Metal bases are usually made thin to minimize bulk and weight, whereas acrylic resin bases may be contoured to provide ideal polished surfaces that contribute to the retention of the denture, restoration of facial contours, and prevention of the accumulation of food at denture borders. Lingual surfaces usually are made concave except in the distal palatal area. Buccal surfaces are made convex at gingival margins, over root prominences, and at the border to fill the area recorded in the impression. Between the border and the gingival contours, the base can be made convex to aid in retention and to facilitate the return of the food bolus to the occlusal table during mastication. Such contours prevent food from being entrapped in the cheek and from working under the denture. This cannot usually be accomplished with metal bases.

However, the advantages of a metal base need not be sacrificed for the sake of esthetics or desirable denture contours when the use of such a base is indicated. Denture bases may be designed to provide almost total metallic coverage yet have resin borders to avoid a display of metal and to add buccal fullness when needed (Figure 9-7). The advantages of thermal conductivity are not necessarily lost by covering a portion of the metal base as long as other parts of the denture are exposed to effect temperature changes through conduction.

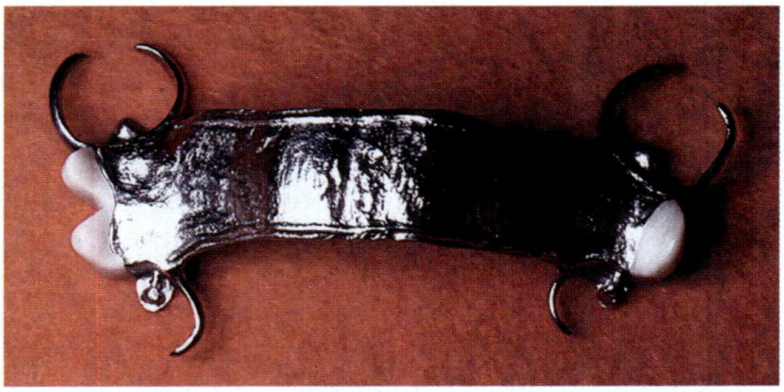

Figure 9-7 Partial metal bases used with palatal strap and resin denture teeth attached directly to the cast metal bases. If needed, a buccal flange of resin could be added to such a base region; however, for these small spans no such flange was needed.

METHODS OF ATTACHING ARTIFICIAL TEETH

Selection of artificial teeth for form, color, and material must precede attachment to the denture. Artificial teeth may be attached to denture bases by the several means that follow: with acrylic resin, with cement, processed directly to metal, cast with the framework, and chemical bonding. Use of acrylic resin to attach artificial teeth to a denture base is the most common method.

Porcelain or Acrylic Resin Artificial Teeth Attached with Acrylic Resin

Artificial porcelain teeth are mechanically retained. The posterior teeth are retained by acrylic resin in their diatoric holes. The anterior porcelain teeth are retained by acrylic resin surrounding their lingually placed retention pins. Artificial resin teeth are retained by a chemical union with the acrylic resin of the denture base, which occurs during laboratory processing procedures.

Attachment of the acrylic resin to the metal base may be accomplished by nailhead retention, retention loops, or diagonal spurs placed at random. Attachment mechanisms should be placed so that they will not interfere with the placement of the teeth on the metal base (see Figure 9-7).

Any junction of acrylic resin with metal should be at an undercut finishing line or should be associated with some retentive undercut. Because only a mechanical attachment exists between metal and acrylic resin, every attempt should be made to prevent separation and seepage, which results in discoloration and uncleanliness. Denture odors are frequently caused by accretions at the junction of the acrylic resin with metal when only a mechanical union exists. Separation occurring between the acrylic resin and metal can eventually lead to some loosening of the acrylic resin base.

Porcelain or Resin Tube Teeth and Facings Cemented Directly to Metal Bases (Figure 9-8)

Some disadvantages of this type of attachment are the difficulties in obtaining satisfactory occlusion, the lack of adequate contours for functional tongue and cheek contact, and the unesthetic display of metal at gingival margins. The latter is prevented when the tooth is butted directly to the residual ridge, but then the retention for the tooth frequently becomes inadequate.

A modification of this method is the attachment of ready-made acrylic resin teeth to the metal base with acrylic resin of the same shade. This is called pressing on a resin tooth and is not the same as using acrylic resin for cementation. It is particularly applicable to anterior replacements, since it is desirable to know in advance of making the casting that the shade and contours of the selected tooth will be acceptable (as was referred to in Figure 9-7). After a labial index of the position of the teeth is made, the lingual portion of the tooth may be cut away or a posthole prepared in the tooth for retention on the casting. Subsequently the tooth is attached to the denture with acrylic resin of the same shade. Because this is done under pressure, the acrylic resin attachment is comparable with the manufactured tooth in hardness and strength.

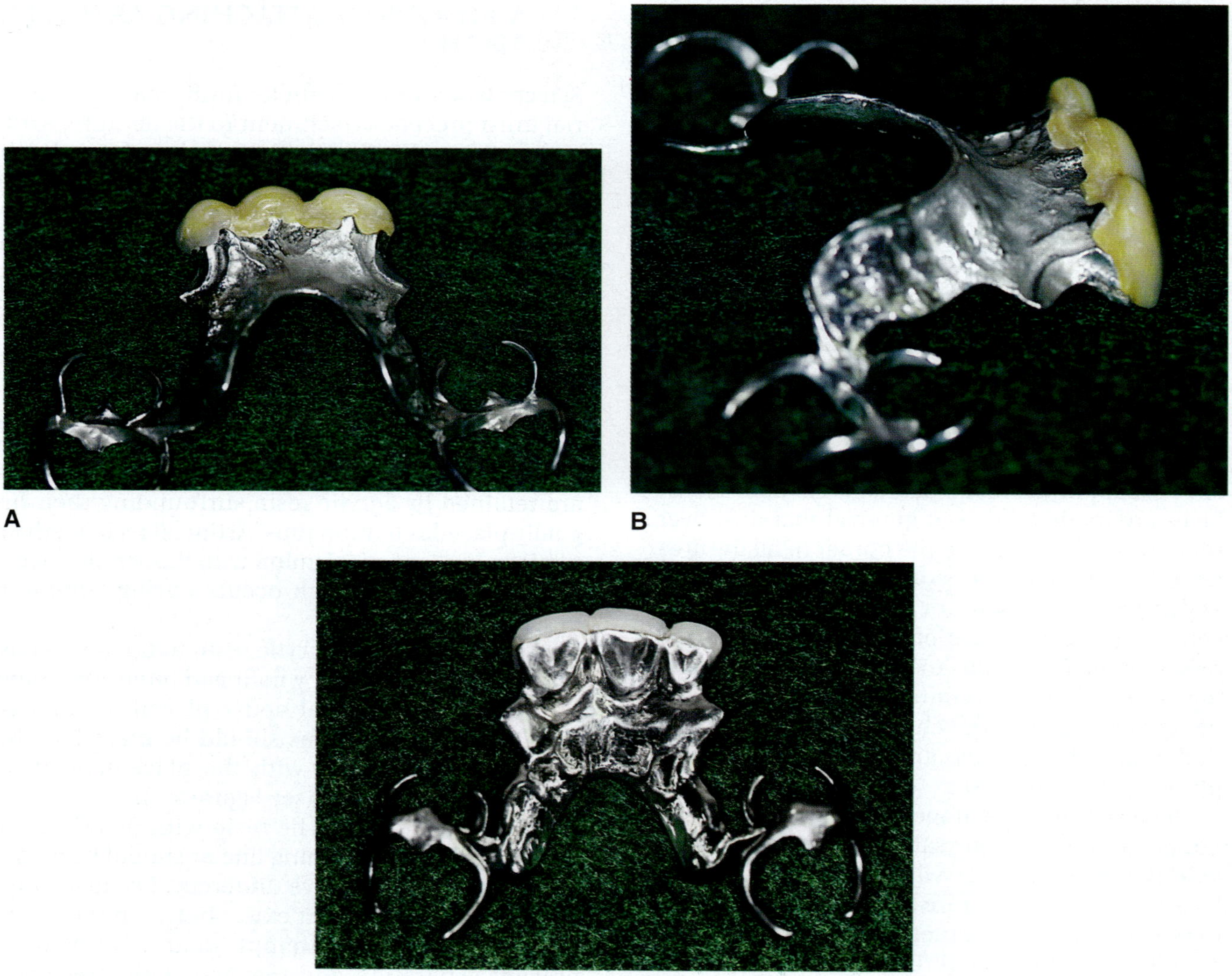

A B C

Figure 9-8 Tissue surface of Class IV removable partial denture in which artificial dentition was added to a metal base. **A,** Teeth were set prior to completion of the framework to allow modification space design to incorporate altered teeth. **B,** Anterior teeth were adjusted to ridge, creating a ridge lap, then framework was waxed to accommodate custom tooth position. **C,** Metal reinforcement adds strength to the artificial teeth and protects against dislodgement.

Tube or side-groove teeth must be selected in advance of waxing the denture framework (Figure 9-9). However, for best occlusal relationships, jaw relation records always should be made with the denture casting in the mouth. This problem may be solved by selecting tube teeth for width but with occlusal surfaces slightly higher than will be necessary. The teeth are ground to fit the ridge with sufficient clearance beneath for a thin metal base and beveled to accommodate a boxing of metal. If an acrylic resin tube tooth is used, the diatoric hole should be made slightly larger. The casting is completed and tried, occlusal relationships are recorded, and then the teeth are ground to harmonious occlusion with the opposing dentition. As is discussed in Chapter 17, artificial posterior teeth on partial dentures can hardly ever be used unaltered but rather should be considered material from which occlusal forms may be created to function harmoniously with the remaining natural occlusion.

Resin Teeth Processed Directly to Metal Bases

Modern cross-linked copolymers enable the dentist or technician to process acrylic resin teeth that have satisfactory hardness and abrasion resistance for many situations. Thus occlusion may be created without resorting to the modification of ready-made artificial teeth (Figure 9-10). Recesses in the denture pattern are either carved by hand or created around manufactured teeth that are used only to form the recess in the pattern. Occlusal relationships may be established in the mouth on the denture framework and transferred to an articulator. The teeth can then be carved and processed in acrylic resin of the proper shade to fit the opposing occlusal record. Better attachment to the metal base than by cementation is thus possible. In addition, unusually long, short, wide, or narrow teeth may be created when necessary to fill spaces not easily filled by the limited selection of commercially available teeth.

Occlusion on acrylic resin teeth may be reestablished to compensate for wear or settling by reprocessing new acrylic resin or using light-activated acrylic resin when this becomes necessary. Distinction always should be made between the need for relining to reestablish occlusion (on a distal extension partial denture) or the need for rebuilding occlusal surfaces on an otherwise satisfactory base (on either a tooth-supported or a tooth- and tissue-supported partial denture).

Reestablishment of occlusion may also be accomplished by placing cast gold or other suitable

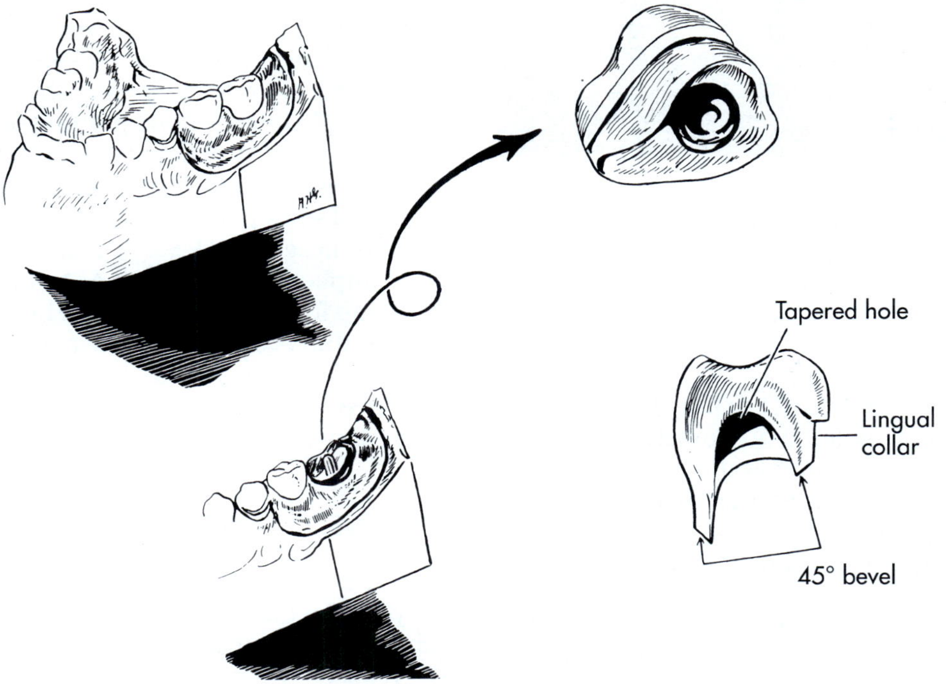

Figure 9-9 Stock porcelain or resin tube tooth, or artificial tooth used as tube tooth, should be ground to accommodate cast coping as illustrated. Hole is drilled from underside of tooth or, if hole is already present, it is made larger. Then tooth is ground to fit ridge with enough clearance for minimum thickness of metal. A 45-degree bevel is then formed around base of tooth, and finally a collar is created on lingual side, extending to interproximal area. Tooth is then lubricated, and wax pattern for denture base is formed around it.

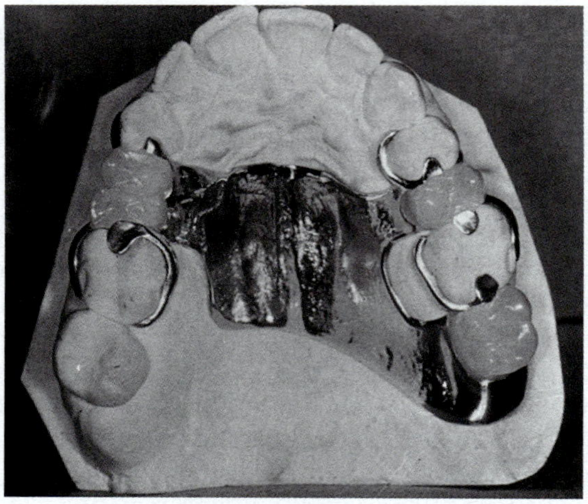

Figure 9-10 Direct attachment of resin teeth to metal bases. These are waxed to fit space and opposing occlusion, then processed or light cured to retention previously provided on metal framework.

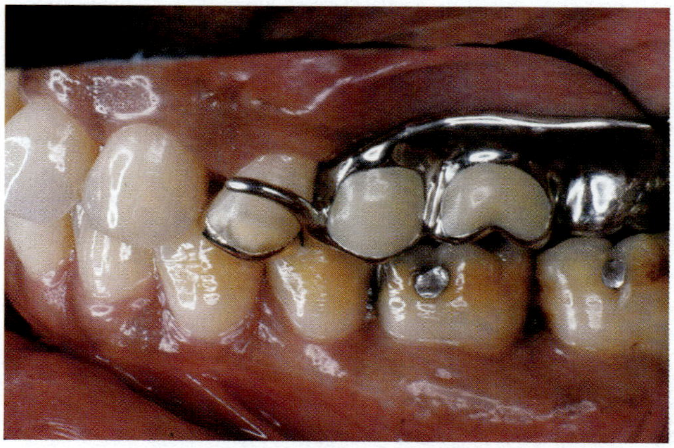

Figure 9-11 Maxillary cast molar designed as integral part of framework. Interocclusal space limitation necessitated using metal rather than another form of artificial posterior teeth. Note overlays on premolar and molar teeth used to resist tooth wear. *(Courtesy Dr. C.J. Andres, Indianapolis, IN.)*

cast alloy restorations on existing resin teeth. Although this may be done on porcelain teeth as well, it is difficult to cut preparations in porcelain teeth unless air abrasive methods are used. Therefore, if later additions to occlusal surfaces are anticipated, acrylic resin teeth should be used, thereby facilitating the addition of new resin or cast gold surfaces. A simple technique to fabricate cast gold occlusal surfaces and attach them to resin teeth is illustrated in Chapter 18.

Metal Teeth

Occasionally a second molar tooth may be replaced as part of the partial denture casting (Figure 9-11). This is usually done when space is too limited for the attachment of an artificial tooth and yet the addition of a second molar is desirable to prevent extrusion of an opposing second molar. Because the occlusal surface must be waxed before casting, perfect occlusion is not possible. Because metal, particularly a chrome alloy, is abrasion resistant, the area of occlusal contact should be held to a minimum to prevent damage to the periodontium of the opposing tooth and the associated discomfort to the patient. Occlusal adjustment on gold occlusal surfaces is readily accomplished, whereas metal teeth made of chrome alloys are difficult to adjust and are objectionably hard for use as occlusal surfaces. Therefore they should be used only to fill a space and to prevent tooth extrusion.

Chemical Bonding

Recent developments in resin bonding have provided a means of direct chemical bonding of acrylic resin to metal frameworks. The investing alveolar and gingival tissue replacement components can be attached without the use of loops, mesh, or surface mechanical locks. Sections of a metal framework that are to support replacement teeth can be roughened with abrasives and then treated with a vaporized silica coating. On this surface, an acrylic resin bonding agent is applied, followed by a thin film of acrylic resin to act as a substrate for later attachment of replacement acrylic resin teeth or for processing of the acrylic resin tissue replacements (Figure 9-12).

A process referred to as tribochemical coating accomplishes a second method of fusing a microscopic layer of ceramic to the metal. This system involves sandblasting the metal framework with a special silica particle material, Rocatec-Plus. Silica from these particles is attached to the framework by impact. A silane is added to this ceramic-like film to form a chemical bond between the silicate layer and the denture base acrylic resin. Denture base acrylic resins formulated with 4-Meta are also available and provide a mechanism of bonding acrylic resin to metal.

NEED FOR RELINING

The distal extension base differs from the tooth-supported base in several respects, one of which is that it must be made of a material that can be relined or rebased when it becomes necessary to reestablish tissue support for the distal extension base. Therefore acrylic resin denture base materials that can be relined are generally used.

Although satisfactory techniques for making distal extension partial denture bases of cast metal are available, the fact that metal bases are difficult if not

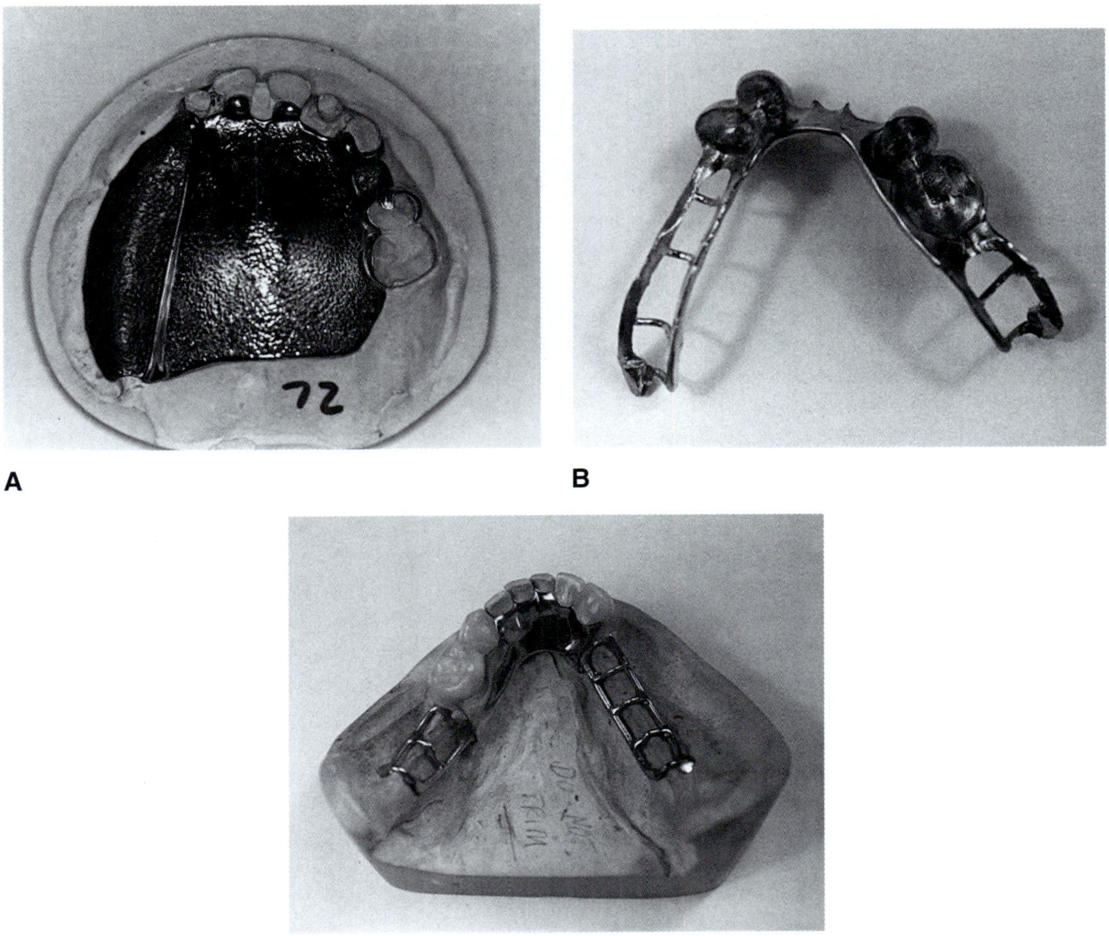

A

B

C

Figure 9-12 Coating of metallic frameworks with vaporized silica facilitates direct application of resin or composite for replacement of basal structures or teeth. **A,** Maxillary metal base silicoated in preparation for addition of replacement teeth. This avoids the need for retentive loops, beads, or meshwork for resin base retention. **B,** Undersurface of removable partial denture fabricated as an overdenture. **C,** Occlusal surface with composite teeth applied directly to silicoated surfaces of the framework, avoiding retention posts or beads and permitting esthetic permanent attachment of the replacement teeth.

impossible to reline limits their use to stable ridges that will change little over a long period.

Loss of support for distal extension bases results from changes in residual ridge form over time. These changes may not be readily visible; however, manifestations can be assessed for this change. One of these is a loss of occlusion between the distal extension denture base and the opposing dentition, increasing as the distance from the abutment increases (Figure 9-13). This change is proved by having the patient close on strips of 28-gauge green casting wax, or any similar wax, and tapping in centric relation only. Indentations in a wax strip of known thickness are quantitative, whereas marks made with articulating ribbon are only qualitative. In other words, indentations in the wax may be interpreted as being light, medium, or heavy, whereas it is difficult if not impossible to interpret a mark made with articulating ribbon as light or heavy. In fact, the heaviest occlusal contact may perforate paper-articulating ribbon and make a lesser mark than areas of lighter contact. Therefore the use of any articulating ribbon is of limited value in checking occlusion intraorally. In making occlusal adjustments, articulating ribbon should be used only to indicate where to relieve after the need for relief has been established by using wax strips of known thickness. For this purpose, 28-gauge green or blue casting wax is generally used, although the thinner 30-gauge or the thicker 26-gauge wax may also be used for better evaluation of the clearance between areas not in contact.

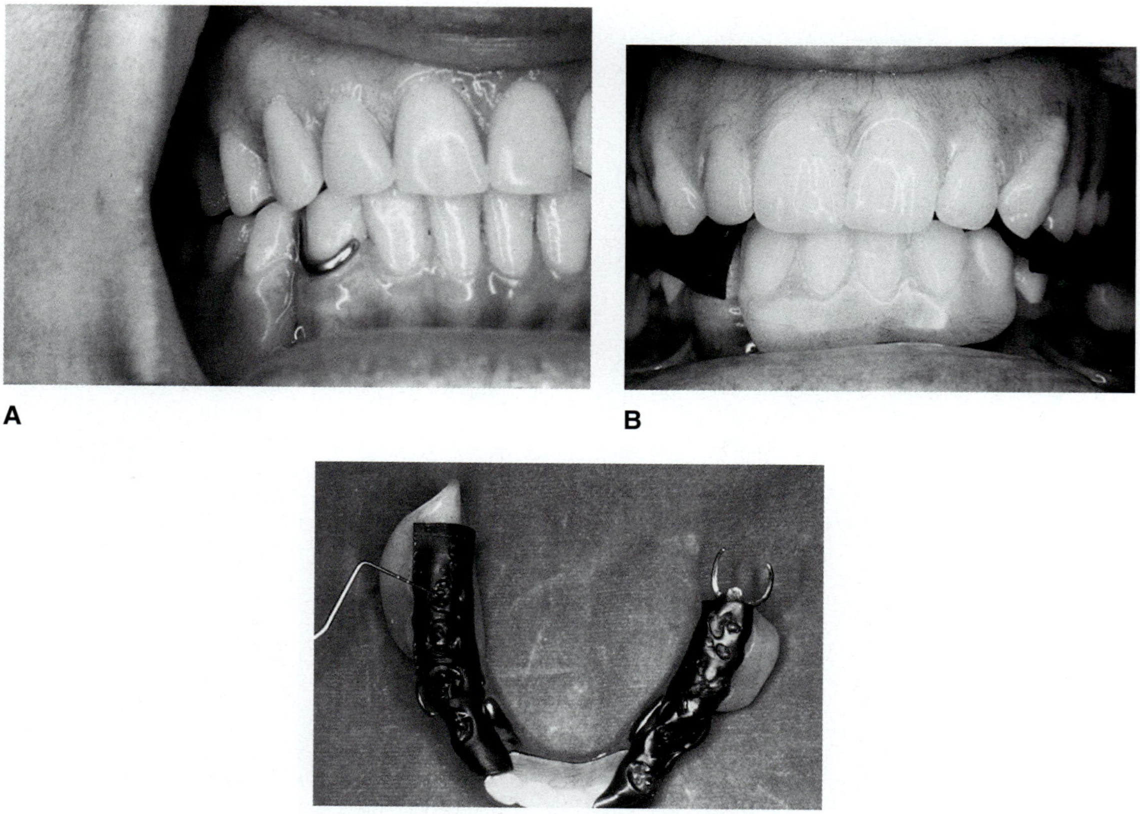

A B C

Figure 9-13 **A,** Distal extension mandibular removable partial denture opposed by maxillary complete denture. There is no contact of opposing posterior teeth. Anterior teeth are in heavy contact at vertical dimension of occlusion. Unless corrected immediately, anterior portion of maxillary residual ridge is destined to undergo rapid resorption. **B,** Another patient with mandibular Class II, mod 2, removable partial denture opposed by maxillary complete denture. Mandibular posterior teeth have been covered with strip(s) of 28-gauge soft green wax, and patient has been assisted in tapping in centric relation. **C,** Mandibular denture is removed, and indentations in interposed wax strips are evaluated. Note relative absence of perforations in wax strips by opposing posterior teeth. Relining and correction of occlusal discrepancies are needed based on this record.

Loss of support for a distal extension base will result in a loss of occlusal contact between the prosthetically supplied teeth and the opposing dentition and a return to heavy occlusal contact between the remaining natural teeth. Usually this is an indication that relining is needed to reestablish the original occlusion by reestablishing supporting contact with the residual ridge. It must be remembered, however, that occlusion on a distal extension base is sometimes maintained at the expense of extrusion of the opposing natural teeth. In such a situation, checking the occlusion alone will not show that settling of the extension base has occurred, because changes in the supporting ridge may have also taken place.

A second manifestation of change also must be observable to justify relining. This second manifestation of change in the supporting ridge is evidence of rotation about the fulcrum line with the indirect retainers lifting from their seats as the distal extension base is pressed against the ridge tissue (Figure 9-14). Originally, if the distal extension base was made to fit the supporting form of the residual ridge, rotation about the fulcrum line is not visible. At the time the denture is initially placed, no anteroposterior rotational movement should exist when alternating finger pressure is applied to the indirect retainer and the distal end of a distal extension base or bases. After changes in the ridge form, which cause some loss of support, rotation occurs about the fulcrum line when alternating finger pressure is applied. This is evidence of changes in the supporting ridge that must be compensated for by relining or rebasing.

If occlusal contact has been lost and rotation about the fulcrum line is evident, relining is indicated. On

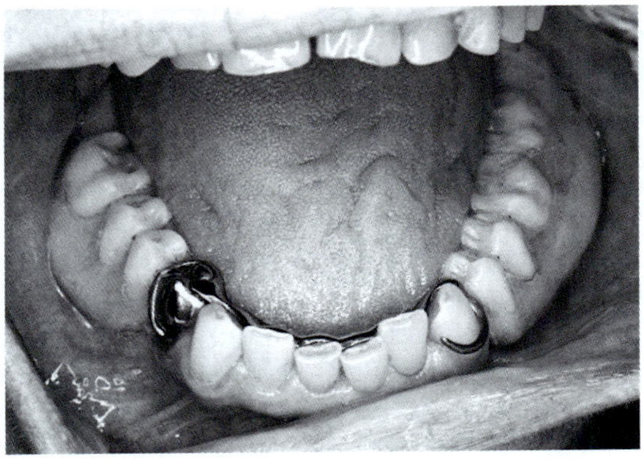

A

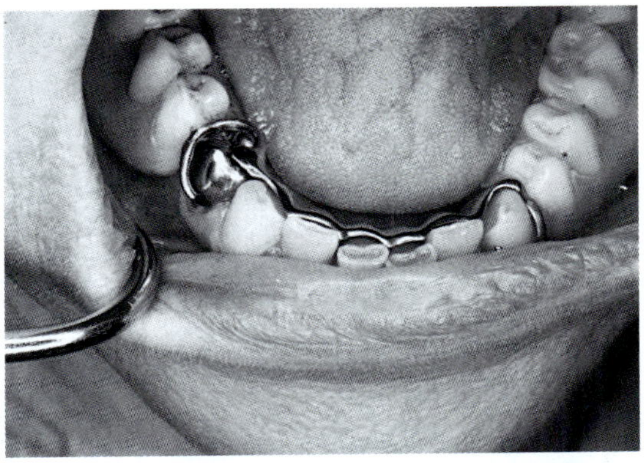

B

Figure 9-14 **A,** Superior border of linguoplate major connector and rests appear to be in their planned relationships to remaining natural teeth in absence of occlusal load. **B,** Slight pressure on denture base activates direct retainers and elevates superior border of linguoplate, resulting in lack of planned contact. If the linguoplate does not immediately return to its designed position when the pressure on the denture base is removed, the denture bases should be relined to reestablish adequate base support by residual ridges.

the other hand, if occlusal contact has been lost without any evidence of denture rotation and if stability of the denture base is otherwise satisfactory, reestablishing the occlusion is the remedy rather than relining. For the latter, the original denture base may be used in much the same manner as the original trial base was used to record occlusal relation. Teeth may then be reoccluded to an opposing cast or to an occlusal template by using light-activated, tooth-colored acrylic resin; tooth-colored composite; cast occlusal surfaces; or new teeth. In any event a new occlusion should be established on the existing bases. Relining in this instance would be the wrong solution to the problem.

Loss of support may also be assessed clinically by other methods. A layer of rather free-flowing irreversible hydrocolloid, wax, or a tissue-conditioning material can be spread on the basal seat portion of the dried denture base(s), and the restoration returned to the patient's mouth. Care is exercised to ensure that the framework is correctly seated (rests and indirect retainers in planned positions). The restoration is removed when the material has set. Notable thickness of material remaining under the bases indicates a lack of intimate contact of the bases with the residual ridges, suggesting a need for relining.

More often, however, loss of occlusion is accompanied by settling of the denture base to the extent that rotation about the fulcrum line is manifest. Because relining is the only remedy short of making completely new bases, use of an acrylic resin base originally facilitates later relining. For this reason, acrylic resin bases are generally preferred for distal extension partial dentures.

The question remains as to when, if ever, metal bases with their several advantages may be used for distal extension partial dentures. It is debatable as to what type of ridge will most likely remain stable under functional loading without apparent change. Certainly the age and general health of the patient will influence the ability of a residual ridge to support function. Minimum and harmonious occlusion, and the accuracy with which the base fits the underlying tissue, will influence the amount of trauma that will occur under function. The absence of trauma plays a big part in the ability of the ridge to maintain its original form.

The best indication for the use of metal distal extension bases is a ridge that has supported a previous partial denture without having become narrowed or flat, or without consisting primarily of easily displaceable tissue. When such changes have occurred under a previous denture, further change may be anticipated because of the possibility that the oral tissues in question are not capable of supporting a denture base without further change. Despite every advantage in their favor, there are some individuals whose ridges respond unfavorably when called on to support any denture base.

In other instances, such as when a new partial denture is to be made because of the loss of additional teeth, the ridges may still be firm and healthy. Because the ridges have previously supported a denture base and have sustained occlusion, bony trabeculae will have become arranged to best support vertical and horizontal loading, cortical bone may have been formed, and tissue will have become favorable for continued support of a denture base.

There are relatively few situations in which the need for relining a distal extension base is not anticipated and metal bases may be considered. There are, however, many instances that may be considered borderline. In these, metal bases may be used with the full understanding on the part of the patient that a new denture may become necessary if unforeseen tissue changes occur. A technique is given in Figure 9-6 that permits replacing metal distal extension bases without having to remake the entire denture. This method should be seriously considered any time a distal extension partial denture is to be made with a metal base or bases.

For reasons previously outlined, the possibility that tissue will remain healthier beneath a metal base than it will beneath an acrylic resin base may justify wider use of metal bases for distal extension partial dentures. Through careful treatment planning, better patient education of the problems involved in making a distal extension base partial denture, and greater care taken in the fabrication of the denture bases, metal may be used to advantage in some situations in which acrylic resin bases are ordinarily used.

STRESS-BREAKERS (STRESS EQUALIZERS)

The previous chapters describing component parts of a partial denture have presumed absolute rigidity of all parts of the partial denture framework except the retentive arm of the direct retainer. All vertical and horizontal forces applied to the artificial teeth are thus distributed throughout the supporting portions of the dental arch. Broad distribution of stress is accomplished through the rigidity of the major and minor connectors. The effect of the stabilizing components is also made possible by the rigidity of the connectors.

In distal extension situations, the use of a rigid connection between the denture base and supporting teeth must account for the base movement without causing either tooth or tissue damage. For such situations, stress on the abutment teeth and residual ridge is minimized through the use of functional basing, broad coverage, harmonious occlusion, and correct choice of direct retainers. Generally, two major types of clasp assemblies are used for distal extensions because of their stress-breaking design. Retentive clasp arms may be cast only if they engage undercuts on the abutment teeth in such a manner that tissueward movement of the extension base transmits only minimum leverage to the abutment. Otherwise, tapered, wrought-wire retentive clasp arms should be used because of their greater flexibility. The tapered, round wrought-wire clasp arm acts somewhat as a stress-breaker between the denture base and the abutment tooth by reducing the effect of the denture base movement on the tooth through its flexibility.

Another concept of stress-breaking exists that insists on separating the action of the retaining elements from the movement of the denture base by allowing independent movement of the denture base (or its supporting framework) and the direct retainers. This form of stress-breaker, also referred to as a stress equalizer, has been used as a means to compensate for inappropriately designed removable partial dentures. Figures 9-15 through 9-21 provide examples of some of the more commonly used stress-breakers.

Regardless of their design, most stress-breakers effectively dissipate vertical stresses, which is the purpose for which they are used. However, this is at the expense of the horizontal stability and the harmful effects of reduced horizontal stability

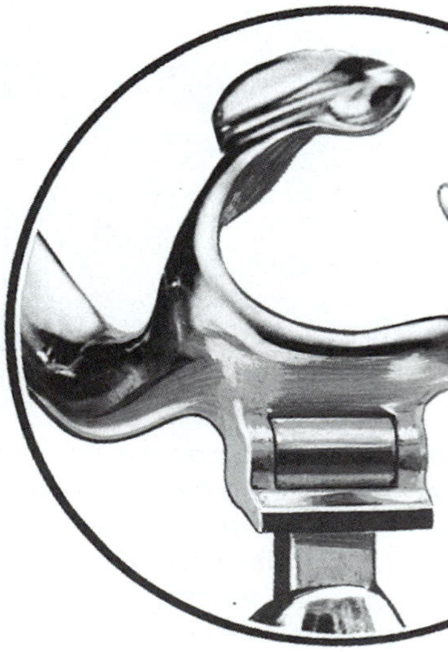

Figure 9-15 D-E hinge-type stress-breaker using vertical stop to limit movement of denture base away from tissues. Trummion design of stress-breaker also prevents lateral movement. *(Courtesy Austenal, Inc., Chicago, IL.)*

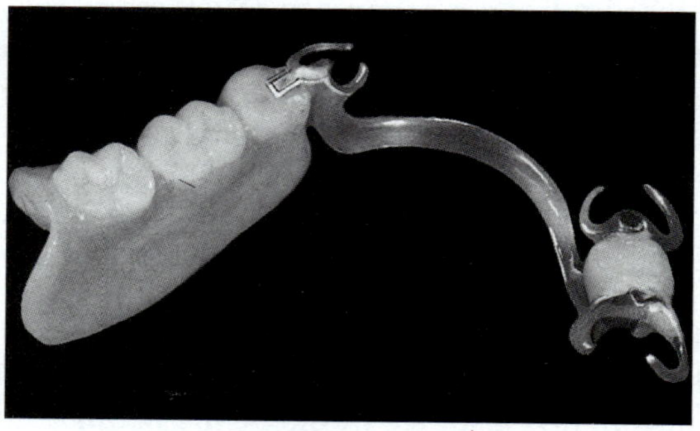

Figure 9-16 Kennedy Class II, modification 1, removable partial denture using hinge stress-breaker of *Baca* design. Hinge and vertical movements are permitted by fact that action is protected by metal sleeve. *(Courtesy Ticonium Division of CMP Industries, Inc., Albany, NY.)*

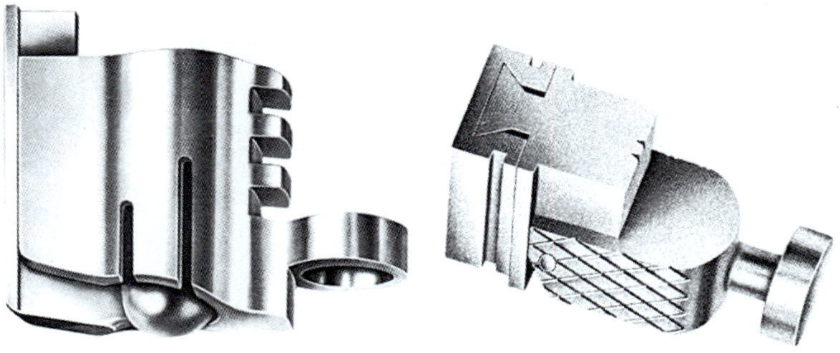

A B

Figure 9-17 **A,** *Dalbo* extracoronal retainer. Limited vertical and hinge movements of denture base are permitted by sleeve-and-spring design of retainer. **B,** *Crismani* intracoronal retainer design permits limited vertical movement of denture base.

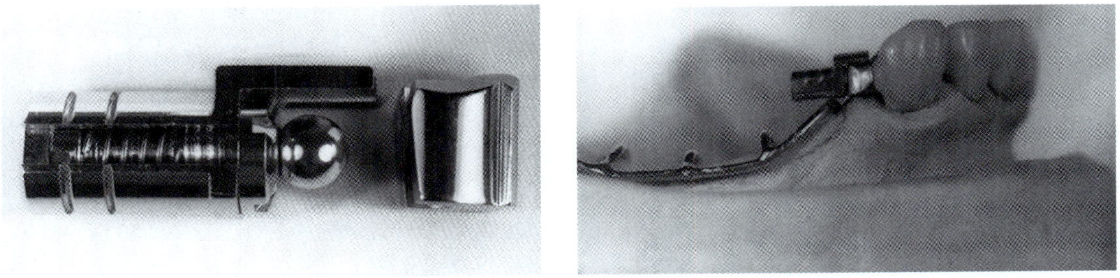

A B

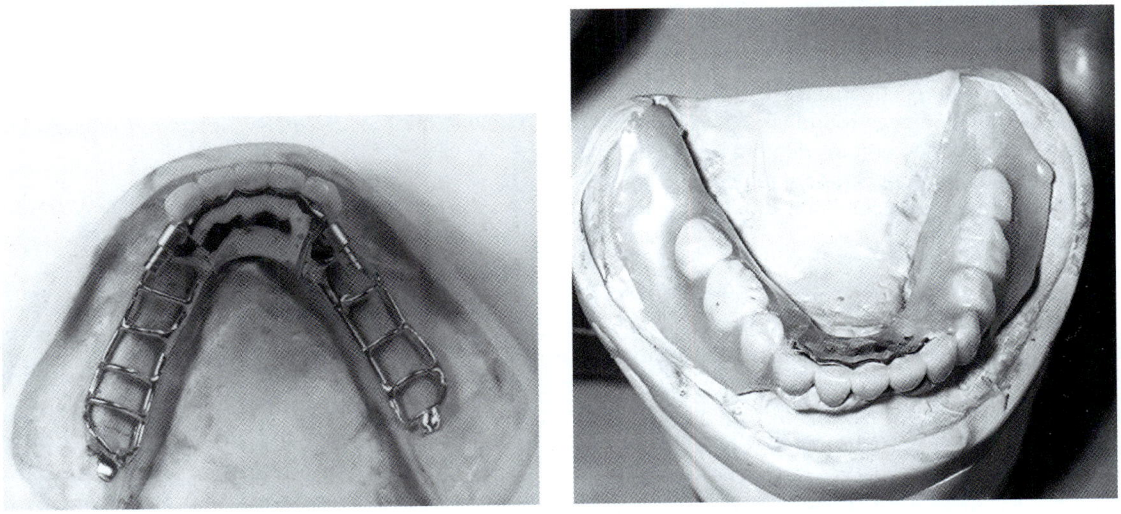

C D

Figure 9-18 Retainers designed to distribute stresses are sometimes selected for use with long distal extension bases. **A,** *ASC-52* retainer is illustrated with a cutaway in the cylinder to reveal a spring-loaded shaft that permits flexion and rebound. Ball portion fits into the female receptacle and is movable in all directions. **B,** Assembled *ASC-52* retainer. Female portion is cast to the canine abutment. Cylinder will be contained within the resin base. **C,** Occlusal view of framework and abutments on cast. Note that the cylinders are parallel to the alveolar ridge-bearing area so that occlusal stresses will not cause torque on the abutments. **D,** Removable partial denture with wax-up bases and replacement teeth, containing the *ASC-52* attachment. Absence of visible clasps enhances esthetics.

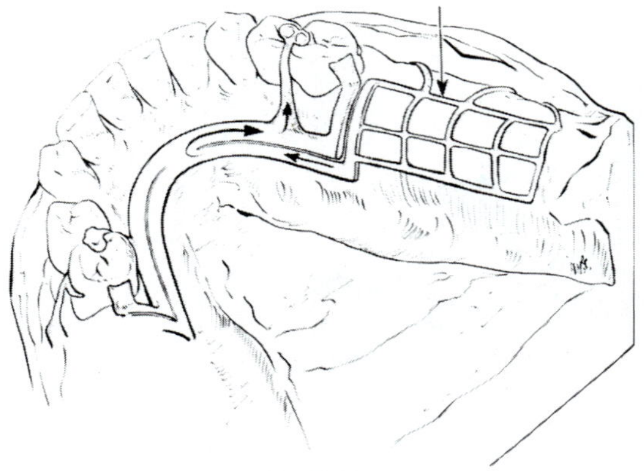

Figure 9-19 Stress-breaking effect of split bar major connector. Vertical and diagonal forces *(arrow)* applied to tissue-supported base must pass anteriorly along lower bar and then back along more rigid upper bar to reach abutment tooth. Thus tipping forces that would otherwise be transmitted directly to abutment tooth are supposedly dissipated by flexibility of lower bar and distance traveled.

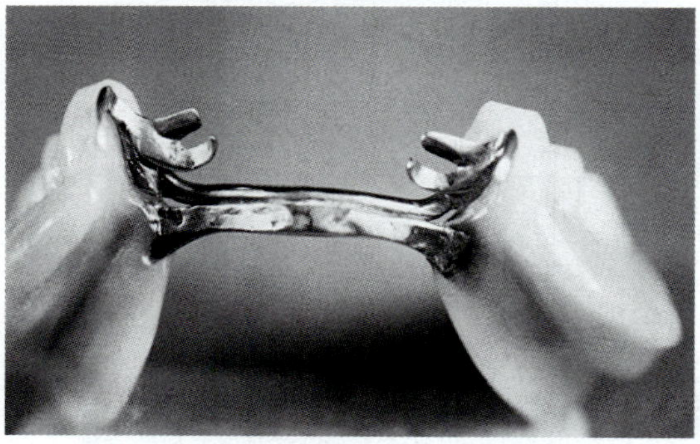

Figure 9-20 Early type of stress equalizer. The direct retainers (clasps) are connected by 16-gauge round wrought wire. Inferiorly placed cast major connector joins denture bases. Heavy wrought wire and cast major connector are joined with solder at midline only. Need for indirect retention still exists even though stress equalizer is used.

(excessive ridge resorption, tissue impingement, and inefficient mastication), which far outweigh the benefits of vertical stress breaking. It is the rigid nature of the more conventional removable partial denture that allows satisfaction of all requirements of support, stability, and retention without overemphasis on only one principle to the detriment of the oral tissue.

The student is referred to two textbooks that describe in detail the use of stress-breakers and articulated partial denture designs: *Precision Attachments in Dentistry,* ed. 3, by H.W. Preiskel; and *Theory and Practice of Precision Attachment Removable Partial Dentures,* by J.L. Baker and R.J. Goodkind.

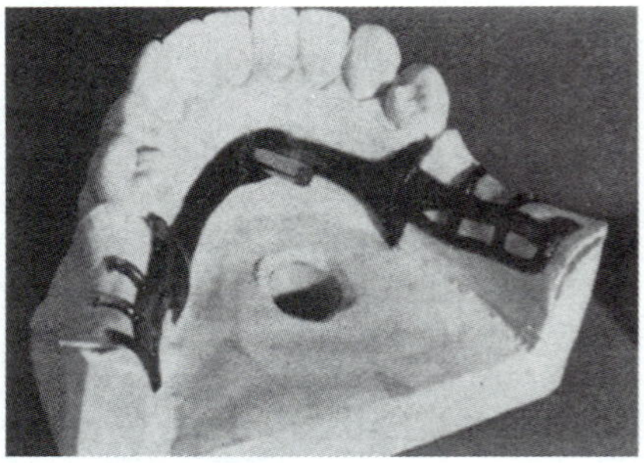

A

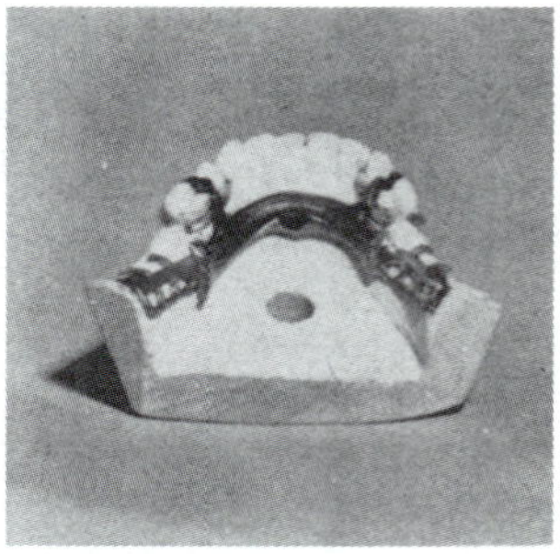

B

Figure 9-21 *Ticonium Hidden-Lock* removable partial denture. **A,** Lower half of framework, consisting of lower half of lingual bar and denture base retainer, is cast first with bi-bevel circle formed in wax pattern by waxing around lightly oiled mandrel, which is removed to provide perfect circle within wax. This half is cast as illustrated. **B,** On second investment cast, original bar is replaced and remainder of framework is waxed to it. This portion consists of clasps, indirect retainers, and remainder of bar. *Hidden L lock* and split bar are made possible because of thin oxide shell that forms during second casting, leaving an almost imperceptible junction line between two sections. Hinge movement occurs at circle in midline. *(Courtesy Ticonium Company, Albany, NY.)*

SELF-ASSESSMENT AIDS

1. What is a denture base?
2. What does the term basal seat mean?
3. Is the primary purpose of a denture base related to masticatory function? If so, how?
4. Describe how the denture base contributes to the factor of appearance.
5. Are the functions of tooth-supported and extension-type bases somewhat different? If so, how do they differ?
6. What are the functions of a tooth-supported partial denture base?
7. Describe the functions of a distal extension partial denture base.
8. The space available for a denture base is controlled by the structures surrounding the space and their movements during function. True or false?

9. Explain the **snowshoe principle** as it applies to denture base design.
10. By what means is an acrylic resin base attached to a framework?
11. A ladderlike minor connector is used to attach an acrylic resin base to frameworks. Should this minor connector be rigid or flexible? Why or why not?
12. Is it important that a minor connector for an extension type of acrylic resin base be located on both the buccal and lingual sides of the residual ridge? Explain.
13. Is an open ladder type of design for connecting an acrylic resin base to a major connector preferable to a closed meshwork design? Why?
14. Give a rule of thumb for how far the minor connector attaching the resin base to the major connector should extend posteriorly.
15. The minor connector for acrylic resin bases must be totally embedded in the acrylic resin base. What thickness of acrylic resin is necessary between the residual ridge and minor connector to allow adjustment of the base if it should become necessary?
16. Nine requirements for an ideal denture base are given in this chapter. List six of them.
17. Metal bases have distinct advantages over acrylic resin bases, such as thermal conductivity and accuracy and permanence of form. What are the other advantages?
18. What are the indications and contraindications for metal bases?
19. Can denture base contours for functional cheek and tongue contact best be accomplished with acrylic resin or metal? Why?
20. Relining of extension bases becomes necessary to reestablish support of the base. Could this be a factor in selecting the material for a denture base? Explain.
21. How can it be determined when a denture base requires relining?
22. What is meant by the word *stress-breaker* in removable partial prosthodontics?
23. By what means can the action of the retaining elements of a stress-breaker be separated from movements of the extension base?
24. Stress-breakers may be divided into two broad groups. Give two examples of each group.

10

PRINCIPLES OF REMOVABLE PARTIAL DENTURE DESIGN

DIFFERENCE IN PROSTHESIS SUPPORT AND THE INFLUENCE ON DESIGN

Some of the biomechanical considerations of removable partial denture design were presented in Chapter 4. The strategy of selecting component parts for a partial denture to help control the movement of the prosthesis under functional load has been highlighted as a method to consider for logical partial denture design. The requirements for movement control are generally functions of whether the prosthesis will be tooth supported or tooth-tissue supported.

For a tooth-supported prosthesis, the movement potential is less because teeth provide resistance to functional loading. Teeth do not vary widely in ability to provide this support; consequently, designs for prostheses are less variable. This is the case even though the amount of supporting bone, crown/root ratios, crown and root morphologies, and tooth number and position in the arch relative to edentulous spaces are well established and may be variables for both tooth and tooth-tissue-supported removable partial dentures. For a tooth-tissue-supported prosthesis, the residual ridge (remaining alveolar bone and overlying connective tissue covered with mucosa) presents a quite variable potential for support. Not only does the underlying alveolar bone demonstrate a highly variable form following extraction, it continues to change with time. As alveolar bone responds to the loss of teeth, the overlying connective tissue and mucosa undergo change that places the soft tissue at risk for pressure-induced inflammatory changes. This variable tissue support potential adds complexity to design considerations when dealing with tooth-tissue-supported prostheses. This is because unlike the efficient support provided by teeth, which results in limited prosthesis movement, the reaction of the ridge tissue to functional forces can be highly variable, leading to variable amounts of prosthesis movement. An understanding of the potential sources of functional force from the opposing arch, which can have an effect on the movement potential of a prosthesis, is helpful.

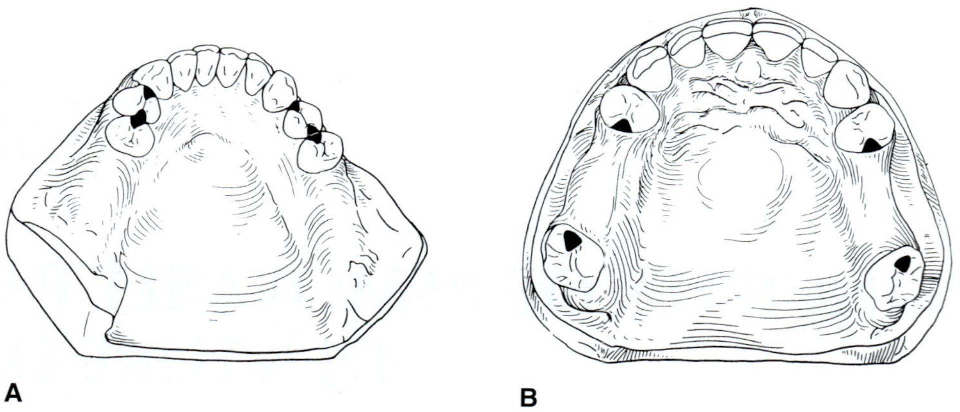

Figure 10-1 **A,** Kennedy Class I partially edentulous arch. Major support for denture bases must come from residual ridges, tooth support from occlusal rests being effective only at anterior portion of each base. **B,** Kennedy Class III, mod 1, partially edentulous arch, which provides total tooth support for prosthesis. Removable partial denture made for this arch is totally supported by rests on properly prepared occlusal rest seats on four abutment teeth.

Factors related to the opposing arch tooth position, the existence and nature of prosthesis support in the opposing arch, and the potential for establishing a harmonious occlusion can greatly influence the partial denture design. Opposing tooth positions that apply forces outside the primary support of the prosthesis can introduce leverage forces that act to dislodge the prosthesis. Such an effect is variable based on the nature of the opposing occlusion since the forces of occlusion differ between natural teeth, removable partial dentures, and complete dentures. In general, removable partial dentures opposing natural teeth will require greater support and stabilization over time because of the greater functional load demands. Therefore occlusal relationships at maximum intercuspation should be broadly dissipated to the supporting units.

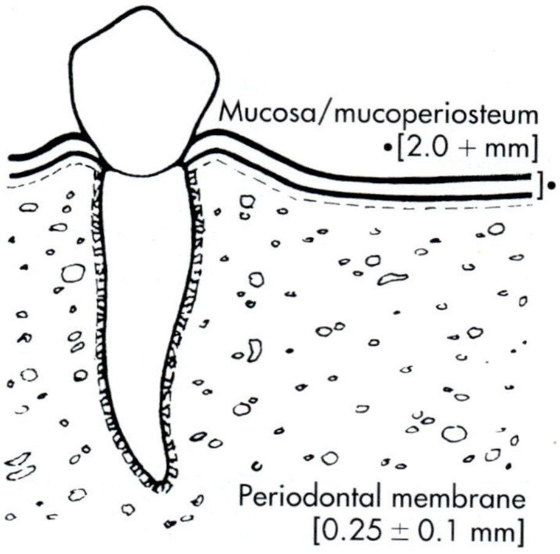

Figure 10-2 Distortion of tissues over edentulous ridge will be approximately 500 μm under 4 newtons of force, whereas abutment teeth will demonstrate approximately 20 μm of intrusion under the same load.

DIFFERENTIATION BETWEEN TWO MAIN TYPES OF REMOVABLE PARTIAL DENTURES

Based on the previous discussion, it is clear that two distinctly different types of removable partial dentures exist. Certain points of difference are present between the Kennedy Class I and Class II types of partial dentures on the one hand and the Class III type of partial denture on the other. The first consideration is the manner in which each is supported. The Class I type and the distal extension side of the Class II type derive their primary support from the tissue underlying the base and secondary support from the abutment teeth (Figures 10-1, *A* and 10-2). The Class III type derives all of its support from the abutment teeth (Figures 10-1, *B* and 10-2).

Second, for reasons directly related to the manner of support, the method of impression registration and jaw record required for each type will vary.

Third, the need for some kind of indirect retention exists in the distal extension type of partial denture, whereas in the tooth-supported, Class III type there is no extension base to lift away from the supporting tissue because of the action of sticky foods and movement of the tissue of the mouth against borders of the denture. This is because a direct retainer on an abutment tooth secures each end of each denture base. Therefore the tooth-supported partial denture does not rotate about a fulcrum as does the distal extension partial denture.

Fourth, the manner in which the distal extension type of partial denture is supported often necessitates the use of a base material that can be relined to compensate for tissue changes. Acrylic resin is generally used as a base material for distal extension bases. The Class III partial denture, on the other hand, being entirely tooth supported, does not require relining except when it is advisable to eliminate an unhygienic, unesthetic, or uncomfortable condition resulting from loss of tissue contact. Metal bases therefore are more frequently used in tooth-supported restorations, since relining is not as likely to be necessary with them.

Differences in Support

The distal extension partial denture derives its major support from the residual ridge with its fibrous connective tissue covering. The length and contour of the residual ridge notably influence the amount of available support and stability (Figure 10-3). Some areas of this residual ridge are firm, with limited displaceability—whereas other areas are displaceable, depending on the thickness and structural character of the tissue overlying the residual alveolar bone. The movement of the base under function determines the occlusal efficiency of the partial denture and also the degree to which the abutment teeth are subjected to torque and tipping stresses.

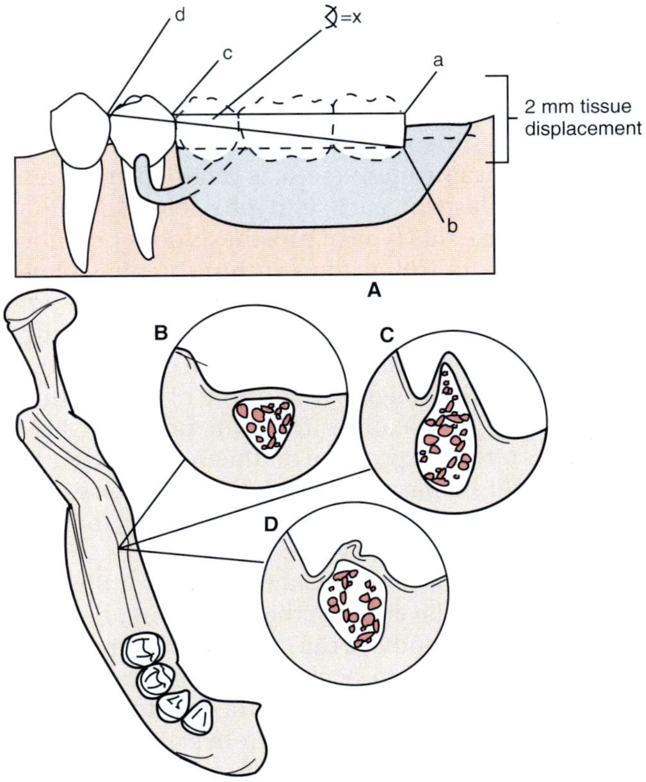

Figure 10-3 **A,** The longer the edentulous area covered by the denture base, the greater the potential lever action on the abutment teeth. If extension base area is 30 mm (ac) and tissue displacement is 2 mm (ab), the amount of movement of the proximal plate on the guiding plane will be approximately 0.25 mm: [$\alpha = \sqrt{(ab)^2 + (ac)^2}$]; arc of the tangent ab/ad = x/cd (2/30 = x/3.75 = 0.25 mm). **B,** Flat ridge will provide good support, poor stability. **C,** Sharp spiny ridge will provide poor support, poor to fair stability. **D,** Displaceable tissue on ridge will provide poor support and poor stability.

Impression Registration

An impression registration for the fabrication of a partial denture must fulfill the following two requirements:

1. The anatomic form and the relationship of the remaining teeth in the dental arch and the surrounding soft tissue must be recorded accurately so that the denture will not exert pressure on those structures beyond their physiological limits. A type of impression material that can be removed from undercut areas without permanent distortion must be used to fulfill this requirement. The elastic impression materials, such as irreversible hydrocolloid (alginate), mercaptan rubber base (Thiokol), silicone impression materials (both condensation and addition reaction), and the polyethers are best suited for this purpose.
2. The supporting form of the soft tissue underlying the distal extension base of the partial denture should be recorded so that firm areas are used as primary stress-bearing areas and readily displaceable tissues are not overloaded. Only in this way can maximum support be obtained for the partial denture base. An impression material capable of displacing tissue sufficiently to register the supporting form of the ridge will fulfill this second requirement. A fluid mouth-temperature wax or any of the readily flowing impression materials (rubber base, silicones, or polyethers in an individual, corrected tray) may be employed for registering the supporting form. Zinc oxide-eugenol paste can also be used when only the extension base area is involved in the impression (see Chapter 15).

No single impression material can satisfactorily fulfill both of the previously mentioned requirements. Recording the anatomic form of both teeth and supporting tissue will result in inadequate support for the distal extension base. This is because the cast will not represent the optimum coordinating forms, which necessitates that the ridge be related to the teeth in a supportive form. This coordination of support maximizes the support capacity for the arch and minimizes movement of the partial denture under function.

Differences in Clasp Design

A fifth point of difference between the two main types of removable partial dentures lies in their requirements for direct retention.

The tooth-supported partial denture, being totally supported by abutment teeth, is retained and stabilized by a clasp at each end of each edentulous space. Because this type of prosthesis does not move under function, (other than within the physiological limitations of the tooth support units) the only requirement of such clasps is that they flex sufficiently during placement and removal of the denture to pass over the height of contour of the teeth in approaching or escaping from an undercut area. During its terminal position on the tooth, a retentive clasp should be passive and should not flex except when engaging the undercut area of the tooth to resist a vertical dislodging force.

Cast retentive arms are generally used for this purpose. These may be either of the circumferential type, arising from the body of the clasp and approaching the undercut from an occlusal direction, or of the bar type, arising from the base of the denture and approaching the undercut area from a gingival direction. Each of these two types of cast clasps has its advantages and disadvantages.

In the combination tooth- and tissue-supported removable partial dentures, because of the anticipated functional movement of the distal extension base, the direct retainer adjacent to the distal extension base must perform still another function in addition to that of resisting vertical displacement. Because of the lack of tooth support distally, the denture base will move tissueward under function proportionate to the quality (displaceability) of the supporting soft tissue, the accuracy of the denture base, and the total occlusal load applied. Because of this tissueward movement, those elements of a clasp that lie in an undercut area mesial to the fulcrum for a distal extension (as is often seen with a distal rest) must be able to flex sufficiently to dissipate stresses that otherwise would be transmitted directly to the abutment tooth as leverage. On the other hand, a clasp used in conjunction with a mesial rest may not transmit as much stress to the abutment tooth because of the reduction in leverage forces, which results from a change in the fulcrum position. This serves the purpose of reducing or "breaking" the stress, hence the term *stress-breakers*, and is a strategy often incorporated into the partial denture designs using various means. Some dentists strongly believe that a stress-breaker is the best means of preventing leverage from being transmitted to the abutment teeth. Others believe just as strongly that a wrought-wire or bar-type retentive arm more effectively accomplishes this purpose with greater simplicity and ease of application. A retentive clasp arm made of wrought wire can flex more readily in all directions than can the cast half-round clasp arm. Thereby, it may more effectively dissipate those stresses that would otherwise be transmitted to the abutment tooth. A discussion of the limitations of stress-breakers has been presented in Chapter 9.

Only the retentive arm of the circumferential clasp, however, should be made of wrought metal. Reciprocation and stabilization against lateral and torquing movement must be obtained through the use of the rigid cast elements, which make up the remainder of the clasp. This is called a *combination clasp*, because it is a combination of both cast and wrought materials incorporated into one direct retainer. It is frequently used on the terminal abutment for the distal extension partial denture and is indicated where a mesiobuccal but no distobuccal undercut exists or where a gross tissue undercut, cervical and buccal to the abutment tooth, exists. It must always be remembered that the factors of length and material contribute to the flexibility of clasp arms. From a materials physical property standpoint, a short wrought-wire arm may be a destructive element because of its reduced ability to flex compared with a longer wrought-wire arm. However, in addition to its greater flexibility compared with the cast circumferential clasp, the combination clasp has further advantages of adjustability, minimum tooth contact, and better esthetics, which justify its occasional use in tooth-supported designs.

The amount of stress transferred to the supporting edentulous ridge(s) and the abutment teeth will depend on: (1) the direction and magnitude of the force; (2) the length of the denture base lever arm(s); (3) the quality of resistance (support from the edentulous ridges and remaining natural teeth); and (4) the design characteristics of the partial denture. As stated in Chapter 7, the location of the rest, the design of the minor connector as it relates to its corresponding guiding plane, and the location of the retentive arm are all factors that influence how a clasp system functions. The greater the surface area contact of each minor connector to its corresponding guiding plane, the more horizontal the distribution of force (Figure 10-4).

ESSENTIALS OF PARTIAL DENTURE DESIGN

Design of the partial denture framework should be systematically developed and outlined on an accurate diagnostic cast based on the following prosthesis concepts: where the prosthesis is supported, how the support is connected, how the prosthesis is retained, how the retention and support are connected, and how the edentulous base support is connected.

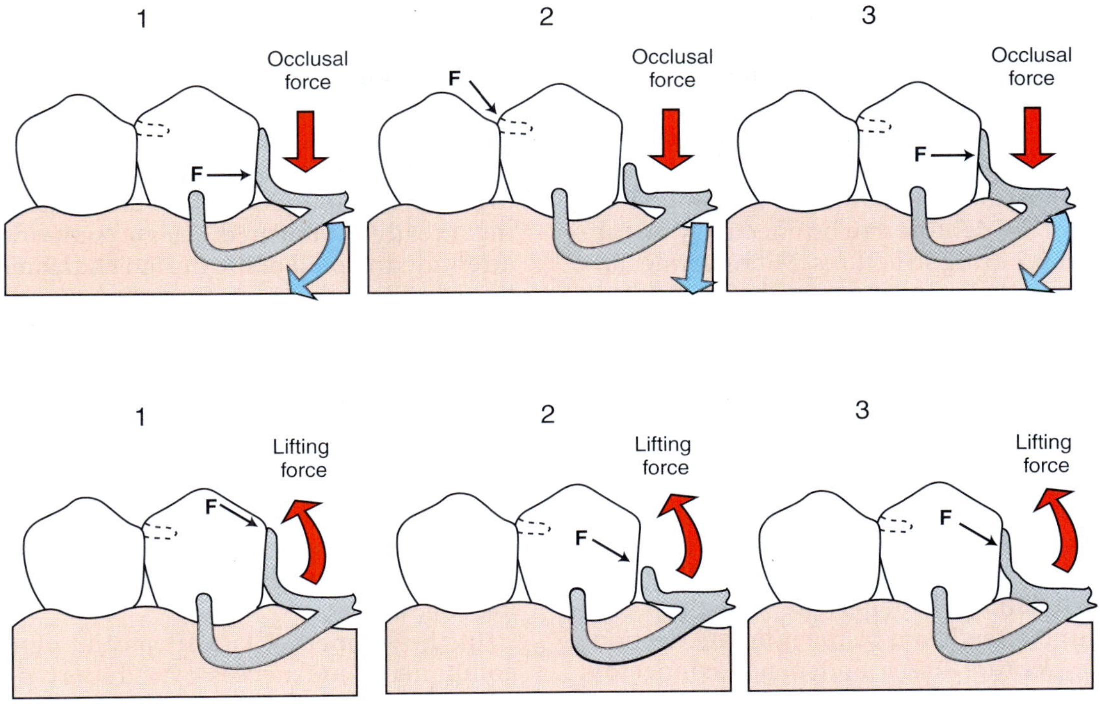

Figure 10-4 *1,* Maximum contact of proximal plate minor connector with guiding plane produces more horizontal distribution of stress to the abutment teeth. *2,* Minimum contact or disengagement of minor connector with guiding plane allows rotation around fulcrum located on mesio-occlusal rest, producing more vertical distribution of stress to ridge area. *3,* Minor connector contact with guiding plane from marginal ridge to junction of middle and gingival thirds of abutment tooth distributes load vertically to ridge and horizontally to abutment tooth. *F* is the location of the fulcrum of movement for the distal extension base.

To develop the design, it is first necessary to determine how the partial denture is to be supported. In an entirely tooth-supported partial denture, the most ideal location for the support units (*rests*) is on prepared rest seats on the occlusal, cingulum, or incisal surface of the abutment adjacent to each edentulous space (see Figure 10-1, *B*). The type of rest and amount of support required must be based on interpretation of the diagnostic data collected from the patient. In evaluating the potential support an abutment tooth can provide, consideration should be given to: (1) periodontal health; (2) crown and root morphologies; (3) crown-to-root ratio; (4) bone index area (how the tooth has responded to previous stress); (5) location of the tooth in the arch; (6) relationship of the tooth to other support units (length of edentulous span); and (7) the opposing dentition. (For more in-depth understanding of these considerations, review Chapters 6 and 12.)

In a tooth- and tissue-supported partial denture, attention to these same considerations must be given to the abutment teeth. However, equitable support must come from the edentulous ridge areas. In evaluating the potential support available from the edentulous ridge areas, consideration must be given to: (1) the quality of the residual ridge, which includes contour, quality of the supporting bone (how the bone has responded to previous stress), and quality of the supporting mucosa; (2) the extent to which the residual ridge will be covered by the denture base; (3) the type and accuracy of the impression registration; (4) the accuracy of the denture base; (5) the design characteristics of the component parts of the partial denture framework; and (6) the anticipated occlusal load. A full explanation of tissue support for extension base partial dentures is found in Chapter 16.

Denture base areas adjacent to abutment teeth are primarily tooth supported. As you proceed away from the abutment teeth, they become more tissue supported. Therefore it is necessary to incorporate characteristics in the partial denture design that will distribute the functional load equitably between the abutment teeth and the supporting tissue of the edentulous ridge. Locating tooth support units (*rests*) on the principal abutment teeth and designing the minor connectors, which are adjacent to the edentulous areas, to contact the guiding planes in such a manner that they disperse the functional load equitably between the available tooth and tissue supporting units will provide designs with controlled distribution of support (see Figure 10-4).

The second step in systematically developing the design for any removable partial denture is to connect the tooth and tissue support units. Designing and locating major and minor connectors in compliance with the basic principles and concepts presented in Chapter 5 facilitate this connection. Major connectors must be rigid so that forces applied to any portion of the denture can be effectively distributed to the supporting structures. Minor connectors arising from the major connector make it possible to transfer functional stress to each abutment tooth through its connection to the corresponding rest and also to transfer the effect of the retainers, rests, and stabilizing components to the remainder of the denture and throughout the dental arch.

The third step is to determine how the removable partial denture is to be retained. The retention must be sufficient to resist reasonable dislodging forces. As stated in Chapter 7, retention is accomplished by mechanical retaining elements (*clasps*) being placed on the abutment teeth and by the intimate relationship of the denture bases and major connectors (maxillary) with the underlying tissue. The key to selecting a successful clasp design for any given situation is to choose one that will: (1) avoid direct transmission of tipping or torquing forces to the abutment; (2) accommodate the basic principles of clasp design by definitive location of component parts correctly positioned on abutment tooth surfaces; (3) provide retention against reasonable dislodging forces (with consideration for indirect retention); and (4) be compatible with undercut location, tissue contour, and esthetic desires of the patient. Location of the undercut is the most important single factor in selecting a clasp. Recontouring or restoring the abutment tooth to accommodate a clasp design better suited to satisfy the criteria for clasp selection, however, can modify undercut location.

The relative importance of retention is highlighted by the results from a clinical trial investigating prosthesis designs (K. Kapur). A 5-year, randomized clinical trial of two basic removable partial denture designs—one with rest, proximal plate, and I-bar (RPI) design and one with circumferential clasp design—demonstrated no discernible changes in nine periodontal health components of the abutment teeth with either of the two designs after 60 months. The overall results indicated that the two designs did not differ in terms of success rates, maintenance, or effects on abutment teeth. Therefore a well-constructed removable partial denture that is supported by favorable abutments and good residual ridges that are both properly prepared and maintained in a patient who exhibits good oral hygiene offers the best opportunity for satisfactory treatment.

The fourth step is to connect the retention units to the support units. If direct and indirect retainers are to function as designed, each must be rigidly attached to the major connector. The criteria for selection, location, and design are the same as those indicated for connecting the tooth and tissue support units.

The fifth and last step in this systematic approach to design is to outline and join the edentulous area to the already established design components. Strict attention to detail of the design characteristics outlined in Chapter 9 is necessary to ensure rigidity of the base material without interfering with tooth placement.

COMPONENTS OF PARTIAL DENTURE DESIGN

All partial dentures have two things in common: (1) they must be supported by oral structures and (2) they must be retained against reasonable dislodging forces.

In the Kennedy Class III partial denture, three components are necessary: support provided by rests, the connectors (stabilizing components), and the retainers.

The partial denture that does not have the advantage of tooth support at each end of each edentulous space still must be supported. But in this situation, the support comes from both the teeth and the underlying ridge tissue rather than from the teeth alone. This is a composite support, and the prosthesis must be fabricated so that the resilient support provided by the edentulous ridge is coordinated with the more stable support offered by the abutment teeth. The essentials—support, connectors, and retainers—must be more carefully designed and executed because of the movement of tissue-supported denture base areas. In addition, provision must be made for three other factors as follows:

1. The best possible support must be obtained from the resilient tissue that covers the edentulous ridges. This is accomplished by the impression technique more than by the partial denture design, although the area covered by the partial denture base is a contributing factor in such support.
2. The method of direct retention must take into account the inevitable tissueward movement of the distal extension base(s) under the stresses of mastication and occlusion. Direct retainers must be designed so that occlusal loading will result in the direct transmission of this load to the long axis of the abutment teeth instead of as leverage.
3. The partial denture, with one or more distal extension denture bases, must be designed to minimize movement of the extension base away from the tissue. This is often referred to as indirect retention and is best described in relation to an axis of rotation through the rest areas of the

principal abutments (see Chapter 8). However, retention from the removable partial denture base itself frequently can be made to help prevent this movement and, in such instances may be discussed as direct-indirect retention.

Tooth Support

The support of the removable partial denture by the abutment teeth is dependent on the alveolar support of those teeth, the crown and root morphology, the rigidity of the partial denture framework, and the design of the occlusal rests. Through clinical and roentgenographic interpretation, the dentist may evaluate the abutment teeth and decide whether they will provide adequate support. In some instances the splinting of two or more teeth is advisable, either by fixed partial dentures or by soldering two or more individual restorations together. In other instances a tooth may be deemed too weak to be used as an abutment, and extraction is indicated in favor of obtaining better support from an adjacent tooth.

Having decided on the abutments, the dentist is responsible for the preparation and restoration of the abutment teeth to accommodate the most ideal design of the partial denture. This includes the form of the occlusal rest seats. These modifications may be prepared either in sound tooth enamel or in restorative materials that will withstand the functional stress and wear of the component parts of the removable partial denture. The technician cannot be blamed for inadequate abutment tooth preparation, such as occlusal rest support. On the other hand, the technician is solely to blame if he or she extends the casting beyond, or fails to include, the total prepared areas. If the dentist has sufficiently reduced the marginal ridge area of the rest seat to prevent interference from opposing teeth, and if a definite occlusal rest seat is faithfully recorded in the master cast and delineated in the penciled design, then no excuse can be made for poor occlusal rest form on the partial denture.

Ridge Support

Support for the tooth-supported removable partial denture or the tooth-supported modification space comes entirely from the abutment teeth by means of rests. Support for the distal extension denture base comes primarily from the overlying soft tissue and the residual alveolar bone of the distal extension base area. In the latter, rest support is effective only at the abutment end of the denture base.

The effectiveness of tissue support depends on six factors: (1) the quality of the residual ridge; (2) the extent to which the residual ridge will be covered by the denture base; (3) the accuracy and type of impression registration; (4) the accuracy of the denture bases; (5) the design characteristics of the component parts of the partial denture framework; and (6) the occlusal load applied.

The quality of the residual ridge cannot be influenced, except to improve it by tissue conditioning, or to modify it by surgical intervention. Such modifications are almost always needed but are not frequently done.

The accuracy of the impression technique is entirely in the hands of the dentist. Maximum tissue coverage for support that encompasses the primary stress-bearing areas should be the primary objectives in any partial denture impression technique. The manner in which this is accomplished should be based on a biological comprehension of what happens beneath a distal extension denture base when an occlusal load is applied.

The accuracy of the denture base is influenced by the choice of materials and by the exactness of the processing techniques. Inaccurate and warped denture bases adversely influence the support of the partial denture. Materials and techniques that will ensure the greatest dimensional stability should be selected.

The total occlusal load applied to the residual ridge may be influenced by reducing the area of occlusal contact. This is done by the use of fewer, narrower, and more effectively shaped artificial teeth (Figure 10-5).

The distal extension removable partial denture is unique in that its support is derived from abutment teeth, which are comparatively unyielding, and from soft tissue overlying bone, which may be comparatively yielding under occlusal forces. Resilient tissues, which are distorted or displaced by occlusal load, are unable to provide support for the denture base comparable with that offered by the abutment teeth. This problem of support is further complicated by the fact that the patient may have natural teeth remaining that can exert far greater occlusal force on the supporting tissue than would result if the patient were completely edentulous. This is clearly evident from the damage often occurring to an edentulous ridge when it is opposed by a few remaining anterior teeth in the opposing arch and especially when the opposing occlusion of anterior teeth has been arranged so that contact exists in both centric and eccentric positions.

Ridge tissues recorded in their resting or nonfunctioning form are incapable of providing the composite support needed for a denture that derives its support from both hard and soft tissue. Three factors must be considered in the acceptance of an impression technique for distal extension removable partial dentures: (1) the material should record the tissue covering the primary stress-bearing areas in their supporting form; (2) tissues within the basal seat area, other than primary stress-bearing areas, must

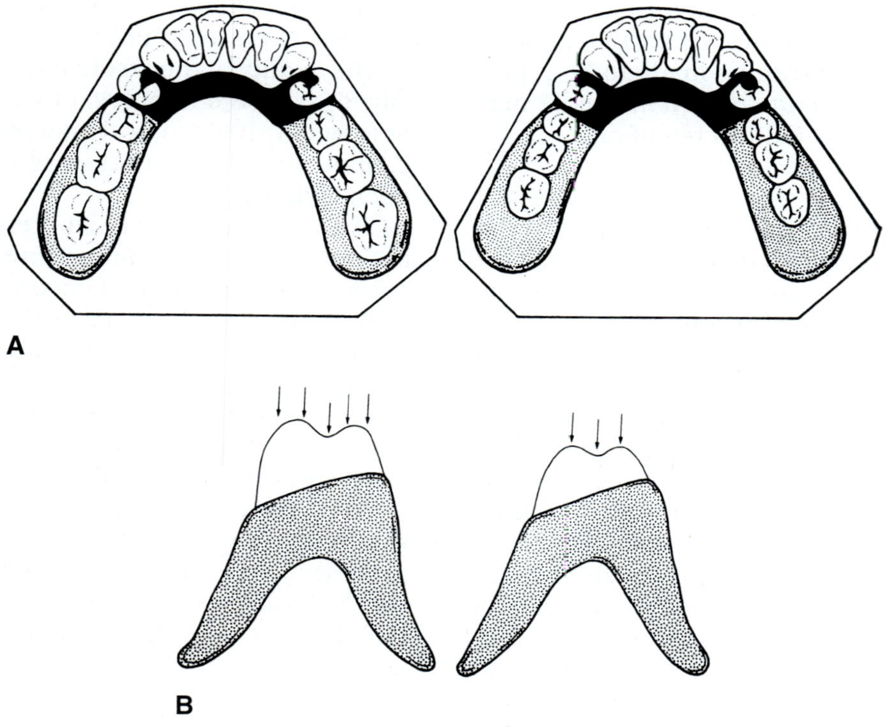

Figure 10-5 **A,** Total occlusal load applied may be reduced by using comparatively smaller posterior teeth represented by right-hand illustration. **B,** Less muscular force will be required to penetrate food bolus with reduced occlusal table, thereby reducing forces to supporting oral structures.

be recorded in their anatomic form; and (3) the total area covered by the impression should be sufficient to distribute the load over as large an area as can be tolerated by the border tissue. This is an application of the principle of the snowshoe.

Anyone who has had the opportunity to compare two master casts for the same partially edentulous arch—one cast having the distal extension area recorded in its anatomic or resting form and the other cast having the distal extension area recorded in its functional form—has been impressed by the differences in the topography (Figure 10-6). A denture base processed to the functional form is generally less irregular and has greater area coverage than does a denture base processed to the anatomic or resting form. Moreover, and of far greater significance, a denture base made to anatomic form exhibits less stability under rotating and/or torquing forces than does a denture base processed to functional form and thus fails to maintain its occlusal relation with the opposing teeth. By having the patient close onto strips of soft wax, it is evident that occlusion is maintained at a point of equilibrium over a longer period of time when the denture base has been made to the functional form. In contrast, evidence exists that there has been a rapid "settling" of the denture base when it has been made to the anatomic form, with an early return of the occlusion to natural tooth contact only. Such a denture not only fails to distribute the occlusal load equitably but also allows rotational movement, which is damaging to the abutment teeth and their investing structures.

Major and Minor Connectors

Major connectors are the units of a partial denture that connect the parts of the prosthesis located on one side of the arch with those on the opposite side. Minor connectors arise from the major connector and join it with other parts of the denture. Thus they serve to connect the tooth and tissue support units together. A major connector should be properly located in relation to gingival and moving tissues and should be designed to be rigid. Rigidity in a major connector is necessary to provide proper distribution of forces to and from the supporting components.

A lingual bar connector should be tapered superiorly with a half-pear shape in cross section and should be relieved sufficiently, but not excessively, over the underlying tissue when such relief is indicated. The addition of a continuous bar retainer or a lingual apron does not alter the basic design of the lingual bar. These are added solely for support, stabilization, rigidity, and protection of the anterior teeth and are neither connectors nor indirect retainers.

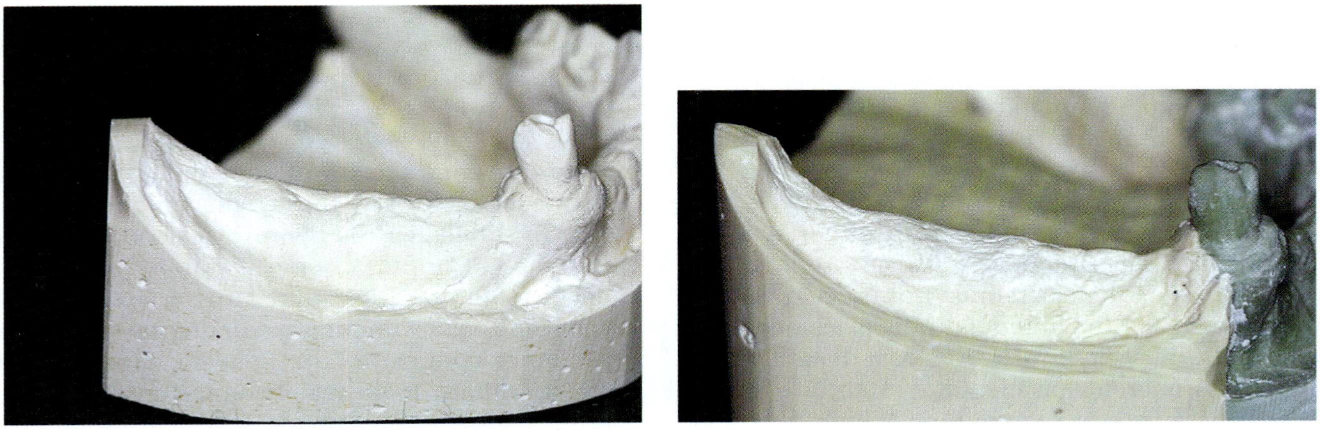

A B

Figure 10-6 **A,** Cast of mandibular partially edentulous arch representing anatomic form of right residual ridge. Impression was made in stock tray using irreversible hydrocolloid. **B,** Impression recording the functional or supporting form of right residual ridge was made in individualized impression tray, permitting placement of tissues and definitive border molding.

The finished inferior border of either a lingual bar or a linguoplate should be gently rounded to prevent irritation to subjacent tissue when the restoration moves even slightly in function.

The use of a linguoplate is indicated when the lower anterior teeth are weakened by periodontal disease. It is also indicated in Kennedy Class I partially edentulous arches when the need for additional resistance to horizontal rotation of the denture is required because of excessively resorbed residual ridges. Still another indication is in those situations in which the floor of the mouth so closely approximates the lingual gingiva of anterior teeth that an adequately inflexible lingual bar cannot be positioned without impinging on the gingival tissue.

Experience with the linguoplate has shown that with good oral hygiene the underlying tissue remains healthy, and there are no harmful effects to the tissue from the metallic coverage per se. However, adequate relief must be provided whenever a metal component crosses the gingival margins and the adjacent gingivae. Excessive relief should be avoided because tissue tends to fill a void, resulting in the overgrowth of abnormal tissue. The amount of relief used therefore should be only the minimum necessary to prevent gingival impingement.

It does not seem that there are many advantages to be found in the use of the continuous bar retainer versus the linguoplate. In rare instances when a linguoplate would be visible through multiple interproximal embrasures, the continuous bar retainer may be preferable for esthetic reasons only. In other instances when a single diastema exists, a linguoplate may be cut out in this area to avoid the display of metal without sacrificing its use.

Rigidity of a palatal major connector is just as important and its location and design just as critical as for a lingual bar. A U-shaped palatal connector is rarely justified except to avoid an inoperable palatal torus that extends to the junction of the hard and soft palates. Neither can the routine use of a narrow, single palatal bar be justified. The combination anterior-posterior palatal strap-type major connector is mechanically and biologically sound if it does not impinge on tissue. The broad, anatomic palatal major connector is frequently preferred because of its rigidity, better acceptance by the patient, and greater stability without tissue damage. In addition, this type of connector may provide direct-indirect retention that may sometimes, but rarely, eliminate the need for separate indirect retainers.

Direct Retainers for Tooth-supported Partial Dentures

Retainers for tooth-supported partial dentures have only two functions: to retain the prosthesis against reasonable dislodging forces without damage to the abutment teeth and to aid in resisting any tendency of the denture to be displaced in a horizontal plane. The prosthesis cannot move tissueward because the rest supports the retentive components of the clasp assembly. There should be no movement away from the tissue and therefore no rotation about a fulcrum because a direct retainer secures the retentive component.

Any type of direct retainer is acceptable as long as the abutment tooth is not jeopardized by its presence. Intracoronal (frictional) retainers are ideal for tooth-supported restorations and offer esthetic advantages that are not possible with extracoronal (clasp) retainers. Nevertheless, the circumferential and bar-type clasp retainers are mechanically effective and are more economically constructed than are intracoronal retainers. Therefore they are used more universally.

Vulnerable areas on the abutment teeth must be protected by restorations with either type of retainer. The clasp retainer must not impinge on gingival tissue. The clasp must not exert excessive torque on the abutment tooth during placement and removal. It must be located the least distance into the tooth undercut for adequate retention, and it must be designed with a minimum of bulk and tooth contact.

The bar clasp arm should be used only when the area for retention lies close to the gingival margin of the tooth and little tissue blockout is necessary. If the clasp must be placed high, if the vestibule is extremely shallow, or if an objectionable space will exist beneath the bar clasp arm because of blockout of tissue undercuts, the bar clasp arm should not be used. In the event of an excessive tissue undercut, consideration should be given to recontouring the abutment and using some type of circumferential direct retainer.

Direct Retainers for Distal Extension Partial Dentures

Retainers for distal extension partial dentures, although retaining the prosthesis, must also be able to flex or disengage when the denture base moves tissueward under function. Thus the retainer may act as a stress-breaker. Mechanical stress-breakers accomplish the same thing, but they do so at the expense of horizontal stabilization. When some kind of mechanical stress-breaker is used, the denture flange must be able to prevent horizontal movement. Clasp designs that allow for flexing of the retentive clasp arm may accomplish the same purpose as mechanical stress-breakers without sacrificing horizontal stabilization and with less complicated techniques.

In evaluating the ability of a clasp arm to act as a stress-breaker, one must realize that flexing in one plane is not enough. The clasp arm must be freely flexible in any direction, as dictated by the stresses applied. Bulky, half-round clasp arms cannot do this, and neither can a bar clasp engaging an undercut on the side of the tooth away from the denture base. Round, tapered clasp forms offer advantages of greater and more universal flexibility, less tooth contact, and better esthetics. Either the combination circumferential clasp, with its tapered wrought-wire retentive arm, or the carefully located and properly designed circumferential or bar clasp can be considered for use on all abutment teeth adjacent to the extension denture bases if the abutment teeth are properly prepared, the tissue support is effectively achieved, and if the patient exercises good oral hygiene.

Stabilizing Components

Stabilizing components of the removable partial denture framework are those rigid components that assist in stabilizing the denture against horizontal movement. The purpose of all stabilizing components should be to distribute stresses equally to all supporting teeth without overworking any one tooth. The minor connectors that join the rests and the clasp assemblies to the major connector serve as stabilizing components.

All minor connectors that contact vertical tooth surfaces (and all reciprocal clasp arms) act as stabilizing components. It is necessary that minor connectors have sufficient bulk to be rigid and yet present as little bulk to the tongue as possible. This means they should be confined to interdental embrasures whenever possible. When minor connectors are located on vertical tooth surfaces, it is best that these surfaces be parallel to the path of placement. When cast restorations are used, these wax-pattern surfaces should be made parallel on the surveyor before casting.

A modification of minor connector design has been proposed that places the minor connector in the center of the lingual surface of the abutment tooth. Proponents of this design claim that it reduces the amount of gingival tissue coverage and provides enhanced bracing and guidance during placement. Disadvantages may include increased encroachment on the tongue space, more obvious borders, and potentially greater space between the connector and the abutment tooth. This proposed variation, however, when combined with thoughtful design principles, may provide some benefit to the periodontal health of the abutment teeth and may be acceptable to some patients.

Reciprocal clasp arms also must be rigid, and they must be placed occlusally to the height of contour of the abutment teeth, where they will be nonretentive. By their rigidity, these clasp arms reciprocate the opposing retentive clasp, and they also prevent horizontal movement of the prosthesis under functional stresses. For a reciprocal clasp arm to be placed favorably, some reduction of the tooth surfaces involved is frequently necessary to increase the suprabulge area.

When crown restorations are used, a lingual reciprocal clasp arm may be inset into the tooth contour by providing a ledge on the crown on which the clasp arm may rest. This permits the use of a wider clasp arm and restores a more nearly normal tooth contour, at the same time maintaining its strength and rigidity (see Chapter 14).

Guiding Plane

The term *guiding plane* is defined as two or more parallel, vertical surfaces of abutment teeth, so shaped to direct a prosthesis during placement and removal. After the most favorable path of placement has been ascertained, axial surfaces of abutment teeth are prepared parallel to the path of placement and therefore become parallel to each other. Guiding planes may be contacted by various components of the partial denture—the body of an extracoronal direct retainer, the stabilizing arm of a direct retainer, the minor connector portion of an indirect retainer—or by a minor connector specifically designed to contact the guiding plane surface.

The functions of guiding plane surfaces are as follows: (1) to provide for one path of placement and removal of the restoration (to eliminate detrimental strain to abutment teeth and framework components during placement and removal); (2) to ensure the intended actions of reciprocal, stabilizing, and retentive components (to provide retention against dislodgment of the restoration when the dislodging force is directed other than parallel to the path of removal and also to provide stabilization against horizontal rotation of the denture); and (3) to eliminate gross food traps between abutment teeth and components of the denture.

Guiding plane surfaces need to be created so that they are as nearly parallel to the long axes of abutment teeth as possible. Establishing guiding planes on several abutment teeth (preferably more than two teeth), which are located at widely separated positions in the dental arch, provides for a more effective use of these surfaces. The effectiveness of guiding plane surfaces is enhanced if these surfaces are prepared on more than one common axial surface of the abutment teeth (Figure 10-7).

As a rule, proximal guiding plane surfaces should be about one half the width of the distance between the tips of adjacent buccal and lingual cusps or about one third of the buccal lingual width of the tooth. They should extend vertically about two thirds of the length of the enamel crown portion of the tooth from the marginal ridge cervically. In preparing guiding plane surfaces, care must be exercised to avoid creating buccal or lingual line angles (Figure 10-8). Assuming that the stabilizing or retentive arm of a direct retainer may originate in the guiding plane region, a line angle preparation would weaken either or both components of the clasp assembly.

A guiding plane should be located on the abutment surface adjacent to an edentulous area. However, excess torquing is inevitable if the guiding planes are used squarely facing each other on a lone

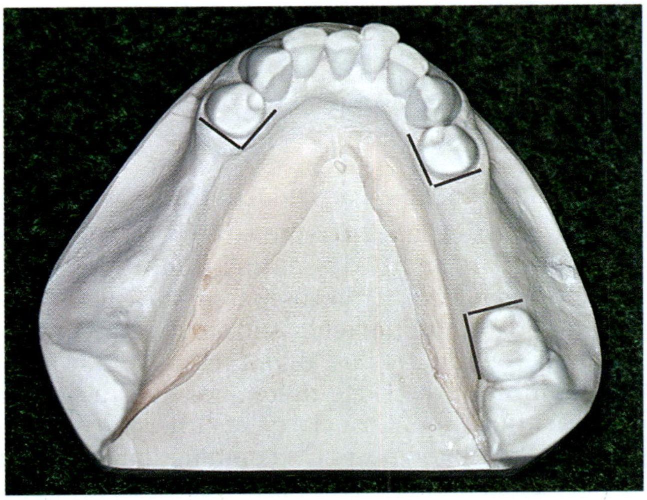

A

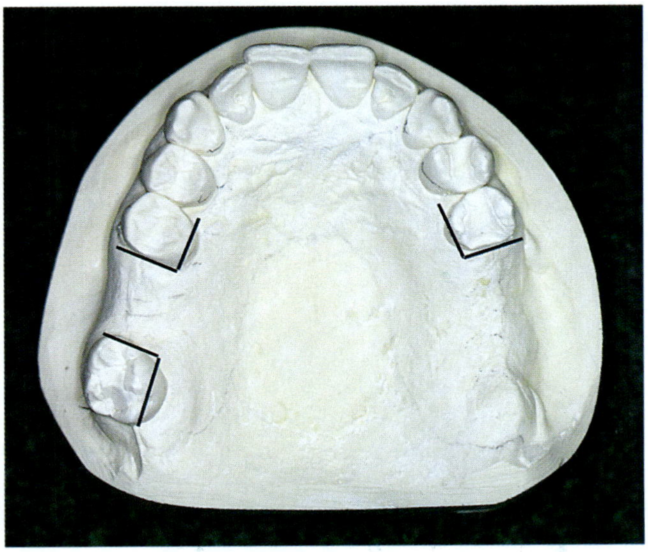

B

Figure 10-7 **A,** Prospective guiding plane surfaces are indicated by lines located on respective surfaces of abutment teeth of this mandibular arch. These surfaces, when used, can be made vertically parallel to path of placement. However, by including guiding plane surfaces, which are not in the same parallel plane horizontally but are divergent, cross-arch resistance to horizontal rotation of denture is enhanced. **B,** Similar guiding plane locations as seen in mandibular arch can be used for maxillary arch. In this Class II Mod 1 partially edentulous arch both proximal and palatal surfaces can be used to maximize stability.

standing abutment adjacent to an extension area (Figure 10-9).

Indirect Retainers

An indirect retainer must be placed as far anterior from the fulcrum line as adequate tooth support permits if it is to function with the direct retainer to restrict movement of a distal extension base away from the basal seat tissue. It must be placed on a rest seat prepared on an abutment tooth that is capable of withstanding the forces placed on it. An indirect retainer cannot function effectively on an inclined tooth surface, nor can a single weak incisor tooth be used for this purpose. Either a canine or premolar tooth should be used for the support of an indirect retainer, and the rest seat must be prepared with as much care as is given any other rest seat. An incisal rest or a lingual rest may be used on an anterior tooth, provided a definite seat can be obtained either in sound enamel or on a suitable restoration.

A second purpose that indirect retainers serve in partial denture design is that of support for major connectors. A long lingual bar or an anterior palatal major connector is thereby prevented from settling into the tissue. Even in the absence of a need for indirect retention, provision for such auxiliary support is sometimes indicated.

Contrary to common use, a cingulum bar or a linguoplate does not in itself act as an indirect retainer. Because these are located on inclined tooth surfaces, they serve more as an orthodontic appliance than as support for the partial denture. When a linguoplate or a cingulum bar is used, terminal rests should always be provided at either end to stabilize the denture and to prevent orthodontic movement of the teeth contacted. Such terminal rests may function as the indirect retainers, but these would function equally well in that capacity without the continuous bar retainer or linguoplate.

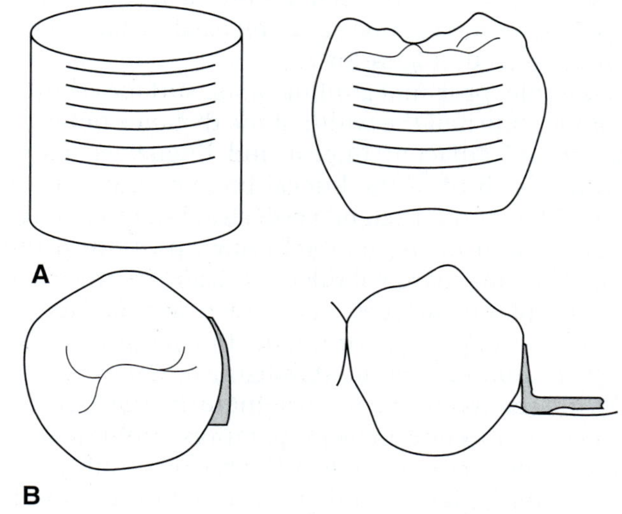

Figure 10-8 A, Guiding plane surface should be like area on cylindric object. It should be continuous surface unbounded by even, rounded line angles. **B,** Minor connector contacting guiding plane surface has same curvature as does that surface. From occlusal view it tapers buccally from thicker lingual portion, thus permitting closer contact of abutment tooth and prosthetically supplied tooth. Viewed from buccal aspect, minor connector contacts enamel of tooth on its proximal surface about two-thirds its length.

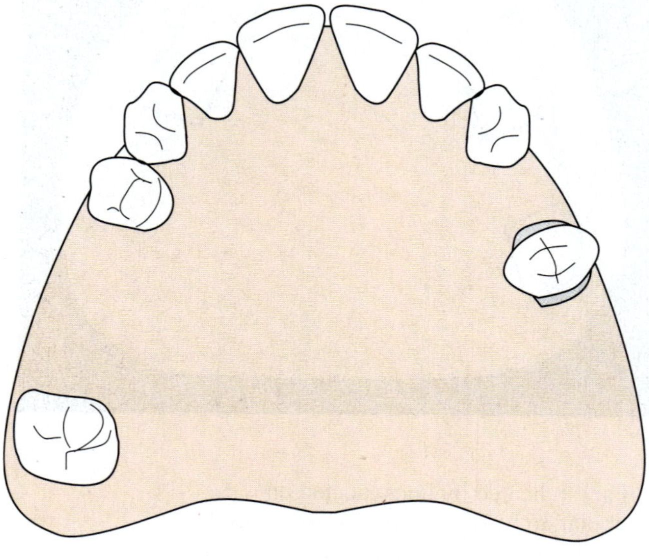

Figure 10-9 Guiding planes squarely facing each other should not be prepared on lone standing abutment. Minor connectors of framework *(gray areas)* would place undue strain on abutment when denture rotated vertically either superiorly or inferiorly.

EXAMPLES OF SYSTEMATIC APPROACH TO DESIGN

Class III Removable Partial Denture

The Kennedy Class III removable partial denture (Figures 10-10 and 10-11), entirely tooth supported, may be made to fit the prepared surfaces of the anatomic form of the teeth and surrounding structures. It does not require an impression of the functional form of the ridge tissue, nor does it require indirect retention. Cast clasps of either the circumferential, the bar type, or the combination clasp may be used depending on how one can modify the surfaces of the abutment teeth (guiding planes, rests, and contours for proper location of clasp arms). Unless a need for later relining is anticipated—as in the situation of recently extracted teeth—the denture base may be made of metal, which has several advantages. The Class III partial denture can frequently be used as a valuable aid to periodontal treatment because of its stabilizing influence on the remaining teeth.

Kennedy Class I, Bilateral, Distal Extension Removable Partial Dentures

The Class I, bilateral, distal extension partial denture is as different from the Class III type as any two dental restorations could be (see Figure 10-1). Because it derives its principal support from the tissue underlying its base, a Class I partial denture made to anatomic ridge form cannot provide uniform and adequate support. Yet, unfortunately, many Class I mandibular removable partial dentures are made from a single irreversible hydrocolloid impression. In such situations, both the abutment teeth and the residual ridges suffer because the occlusal load placed on the remaining teeth is increased by the lack of adequate posterior support.

Many dentists, recognizing the need for some type of impression registration that will record the supporting form of the residual ridge, attempt to record this form with a metallic oxide, rubber base, or one of the silicone impression materials. Such materials actually only record the anatomic form of the ridge, except when special design of the impression trays permits recording the primary stress-bearing areas under a simulated load. Others prefer to place a base, which is made to fit the anatomic form of the ridge, under some pressure at the time that it is in contact with the remaining teeth, thus obtaining functional support. Still others who believe that a properly compounded mouth-temperature wax will displace only tissue that is incapable of providing support to the denture base use a wax secondary impression to record the supporting, or functional, form of the edentulous ridge. Any impression record will be influenced by the consistency of the impression material and the amount of hydraulic pressure exerted by its confinement within the impression tray.

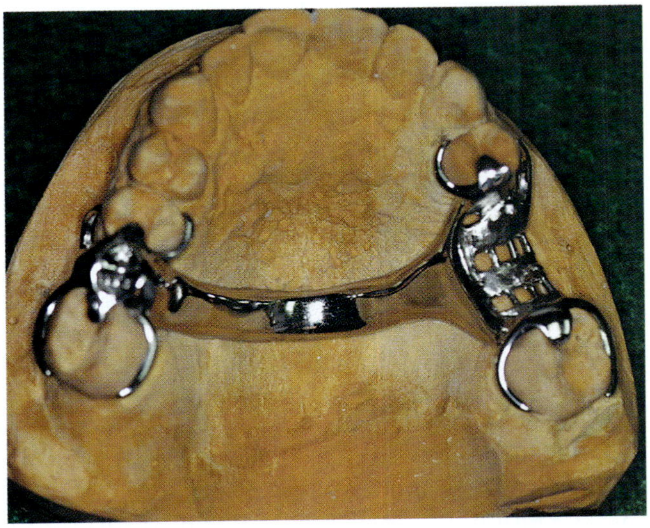

Figure 10-10 Removable partial denture in maxillary Class III, Mod 1 arch. Design consists of single palatal connecting a single tooth space to a 2-tooth space. The impression for such modification spaces does not require tissues to be captured in a supportive form. A palatal strap major connector is less bulky and for most patients would be more comfortable than a thicker bar design.

Kennedy Class II Removable Partial Dentures

The Kennedy Class II partial denture (Figures 10-12 and 10-13) actually may be a combination of both tissue-supported and tooth-supported restorations. The distal extension base must have adequate tissue support, whereas tooth-supported bases elsewhere in the arch may be made to fit the anatomic form of the underlying ridge. Indirect retention must be

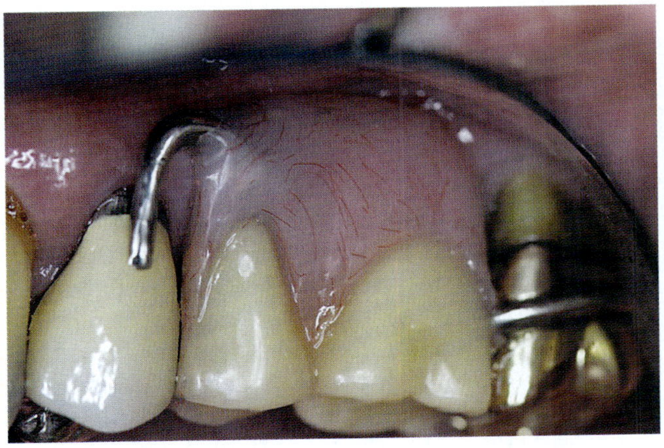

Figure 10-11 Modification space for a maxillary Class III arch in which both I-bar and circumferential clasp retainers are used. This modification space only requires an anatomic form impression technique.

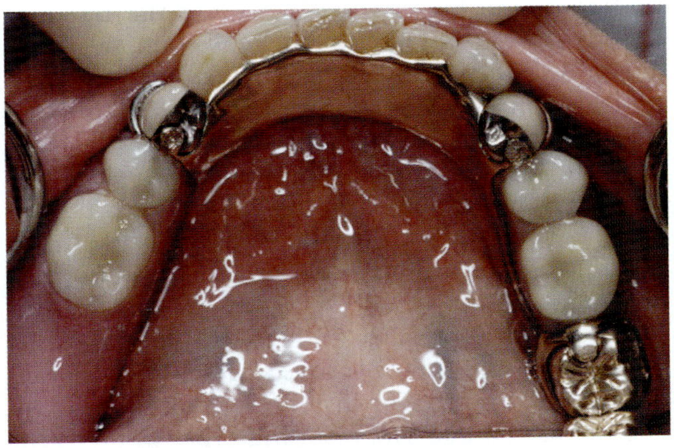

Figure 10-12 Mandibular Class II removable partial denture with distal extension base. Surveyed crowns were used for all three abutments. Because of tissue undercut cervical to buccal surface of left right premolar and lack of distobuccal undercut, wrought-wire (*tapered*) retainer arm was used.

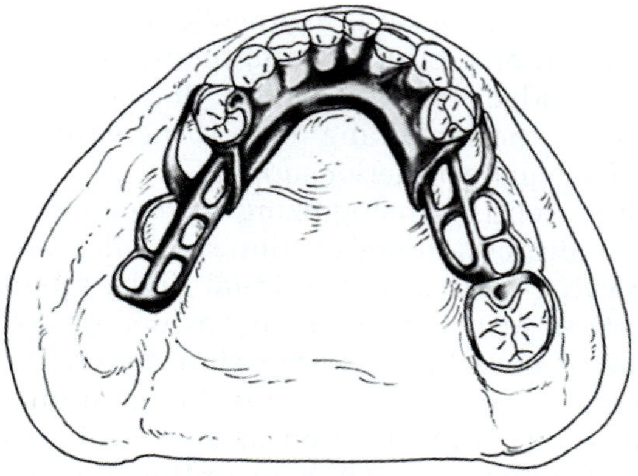

Figure 10-13 Mandibular Class II, mod 1, partially edentulous arch. Note that bar-type retentive arms are used on both premolar abutments, engaging distobuccal undercuts at their terminal ends. Lever-like forces may not be as readily imparted to right premolar, as opposed to cast circumferential direct retainer engaging mesiobuccal undercut.

provided for; however, occasionally the anterior abutment on the tooth-supported side will satisfy this requirement. If additional indirect retention is needed, provisions must be made for it.

Cast clasps are generally used on the tooth-supported side. However, a clasp design using wrought wire may reduce the application of torque on the abutment tooth adjacent to the distal extension and should be considered (see Figure 10-15). The use of a cast circumferential clasp engaging a mesiobuccal undercut on the anterior abutment of the tooth-supported modification space may result in a Class I leverlike action if the abutment teeth have not been properly prepared and/or if the tissue support from the extension base area is not adequate. It seems rational under these circumstances to use a bar-type retainer engaging a distobuccal undercut (see Figure 10-16). Should the bar-type retainer be contraindicated because of a severe tissue undercut or the existence of only a mesiobuccal undercut on the anterior abutment, then a combination direct retainer with the retentive arm made of tapered wrought wire should be used. A thorough understanding of the advantages and disadvantages of various clasp designs is necessary to determine the type of direct retainer that is to be used for each abutment tooth.

The steps in the fabrication of the Class II partial denture closely follow those of the Class I partial denture, except that the distal extension base is usually made of an acrylic resin material, whereas the base for any tooth-supported area is frequently made of metal. This is permissible because the residual ridge beneath tooth-supported bases is not called on to provide support for the denture, and later rebasing is not as likely to be necessary.

ADDITIONAL CONSIDERATIONS INFLUENCING DESIGN

Every effort should be made to gain the greatest support possible for removable prostheses by use of abutments bounding edentulous spaces. This will not only relieve the residual ridges of some of their obligation for support but also may allow the design of the framework to be greatly simplified. To this end, use of splint bars, internal clip attachments, overlay abutments, overlay attachments, a component partial, and implants should be considered.

Use of a Splint Bar for Denture Support

In the Chapter 14 discussion of missing anterior teeth, mention is made that missing anterior teeth are best replaced with a fixed partial denture. The following is quoted from that chapter: "From a biomechanical standpoint, . . . a removable partial denture should replace only the missing posterior teeth after the remainder of the arch has been made intact by fixed restorations."

Occasionally a situation is found in which it is necessary that several missing anterior teeth be replaced with the removable partial denture rather than by fixed restorations. This may be because of the length of the edentulous span, the loss of a large amount of the residual ridge by resorption, accident, surgery, or the result of a situation in which too much vertical space prevents the use of a fixed partial denture or in which esthetic requirements can better be met through the use of teeth added to the denture framework. In such instances it is necessary to provide the best possible support for the replaced anterior teeth. Ordinarily, this is done through the placement of occlusal or lingual rests, or both, on the adjacent natural teeth, but when the edentulous span is too large to ensure adequate support from the adjacent teeth, other methods must be used. This is included here only because it influences the design of the major connector that must be used.

An anterior splint bar may be attached to the adjacent abutment teeth in such a manner that fixed splinting of the abutment teeth results, with a smooth, contoured bar resting lightly on the gingival tissue to support the removable partial denture (Figure 10-14). As with any fixed partial denture, the type of abutment retainers and the decision to use multiple abutments will depend on the length of the span and the available support and stability of the teeth being used as abutments. Regardless of the type of abutment retainers used, the connecting bar may be cast of a rigid alloy, or a commercially available bar may be

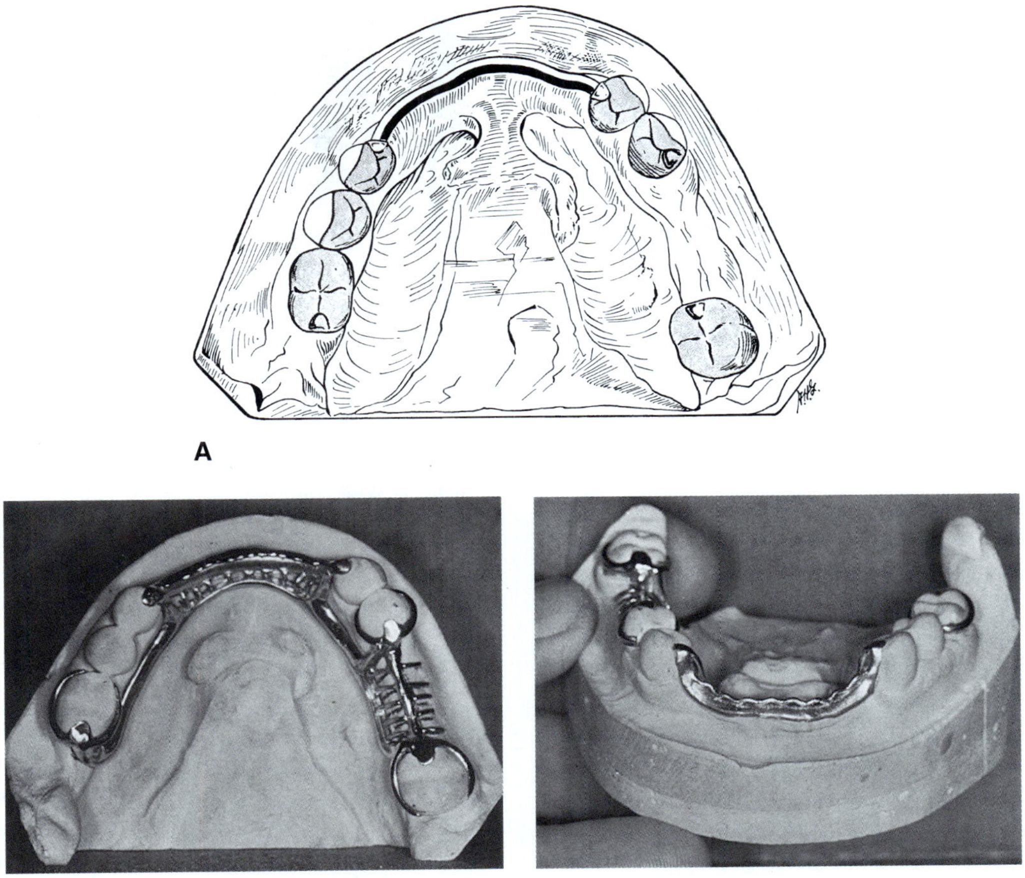

A

B C

Figure 10-14 **A,** Splint bar attached to double abutments on either side of arch. Although this may be made of hard gold alloy, its rigidity is better assured by making bar of base-metal alloy. Bar can be made to fit into recesses prepared in abutments, attaching it by electric soldering. **B** and **C,** Denture framework designed to fit and be supported by splint bar. **B** has no major connector at edentulous areas

used and cast to the abutments or attached to the abutments by soldering.

The length of the span influences the size of a splint bar. Long spans require more rigid bars (10 gauge) than short spans (13 gauge). If the bar is to be soldered, it is best that recesses be formed in the proximal surfaces of the abutments and that the connecting bar, which rests lightly on the tissue, be cast or made to fit into these recesses and then attached by soldering.

Because of the greater rigidity of the chromium-cobalt alloys, the splint bar is preferably cast in one of these materials and then attached to the abutments by soldering. The complete assembly (abutments and connecting bar) is then cemented permanently to the abutment teeth, the same as a fixed partial denture. The impression for the partial denture is then made, and a master cast is obtained that accurately reproduces the contours of the abutments and the splint bar. The denture framework is then made to fit the abutments and the bar by extending the major connector or minor connectors to cover and rest upon the splint bar. Retention for the attachment of a resin base, or any other acceptable means of attaching the replaced anterior teeth, is incorporated into the denture design (Figure 10-14, *B* and *C*). In those situations, wherein the removable partial denture will be tooth supported, the splint bar may be curved to follow the crest of the residual ridge, as seen in Figure 10-17, *A*. However, in a distal extension situation—because of the vertical rotation of the denture—caution must be exercised to form the splint bar so that excessive torque will not accrue to its supporting abutments (Figure 10-15). The proximal contours of abutments adjacent to splint bars should be parallel to the path of placement.

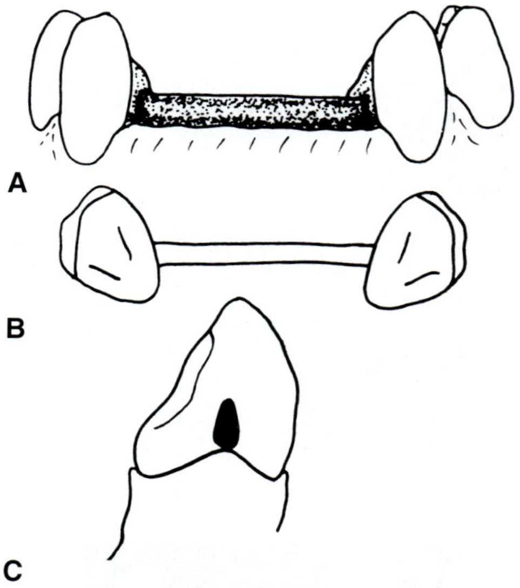

Figure 10-15 **A,** Insofar as possible, the splint bar should be round or ovoid. Provision must be made in construction and location of bar so that dental floss may be threaded underneath bar to allow proper cleaning by patient. **B,** As viewed from above, bar is in straight line between abutments. This is especially critical for distal extension removable partial dentures to avoid excess torque on abutments as denture rotates in function. **C,** Sagittal section through bar demonstrates rounded form of bar making point contact with residual ridge. Entire tissue surface of bar is easily accessible for cleaning with dental floss. Pear-shaped bar *(in cross section)* will permit rotation of removable partial denture without appreciable resistance or torque.

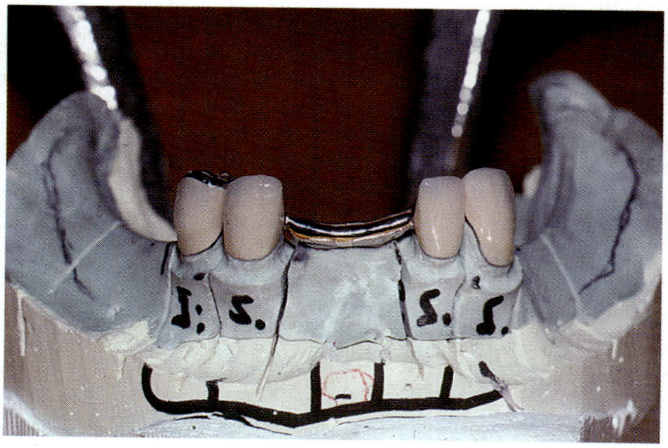

Figure 10-16 Lower canines and lateral incisors splinted together with splint bar. Longevity of these teeth is greatly enhanced by splinting, and enhanced stability of the removable partial denture is provided. Tissue surfaces are minimally contacted by rounded form of lower portion of bar. Anterior and posterior slopes of splint bar must be compatible with path of placement of denture.

This serves three purposes: (1) it permits a desirable arrangement of artificial teeth; (2) it aids in resisting horizontal rotation of the restoration; and (3) they act as guiding planes to direct the partial denture to and from its terminal position.

The splint bar must be positioned anteroposteriorly just lingual to the residual ridge to allow an esthetic arrangement of artificial teeth. The resulting partial denture will have esthetic advantages of removable anterior replacements and positive support, retention, and stability from the underlying splint bar (Figure 10-16).

Internal Clip Attachment

The internal clip attachment differs from the splint bar in that the internal clip attachment provides both support and retention from the connecting bar (Figure 10-17).

Several preformed connecting bars are commercially available in plastic patterns. These can be customized for length and cast in the metal alloy of choice. Internal clip attachments are also commercially available in various metal alloys and durable nylon. To fabricate a custom-made connecting bar and clip, the bar should be cast from 10- or 13-gauge sprue wax. The cast bar should rest lightly or be located slightly above the tissue. Retention is provided by one of the commercial preformed metal or nylon clips, which is contoured to fit the bar and is retained in a preformed metal housing or partially embedded by means of retention spurs or loops into the overlying resin denture base.

The internal clip attachment thus provides support, stability, and retention for the anterior modification area and may serve to eliminate both occlusal rests and retentive clasps on the adjacent abutment teeth.

Overlay Abutment as Support for a Denture Base

Every consideration should be directed to preventing the need for a distal extension removable partial denture. In many instances it is possible to salvage the roots and a portion of the crown of a badly broken-down molar through endodontic treatment. A periodontally involved molar, otherwise indicated for extraction, may sometimes be salvaged by periodontal and endodontic treatment accompanied by reduction of the clinical crown almost level with the gingival tissue. In another situation an unopposed molar may have extruded to such an extent that restoring the tooth with a crown is inadequate to develop a harmonious occlusion. Then too, it is not unusual to encounter a molar that is so grossly tipped anteriorly that it cannot serve as an abutment unless the clinical crown is reduced drastically.

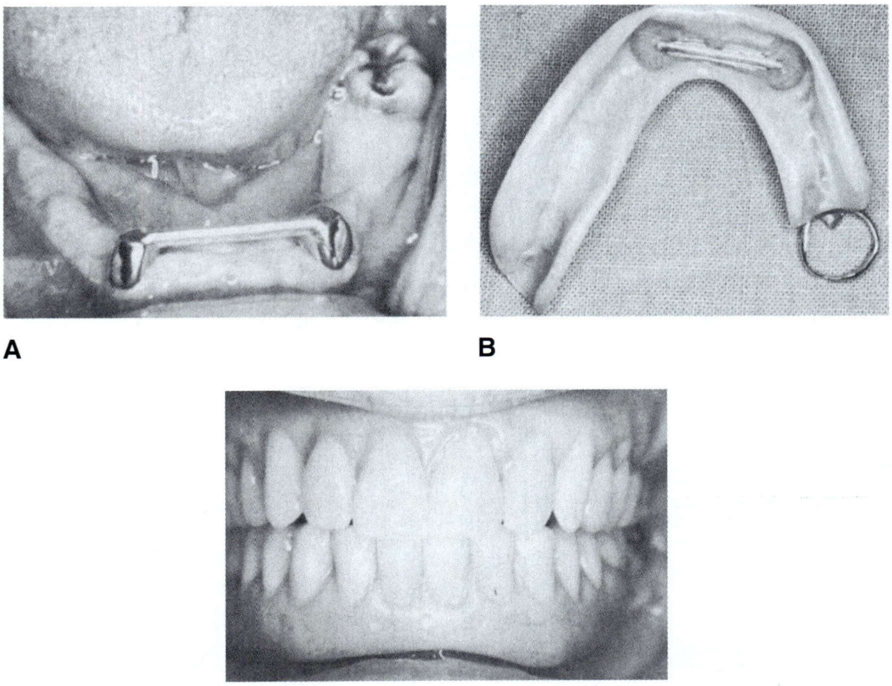

A B C

Figure 10-17 **A,** Canines have been endodontically treated and are splinted together with round, straight connecting bar, slightly elevated from residual ridge. Retaining left molar as abutment will immeasurably contribute to stability of removable partial denture. **B,** Tissue surface of completed mandibular restoration containing internal clip attachment. **C,** Complete denture and removable partial denture have been initially placed for patient. *(Courtesy Dr. Bernard Wilkie, Charlotte, NC.)*

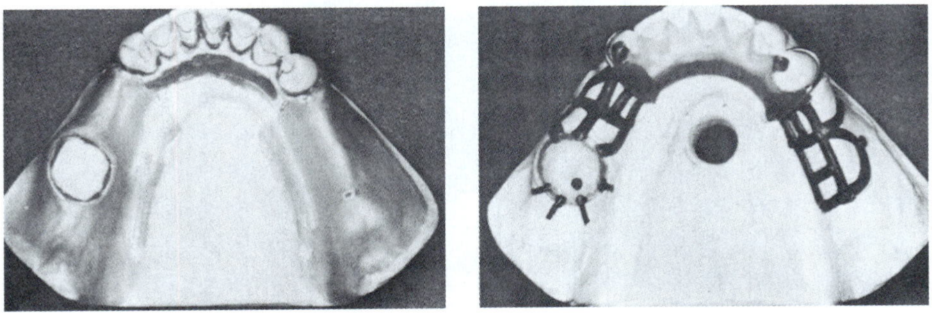

A B

Figure 10-18 **A,** Master cast has been prepared for duplicating in refractory investment to develop wax pattern for removable partial denture framework, supported by overlay on second molar abutment. Molar could not be restored by conventional means. It was endodontically treated, and crown was reduced to slightly elevated dome shape. Pulp chamber was filled with silver amalgam alloy. **B,** Wax pattern has been developed on investment cast, and provision has been made to attach properly extended resin denture base. Bilateral distal extension denture has been avoided by planning overlay prosthesis.

Such teeth should be considered for possible support for an otherwise distal extension denture base. Endodontic treatment and preparation of the coronal portion of the tooth as a slightly elevated dome-shaped abutment often offer an alternative to a distal extension base (Figure 10-18). The student is referred to the Selected Reading Resources section (textbooks and abutment retainers) for sources of information on overdenture abutments and overlay-type prostheses.

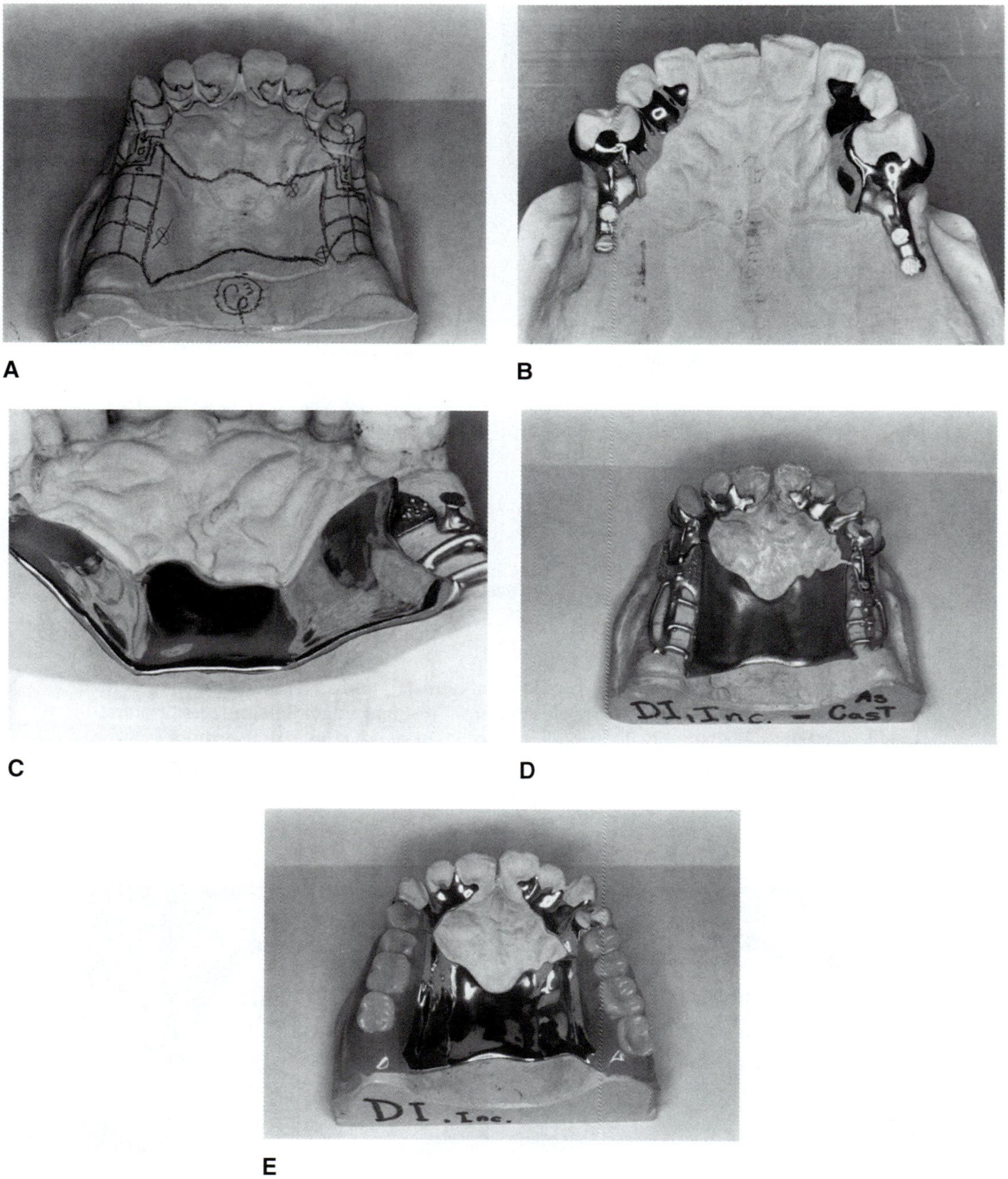

Figure 10-19 **A,** Design of component part removable partial denture. **B,** Tooth support component individually fabricated and fit to the master cast. **C,** Tissue support component individually fabricated and fit to the master cast. **D,** Tooth and tissue support components assembled on cast. **E,** Components joined with high-impact resin. *(Courtesy B.T. Cecconi, San Antonio, Tex.)*

Use of a Component Partial to Gain Support

A component partial is a removable partial denture in which the framework is designed and fabricated in separate parts. The tooth support and tissue-supported components are individually fabricated, and the two are joined with a high-impact acrylic resin to become a single, rigid functioning unit (Figure 10-19).

SELF-ASSESSMENT AIDS

1. The text suggests at least nine factors that will influence the design of a removable partial denture. Please list them.
2. How is the design of a denture influenced by the classification of the arch being restored?
3. There are really only two types of removable partial dentures. What are they?

4. Because there are two basic types of removable partial dentures, it is evident that a dentist must consider: (1) the manner in which each is supported; (2) the method of impression registration; (3) the need or lack of need for indirect retention; and (4) the use of a base material that can be readily relined. Write a meaningful essay of 100 words or less about each of these listed considerations.
5. What is a guiding plane?
6. What are the three main functions of guiding plane surfaces contacted by minor connectors?
7. Should guiding planes prepared on enamel surfaces of abutment teeth be rounded or flat? Why?
8. Give a rule of thumb for the dimensions of proximal guiding planes.
9. Direct retainers for tooth-supported dentures differ in design from those used in extension base-type dentures. What requirement, in relation to an undercut, exists for the direct retainer (clasp) on a terminal abutment of an extension denture when the denture base is forced into heavier contact with the residual ridge?
10. Name the component(s) of a removable partial denture that must be rigid. Name the component(s) in which flexibility is desirable.
11. Would you agree that a fixed partial denture, where indicated, should be the restoration of choice, in lieu of a removable partial denture? Give an example and explain.
12. What method should usually be used to replace single missing teeth or missing anterior teeth? Justify your answer.
13. When confronted with a Kennedy Class I arch in which all molars and first premolars are missing, should one consider replacing the first premolars with fixed partial dentures rather than restoring the spaces with a removable restoration? Why?
14. The amount of stress transferred to the supporting edentulous ridges and the abutment teeth in extension base partial dentures is dependent on four factors. One is the length of the lever arm(s) or denture bases. Identify the other three and describe how each influences this stress transfer.
15. A systematic approach to developing the design for any removable partial denture was presented and discussed. Outline the steps presented in this approach.
16. In evaluating the potential support that abutment teeth can provide, what specific characteristics of the teeth should you consider?
17. In evaluating the potential tissue support that the edentulous ridges can provide in extension base situations, what specific characteristics should be considered?
18. In developing the design for an extension base removable partial denture, what component parts are used to connect the supporting units? What specific characteristics should each of these components have to effectively distribute functional stresses to the supporting units?
19. In developing a design for an extension base removable partial denture, when does one determine how the denture is to be retained? What are the keys to selecting successful clasp designs?
20. How does one know if indirect retention needs to be incorporated into the design? If needed, where should it be located, and what component parts would be included in the design to serve as indirect retainers?
21. What is the final step in the proposed systematic approach to design? Should this design characteristic have any special requirements? If so, what are they?
22. What is a splint bar?
23. Draw a splint bar from a frontal, horizontal, and sagittal view. Label the dimensions and relationship of the bar to the tissue and the abutments.
24. What purposes are served by use of splint bars where indicated?
25. A decision has been made to use a splint bar from canine to canine. Will this decision influence the design of the framework? If so, how?
26. For what reasons must a splint bar be convex, rather than concave, adjacent to the residual ridge?
27. Is a 13-gauge splint bar adequate for a span from canine to canine? Why or why not?
28. Define and describe an internal clip attachment.
29. The internal clip attachment must be used in conjunction with some type of bar supported by abutment teeth. What is the cross-sectional shape of such a bar? What advantages accrue from using such a design for a restoration?
30. You are confronted with a mandibular arch with only the six anterior teeth and two second molars remaining. The maxillary arch is edentulous. The anterior teeth are restorable individually and show no mobility or periodontal involvement. The molars, however, are grossly involved with caries; in fact most of the clinical crown is gone. They also show a Miller mobility classification of 1 and exhibit a 5- to 6-mm gingival crevicular depth. They can be treated periodontally and endodontically. In such a situation, if finances were not a factor, would you: (1) Extract both molars? (2) Prepare the molars for an overlay prosthesis? (3) Extract all the mandibular teeth and treat the patient with complete dentures?
31. If the molars mentioned in the preceding section were prepared for an overlay prosthesis, state the reasons for doing so in terms of benefits to the patient.

11

SURVEYING

When preparing a fixed partial denture (FPD), the orientation of the diamond bur is controlled to remove an amount of tooth structure necessary to satisfy the requirements of the path-of-insertion for the prosthesis. Accomplishment of parallel preparations is ultimately verified by complete seating of the prosthesis, but could be verified on the master cast or dies by the use of the surveyor. Once the FPD is fabricated and completely seated, it is ensured full engagement of the entire circumference of and occlusal support from the abutment retainers. If adequate resistance form and fit of the prosthesis is provided, the chance for functional stability equal to natural teeth is good. This could not be ensured unless the relationship of the fixed prosthesis and prepared teeth was carefully controlled.

For a removable prosthesis, the necessity for appropriately planned and executed tooth preparation—followed by verification of a well-fitting prosthesis that engages the teeth as planned—is equally important. As briefly mentioned in Chapter 7, a dental surveyor is vitally important to the planning, execution, and verification of appropriate mouth modifications for a removable partial denture. Though not necessarily impacting the occlusal rest preparations on abutment teeth, the use of the surveyor is critical for planning the modifications of all tooth surfaces that will be involved with the support, stabilization, and retention of the prosthesis. In this role, the use of a surveyor to determine the needed mouth preparation is vitally important to helping provide stable and comfortable removable prostheses.

A *dental surveyor* has been defined as an instrument used to determine the relative parallelism of two or more surfaces of the teeth or other parts of the cast of a dental arch. Therefore the primary purpose of surveying is to identify the modifications of oral structures that are necessary to fabricate a removable partial denture that will have a successful prognosis. It is the modification of tooth surfaces, to accommodate placement of the component parts of the partial denture in their designated ideal position on abutment teeth, that facilitates this prognosis.

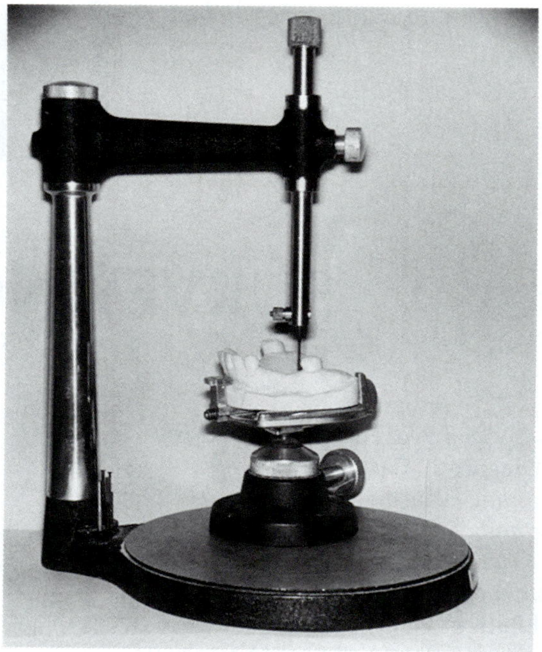

Figure 11-1 Ney surveyor is widely used because of its simplicity and durability. Dental students should be required to own such a surveyor. By becoming familiar with and dependent on its use, they are more likely to continue using the surveyor in practice as a necessary piece of equipment toward more adequate diagnosis, effective treatment planning, and performance of many other aspects of prosthodontic treatment. *(Courtesy JM Ney Company, Hartford, Conn.)*

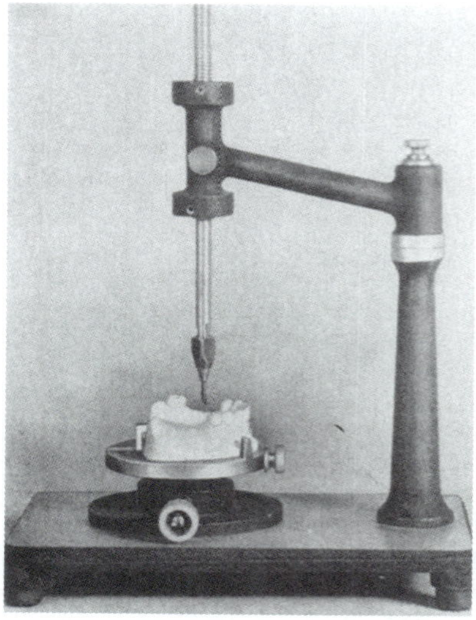

Figure 11-2 Jelenko surveyor. Note spring-mounted paralleling tool and swivel at top of vertical arm. Horizontal arm may be fixed in any position by tightening nut at top of vertical arm. *(Courtesy JF Jelenko & Company, New York, NY.)*

Any one of several moderately priced surveyors on the market will adequately accomplish the procedures necessary to develop the design and construction of a partial denture. In addition, these surveyors may be used to parallel internal rests and intracoronal retainers. With a handpiece holder added, they also may be used to machine internal rests and to make the guiding plane surfaces of abutment restorations parallel.

DESCRIPTION OF DENTAL SURVEYOR

The most widely used surveyors are the Ney (Figure 11-1) and the Jelenko (Figure 11-2). Both of these are precision-made instruments. They differ principally in that the Jelenko arm swivels, whereas the Ney arm is fixed. The technique for surveying and trimming blockout is therefore somewhat different. Other surveyors also differ in this respect, and the dentist may prefer one over another for this reason.

The principal parts of the Ney surveyor follow:

1. Platform on which the base is moved
2. Vertical arm that supports superstructure
3. Horizontal arm from which surveying tool suspends
4. Table to which the cast is attached
5. Base on which the table swivels
6. Paralleling tool or guideline marker (this tool contacts the convex surface to be studied in a tangential manner; the relative parallelism of one surface to another may thus be determined; by substituting a carbon marker, the height of contour then may be delineated on the surfaces of the abutment teeth and also on areas of interference requiring reduction on blockout)
7. Mandrel for holding special tools (Figure 11-3)

The principal parts of the Jelenko surveyor are essentially the same as those for the Ney surveyor except that by loosening the nut at the top of the vertical arm, the horizontal arm may be made to swivel. The objective of this feature, originally designed by Dr. Noble Wills, is to permit freedom of movement of the arm in a horizontal plane rather than to depend entirely on the horizontal movement of the cast. To some this is confusing, because two horizontal movements must be coordinated. For those who prefer to move the cast only in a horizontal relationship to a fixed vertical arm, the nut may be tightened and the horizontal arm used in a fixed position. The jointed horizontal arm of the Williams surveyor differs from both the Ney and Jelenko surveyors. This feature permits the vertical arm to be moved to scribe the survey lines without moving the cast.

Another difference between the Ney and Jelenko surveyors is that the vertical arm on the Ney surveyor is retained by friction within a fixed bearing. The shaft may be moved up or down within this bearing, but it remains in any vertical position until again

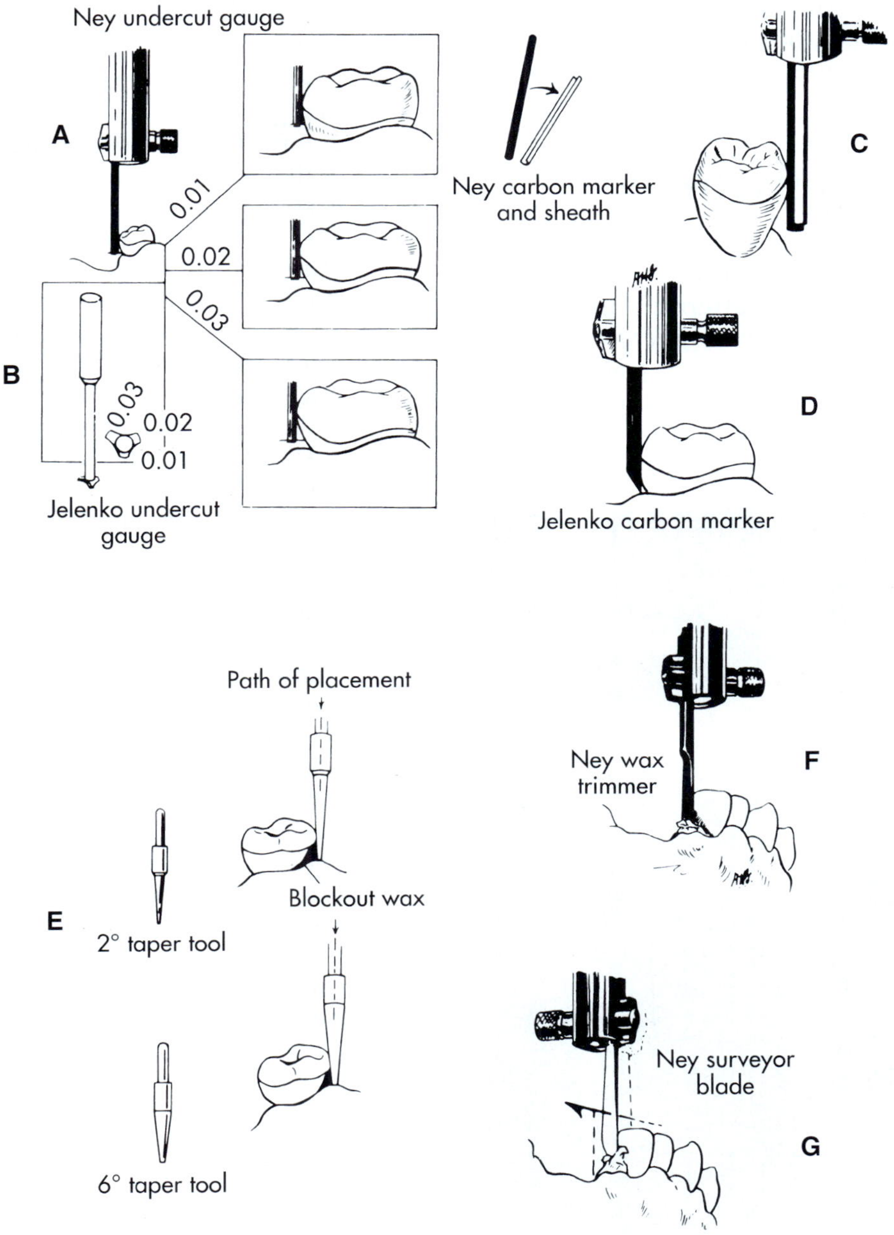

Figure 11-3 Various tools that may be used with dental surveyor. **A,** Ney undercut gauges. **B,** Jelenko undercut gauge. **C,** Ney carbon marker with metal reinforcement sheath. **D,** Jelenko carbon marker. **E,** Tapered tools, 2- and 6-degree, for trimming blockout when some nonparallelism is desired. **F,** Ney wax trimmer for paralleling blockout. **G,** Surveying blade being used for trimming blockout.

moved. The shaft may be fixed in any vertical position desired by tightening a setscrew. In contrast, the vertical arm of the Jelenko surveyor is spring mounted and returns to the top position when it is released. It must be held down against spring tension when it is in use, which to some is a disadvantage. The spring may be removed, but the friction of the two bearings supporting the arm does not hold it in position as securely as does a bearing designed for that purpose. These minor differences in the two surveyors lead to personal preferences but do not detract from the effectiveness of either surveyor when each is properly used.

Because the shaft on the Ney surveyor is stable in any vertical position—yet may be moved vertically with ease—it lends itself well for use as a drill press when a handpiece holder is added (Figure 11-4). The handpiece may thus be used to cut recesses in cast restorations with precision using burs or carborundum points of various sizes.

Several other types of surveyors have been designed and are in use today. Many of these are more elaborate and costly, yet possess little advantage over the simpler type of surveyors.

PURPOSES OF SURVEYOR

The surveyor may be used for surveying the diagnostic cast, recontouring abutment teeth on the diagnostic cast, contouring wax patterns, measuring a specific depth of undercut, surveying ceramic veneer crowns, placing intracoronal retainers, placing internal rests, machining cast restorations, and surveying and blocking out the master cast.

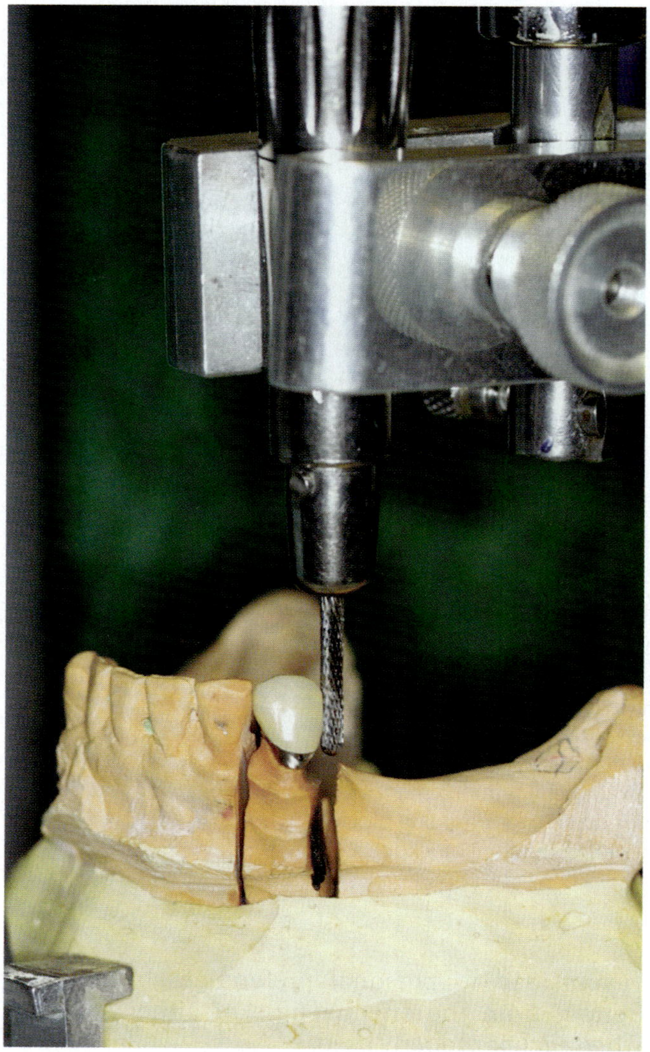

Figure 11-4 Lab handpiece clamp. Handpiece holders attach to the vertical spindle of surveyors and may be used to create and refine any parallel surface on a surveyed crown, as a drill press to prepare internal rests and recesses in patterns and/or castings, and to establish lingual surfaces above ledge, which are parallel to path of placement in abutment restorations.

Surveying the Diagnostic Cast

Surveying the diagnostic cast is essential to effective diagnosis and treatment planning. The objectives are as follows:

1. To determine the most desirable path of placement that will eliminate or minimize interference to placement and removal (Figure 11-5). The path of placement is the direction in which a restoration moves from the point of initial contact of its rigid parts with the supporting teeth to its terminal resting position, with rests seated and the denture base in contact with the tissue. The path of removal is exactly the reverse because it is the direction of restoration movement from its terminal resting position to the last contact of its rigid parts with the supporting teeth. When the restoration is properly designed to have positive guiding planes, the patient may place and remove the restoration with ease in only one direction. This is possible only because of the guiding influence of tooth surfaces (guiding planes) made parallel to that path of placement.
2. To identify proximal tooth surfaces that are, or need to be, made parallel so that they act as guiding planes during placement and removal.
3. To locate and measure areas of the teeth that may be used for retention.
4. To determine whether tooth and bony areas of interference will need to be eliminated surgically or by selecting a different path of placement.
5. To determine the most suitable path of placement that will permit locating retainers and artificial teeth to the best esthetic advantage.
6. To permit an accurate charting of the mouth preparation to be made. This includes the preparation of proximal tooth surfaces to provide guiding

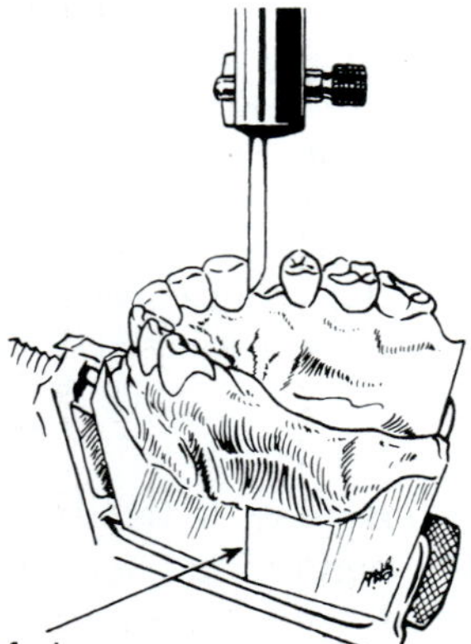

Figure 11-5 Tilt of cast on adjustable table of surveyor in relation to vertical arm establishes path of placement and removal that removable partial denture will take. *All mouth preparations must be made to conform to this determined path of placement,* which has been recorded by scoring base of cast or by tripoding.

planes and the reduction of excessive tooth contours to eliminate interference and to permit a more acceptable location of reciprocal and retentive clasp arms. By marking these areas on the diagnostic cast in red, using an undercut gauge to estimate the amount of tooth structure that may safely (without exposing dentin) be removed, and then trimming the marked areas on the stone cast with the surveyor blade, the angulation and extent of tooth reduction may be established before preparing the teeth in the mouth (Figure 11-6). With the diagnostic cast on the surveyor at the time of mouth preparation, reduction of tooth contours may be accomplished with acceptable accuracy.

7. To delineate the height of contour on abutment teeth and to locate areas of undesirable tooth undercut that are to be avoided, eliminated, or blocked out. This will include areas of the teeth to be contacted by rigid connectors, the location of nonretentive reciprocal and stabilizing arms, and the location of retentive clasp terminals.
8. To record the cast position in relation to the selected path of placement for future reference. This may be done by locating three dots or parallel lines on the cast, thus establishing the horizontal plane in relation to the vertical arm of the surveyor (see Figures 11-5 and 11-15).

Contouring Wax Patterns

The surveyor blade is used as a wax carver during this phase of mouth preparation so that the proposed path of placement may be maintained throughout the preparation of cast restorations for abutment teeth (Figure 11-7).

Guiding planes on all proximal surfaces of wax patterns adjacent to edentulous areas should be made parallel to the previously determined path of placement. Similarly, all other tooth contours that will be contacted by rigid components should be made parallel. The surfaces of restorations on which reciprocal and stabilizing components will be placed should be contoured to permit their location well below occlusal surfaces and on nonretentive areas. Those surfaces of restorations that are to provide retention for clasp arms should be contoured so that retentive clasps may be placed in the cervical third of the crown and to the best esthetic advantage. Generally, a small amount of undercut from 0.01 to 0.02 inch (0.25–0.50) or less is sufficient for retentive purposes.

Surveying Ceramic Veneer Crowns

Ceramic veneer crowns are often used to restore abutment teeth on which extracoronal direct retainers will be placed. The surveyor is used to contour all areas of the wax pattern for the veneer crown except the buccal or labial surface. It must be remembered that one of the principal goals in using a porcelain veneer restoration is to develop an esthetic replica of a natural tooth. It is unlikely that the ceramic veneer portion can be fabricated exactly to the form required for the planned placement of retentive clasp arms

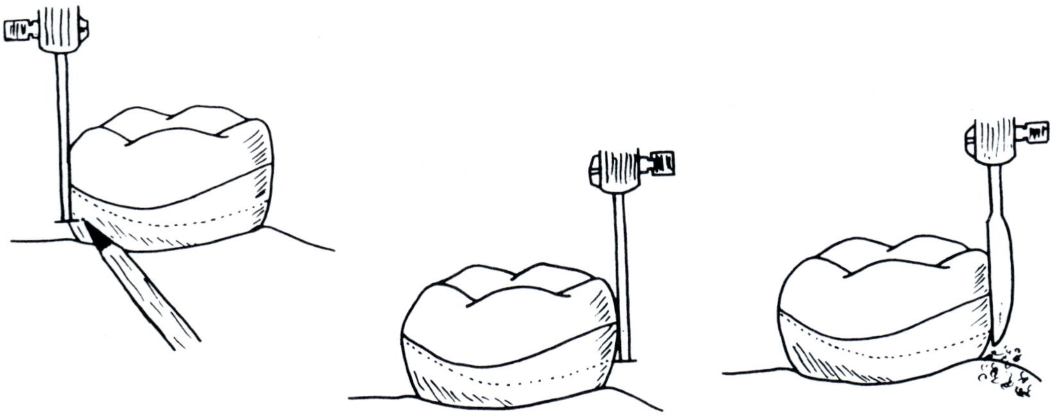

A B C

Figure 11-6 **A,** Solid line represents height of contour on abutment at selected orientation of diagnostic cast to vertical spindle of surveyor. Dotted line represents desirable height of contour to optimally locate component of direct retainer assembly. A 0.01-inch (0.25 mm) undercut gauge is used to mark location of tip of retentive arm of direct retainer. **B,** By reducing axial contour of tooth only 0.01 inch, optimum height of contour can be achieved without exposing dentin. **C,** Stone tooth is trimmed with surveyor blade to desired height of contour. Trimmed area is marked in red pencil and serves as blueprint for similar recontouring in mouth. If one can safely assume that enamel is 1- to 1.5-mm thick in area of contemplated reduction, only 0.25 mm of enamel need be removed to achieve optimum height of contour.

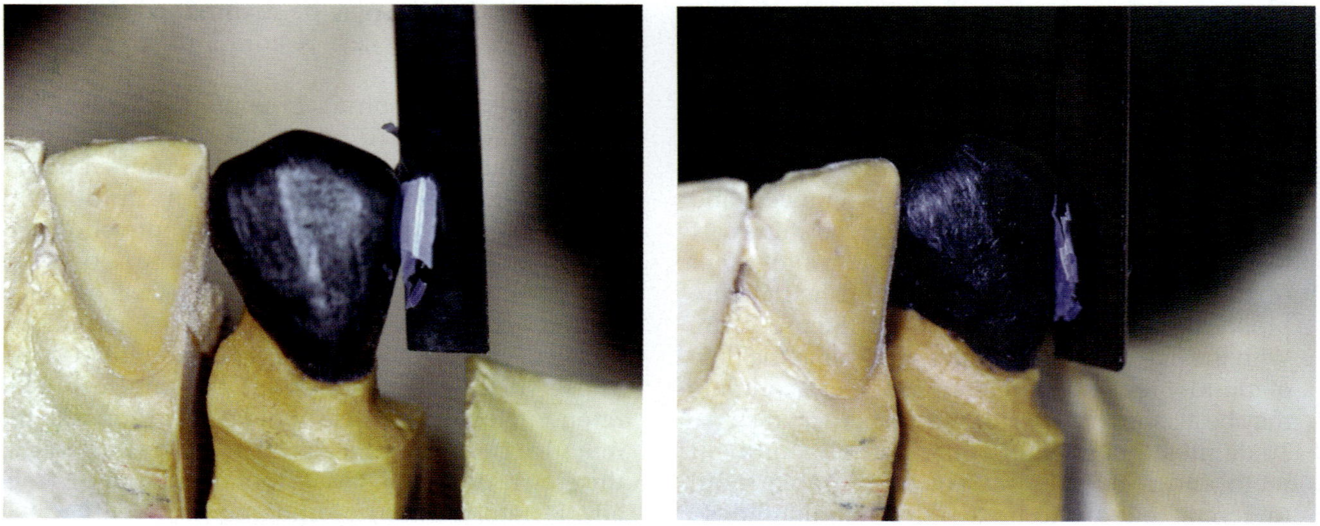

A

B

Figure 11-7 After the cast has been oriented to the surveyor at the predetermined path of placement, designated axial surfaces of the wax pattern are altered with the surveyor blade to meet specific requirements for placement of framework components. **A,** Wax pattern is carved with surveyor blade to produce a distal guide plane surface parallel to the selected path of insertion. **B,** Same pattern is modified from the distal guide plane along the buccal surface to align the surface with the height of contour most favorable to the direct retainer specifications.

without some reshaping with stones. Before the final glaze is accomplished, the abutment crowns should be returned to the surveyor on a full-arch cast to ensure the correct contour of the veneered portions or to locate those areas that need recontouring (Figure 11-8). The final glaze is accomplished only after the crowns have been recontoured.

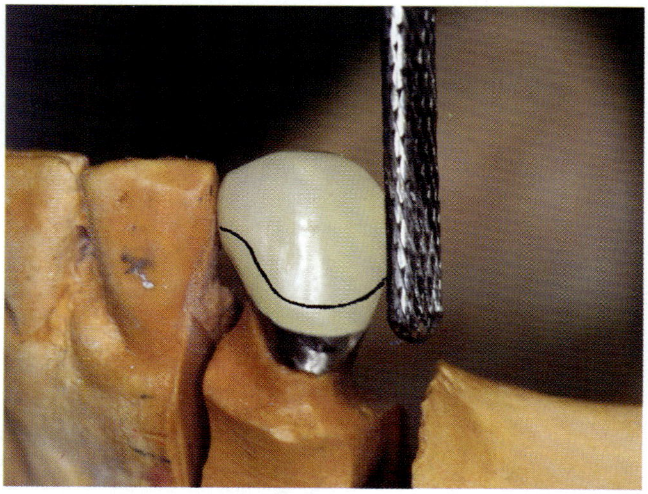

Figure 11-8 Resultant metal-ceramic surveyed crown from Figure 11-7, which is being refined to maintain the distal guide plane and buccal height of contour previously designed. Final glaze has not been placed on veneer crown and required alterations of surfaces to conform to ideal placement of retainer (*solid line*) can be performed by machining. Final glaze is produced only after necessary recontouring is accomplished.

Placement of Intracoronal Retainers (Internal Attachments)

In the placement of intracoronal retainers, the surveyor is used as follows:

1. To select a path of placement in relation to the long axes of the abutment teeth that will avoid areas of interference elsewhere in the arch
2. To cut recesses in the stone teeth on the diagnostic cast for estimating the proximity of the recess to the pulp (used in conjunction with roentgenographic information to estimate pulp size and location) and to facilitate the fabrication of metal or resin jigs to guide the preparations of the recesses in the mouth
3. To carve recesses in wax patterns, to place internal attachment trays in wax patterns, or to cut recesses in castings with the handpiece holder (whichever method is preferred)
4. To place the keyway portion of the attachment in the casting before investing and soldering; each keyway must be located parallel to the other keyways elsewhere in the arch

The student is referred to the Selected Reading Resources section of the textbook for sources of information on intracoronal retainers (internal attachments).

Placement of Internal Rest Seats

The surveyor may be used as a drill press, with a dental handpiece attached to the vertical arm by a handpiece holder. Internal rest seats may be carved in the wax patterns and further refined with the handpiece after casting, or the entire rest seat may be cut in the cast restoration with the handpiece. It is best to carve the outline form of the rest seat in wax and merely refine the casting with the handpiece.

An internal rest differs from an internal attachment in that some portion of the prosthesis framework is waxed and cast to fit into the rest seat rather than a matched key and keyway attachment used (see Figure 6-13). The former is usually nonretentive but provides a definite seat for a removable partial denture or a cantilever rest for a broken-stress fixed partial denture. When they are used with fixed partial dentures, nonparallel abutment pieces may be placed separately.

The internal rest in partial denture construction provides a positive occlusal support that is more favorably located in relation to the rotational axis of the abutment tooth than the conventional spoon-shaped occlusal rest. It also provides horizontal stabilization through the parallelism of the vertical walls, thereby serving the same purpose as stabilizing and reciprocal arms placed extracoronally. Because of the movement of a distal extension base, more torque may be applied to the abutment tooth by an interlocking type of rest, and for this reason its use in conjunction with a distal extension partial denture is considered to be contraindicated. The ball-and-socket, spoon-shaped occlusal, or noninterlocking rest should be used in distal extension partial denture designs. The use of the dovetailed or interlocking internal rest should be limited to tooth-supported removable restorations, except when it is used in conjunction with some kind of stress-breaker between the abutments and the movable base. The use of stress-breakers has been discussed in Chapter 9.

Internal rest seats may be made in the form of a nonretentive box, a retentive box fashioned after the internal attachment, or a semiretentive box. In the latter the walls are usually parallel and nonretentive, but a recess in the floor of the box prevents proximal movement of the male portion. Internal rest seats are cut with dental burs of various sizes and shapes. Tapered or cylindrical fissure burs are used to form the vertical walls, and small round burs are used to cut recesses in the floor of the rest seat.

Machining Cast Restorations

With handpiece holder attached (see Figure 11-4), axial surfaces of cast and ceramic restorations may be refined by machining with a suitable cylindrical carborundum point. Proximal surfaces of crowns and inlays, which will serve as guiding planes, and vertical surfaces above crown ledges may be improved by machining, but only if the relationship of one crown to another is correct (see Figure 14-8). Unless the seating of removable dies is accurate and they are held in place with additional stone or plaster, cast restorations should first be tried in the mouth and then transferred, by means of a plaster or acrylic resin index impression, to a reinforced stone cast for machining purposes. The new cast is then positioned on the surveyor, conforming to the path of placement of the partial denture, and vertical surfaces are machined with a true-running cylindrical carborundum point.

Although machined parallelism may be considered ideal and beyond the realm of everyday application, its merits more than justify the additional steps required to accomplish it. When such parallelism is accomplished and reproduced in a master cast, it is essential that subsequent laboratory steps be directed toward the use of these parallel guiding plane surfaces.

Surveying the Master Cast

Because surveying the master cast follows mouth preparation, the path of placement, the location of retentive areas, and the location of remaining interference must be known before proceeding with the final design of the denture framework. The objectives of surveying the master cast are as follows:

1. To select the most suitable path of placement by following mouth preparations that satisfy the requirements of guiding planes, retention, noninterference, and esthetics
2. To permit measurement of retentive areas and to identify the location of clasp terminals in proportion to the flexibility of the clasp arm being used; flexibility will depend on many of the following factors: the alloy used for the clasp, the design and type of the clasp, whether its form is round or half round, whether it is of cast or wrought material, and the length of the clasp arm from its point of origin to its terminal end; retention will then depend on (a) the flexibility of the clasp arm, (b) the magnitude of the tooth undercut, and (c) the depth the clasp terminal is placed into this undercut
3. To locate undesirable undercut areas that will be crossed by rigid parts of the restoration during placement and removal; these must be eliminated by blockout
4. To trim blockout material parallel to the path of placement before duplication (Figure 11-9)

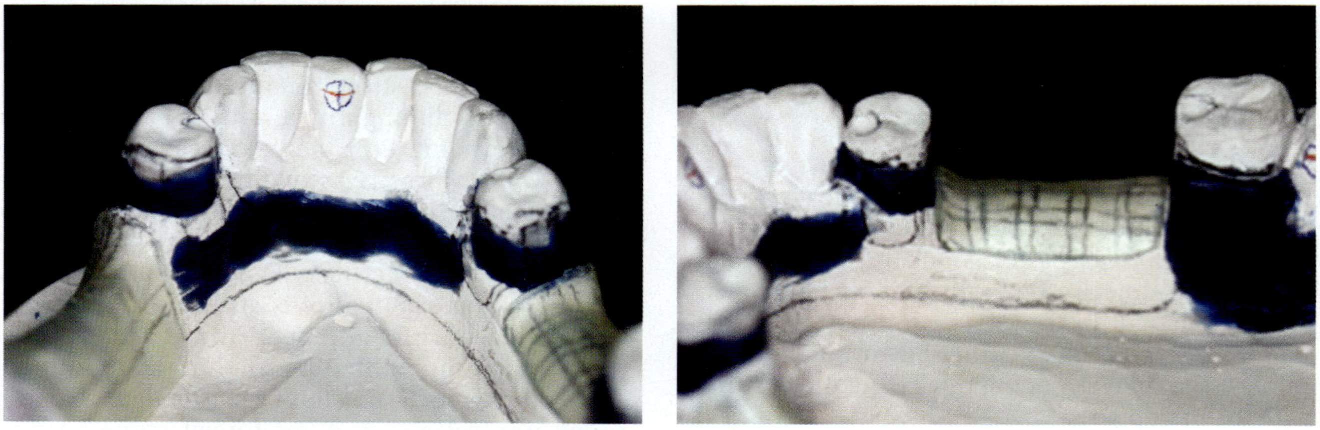

Figure 11-9 Master casts are modified by addition of wax relief to nonbearing regions and by placement of blockout wax parallel to the path of insertion at regions beneath the height of contour where framework contact is not planned (i.e., all areas except retentive clasp tips). **A,** Blockout wax is provided for tooth contours beneath the height of contour on teeth #s 21 and 28. **B,** Similar blockout accomplished for mandibular molar #31. Blockout is carved with straight surveyor blade to assure parallelism with the identified path of insertion.

The partial denture must be designed so that (1) it will not stress abutment teeth beyond their physiologic tolerance; (2) it can be easily placed and removed by the patient; (3) it will be retained against reasonable dislodging forces; and (4) it will not create an unfavorable appearance. It is necessary that the diagnostic cast be surveyed with these principles in mind. Mouth preparation should therefore be planned in accordance with certain factors that will influence the path of placement and removal.

FACTORS THAT DETERMINE PATH OF PLACEMENT AND REMOVAL

The factors that will determine the path of placement and removal are guiding planes, retentive areas, interference, and esthetics.

Guiding Planes

Proximal tooth surfaces that bear a parallel relationship to one another must either be found or be created to act as guiding planes during placement and removal of the prosthesis. Guiding planes are necessary to ensure the passage of the rigid parts of the prosthesis past existing areas of interference. Thus the denture can be easily placed and removed by the patient without strain on the teeth contacted or on the denture itself and without damage to the underlying soft tissue.

Guiding planes are also necessary to ensure predictable clasp assembly function, including retention and stabilization. For a clasp to be retentive, its retentive arm must be forced to flex. Hence, guiding planes are necessary to give a positive direction to the movement of the restoration to and from its terminal position.

Retentive Areas

Retentive areas must exist for a given path of placement and must be contacted by retentive clasp arms, which are forced to flex over a convex surface during placement and removal. Satisfactory clasp retention is no more than the resistance of metal to deformation. For a clasp to be retentive, its path of escapement must be other than parallel to the path of removal of the denture itself; otherwise, it would not be forced to flex and thereby generate the resistance known as retention. Clasp retention therefore depends on the existence of a definite path of placement and removal.

Although desirable, retention at each principal abutment may not be balanced in relation to the tooth on the opposite side of the arch (exactly equal and opposite in magnitude and relative location); however, positive cross-arch reciprocation to retentive elements must be present. Retention should be sufficient only to resist reasonable dislodging forces. In other words, it should be the minimum acceptable for adequate retention against reasonable dislodging forces.

Fairly even retention may be obtained by one of two means. One is to change the path of placement to increase or decrease the angle of cervical convergence of opposing retentive surfaces of abutment teeth. The other is to alter the flexibility of the clasp arm by changing its design, its size and length, or the material of which it is made.

Interference

The prosthesis must be designed so that it may be placed and removed without encountering tooth or soft tissue interference. A path of placement may be selected that encounters interference only if the interference can be eliminated during mouth preparation or on the master cast by a reasonable amount of blockout. Interference may be eliminated during mouth preparation by surgery, extraction, modifying interfering tooth surfaces, or altering tooth contours with restorations.

Generally, interference that cannot be eliminated for one reason or another will take precedence over the factors of retention and guiding planes. Sometimes certain areas can be made noninterfering only by selecting a different path of placement at the expense of existing retentive areas and guiding planes. These must then be modified with restorations that are in harmony with the path dictated by the existing interference. On the other hand, if areas of interference can be eliminated by various reasonable means, they should be. By so doing, the axial contours of existing abutments may frequently be used with little alteration.

Esthetics

By one path of placement the most esthetic location of artificial teeth is made possible, and less clasp metal and base material may be displayed.

The location of retentive areas may influence the path of placement selected, and therefore retentive areas always should be selected with the most esthetic location of clasps in mind. When restorations are to be made for other reasons, they should be contoured to permit the least display of clasp metal. Generally, less metal will be displayed if the retentive clasp is placed at a more distogingival area of tooth surface made possible either by the path of placement selected or by the contour of the restorations.

Esthetics also may dictate the choice of path selected when missing anterior teeth must be replaced with the partial denture. In such situations a more vertical path of placement is often necessary so that neither the artificial teeth nor the adjacent natural teeth will have to be modified excessively (Figure 11-10). In this instance, esthetics may take precedence over other factors. This necessitates the preparation of abutment teeth to eliminate interference and to provide guiding planes and retention in harmony with that path of placement dictated by esthetic factors.

Because the primary consideration should be the preservation of the remaining oral tissues, esthetics should not be allowed to jeopardize the success of the partial denture. The replacement of missing anterior teeth therefore should be accomplished by means of fixed partial dentures whenever possible, especially if the mechanical and functional effectiveness of the partial denture will require significant tooth preparation.

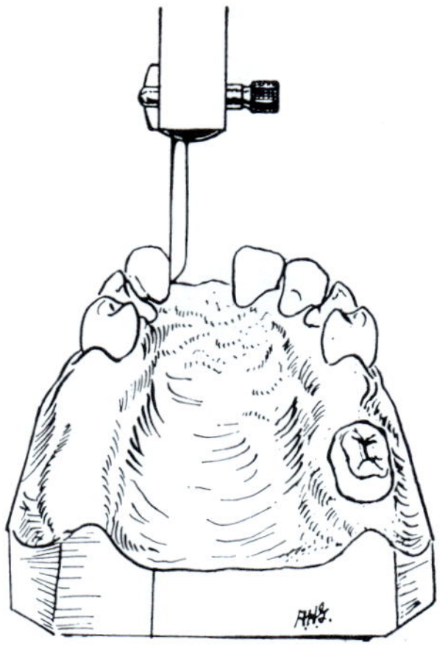

Figure 11-10 When anterior teeth must be replaced with removable partial denture, vertical path of placement may be necessary to avoid excessively altering abutment teeth and supplied teeth.

STEP-BY-STEP PROCEDURES IN SURVEYING A DIAGNOSTIC CAST

Attach the cast to the adjustable surveyor table by means of the clamp provided. Position the adjustable table so that the occlusal surfaces of the teeth are approximately parallel to the platform (Figure 11-11). Such an orientation is a tentative but practical way to start considering the factors that influence the path of placement and removal.

Guiding Planes

Determine the relative parallelism of proximal surfaces of all of the potential abutment teeth by contacting the proximal tooth surfaces with the surveyor blade or diagnostic stylus. Alter the cast position anteroposteriorly until these proximal surfaces are in as close to parallel relation to one another as possible, or near enough that they can be made parallel by recontouring. For posterior modification spaces, this will determine the anteroposterior tilt of the cast in relation to the vertical arm of the surveyor (Figure 11-12). Although the surveyor table is universally adjustable, it should be thought of as having only two axes, thus allowing only anteroposterior and lateral tilting.

In making a choice between having contact with a proximal surface at the cervical area only or contact at the marginal ridge only, the latter is preferred because a plane may then be established by

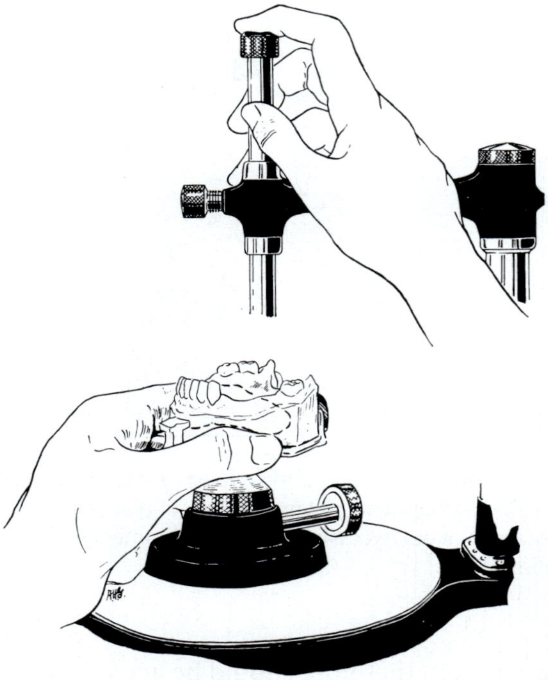

Figure 11-11 Recommended method for manipulating dental surveyor. Right hand is braced on horizontal arm of surveyor, and fingers are used, as illustrated, to raise and lower vertical shaft in its spindle. Left hand holding cast on adjustable table slides horizontally on platform in relation to vertical arm. Right hand must be used also to loosen and tighten tilting mechanism as suitable anteroposterior and lateral tilt of cast in relation to surveyor is being determined.

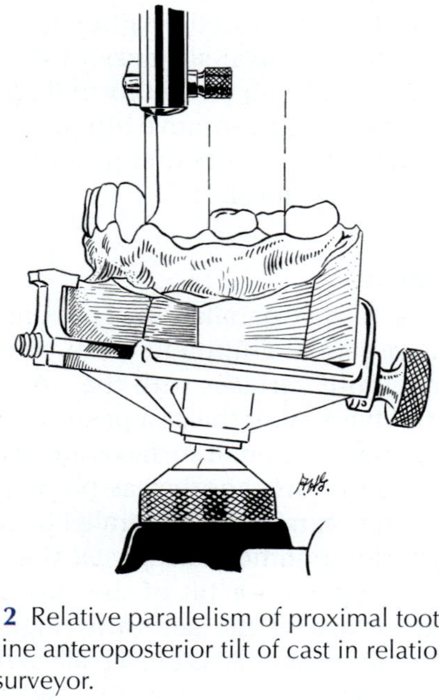

Figure 11-12 Relative parallelism of proximal tooth surfaces will determine anteroposterior tilt of cast in relation to vertical arm of surveyor.

recontouring (Figure 11-13). It is obvious that when only gingival contact exists, a restoration is the only means of establishing a guiding plane. Therefore, if a tilt that does not provide proximal contact is apparent, the proximal surface must be established with some kind of restoration.

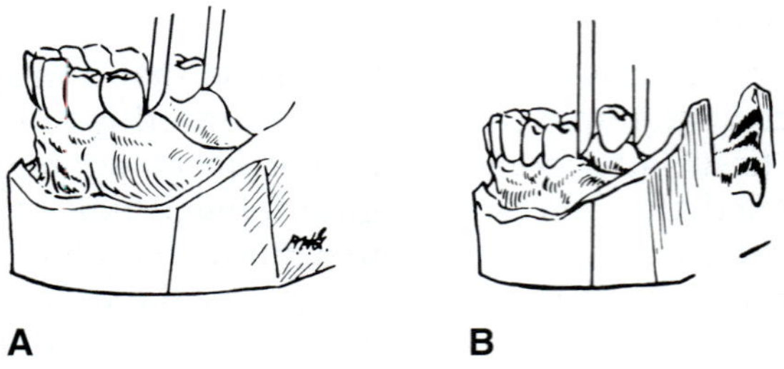

Figure 11-13 In selecting most desirable anteroposterior tilt of cast in relation to surveyor blade, choice must be made between positions illustrated in **A** and **B**. In **A,** distal surface of left premolar abutment would have to be extended by means of a restoration. In **B,** right premolar could be altered slightly to provide acceptably parallel guiding plane. Unless restorations are necessary for other reasons, tilt shown in **B** is preferred.

The end result of selecting a suitable anteroposterior tilt should be to provide the greatest combined areas of parallel proximal surfaces that may act as guiding planes. Other axial surfaces of abutment teeth may also be used as guiding planes. This is realized most often by having the stabilizing component of the direct retainer assembly contacting in its entirety the axial surface of the abutment, which has been found or made parallel to the path of placement (see Figure 14-6). In this instance, both a lateral and an anteroposterior tilt of the cast must be considered when using guiding planes.

Retentive Areas

By contacting buccal and lingual surfaces of abutment teeth with the surveyor blade, the amount of retention existing below their height of convexity may be determined. This is best accomplished by directing a small source of light toward the cast from the side away from the dentist. The angle of cervical convergence is best observed as a triangle of light between the surveyor blade and the apical portion of the tooth surface being studied (see Figure 7-6).

Alter the cast position by tilting it laterally until similar retentive areas exist on the principal abutment teeth. If only two abutment teeth are involved, as in a Kennedy Class I partially edentulous arch, they are both principal abutments. However, if four abutment teeth are involved (as they are in a Kennedy Class III, modification 1 arch), they are all principal abutments, and retentive areas should be located on all four. But if three abutment teeth are involved (as they are in a Kennedy Class II, modification 1 arch), the posterior abutment on the tooth-supported side and the abutment on the distal extension side are considered to be the principal abutments, and retention needs to be equalized accordingly. The third abutment may be considered to be secondary, and less retention is expected from it than from the other two. An exception is when the posterior abutment on the tooth-supported side has a poor prognosis and the denture is designed to ultimately be a Class I. In such a situation, the two stronger abutments are considered to be principal abutments.

In tilting the cast laterally to establish reasonable uniformity of retention, it is necessary that the table be rotated about an imaginary longitudinal axis without disturbing the anteroposterior tilt previously established. The resulting position is one that provides or makes possible parallel guiding planes and provides for acceptable retention on the abutment teeth. It should be noted that achievement of this most desirable position will always require some tooth modification. Note that possible interference to this tentative path of placement has not, as yet, been taken into consideration.

Interference

If a mandibular cast is being surveyed, check the lingual surfaces that will be crossed by a lingual bar major connector during placement and removal. Bony prominences and lingually inclined premolar teeth are the most common causes of interference to a lingual bar connector.

If the interference is bilateral, surgery or recontouring of lingual tooth surfaces, or both, may be unavoidable. If it is only unilateral, a change in the lateral tilt may prevent an area of tooth or tissue interference. In changing the path of placement to prevent interference, previously established guiding planes and an ideal location for retentive elements may be lost. Then the decision must be made whether to remove the existing interference by whatever means necessary or to resort to restorations on the abutment teeth, thereby changing the proximal and retentive areas to conform to the new path of placement.

In a like manner, bony undercuts that will offer interference to the seating of denture bases must be evaluated and the decision made to remove them surgically; to change the path of placement at the expense of modifying or restoring teeth to achieve guiding planes and retention; or to design denture bases to prevent such undercut areas. The latter may be done by shortening buccal and labial flanges and distolingual extension of denture bases. However, it should be remembered that the maximum area available for support of the denture base should be used whenever possible.

Interference to major connectors rarely exists in the maxillary arch. Areas of interference are usually found on buccally inclined posterior teeth and those bony areas on the buccal aspect of edentulous spaces. As with the mandibular cast, the decision must be made whether to eliminate them, to change the path of placement at the expense of modifying or restoring teeth to achieve the required guiding planes and retention, or to design the connectors and bases to avoid them.

Other areas of possible interference to be evaluated are those surfaces of abutment teeth that will support or be crossed by minor connectors and clasp arms. Although interference to vertical minor connectors may be blocked out, doing so may cause discomfort to the patient's tongue and may create objectionable spaces, which could result in the trapping of food. Also it is desirable that tooth surfaces contacted by vertical connectors be used as auxiliary guiding planes whenever possible. Too much relief is perhaps better than too little because of the possibility of irritation to soft tissue. It is always better that the relief be placed with some objective in mind. If possible, a minor connector should pass vertically along a tooth surface that is either parallel to the path of placement (which is considered ideal) or tapered occlusally. If tooth undercuts that necessitate the use of an objectionable amount of blockout exist, they may be eliminated or minimized by slight changes in the path of placement and/or eliminated during mouth preparation. The need for such alteration should be indicated on the diagnostic cast in red pencil after final acceptance of a path of placement.

Tooth surfaces on which reciprocal and stabilizing clasp arms will be placed should be studied to see if sufficient areas exist above the height of convexity for the placement of these components. The addition of a clasp arm to the occlusal third of an abutment tooth adds to its occlusal dimension and therefore to the occlusal loading of that tooth. Nonretentive and stabilizing clasp arms are best located between the middle third and gingival third of the crown rather than on the occlusal third.

Reshaping tooth surfaces during mouth preparation can eliminate areas of interference to proper placement of clasp arms. These areas should be indicated on the diagnostic cast. Areas of interference to the placement of clasps may necessitate minor changes in the path of placement or changes in the clasp design. For example, a bar clasp arm originating mesially from the major connector to provide reciprocation and stabilization might be substituted for a distally originating circumferential arm.

Areas of interference often overlooked are the distal line angles of premolar abutment teeth and the mesial line angles of molar abutments. These areas frequently offer interference to the origin of circumferential clasp arms. If not detected at the time of initial survey, they are not included in the plan for mouth preparation. When such an undercut exists, the following three alternatives may be considered:

1. They may be blocked out the same as any other area of interference. This is by far the least satisfactory method, because the origin of the clasp

must then stand away from the tooth in proportion to the amount of blockout used. Although this is perhaps less objectionable than its being placed occlusally, it may be objectionable to the tongue and the cheek and may create a food trap.

2. Approaching the retentive area from a gingival direction with a bar clasp arm may circumvent them. This is often a satisfactory solution to the problem if other contraindications to the use of a bar clasp arm are not present, such as a severe tissue undercut or a retentive area that is too high on the tooth.
3. Reducing the offending tooth contour during mouth preparation may eliminate them. This permits the use of a circumferential clasp arm originating well below the occlusal surface in a satisfactory manner. If the tooth is to be modified during mouth preparation, it should be indicated on the diagnostic cast with a colored pencil.

When the retentive area is located objectionably high on the abutment tooth or the undercut is too severe, interference may also exist on tooth surfaces that support retentive clasps. Such areas of extreme or high convexity must be considered as areas of interference and should be reduced accordingly. These areas are likewise indicated on the diagnostic cast for reduction during mouth preparation.

Esthetics

The path of placement thus established must still be considered from the standpoint of esthetics, both as to the location of clasps and the arrangement of artificial teeth.

Clasp designs that will provide satisfactory esthetics usually may be selected for any given path of placement. In some instances gingivally placed bar clasp arms may be used to advantage; in others, circumferential clasp arms located cervically may be used. This is especially true when other abutment teeth located more posteriorly may bear the major responsibility for retention. In still other instances, a tapered wrought-wire retentive clasp arm may be placed to better esthetic advantage than a cast clasp arm. The location of clasp arms for esthetic reasons does not ordinarily justify altering the path of placement at the expense of mechanical factors. However, it should be considered concurrently with other factors, and if a choice between two paths of insertion of equal merit permits a more esthetic placement of clasp arms by one path than the other, that path should be given preference.

When anterior replacements are involved, the choice of path is limited to a more vertical one for reasons previously stated. In this instance alone, esthetics must be given primary consideration, even at the expense of altering the path of placement and making all other factors conform. This factor should be remembered when considering the other three factors so that compromises can be made at the time of consideration for other factors.

FINAL PATH OF PLACEMENT

The final path of placement will be the anteroposterior and lateral position of the cast, in relation to the vertical arm of the surveyor that best satisfies all four factors: guiding planes, retention, interference, and esthetics.

All proposed mouth changes should be indicated on the diagnostic cast in red pencil, with the exception of restorations to be done. These may also be indicated if desired on an accompanying chart. Extractions and surgery are given priority to allow time for healing. The remaining red marks represent the actual modifications of the teeth that remain to be done, which consist of the preparation of proximal surfaces, the reduction of buccal and lingual surfaces, and the preparation of rest seats. Except when they are placed in the wax pattern for a cast restoration, the preparation of rest seats should always be deferred until all other mouth preparations have been completed.

The actual location of rests will be determined by the proposed design of the denture framework. Therefore the tentative design should be sketched on the diagnostic cast in pencil after deciding on the path of placement. This is done not only to locate rest areas but also to record graphically the plan of treatment before mouth preparation. In the intervening time between patient visits, other partial denture restorations may have been considered. The dentist should have the plan of treatment readily available at each succeeding appointment to avoid confusion and to be a reminder about what is to be done and the sequence that will be required.

The plan for treatment should include (1) the diagnostic cast with the mouth preparation and the denture design marked on it; (2) a chart showing the proposed design and the planned treatment for each abutment; (3) a working chart showing the total treatment involved that will permit a quick review and a check-off of each step as the work progresses; and (4) a record of the fee quoted for each phase of treatment that can be checked off as it is recorded on the patient's permanent record.

Red pencil marks on the diagnostic cast are used to indicate the location of areas to be modified and the location of rests (Figure 11-14). Although it is not necessary that rest areas be prepared on the diagnostic cast, it is advisable for the beginning student to have done so before proceeding to alter the abutment teeth. This applies equally to crown and inlay preparations on abutment teeth. It is advisable,

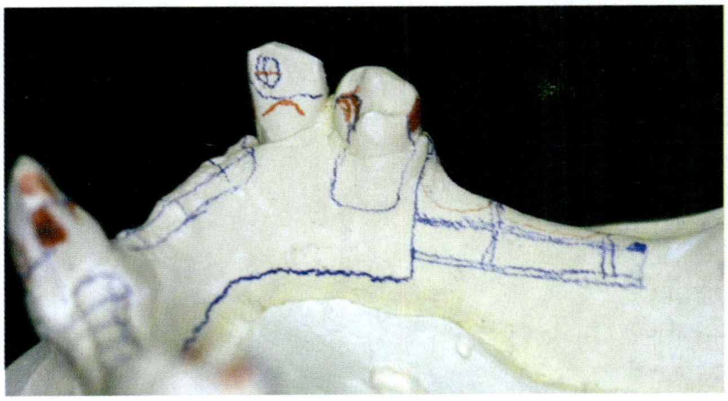

A

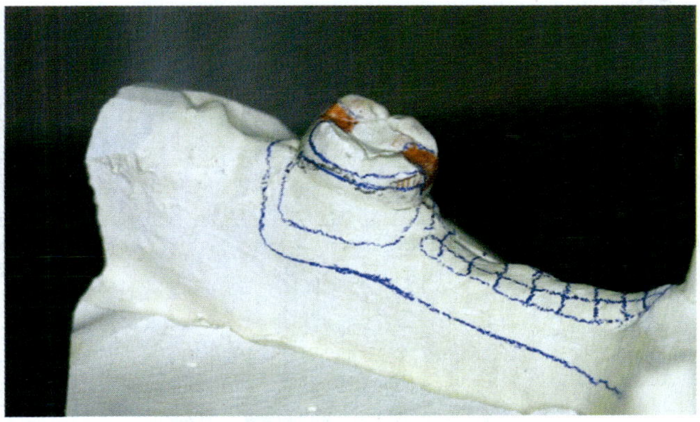

B

Figure 11-14 Diagnostic casts can serve as a visual guide for tooth preparation. **A,** Surveyed casts shows areas requiring tooth reduction in red (mesio-occlusal rest and distal guide plane #28, cingulum rest #27) as well as path of insertion tripod marks. **B,** This mesially tipped molar has been diagnosed to have a ring clasp. Red markings show the necessary mesio-occlusal and disto-occlusal rests required, as well as the mesial guide plane. Also shown is the reduction necessary to lower the lingual height of contour at the mesio-lingual line angle. All of the required axial contour adjustments are determined through the appropriate use of a surveyor.

however, for even the most experienced dentist to have trimmed the stone teeth with the surveyor blade wherever tooth reduction is to be done. This identifies not only the amount to be removed in a given area but also the plane in which the tooth is to be prepared. For example, a proximal surface may need to be recontoured in only the upper third or the middle third to establish a guiding plane that will be parallel to the path of placement. This is not usually parallel to the long axis of the tooth, and if the rotary instrument is laid against the side of the tooth, the existing surface angle will be maintained, rather than having to establish a new plane that is parallel to the path of placement.

The surveyor blade, representing the path of placement, may be used to advantage to trim the surface of the abutment tooth whenever a red mark appears. The resulting surface represents the amount of tooth to be removed in the mouth and indicates the angle at which the handpiece must be held. The cut surface on the stone tooth is not marked with red pencil again, but it is outlined in red pencil to positively locate the area that is to be prepared.

RECORDING RELATION OF CAST TO SURVEYOR

Some method of recording the relation of the cast to the vertical arm of the surveyor must be used so that it may be returned to the surveyor for future reference, especially during mouth preparation. The same applies to the need for returning any working cast to the surveyor for shaping wax patterns, trimming blockout on the master cast, or locating clasp arms in relation to undercut areas.

Obviously the trimmed base will vary with each cast; therefore recording the position of the surveyor table is of no value. If it were, calibrations could be incorporated on the surveyor table that would allow the reestablishment of the same position. Instead, the position of each cast must be established separately, and any positional record applies only to that cast.

Of several methods, two seem to be the most convenient and accurate. One method is to place three widely divergent dots on the tissue surface of the cast using the tip of a carbon marker, with the vertical arm of the surveyor in a locked position. Preferably, these dots should not be placed on areas of the cast involved in the framework design. The dots should be encircled with a colored pencil for easy identification. On returning the cast to the surveyor, it may be tilted until the tip of the surveyor blade or diagnostic stylus again contacts the three dots in the same plane. This will produce the original position of the cast and therefore the original path of placement. This is known as *tripoding* the cast (Figure 11-15). Some dentists prefer to make tiny pits in the cast at the location of the tripoding dots to preserve the orientation of the cast and to transfer this relationship to the refractory cast.

A second method is to score two sides and the dorsal aspect of the base of the cast with a sharp instrument held against the surveyor blade (see Figure 11-15). By tilting the cast until all three lines are again parallel to the surveyor blade, the original cast position can be reestablished. Fortunately, the

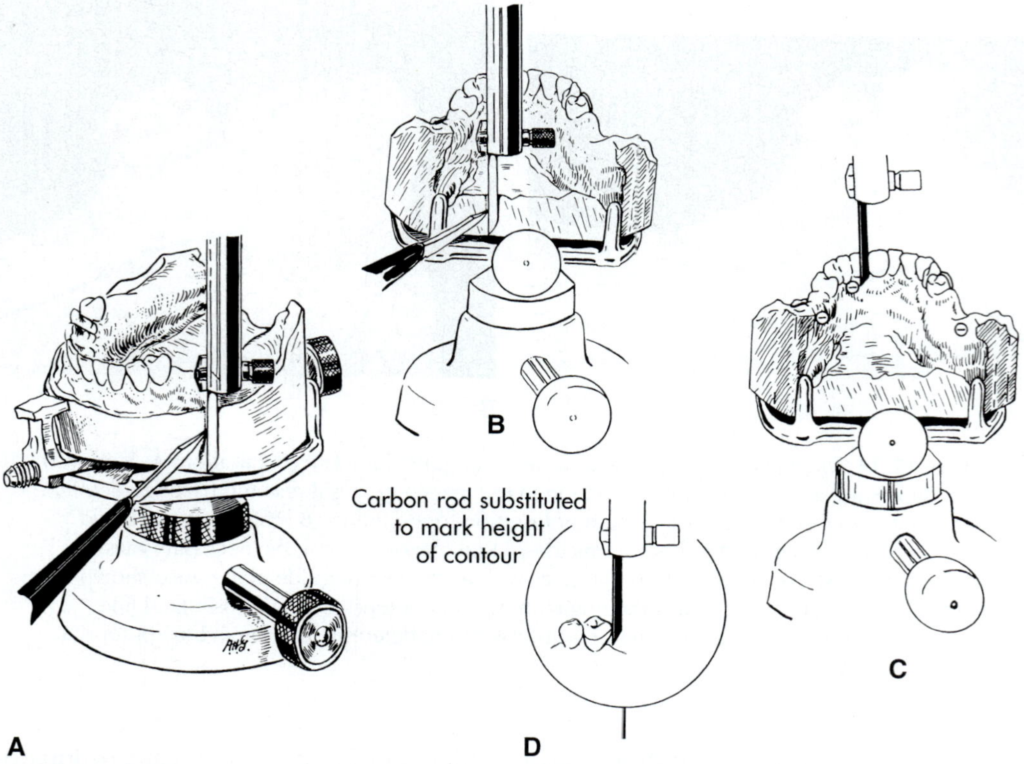

Figure 11-15 **A** and **B,** Path of placement is determined, base of cast is scored to record its relation to surveyor for future repositioning. **C,** Alternate method to record relation of cast to surveyor is known as tripoding. Carbon marker is placed in vertical arm of surveyor, and arm is adjusted to height by which cast can be contacted in three divergent locations. Vertical arm is locked in position, and cast is brought into contact with tip of carbon marker. Three resultant marks are encircled with colored lead pencil for ease of identification. Reorientation of cast to surveyor is accomplished by tilting cast until plane created by three marks is at right angle to vertical arm of surveyor. **D,** Height of contour is then delineated by carbon marker.

scratch lines will be reproduced in any duplication, thereby permitting any duplicate cast to be related to the surveyor in a similar manner. Whereas a diagnostic cast and a master cast cannot be made interchangeable, a refractory cast, being a duplicate of the master cast, can be repositioned on the surveyor at any time. The technician must be cautioned not to trim the sides of the cast on the cast trimmer and thereby lose the reference marks for repositioning.

It must be remembered that repositioning a cast on a surveyor at any time can involve a certain amount of human error. It has been estimated that an error of 0.2 mm can be anticipated in reorienting a cast with three reference points on its base. This reorientation error can influence the placement of appropriate blockout wax and may result in ineffective placement of direct retainers into prescribed undercuts and improper contacts of minor connectors to guiding planes. Therefore reorientation of the cast to surveyor by any method must be done with great care.

SURVEYING THE MASTER CAST

The master cast must be surveyed as a new cast, but the prepared proximal guiding plane surfaces will indicate the correct anteroposterior tilt. Some compromises may be necessary, but the amount of guiding plane surface remaining after blockout should be the maximum for each tooth. Areas above the point of contact with the surveyor blade are not considered to be part of the guiding plane area and neither are gingival undercut areas, which will be blocked out.

The lateral tilt will be the position that provides equal retentive areas on all principal abutments in relation to the planned clasp design. Factors of flexibility, including the need for extra flexibility on distal extension abutments, must be considered in deciding what will provide equal retention on all abutment teeth. For example, cast circumferential or cast bar retention on the tooth-supported side of a Class II design should be balanced against the 18-gauge wrought-wire retention on a distal abutment only if

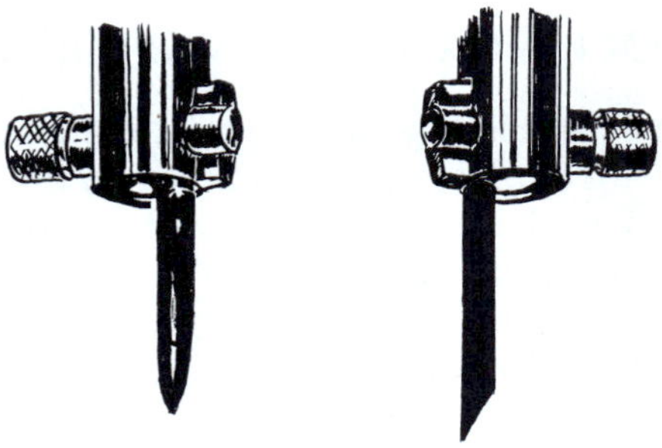

Figure 11-16 Worn carbon marker *(left)* should be discarded because it will invariably misleadingly mark height of contour for given orientation of cast to vertical spindle of surveyor. Unworn carbon *(right)* with angled end is preferable for marking heights of contour on abutment teeth and performing survey of soft tissue areas.

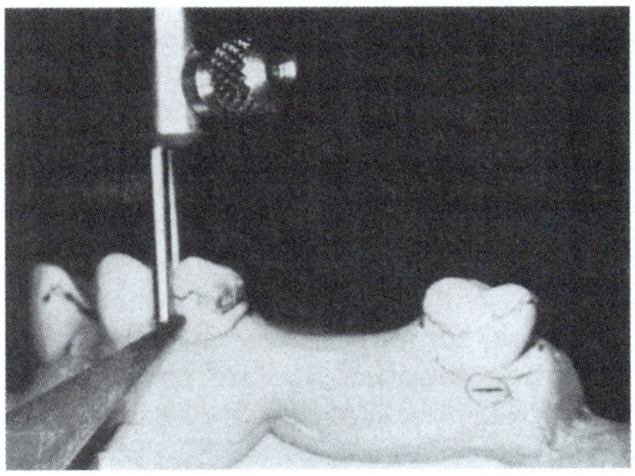

A

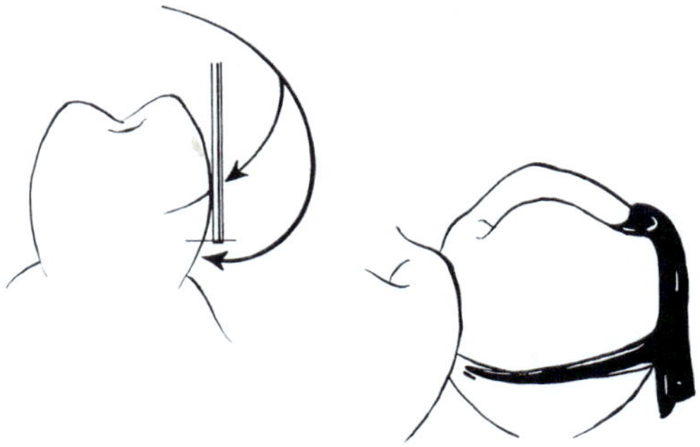

B

Figure 11-17 **A,** Undercut gauge will measure depth of undercut below height of contour. I-bar direct retainer will contact the tooth from the point of the undercut to the height of contour. Depth to which retentive clasp arm can be placed depends not only on its length, taper, diameter, and alloy from which it is made but also on type of clasp. Circumferential clasp arm is more flexible than is bar clasp arm of same length (Chapter 7). **B,** Specific measurement of undercut gingiva to height of contour may be ascertained by use of undercut gauge attached to surveyor. Simultaneous contact of shank of undercut gauge at height of contour and contact of lip of specific undercut gauge on tooth in infrabulge area establishes definitive degree and location of undercut. Therefore tip of retentive arm of direct retainer may be placed in planned depth of undercut.

the more rigid cast clasp engages a lesser undercut than the wrought-wire clasp arm. Therefore the degree of undercut alone does not ensure relatively equal retention unless clasp arms of equal length, diameter, form, and material are used.

Gross interference will have been eliminated during mouth preparation. Thus for a given path of placement providing guiding planes and balanced retention, any remaining interference must be eliminated with blockout. If mouth preparation has been adequately planned and executed, the undercuts remaining to be blocked out should be minimal.

The base of the cast is now scored, or the cast is tripoded as described previously. The surveyor blade or diagnostic stylus then may be replaced with a carbon marker, and the height of convexity of each abutment tooth and soft tissue contours may be delineated. Similarly, any areas of interference to the rigid parts of the framework during seating and removal should be indicated with the carbon marker to locate areas to be blocked out or relieved.

Carbon markers that become the slightest bit worn from use should be discarded. A worn (tapered) carbon marker will indicate heights of contour more occlusally located than they actually exist. The carbon marker must be parallel to the vertical spindle of the surveyor (Figure 11-16). The diagnostic stylus should always be checked to be sure that it is not bent or distorted.

MEASURING RETENTION

The surveyor is used with the master cast for two purposes: (1) to delineate the height of contour of the abutment teeth both to locate clasp arms and to identify the location and magnitude of retentive undercuts; and (2) to trim blockout of any remaining interference to placement and removal of the denture. The areas involved are those that will be crossed by rigid parts of the denture framework.

The exact undercut that retentive clasp terminals will occupy must be measured and marked on the master cast (Figure 11-17). Undercuts may be measured with an undercut gauge, such as those provided with the Ney and Jelenko surveyors. The amount of undercut is measured in hundredths of an inch, with the gauges allowing measurements up to 0.03 inch. Theoretically the amount of undercut used may vary with the clasp to be used up to a full 0.03 inch. However, undercuts of 0.01 inch are often adequate for retention by cast retainers. Tapered wrought-wire retention may safely use up to 0.02 inch without

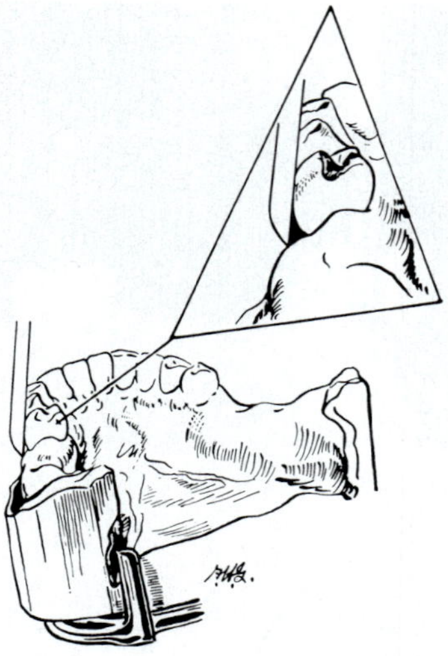

Figure 11-18 Tooth undercut is best viewed against good source of light passing through triangle, which is bounded by surface of abutment tooth, surveyor blade, and gingival tissues.

inducing undesirable torque on the abutment tooth, provided the wire retentive arm is long enough (at least 8 mm). The use of 0.03 inch is rarely, if ever, justified with any clasp. When greater retention is required, such as when abutment teeth remain on only one side of the arch, multiple abutments should be used rather than increasing the retention on any one tooth.

When a source of light is directed toward the tooth being surveyed, a triangle of light is visible. This triangle is bounded by the surface of the abutment tooth on one side and the blade of the surveyor on the other, the apex being the point of contact at the height of convexity and the base of the triangle being the gingival tissue (Figure 11-18). Retention will be determined by (1) the magnitude of the angle of cervical convergence below the point of convexity; (2) the depth at which the clasp terminal is placed in the angle; and (3) the flexibility of the clasp arm. The intelligent application of various clasp designs and their relative flexibility are of greater importance than the ability to measure an undercut with precise accuracy.

The final design may now be drawn on the master cast with a fine crayon pencil, preferably one that will not come off during duplication. Graphite is usually lifted in duplication, but some crayon pencil marks will withstand duplication without blurring or transfer.* Sizing or spraying the master cast to protect such pencil marks is usually not advisable unless done with extreme care to avoid obliterating the surface detail.

*Such as the Dixon Thinex pencil.

BLOCKING OUT THE MASTER CAST

After the establishment of the path of placement and the location of undercut areas on the master cast, any undercut areas that will be crossed by rigid parts of the denture (which is every part of the denture framework but the retentive clasp terminals) must be eliminated by blockout.

In the broader sense of the term, blockout includes not only the areas crossed by the denture framework during seating and removal but also (1) those areas not involved that are blocked out for convenience; (2) ledges on which clasp patterns are to be placed; (3) relief beneath connectors to prevent tissue impingement; and (4) relief to provide for attachment of the denture base to the framework.

Ledges or shelves (shaped blockout) for locating clasp patterns may or may not be used (Figure 11-19). However, this should not be confused with the actual blocking out of undercut areas that would offer interference to the placement of the denture framework. Only the latter is made on the surveyor, with the surveyor blade or diagnostic stylus being used as a paralleling device.

Hard inlay wax may be used satisfactorily as a blockout material. It is easily applied and is easily trimmed with the surveyor blade. Trimming is facilitated by slightly warming the surveyor blade with an alcohol torch. Whereas it is true that any wax will melt more readily than a wax-clay mixture if the temperature of the duplicating material is too high, it should be presumed that the duplicating material will not be used at such an elevated temperature. If the temperature of the duplicating material is high enough to damage a wax blockout, other distortions resulting in an inaccurate duplication will likely occur.

Parallel blockout is necessary for areas that are cervical to guiding plane surfaces and over all undercut areas that will be crossed by major or minor connectors. Other areas that are to be blocked out for convenience and to avoid difficulties in duplication should be blocked out with hard baseplate wax or oil-base modeling clay (artist's modeling clay). Such areas are the labial surfaces and labial undercuts not involved in the denture design and the sublingual and distolingual areas beyond the limits of the denture design. These are blocked out arbitrarily with hard baseplate wax or clay, but because they have no relation to the path of placement, they do not require the use of the surveyor. Modeling clay that is water-soluble should not be used when duplication procedures are involved.

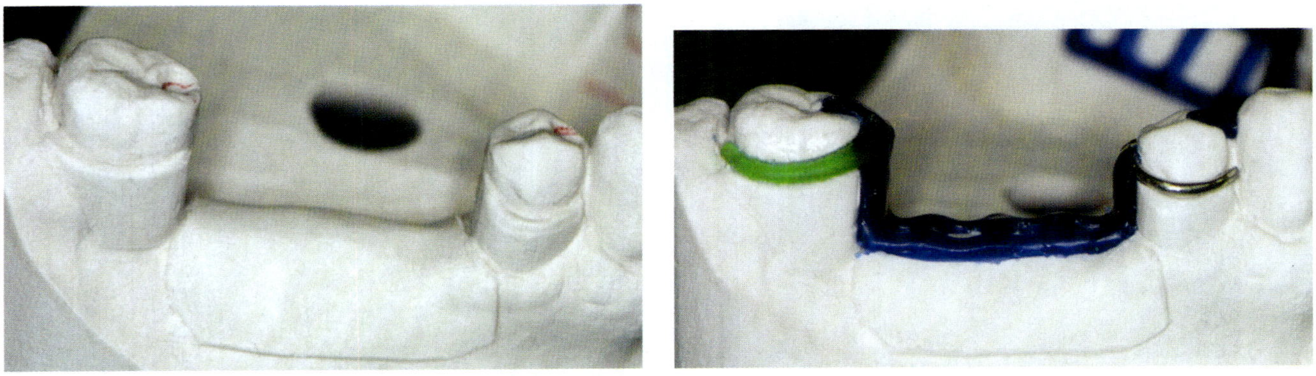

Figure 11-19 **A,** Wax ledges on buccal surfaces of premolar and molar abutments have been duplicated in refractory the cast for exact placement of clasp molar pattern and the premolar wrought wire clasp. **B,** Pattern and wrought wire in position at wax pattern stage. The molar ledge has been placed slightly below the outline of cast clasp arm to allow the gingival edge of clasp arm to be polished and still remain in its planned relationship to tooth when denture is seated. It should also be noted that wax ledge definitively establishes planned placement of direct retainer tip into measured undercut.

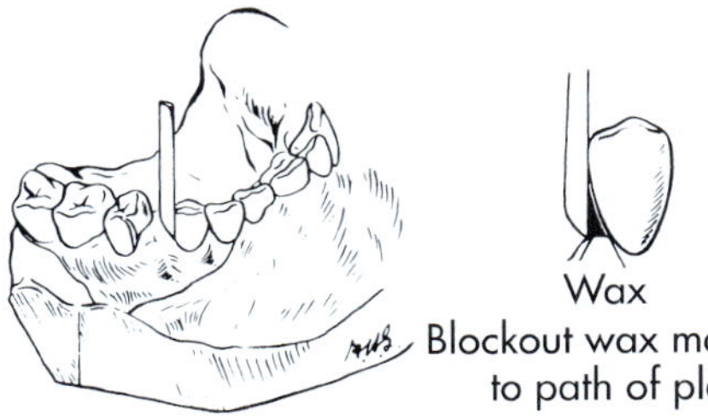

Figure 11-20 All guiding plane areas must be parallel to path of placement, and all other areas that will be contacted by rigid parts of denture framework must be made free of undercut by parallel blockout. Relief must also be provided for the gingival crevice and gingival margin.

Areas to be crossed by rigid connectors, on the other hand, should be trimmed with the surveyor blade or some other surveyor tool parallel to the path of placement (Figure 11-20). This imposes a considerable responsibility on the technician. If the blockout is not sufficiently trimmed to expose guiding plane surfaces, the effect of these guiding planes, which were carefully established by the dentist, will be nullified. If, on the other hand, the technician is overzealous in paralleling the blockout, the stone cast may be abraded by heavy contact with the surveyor blade. Although the resulting cast framework would seat back onto the master cast without interference, interference to placement in the mouth would result. This would necessitate relieving the casting at the chair, which is not only an embarrassing and time-consuming operation but also one that may have the effect of obliterating guiding plane surfaces.

RELIEVING THE MASTER CAST

Tissue undercuts that must be blocked out are paralleled in much the same manner as tooth undercuts. The difference between blockout and relief must be clearly understood (Figures 11-21 and 11-22). For example, tissue undercuts that would offer interference to the seating of a lingual bar connector are blocked out with blockout wax and trimmed parallel to the path of placement. This does not in itself necessarily afford relief to prevent tissue impingement. In addition to such blockout, a relief of varying thickness must sometimes be used—depending on the location of the connector, the relative slope of the alveolar ridge, and the predictable effect of denture rotation. It must be assumed that indirect retainers, as such, or indirect retention is provided in the design of the denture to prevent rotation of the lingual bar inferiorly. A vertical downward rotation of the denture bases around posterior abutments places the bar increasingly farther from the lingual aspect of the alveolar ridge when this surface slopes inferiorly and posteriorly (Figure 11-23). Adequate relief of soft tissues adjacent to the lingual bar is obtained by the initial finishing and polishing of the framework in these instances. However, excessive upward vertical rotation of a lingual bar will impinge on lingual tissues if the alveolar ridge is nearly vertical or undercut to the path of placement (Figure 11-24). The region of the cast involving the proposed placement of the lingual bar should, in this situation, be first relieved by parallel blockout and then by a 32-gauge wax strip. Low-fusing casting wax, such as

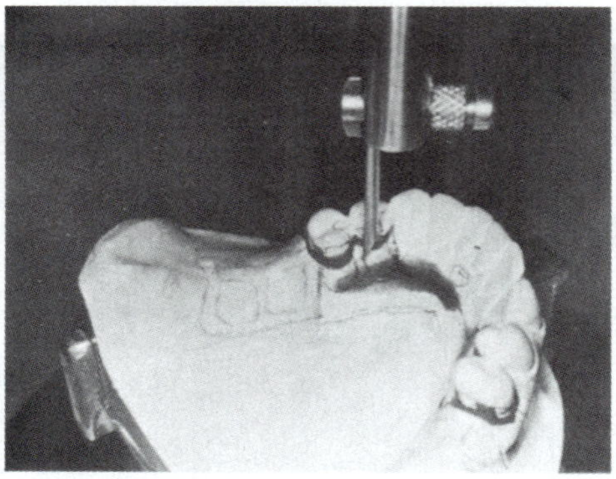

A

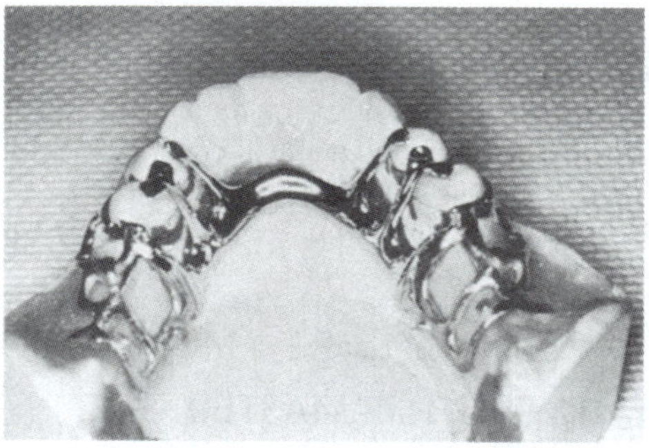

B

Figure 11-21 Relationship of parallel blockout and relief to removable partial denture framework. **A,** Interproximal spaces to be occupied by minor connectors are blocked out parallel to path of placement. In like manner, tissue undercuts intimate to lingual bar and minor connectors are blocked out parallel to path of placement rather than using an arbitrary blockout. Arbitrary blockout in lingual bar region could create unnecessary spaces for entrapment of food. Blockout of tissue surface inferior to buccal surface of right second premolar is required. Because this slight undercut coincided with placement of bar-type direct retainer arm, it was blocked out parallel to path of placement to avoid tissue damage when denture rotated or when restoration was being removed or placed. **B,** Finished removable partial denture framework accurately fits blocked-out master cast. Adjustment of framework by grinding to fit master cast or mouth is largely eliminated when blockout of cast has been meticulously carried out.

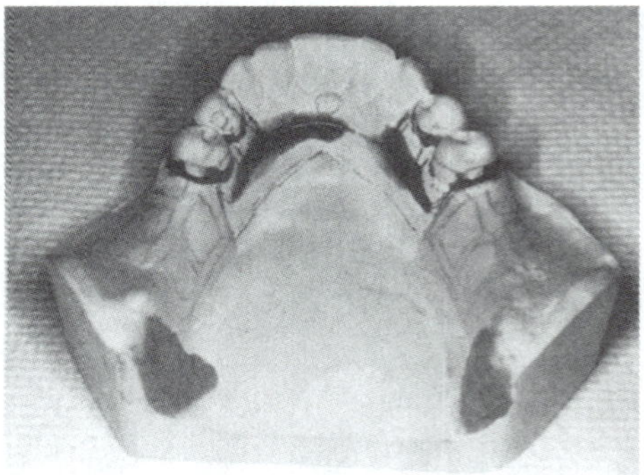

Figure 11-22 Relief and blockout of master cast before duplication. All undercuts involved in denture design (except tips of retentive clasp arms) have been blocked out parallel to path of placement. Residual ridges have been relieved with 20-gauge sheet wax to provide space for denture base material to totally enclose denture base minor connector. Small window has been created in wax adjacent to distogingival surface of each posterior abutment. Framework will occupy this space and will definitively establish most anterior extent of denture bases in these regions. Severe undercuts in retromylohyoid regions of cast have been arbitrarily blocked out to prevent possible distortion of duplicating mold when master cast is removed.

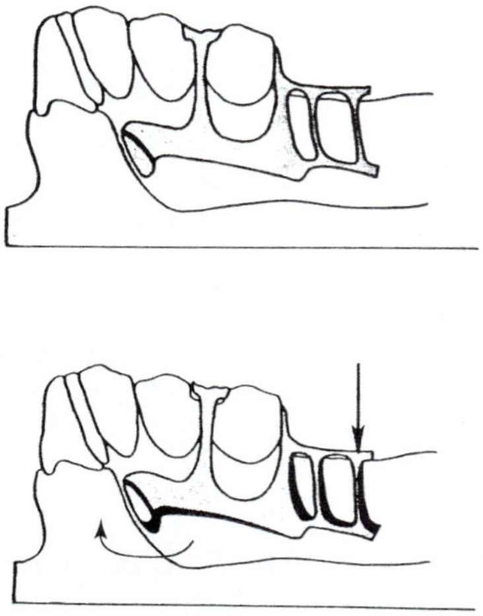

Figure 11-23 Sagittal section of cast and denture framework. Lingual alveolar ridge slopes inferiorly and posteriorly *(upper figure)*. When force is directed to displace denture base downward, lingual bar rotates forward and upward but does not impinge on soft tissue of alveolar ridge *(lower figure)*. Therefore in such instances, adequate relief to avoid impingement is gained when tissue side of lingual bar is highly polished during finishing process.

Kerr's green casting wax, should not be used because it is too easily thinned during adaptation and may be affected by the temperature of the duplicating material. Pink casting wax should be used, even though it is difficult to adapt uniformly. A pressure-sensitive, adhesive-coated casting wax is preferred because it adapts readily and adheres to the cast surface. Any wax, even the adhesive type, should be sealed all around its borders with a hot spatula to prevent its lifting when the cast is moistened before or during duplication.

Horizontal rotational tendencies of mandibular distal extension removable partial dentures account for many of the tissue irritations seen adjacent to a lingual mandibular major connector. These irritations can usually be avoided by blocking out all undercuts adjacent to the bar parallel to the path of placement and then including adequate stabilizing components in the design of the framework to resist horizontal rotation. Judicious relief of the tissue side of the lingual bar with rubber wheels at the site of

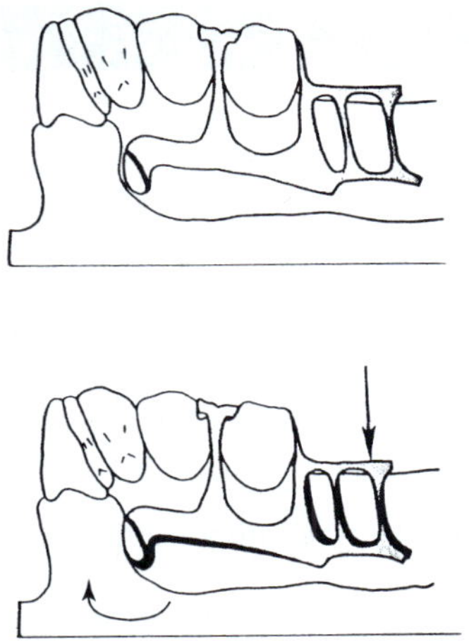

Figure 11-24 Undercut alveolar ridge was blocked out parallel to path of placement in fabricating lingual bar (*upper figure*). Application of vertical force to create rotation of lingual bar upward can cause impingement of lingual tissue on alveolar ridge (*lower figure*). To avoid impingement in these instances, not only should master cast be blocked out parallel to path of placement but also an additional relief of 32-gauge sheet wax should be used in blocking out cast in such undercut areas.

the irritation will most often correct the discrepancy. Under no circumstances should grinding any portion jeopardize the rigidity of the major connector.

Still other areas requiring relief are the areas where component parts cross the gingiva and gingival crevices. All gingival areas bridged by the denture framework should be protected from possible impingement resulting from rotation of the denture framework. Hard inlay wax may be used to block out gingival crevices (see Fig. 11-21).

PARALLEL BLOCKOUT, SHAPED BLOCKOUT, ARBITRARY BLOCKOUT, AND RELIEF

Table 11-1 differentiates between parallel blockout, shaped blockout, arbitrary blockout, and relief. The same factors apply to both the maxillary and mandibular arches, except that relief is ordinarily not used beneath palatal major connectors, as it is with mandibular lingual bar connectors, except when maxillary tori cannot be circumvented or when resistive median palatal raphae are encountered.

TABLE 11-1. Differentiations Between Parallel Blockout, Shaped Blockout, Arbitrary Blockout, and Relief

Site	Material	Thickness
PARALLEL BLOCKOUT		
Proximal tooth surfaces to be used as guiding planes	Hard baseplate wax or blockout material	Only undercut remaining gingival to contact of surveyor blade with tooth surface
Beneath all minor connectors	Hard baseplate wax or blockout material	Only undercut remaining gingival to contact of surveyor blade with tooth surface
Tissue undercuts to be crossed by rigid connectors	Hard baseplate wax or blockout material	Only undercut remaining below contact of surveyor blade with surface of cast
Tissue undercuts to be crossed by origin of bar clasps	Hard baseplate wax or blockout material	Only undercut remaining below contact of surveyor blade with surface of cast
Deep interproximal spaces to be covered by minor connectors or linguoplates	Hard baseplate wax or blockout material	Only undercut remaining below contact of surveyor blade with surface of cast
Beneath bar clasp arms to gingival crevice	Hard baseplate wax or blockout material	Only undercut area involved in attachment of clasp arm to minor connector
SHAPED BLOCKOUT		
On buccal and lingual surfaces to locate plastic or wax patterns for clasp arms	Hard baseplate wax	Ledges for location of reciprocal clasp arms to follow height or convexity so that they may be placed as cervical as possible without becoming retentive

Continued

TABLE 11-1. Differentiations Between Parallel Blockout, Shaped Blockout, Arbitrary Blockout, and Relief—cont'd

Site	Material	Thickness
		Ledges for location of retentive clasp arms to be placed as cervical as tooth contour permits; point of origin of clasp to be occlusal or incisal to height of convexity, crossing survey line at terminal fourth, and to include undercut area previously selected in keeping with flexibility of clasp type being used
ARBITRARY BLOCKOUT		
All gingival crevices	Hard baseplate wax	Enough to just eliminate gingival crevice
Gross tissue undercuts situated below areas involved in design of denture framework	Hard baseplate wax or oil-base clay	Leveled arbitrarily with wax spatula
Tissue undercuts distal to cast framework	Hard baseplate wax or oil-base clay	Smoothed arbitrarily with wax spatula
Labial and buccal tooth and tissue undercuts not involved in denture design	Hard baseplate wax or oil-base clay	Filled and tapered with spatula to within upper third or crown
RELIEF		
Beneath lingual bar connectors or the bar portion of the linguoplates when indicated (see text)	Adhesive wax sealed to cast; should be wider than major connector to be placed on it	32-gauge wax if slope of lingual alveolar ridge is parallel to path of placement; 32-gauge wax after parallel blockout of undercuts if slope of lingual alveolar ridge is undercut to path of placement
Areas in which major connectors will contact thin tissue, such as hard areas so frequently found on lingual or mandibular ridges and elevated palatal raphes	Hard baseplate wax	Thin layer flowed on with hot wax spatula; however, if maxillary torus must be covered, the thickness of the relief must represent the difference in the degree of displacement of the tissues covering the torus and the tissues covering the residual ridges
Beneath framework extensions onto ridge areas for attachment of resin bases	Adhesive wax, well adapted to and sealed to cast beyond the involved area	20-gauge wax

SELF-ASSESSMENT AIDS

1. Define a dental cast surveyor.
2. What are the basic parts of a surveyor?
3. What does height of contour mean? How does it relate to a direct retainer assembly?
4. Because no component of a removable partial denture may engage an undercut except a portion of the retentive arm of a direct retainer, then both desirable and undesirable undercuts must be known in designing a restoration. True or false?
5. When planning the design of a partial denture, four factors must be considered in determining the path of placement and removal. Two of these factors are retention and esthetics. Name the two other factors.
6. With the diagnostic cast securely clamped to the adjustable table and the diagnostic stylus in the vertical spindle, what orientation of the occlusal plane to the base of the surveyor is recommended as a provisional study position?
7. When considering a design for a Class III, modification 1 arch, which directional tilt of the cast will indicate the greatest area of parallel proximal surfaces to act as guiding planes—anteroposterior or lateral?

8. Suppose, in the previous situation, that the diagnostic stylus touches only gingival areas of the proximal surfaces. What are the options to obtain guiding plane surfaces?
9. When possible retentive areas are being ascertained, the cast is tilted laterally. How can one avoid changing the established anteroposterior tilt of the cast?
10. Uniformity of retention bilaterally is desirable. In what manner does the angle of cervical convergence contribute to obtaining uniform retention?
11. What are the most common causes of interference to the placement of a mandibular major connector?
12. Why should soft tissue contours be surveyed along with teeth?
13. What advantages accrue in having the tip of the carbon marker touch gingival areas intermittently when marking the heights of contour of abutment teeth?
14. After the diagnostic cast has been surveyed, how can the relationship of the cast to the vertical spindle of the surveyor in three dimensions be recorded?
15. What is the disadvantage of using a carbon marker that is even slightly worn?
16. What is an undercut gauge? How can it be used to measure the depth of undercut in the angle of cervical convergence?
17. Heights of contour in many instances will be more optimally located for direct retainer assemblies if axial surfaces are recontoured. How may an undercut gauge assist in determining whether they can be recontoured without exposing dentin?
18. Diagnostic casts are quite often altered during design on the surveyor or in other uses. Why is it a good idea to have duplicate diagnostic casts?
19. The designed diagnostic cast can readily serve as a blueprint to accomplish contouring of abutment teeth during mouth preparation procedures. How may the contoured areas on the diagnostic cast be indicated to avoid overlooking these areas when preparing them in the mouth?
20. After mouth preparation procedures are completed and a master cast has been made, it must be surveyed to definitively locate components. What are the guides to relate the cast to the surveyor?
21. The terminal portion of the retentive arm of a direct retainer should engage a planned and measured undercut. Using the same degree of undercut bilaterally will not necessarily ensure relative equal retention. What factor other than the degree of undercut must be considered?
22. After the path of placement is established, undercut areas that will be crossed by rigid parts must be eliminated. How is this accomplished? With what materials?
23. By what means can the definitive locations of components of the framework be transferred from the master cast to the duplicate investment cast on which the pattern for the framework will be developed?
24. Explain the differences between shaped blockout, arbitrary blockout, relief of the master cast, and parallel blockout.
25. Why should undercuts on the master cast not involved with the framework be blocked out?
26. How do you handle the blockout of gingival crevices that will be crossed by a component of the framework?
27. What relief of a mandibular master cast is required for the lingual aspect of the alveolar ridge that will be covered by a lingual bar or linguoplate when the ridge slopes inferiorly and posteriorly? The ridge is parallel to the path of placement? The ridge is undercut to the path of placement?
28. Why should a master cast be relieved?
29. What determines the amount of palatal relief required when a major connector must traverse the median palatal raphe in a Class I arch?
30. What are the requirements for relief on a master cast for minor connectors that will attach acrylic resin bases to the major connector?
31. What uses are there for a dental cast surveyor other than surveying casts for designs and preparation of master casts for duplication in a refractory investment?
32. How can a dental cast surveyor help develop the optimum contour for crowns?
33. By what means can some dental cast surveyors be converted into a convenient drill press or machining tool?
34. Ceramo-metal restorations in many instances require machining before the final glazing procedures to make sure that originally planned contours are accomplished. How can this be done?
35. Internal rests on crowns may be machined with the surveyor as a drill press, or they may be made by another method involving the dental cast surveyor. What is this other method?
36. Why would a dental cast surveyor be required to place some types of manufactured internal attachments?
37. What are some sequelae of marring a master cast during surveying or blockout procedures?
38. What are some applications for use of the dental cast surveyor in planning for a fixed partial denture?

II

Clinical and Laboratory

12

DIAGNOSIS AND TREATMENT PLANNING

PURPOSE AND UNIQUENESS OF TREATMENT

The purpose of dental treatment is to respond to a patient's needs, both the needs perceived by the patient and those demonstrated through a clinical examination and patient interview. Although there are similarities between partially edentulous patients (such as classification designations), significant differences exist making each patient, and the ultimate treatment, unique.

The delineation of each patient's uniqueness occurs through the patient interview and diagnostic clinical examination process. This includes four distinct processes: (1) understanding the patient's desires or chief concerns/complaints regarding their condition (including its history) through a systematic interview process, (2) ascertaining the patient's dental needs through a diagnostic clinical exam, (3) developing a treatment plan that reflects the best management of the desires and needs (with influences unique to their medical condition or oral environment), and (4) appropriately sequenced execution of the treatment with planned follow up. The ultimate treatment is individualized to address disease management and the unique coordinated restorative and prosthetic needs of the patient. Provision of the best care for a patient may involve no treatment, limited treatment, or extensive treatment, and the dentist must be prepared to help patients decide the best treatment option given their individual circumstances.

PATIENT INTERVIEW

Although oral health is an important aspect of overall health, it is an elective health pursuit for most individuals. Consequently, the patient comes for professional examination because of some perception of (1) an abnormality that requires correction or (2) to maintain optimum oral health. For either situation, but especially the patient with some chief complaint (often with an important history related to that complaint), it is mandatory that the dentist clearly understand what brings the patient in for this valuation. Failure to do so risks the chance that the patient will be unhappy with the treatment result, as it might not address the very reason they came for help. With experience, this subtle point becomes a major component of a clinician's management focus.

A fundamental objective of the patient interview, which accompanies the diagnostic examination, is to gain a clear understanding of why the patient is coming for examination, and involves having the patient describe the history related to the chief complaint. For complicated clinical problems, the interview and diagnostic examination require two appointments to allow complete gathering of all the diagnostic information for formulation of a complete plan of treatment.

The interview, an opportunity to develop rapport with the patient, involves listening to and understanding the patient's chief complaint or concern about their oral health. This can include clinical symptoms of pain (provoked or unprovoked), difficulty with function, concern about their appearance, problems with an existing prosthesis, or any combination of symptoms related to their teeth, periodontium, jaws, or previous dental treatment. It is important to listen carefully to what the patient has stated is their reason for coming for examination. This is because all the subsequent information gathered will be used to discuss these concerns and to relate whether the proposed treatment will impact them in any way. Such a discussion at the outset of patient care helps to outline realistic expectations.

Although formats for sequencing the patient interview (and clinical examination) vary, to ensure thoroughness the dentist should follow a sequence that includes:

1. Chief complaint and its history
2. Medical history review
3. Dental history review; especially related to previous prosthetic experience(s)
4. Patient expectations

It is from the above interaction that patient uniqueness, as mentioned above, is best defined. The expectations described by the patient are critical to an understanding of whether a removable partial denture will satisfy the stated treatment goal(s). The fact that removable partial dentures by necessity require material bulk and often use oral soft tissue for support may be hard to comprehend by patients with no such prosthetic history. Helping them understand the normal phase of accommodation to such a prosthesis is an important discussion point when choosing a prosthesis. For those patients with an unfavorable past prosthesis experience, it is necessary to determine if the design, fit, occlusion, or lack of maintenance of the prosthesis can be improved to provide a more positive experience before starting treatment.

INFECTION CONTROL

The American Dental Association follows the Centers for Disease Control and Prevention (CDC) recommended infection control procedures for dentistry. The recommendations were last published in the CDC Morbidity and Mortality Weekly Report (MMWR) in 1993 and are currently being updated. Although infection control principles do not change significantly, continued monitoring of the effectiveness of guidelines along with new technologies, materials, and equipment require continuous evaluation of current infection control practices. The recommendations provide guidance for measures to be taken that will reduce the risks of disease transmission, among both dental healthcare workers (DHCWs) and their patients. The recommended infection control practices are applicable to all settings in which dental treatment is provided and are listed in Box 12-1.

BOX 12-1 Recommended Infection Control Practices for Dental Treatment

- Gloves should be worn in treating all patients.
- Masks should be worn to protect oral and nasal mucosa from splatter of blood and saliva.
- Eyes should be protected with some type of covering to protect from splatter of blood and saliva.
- Sterilization methods known to kill all life forms should be used on dental instruments. Sterilization equipment includes steam autoclave, dry heat oven, chemical vapor sterilizers, and chemical sterilants.
- Attention should be given to cleanup of instruments and surfaces in the operatory. This includes scrubbing with detergent solutions and wiping down surfaces with iodine or chlorine (diluted household bleach solutions).
- Contaminated disposable materials should be handled carefully and discarded in plastic bags to minimize human contact. Sharp items, such as needles and scalpel blades, should be contained in puncture-resistant containers before disposal in the plastic bags.

Dental patients and DHCWs potentially may be exposed to a variety of microorganisms. The exposure can occur via blood and/or oral or respiratory secretions. The microorganisms may include viruses and bacteria that infect the upper respiratory tract in general and also cytomegalovirus, hepatitis B virus (HBV), hepatitis C virus (HCV), herpes simplex virus types 1 and 2, human immunodeficiency virus (HIV), *Mycobacterium tuberculosis*, staphylococci, and streptococci. The transmission of infections in the dental operatory can occur through several routes. These include direct contact (blood, oral fluids, or other secretions), indirect contact (contaminated instruments, operatory equipment, or environmental surfaces), or contact with airborne contaminants present in either droplet spatter or aerosols of oral and respiratory fluids. For infection to occur via any of these routes, the "chain of infection" must be present. This includes a susceptible host, a pathogen with sufficient infectivity and numbers to cause infection, and a portal through which the pathogen may enter the host. For infection control procedures to be effective, one or more of these "links" in the chain must be broken.

Studies from the CDC report that clothing exposed to the acquired immunodeficiency syndrome (AIDS) virus may be safely used after a normal laundry cycle. A high temperature (140° to 160° F, 60° to 70° C) wash cycle with normal bleach concentrations, followed by machine drying (212° F, 100° C, or higher) is preferable if clothing is visibly soiled with blood or other body fluids. Dry cleaning and steam pressing will also kill the AIDS virus, according to these studies. Patients with oral lesions suggestive of infectious diseases or patients with a known history of HBV, AIDS, AIDS-related complex, or other infectious diseases should be referred for appropriate medical care. In addition to environmental surface and equipment disinfection, all instruments, stones, burs, and other reusable items should be disinfected in 2% glutaraldehyde for 10 minutes, cleaned of debris, rinsed, and patted dry before initiating the sterilizing process. Heat-sensitive items can be sterilized using ethylene oxide (gas).

For items that have been used in the mouth, including laboratory materials (e.g., impressions, bite registrations, fixed and removable prostheses, orthodontic appliances), cleaning and disinfection are required before being manipulated in a laboratory (whether on-site or at a remote location). Any item manipulated in the laboratory should also be cleaned and disinfected before placement in the patient's mouth. Fresh pumice with iodophor should be used for each polishing procedure, and the pumice pan should be washed, rinsed, and dried after each procedure. Since materials are constantly evolving, DHCWs are advised to follow manufacturers' suggested procedures for specific materials relative to disinfection procedures. As a guide, use of a chemical germicide having at least an intermediate level of activity (e.g., "tuberculocidal hospital disinfectant") is appropriate for such disinfection. Careful communication between dental office and dental laboratory regarding the specific protocol for handling and decontamination of supplies and materials is important to prevent any cross contamination.

CLINICAL EXAMINATION

OBJECTIVES OF PROSTHODONTIC TREATMENT

The objectives of any prosthodontic treatment may be stated as: (1) the elimination of disease; (2) the preservation, restoration, and maintenance of the health of the remaining teeth and oral tissues (which will enhance the removable partial denture design); and (3) the selected replacement of lost teeth for the purpose of restoration of function in a manner that ensures optimum stability and comfort in an esthetically pleasing manner. Preservation is a principle that protects dentists from placing too high a premium on cosmetic concerns. It is the dentist's obligation to emphasize the importance of restoring the total mouth to a state of health and of preserving the remaining teeth and surrounding tissues.

Diagnosis and treatment planning for oral rehabilitation of partially edentulous mouths must take into consideration the following: control of caries and periodontal disease, restoration of individual teeth, provision of harmonious occlusal relationships, and the replacement of missing teeth by fixed (using natural teeth and/or implants) or removable prostheses. Because these procedures are integrally related, the appropriate selection and sequencing of treatment should precede all irreversible procedures.

The treatment plan for the removable partial denture, which is often the final step in a lengthy sequence of treatment, should precede all but emergency treatment. This allows abutment teeth and other areas in the mouth to be properly prepared to support, stabilize, and retain the removable partial denture. This means that diagnostic casts, for designing and planning removable partial denture treatment, must be made before definitive treatment is undertaken. After evaluation of the major factors that create functional forces and those that resist it are understood, the removable partial denture design is drawn on the diagnostic cast, along with a detailed chart of mouth conditions and proposed treatment. This becomes the master plan for the mouth preparations and the design of the removable partial denture to follow.

As pointed out in Chapter 1, failures of removable partial dentures can usually be attributed to factors that result in poor stability. These can result from inadequate diagnosis and a failure to properly evaluate the conditions present. This results in a failure to prepare the patient and the oral tissue properly before fabrication of the master cast. The importance of the examination, the consideration of favorable and unfavorable aspects relative to movement control, and the importance of planning the elimination of unfavorable influences cannot be overemphasized (see Chapter 2).

As mentioned earlier, complex treatment planning often require two appointments. The first will likely include a preliminary oral examination (to determine the need for management of acute needs), a prophylaxis, full-mouth radiographs, diagnostic casts, and mounting records if baseplates are not required. The follow-up appointment includes mounting of the diagnostic casts (when baseplates and occlusion rims are needed), a definitive oral evaluation, review of the radiographs to augment and correlate with clinical findings, and, where required, arrangement of additional consultations. Following collection and synthesis of all the patient and clinical information, including surveying of the casts, a treatment plan (often with options) is presented.

ORAL EXAMINATION

A complete oral examination should precede any treatment decision. It should include a visual and digital evaluation of the teeth and surrounding tissue with mouth mirror, explorer, periodontal probe, vitality tests of critical teeth, and an examination of casts correctly oriented on a suitable articulator. The clinical findings are augmented by and correlated with a complete intraoral radiographic survey.

During the examination, the objective to be kept foremost in mind should be the consideration of possibilities for restoring and maintaining the remaining oral structures in a state of health for the longest period of time. This is best accomplished by an evaluation of factors that generate functional forces and those that resist them. The stability of tooth and prosthesis position is the goal of such an evaluation. The following sequence of examination allows attention to be paid to aspects of each of these critical features of evaluation for removable partial denture service.

Sequence for Oral Examination

An oral examination should be accomplished in the following sequence: visual examination, pain relief and temporary restorations, radiographs, oral prophylaxis, evaluation of teeth and periodontium, vitality tests of individual teeth, determination of the floor of the mouth position, and impressions of each arch.

Relief of Pain and Discomfort and Placement of Temporary Restorations

A preliminary examination is conducted to determine the need for management of acute needs and whether a prophylaxis is required to conduct a thorough oral examination. It is advisable not only to relieve discomfort arising from tooth defects but also to determine as early as possible the extent of caries and to arrest further caries activity until definitive treatment can be instituted. By restoring tooth contours with temporary restorations, the impression will not be torn on removal from the mouth, and a more accurate diagnostic cast may be obtained.

A Thorough and Complete Oral Prophylaxis

An adequate examination can be accomplished best with the teeth free of accumulated calculus and debris. Also, accurate diagnostic casts of the dental arches can be obtained only if the teeth are clean; otherwise the teeth reproduced on the diagnostic casts are not a true representation of tooth and gingival contours. Cursory examination may precede an oral prophylaxis, but a complete oral examination should be deferred until the teeth have been thoroughly cleaned.

Complete Intraoral Radiographic Survey (Figure 12-1)

The objectives of a radiographic examination are (a) to locate areas of infection and other pathosis that may be present; (b) to reveal the presence of root fragments, foreign objects, bone spicules, and irregular ridge formations; (c) to display the presence and extent of caries and the relation of carious lesions to the pulp and periodontal attachment; (d) to permit evaluation of existing restorations for evidence of recurrent caries, marginal leakage, and overhanging gingival margins; (e) to reveal the presence of root canal fillings and to permit their evaluation as to future prognosis (the design of the removable partial denture may hinge on the decision to retain or extract an endodontically treated tooth); (f) to permit an

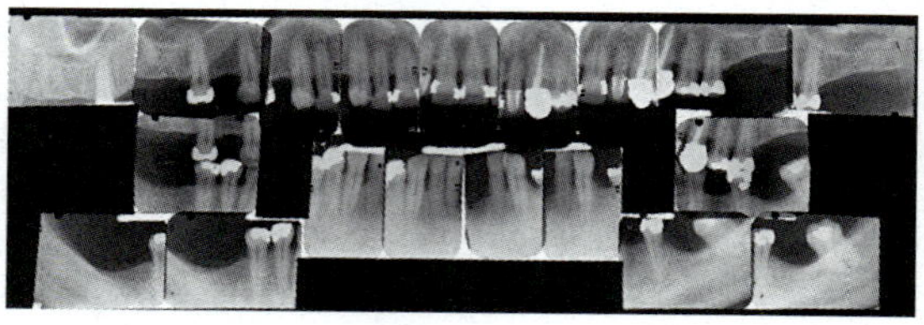

Figure 12-1 Complete intraoral radiographic survey of remaining teeth and adjacent edentulous areas reveals much information vital to effective diagnosis and treatment planning. Response of bone to previous stress is of particular value in establishing prognosis of teeth that are to be used as abutments.

evaluation of periodontal conditions present and to establish the need and possibilities for treatment; and (g) to evaluate the alveolar support of abutment teeth, their number, the supporting length and morphology of their roots, the relative amount of alveolar bone loss suffered through pathogenic processes, and the amount of alveolar support remaining.

Impressions for Making Accurate Diagnostic Casts to Be Mounted for Occlusal Examination

The casts preferably will be articulated on a suitable instrument. The importance of accurate diagnostic casts and their use will be discussed later in this chapter.

Examination of Teeth, Investing Structures, and Residual Ridges

The teeth, periodontium, and residual ridges can be explored by instrumentation and visual means. History and diagnosis charts should be filled out at this time and also a simple working chart for future reference (Figures 12-2 and 12-3).

Visual examination will detect many of the signs of dental disease. Consideration of caries susceptibility is of primary importance. The number of restored teeth present, signs of recurrent caries, and evidence of decalcification should be noted. Only those patients with demonstrated good oral hygiene habits and low caries susceptibility should be considered good risks

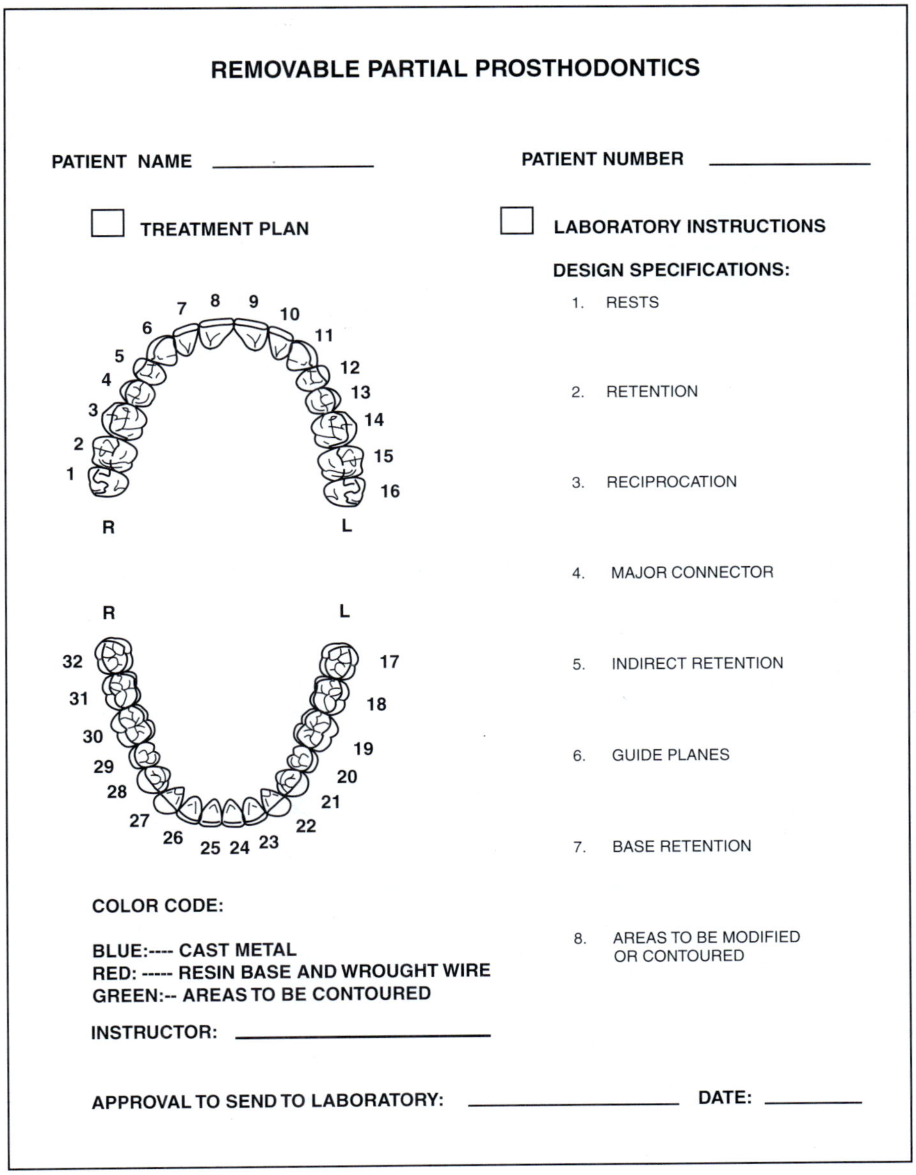

REMOVABLE PARTIAL PROSTHODONTICS

PATIENT NAME ________ PATIENT NUMBER ________

☐ TREATMENT PLAN

☐ LABORATORY INSTRUCTIONS

DESIGN SPECIFICATIONS:

1. RESTS
2. RETENTION
3. RECIPROCATION
4. MAJOR CONNECTOR
5. INDIRECT RETENTION
6. GUIDE PLANES
7. BASE RETENTION
8. AREAS TO BE MODIFIED OR CONTOURED

COLOR CODE:

BLUE:---- CAST METAL
RED: ----- RESIN BASE AND WROUGHT WIRE
GREEN:-- AREAS TO BE CONTOURED

INSTRUCTOR: ________

APPROVAL TO SEND TO LABORATORY: ________ DATE: ________

A

Figure 12-2 A, Diagnosis record for recording pertinent data.

Continued

PATIENT'S NAME John Doe CHART NO. 383838

STUDENT'S NAME Joe Smith JR. X SR. ____ STUDENT NO. 1234

STARTING DATE 1/14/99 INSTRUCTOR SIGNATURE PGreen

COMPLETION DATE ____ INSTRUCTOR SIGNATURE ____

REMOVABLE PARTIAL DENTURE

MAX RPD **MAND. RPD**

DIAGNOSIS

1. Are you wearing or have you worn an oral prosthesis? No____ Yes ✓. If so, what type? metal + plastic
2. If a previously worn prosthesis was not entirely satisfactory, what in your opinion were the problems with it? no retention, + teeth badly worn
3. What was the cause of loss of the natural teeth? Perio X, Caries X, Trauma____.

INTRAORAL FINDINGS

1. Oral hygiene index: Good X Fair____ 2. Caries Index: High____ Moderate____ Low X.
3. Do centric occlusion and centric relation coincide? Yes X No____.
4. Are there frenula or muscle attachments that might interfere with maximum fit and comfort? Yes____ No X.
5. Is type and quality of saliva normal? Yes X No____. Comments____
6. Examine the following areas for possible interference with optimal fit and comfort.

   Mylohyoid Ridge Normal ✓ Other:____ Alveolar Ridges Tissues Normal ✓

   Tuberosity Normal ✓ Other:____ Supporting Alveolar Bone Normal ✓

   Tori Present Yes____ No X
7. Is any surgical procedure indicated to improve the prognosis? No ✓ Note____

DIAGNOSTIC CAST ANALYSIS

On the Articulator

1. Is there adequate interridge space for the contemplated prosthesis? Yes ✓ No____
2. Is the occlusal plane retrievable? Yes ✓ Doubtful____
3. Is there adequate inter-occlusal space for contemplated rest seats and rests where they will be needed?

   Yes ✓ Note____
4. Are there anomalies which were not evident intra-orally? No ✓ Note____

On The Surveyor

1. Which teeth are the most suitable abutments? Abutment #1 20 Abutment #2 28 Abutment #3____

   Abutment #4____ Other____.
2. Do the abutments have adequate retentive undercuts in a favorable location on the tooth? Yes X No____.
3. Can suitable guiding planes be developed on the probable abutments? Yes X No____
4. Will tooth alterations be required? No____ Yes X

RADIOGRAPHIC INTERPRETATION

1. What is the crown root ratio of each abutment? Abutment #1 1:3 Abutment #2 1:3 Abutment #3____

   Abutment #4____
2. Does the supporting bone appear to be of good quality? Yes X No____.

QUALITY PRESS, INC.

B

Figure 12-2 Cont'd B, Treatment record chart for recording treatment plan and treatment progress.

Name: *John Doe* Date: *July 1, 1999*

Summary Plan:

Maxillary Conventional Complete denture

Mandibular Class II mod. 1 removable partial denture

Porcelain fused to metal abutment Crowns #18, #29

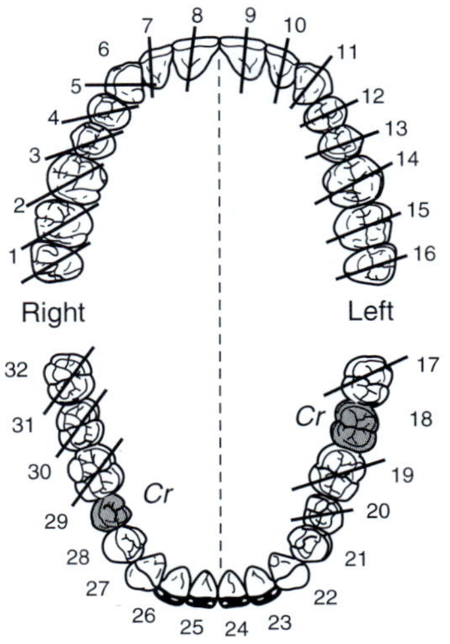

Procedures:

Tissue conditioning maxillary arch

Primary impression-both arches; make impression trays

Preparations. Contour and rest seats #21, #28. Abutment crown preparations #18, #29

Try-in abutment crowns; pick-up for cast for framework casting

Try-in abutment crowns and framework

Fluid wax functional impression: Make altered cast

Jaw relation records; shade and mold selection

Tooth arrangement

Try-in trial set-up; verify jaw relations

Placement: Mandibular crowns, partial denture, maxillary complete denture

Follow-up care

Red line each completed unit

Figure 12-3 Simple working chart. Restorations for individual teeth, crowns, and fixed partial dentures to be made may be marked on chart and checked off as completed during mouth preparations.

without resorting to prophylactic measures, such as the restoration of abutment teeth. At the time of the initial examination, periodontal disease, gingival inflammation, the degree of gingival recession, and mucogingival relationships should be observed. Such an examination will not provide sufficient information to allow a definitive diagnosis and treatment plan. For this purpose, a complete periodontal charting should be performed that includes pocket depths, assessment of attachment levels, furcation involvement, mucogingival problems, and tooth mobility. The extent of periodontal destruction must be determined with both appropriate radiographs and use of the periodontal probe.

The number of teeth remaining, the location of the edentulous areas, and the quality of the residual ridge will have a definite bearing on the proportionate amount of support that the removable partial denture will receive from the teeth and the edentulous ridges. Tissue contours may appear to present a well-formed edentulous residual ridge; however, palpation often indicates that supporting bone has been resorbed and has been replaced by displaceable, fibrous connective tissue. Such a situation is common in maxillary tuberosity regions. The removable partial denture cannot be supported adequately by tissue that is easily displaced. In preparing the mouth, this tissue should be recontoured or removed surgically unless otherwise contraindicated.

A small but stable residual ridge is preferable to a larger, unstable ridge for providing support for the denture. The presence of tori or other bony exostoses must be detected and an evaluation must be made of their presence in relation to framework design. Failure to palpate the tissue over the median palatal raphe to ascertain the difference in its displaceability as compared with the displaceability of the soft tissues covering the residual ridges can lead to a rocking, unstable, uncomfortable denture and to a dissatisfied patient. Adequate relief of the palatal major connectors must be planned, and the amount of relief required is directly proportionate to the difference in displaceability of the tissue over the midline of the palate and the tissue covering the residual ridges.

During the examination, not only each arch but also its occlusal relationship with the opposing arch must be considered separately. A situation that looks simple when the teeth are apart may be complicated when the teeth are in occlusion. For example, an extreme vertical overlap may complicate the attachment of anterior teeth to a maxillary denture. Extrusion of a tooth or teeth into an opposing edentulous area may complicate the replacement of teeth in the edentulous area or may create occlusal interference, which will complicate the location and design of clasp retainers and occlusal rests. Such findings subsequently will be evaluated further by careful analysis of mounted diagnostic casts.

A breakdown of the fee may be recorded on the back of this chart for easy reference if adjustments or substitutions become necessary by changes in the diagnosis as the work progresses.

Vitality Tests of Remaining Teeth

Vitality tests should be given particularly to teeth to be used as abutments and those having deep restorations or deep carious lesions. This should be done with both thermal and electronic means.

Determination of Height of the Floor of the Mouth to Locate Inferior Borders of Lingual Mandibular Major Connectors

Mouth preparation procedures are influenced by a choice of major connectors (see Figure 5-7). This determination must precede altering contours of abutment teeth.

The fee for examination, which should include the cost of the radiographic survey and the examination of articulated diagnostic casts, should be established before the examination and should not be related to the cost of treatment. It should be understood that the fee for examination is based on the time involved and the service rendered and that the material value of the radiograph and diagnostic casts is incidental to the effectiveness of the examination.

The examination record should always be available in the office for future consultation. If consultation with another dentist is requested, respect for the hazards of unnecessary radiation justifies loaning the dentist the radiograph for this purpose. However, duplicate films should be retained in the dentist's files.

DIAGNOSTIC CASTS

A diagnostic cast should be an accurate reproduction of all the potential features that aid diagnosis. These include the teeth locations, contours, and occlusal plane relationship; the residual ridge contour, size, and mucosal consistency; and the oral anatomy delineating the prosthesis extensions (vestibules, retromolar pads, pterygomaxillary notch, hard and/or soft palatal junction, floor of the mouth, and frena). Additional information provided by appropriate cast mounting includes occlusal plane orientation and the impact on the opposing arch; tooth-to-palatal soft tissue relationship; and tooth-to-ridge relationship, both vertically and horizontally.

A diagnostic cast is usually made of dental stone because of its strength, and it is less easily abraded than is dental plaster. Generally the improved dental stones (die stones) are not used for diagnostic casts because of their cost. Their greater resistance to abrasion does, however, justify their use for master casts.

The impression for the diagnostic cast is usually made with an irreversible hydrocolloid (alginate) in a stock (perforated or rim lock) impression tray. The size of the arch will determine the size of the tray to be used. The tray should be sufficiently oversized to ensure an optimum thickness of impression material to prevent distortion or tearing on removal from the mouth. The technique for making impressions is covered in more detail in Chapter 15.

Purposes of Diagnostic Casts

Diagnostic casts serve several purposes as an aid to diagnosis and treatment planning. Some of these are as follows:

1. Diagnostic casts are used to supplement the oral examination by permitting a view of the occlusion from the lingual and buccal aspects. Analysis of the existing occlusion is made possible when opposing casts are occluded along with a study of the possibilities for improvement—either by occlusal adjustment or occlusal reconstruction, or both. The degree of overclosure, the amount of interocclusal space available, and the possibilities of interference to the location of rests may also be determined. As stated previously, opportunities for improvement of the occlusal scheme, by either occlusal adjustment or occlusal reconstruction, are best evaluated by analysis and modification of mounted diagnostic casts. Such procedures often include diagnostic waxing to determine the possibility of enhancing the occlusion before definitive treatment is begun (Figure 12-4). In other words, diagnostic casts permit the dentist to plan ahead to avoid undesirable compromises in the treatment being given a patient.
2. Diagnostic casts are used to permit a topographic survey of the dental arch that is to be restored by means of a removable partial denture. The cast of the arch in question may be surveyed individually with a cast surveyor to determine the parallelism or lack of parallelism of tooth surfaces involved and to establish their influence on the design of the removable partial denture. The principal considerations in studying the parallelism of tooth and tissue surfaces of each dental arch are to determine the need for mouth preparation including (a) proximal tooth surfaces, which can be made parallel to serve as guiding planes; (b) retentive and nonretentive

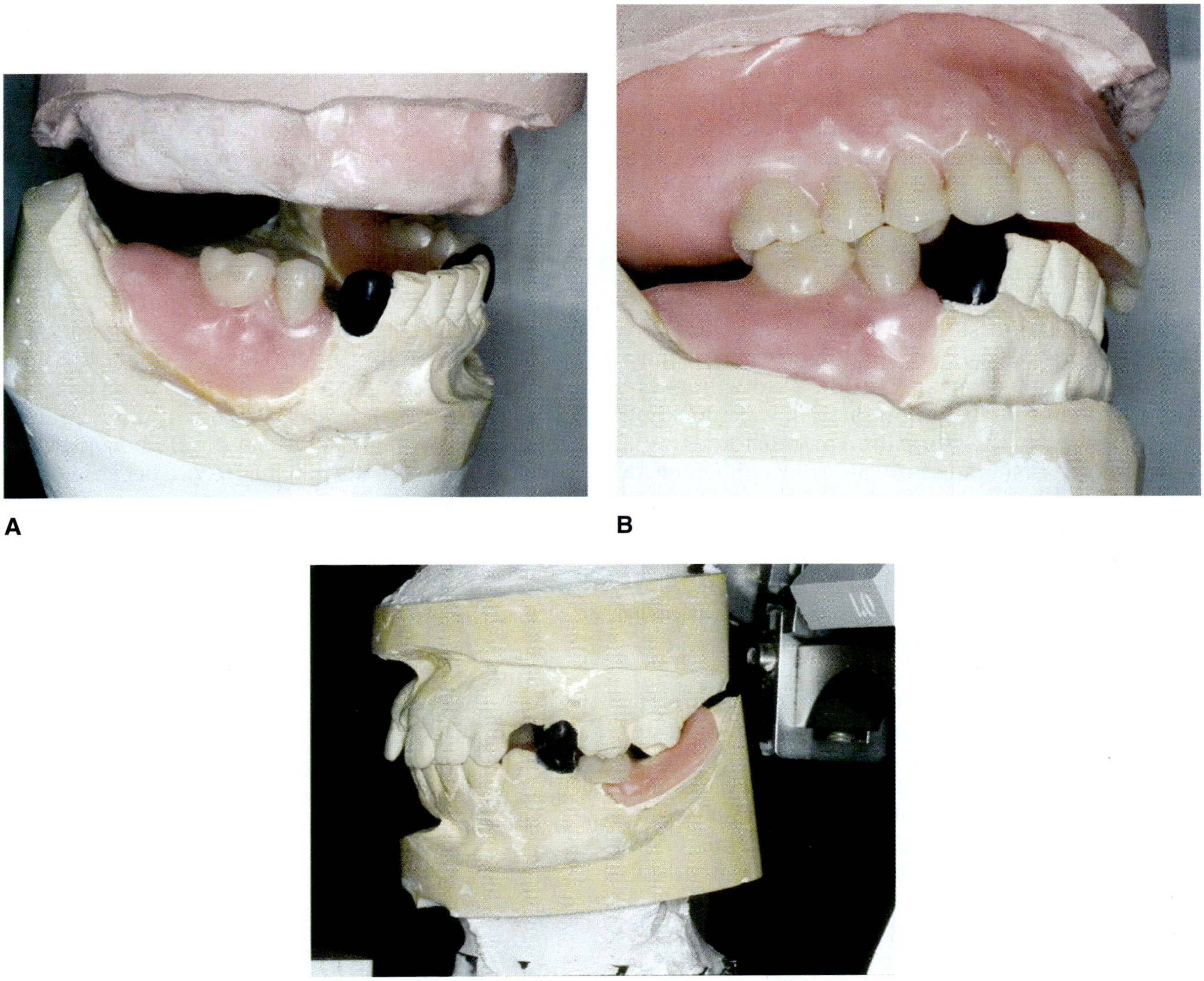

A B C

Figure 12-4 **A,** Following mounting of the diagnostic casts (edentulous maxilla and Kennedy Class I mandibular cast) tooth arrangement can be finalized, along with diagnostic waxing of surveyed crowns. Evaluation of the mandibular occlusal plane requirements can be accomplished. **B,** Following appropriate positioning of the maxillary anterior teeth in an ideal position, the maxillary posterior teeth are aligned for esthetics (especially maxillary first premolar) and function. Intercuspation of the mandibular posterior teeth in this mounting has resulted in a space posterior to surveyed crown #27. If such a finding were objectionable, alternative arrangements could be investigated. This is not possible unless a diagnostic workup is completed. **C,** Occlusion of mandibular removable partial denture will be enhanced by improving the maxillary posterior occlusal plane of the super-erupted molars.

areas of the abutment teeth; (c) areas of interference to placement and removal; and (d) esthetic effects of the selected path of insertion. From such a survey, a path of placement may be selected that will satisfy requirements for parallelism and retention to the best mechanical, functional, and esthetic advantage. Then mouth preparations may be planned accordingly.

3. Diagnostic casts are used to permit a logical and comprehensive presentation to the patient of present and future restorative needs and the hazards of future neglect. Occluded and individual diagnostic casts can be used to point out to the patient (a) evidence of tooth migration and the existing results of such migration; (b) effects of further tooth migration; (c) loss of occlusal support and its consequences; (d) hazards of traumatic occlusal contacts; and (e) cariogenic and periodontal implications of further neglect. Treatment planning actually may be accomplished

with the patient present so that economic considerations may be discussed. Such use of diagnostic casts permits a justification of the proposed fee through the patient's understanding of the problems involved and of the treatment needed. Inasmuch as mouth rehabilitation procedures are frequently lengthy and often irreversible, there must be complete accord between dentist and patient before extensive treatment is begun, and financial arrangements must be consummated during the planning phase.

4. Individual impression trays may be fabricated on the diagnostic casts, or the diagnostic cast may be used in selecting and fitting a stock impression tray for the final impression. If wax blockout is to be used in the fabrication of individual trays, a duplicate cast made from an irreversible hydrocolloid (alginate) impression of the diagnostic cast should be used for this purpose. The diagnostic cast is too valuable for future reference to risk damage resulting from the making of an impression tray. On the other hand, if oil base clay blockout is used, the diagnostic cast may be used without fear of damage.
5. Diagnostic casts may be used as a constant reference as the work progresses. Penciled marks indicating the type of restorations, the areas of tooth surfaces to be modified, the location of rests, and the design of the removable partial denture framework along with the path of placement and removal, all may be recorded on the diagnostic cast for future reference (Figure 12-5). These steps may be checked off the work sheet as they are completed. Areas of abutment teeth to be modified may first be changed on the duplicate diagnostic cast by trimming the stone cast with the surveyor blade. A record is thus made of the location and degree of modification to be done in the mouth. This must be done in relation to a definite path of placement. Any mouth preparations to be accomplished with new restorations necessitate that restored teeth be shaped in accordance with a previously determined path of placement. Even so, the shaping of abutment teeth on the duplicate diagnostic cast serves as a guide to the form of the abutment. This is particularly true if the contouring of wax patterns is to be delegated to the technician, as it may be in a busy practice.
6. Unaltered diagnostic casts should become a permanent part of the patient's record because records of conditions existing before treatment are just as important as are preoperative radiographs. Therefore diagnostic casts should be duplicated, one cast serving as a permanent record and the duplicate cast used in situations that may require alterations.

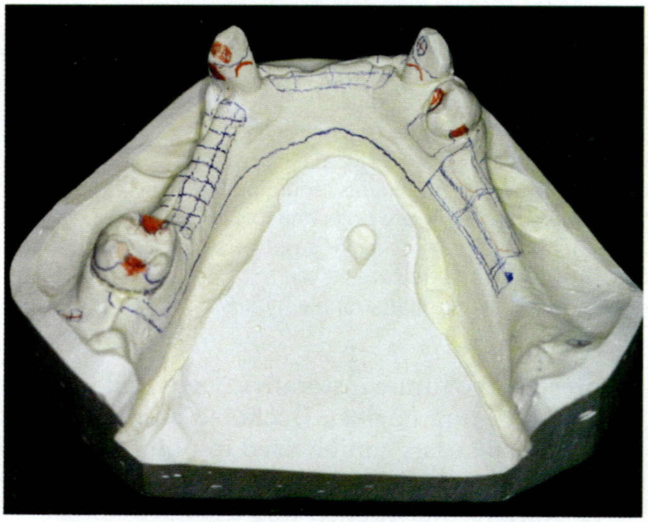

Figure 12-5 Proposed mouth changes and design of removable partial denture framework are indicated in pencil on diagnostic cast in relation to previously determined path of placement. This serves as a means for communicating with the patient and as a chair-side guide to tooth modification.

Mounting Diagnostic Casts

For diagnostic purposes, casts should be related on an anatomically appropriate articulator to best understand the role occlusion may have in the design and functional stability of the removable partial denture. This becomes increasingly more important as the prosthesis replaces more teeth. If the patient presents with a harmonious occlusion and the edentulous span is a tooth-bound space, simple hand articulation is generally all that is required. However, when the natural dentition is not harmonious and/or when the replacement teeth must be positioned within the normal movement patterns of the jaws, the diagnostic casts must be related in an anatomically appropriate manner for diagnosis. This means placement of the maxillary cast in a position relative to the opening axis on the articulator, which is similar to the maxilla's position to the temporomandibular joint (TMJ) of the patient (Figure 12-6). The mandibular cast is then placed beneath the maxillary cast in a horizontal position dictated by mandibular rotation without tooth contact, at a minimal vertical opening.

The Glossary of Prosthodontic Terms* describes an articulator as a mechanical device that represents the temporomandibular joints and jaw members, to which maxillary and mandibular casts may be attached. Because the dominant influence on mandibular movement in a partially edentulous mouth is the occlusal plane and the cusps of the remaining teeth, an anatomic reproduction of condylar paths is probably

*From J Prosthet Dent 81:45-110, 1999.

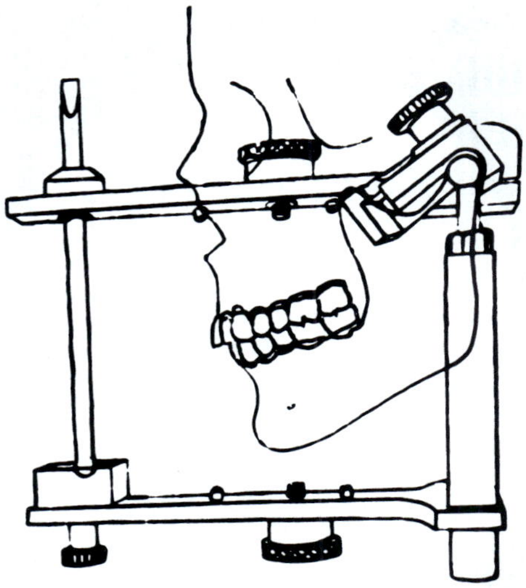

Figure 12-6 Use of face-bow makes possible the recording of the spatial relationship of the maxillae to some anatomic reference points and to transfer this relationship to an articulator.

not necessary. Still, movement of the casts in relation to one another as influenced by the occlusal plane and the cusps of the remaining teeth, when mounted at a reasonably accurate distance from the axis of condylar rotation, permits a relatively valid analysis of occlusal relations. This is more anatomically accurate than a simple hinge mounting.

It is better that the casts be mounted in relation to the axis-orbital plane to permit better interpretation of the plane of occlusion in relation to the horizontal plane. Although it is true that an axis-orbital mounting has no functional value on a nonarcon instrument because that plane ceases to exist when opposing casts are separated, the value of such a mounting lies in the orientation of the casts in occlusion. (An arcon articulator is one in which the condyles are attached to the lower member as they are in nature, the term being a derivation coined by Bergström from the words articulation and condyle. Many of the more widely used articulators, such as the Hanau H series, Dentatus, and improved Gysi, have the condyles attached to the upper member and are therefore nonarcon instruments.)

Sequence for Mounting Maxillary Cast to Axis-Orbital Plane

These initial steps allow recording of the maxilla-TMJ relationship:

1. Identify the anterior and posterior reference points for the face-bow (e.g., EAM and Orbitale)
2. Prepare the bite fork and occlusion rim
3. Place the bite fork centered to the arch, indexing it to the teeth with wax or elastomer
4. Place the face-bow over the bite fork rod anteriorly
5. Place the bow evenly into the ears posteriorly
6. Secure the bow anteriorly
7. Position the bow anteriorly to the third point of reference (establish the horizontal plane)
8. Secure the bite fork vertical rod, then horizontal rod (holding the bow securely to prevent torque)
9. Release bow anteriorly to allow spread and disengage from the ears
10. Remove the fork downward and out of the mouth with attached bow
11. Carefully check the security of the attachments

The next steps allow transfer of the recorded relationship to the articulator:

1. Position the posterior reference points on the articulator (usually a posterior attachment point)
2. Secure the posterior points by securing the bow anteriorly
3. Vertically relate the secured bow to the articulator anterior reference point
4. Seat the maxillary cast into the bite fork registration (wax or elastomer)
5. Close the articulator and check clearance for mounting plaster (modify cast as needed)
6. Mount with low expansion plaster

The face-bow is a relatively simple device used to obtain a transfer record for orienting a maxillary cast on an articulating instrument. Originally the face-bow was used only to transfer a radius from condyle reference points so that a given point on the cast would be the same distance from the condyle as it is on the patient. The addition of an adjustable, infraorbital pointer to the face-bow and the addition of an orbital plane indicator to the articulator make possible the transfer of the elevation of the cast in relation to the axis-orbital plane. This permits the maxillary cast to be correctly oriented in the articulator space comparable with the relationship of the maxilla to the axis-orbital plane on the patient. To accommodate this orientation of the maxillary cast and still have room for the mandibular cast, the posts of the conventional articulator must be lengthened. The older Hanau model H articulator usually will not permit a face-bow transfer using an infraorbital pointer.

A face-bow may be used to transfer a comparable radius from arbitrary reference points or it may be designed so that the transfer can be made from hinge axis points. The latter type of transfer necessitates that a hinge-bow attached to the mandible be used initially to determine the hinge axis points, to which the face-bow is then adjusted for making the hinge axis transfer.

A face-bow transfer of the maxillary cast, which is oriented to the axis-orbital plane in a suitable articulator, is an uncomplicated procedure. The Hanau series Wide-Vue 183-2, all 96H2-0 models, the Whip-Mix articulator, and the Dentatus model ARH will accept this transfer. The Hanau earpiece face-bow models 153 and 158, the Hanau facia face-bow 132-2SM, and the Dentatus face-bow type AEB incorporate the infraorbital plane to the articulator. None of these are hinge axis bows but are used instead at an arbitrary point.

The location of the arbitrary point or axis has long been the subject of controversy. Gysi and others have placed it 11 to 13 mm anterior to the upper third of the tragus of the ear on a line extending from the upper margin of the external auditory meatus to the outer canthus of the eye. Others have placed it 13 mm anterior to the posterior margin of the center of the tragus of the ear on a line extending to the corner of the eye. Bergström has located the arbitrary axis 10 mm anterior to the center of a spherical insert for the external auditory meatus and 7 mm below the Frankfort horizontal plane.

In a series of experiments reported by Beck, it was shown that the arbitrary axis suggested by Bergström falls consistently closer to the kinematic axis than do the other two. It is desirable that an arbitrary axis be placed as close as possible to the kinematic axis. Although most authorities agree that any of the three axes will permit a transfer of the maxillary cast with reasonable accuracy, it would seem that the Bergström point compares most favorably with the kinematic axis.

The lowest point on the inferior orbital margin is taken as the third point of reference for establishing the axis-orbital plane. Some authorities use the lower-margin point of the bony orbit in line with the center of the pupil of the eye. For the sake of consistency, the right infraorbital point is generally used and the face-bow assembled in this relationship. All three points (right and left axes and infraorbital point) are marked on the face with an ink dot before making the transfer.

Casts are prepared for mounting on an articulator by placing three index grooves in the base of the casts. Two V-shaped grooves are placed in the posterior section of the cast and one groove in the anterior portion (Figure 12-7).

An occlusion rim properly oriented on a well-fitting record base should be used in face-bow procedures involving the transfer of casts representative of the Class I and II partially edentulous situations. Without occlusion rims, such casts cannot be located accurately in the imprints of the wax covering the face-bow fork. Tissues covering the residual ridges may be displaced grossly when the patient closes into the wax on the face-bow fork. Therefore the wax imprints of the soft tissues will not be true negatives of the edentulous regions of the diagnostic casts.

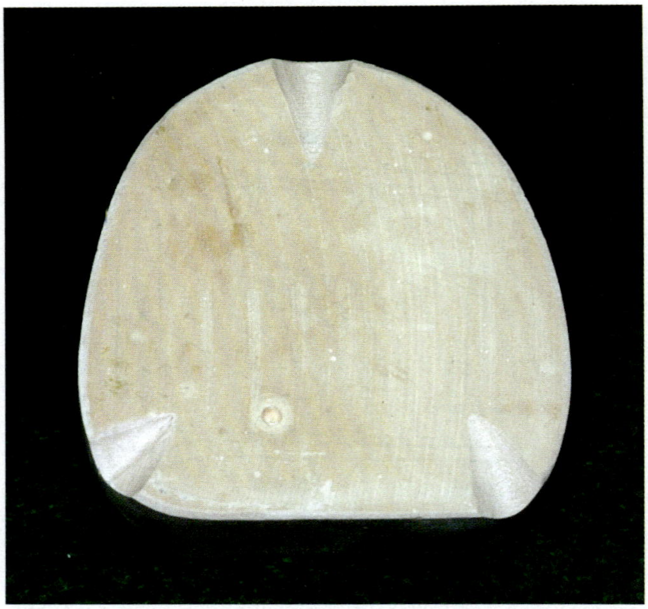

Figure 12-7 Base of cast has been prepared for mounting by placing three triangular grooves to allow indexing when mounted. Grooves are prepared with a 3-inch stone mounted in laboratory lathe. This is helpful for reorienting the cast on the articulator, which should be done after processing to correct for processing errors, without the need for another face-bow transfer record.

For the purpose of illustration a face-bow using the external auditory meatus as the posterior reference point, the Whip Mix face-bow technique (DB 2000), will be shown. The face-bow fork is covered with a polyether, polyvinyl Siloxane or a roll of softened baseplate wax with the material distributed equally on the top and on the underneath side of the face-bow fork. Then the fork should be pressed lightly on the diagnostic casts with the midline of the face-bow fork corresponding to the midline of the central incisors (Figure 12-8). This will leave imprints of the occlusal and incisal surfaces of the maxillary casts and occlusion rim on the softened baseplate wax and is an aid in correctly orienting the face-bow fork in the patient's mouth. The face-bow fork is placed in position in the mouth, and the patient is asked to close the lower teeth into the wax to stabilize it in position. It is removed from the mouth and chilled in cold water and then replaced in position in the patient's mouth. An alternative method of stabilizing the face-bow fork and recording bases is to enlist the assistance of the patient.

If an earpiece face-bow is to be used, the patient should be reminded that the plastic earpieces in the auditory canals will greatly amplify

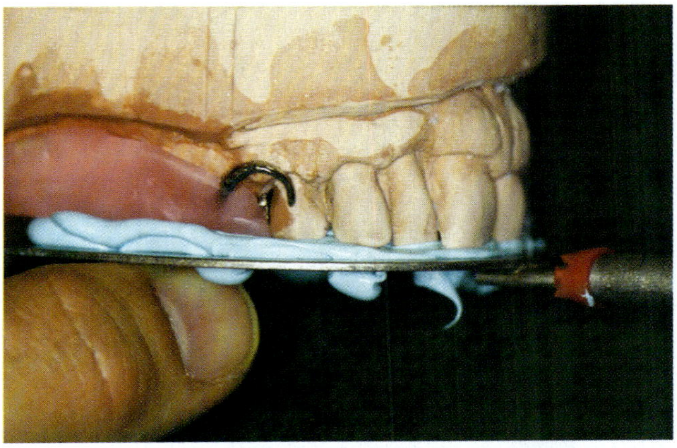

Figure 12-8 Orienting face-bow fork to maxillary cast and occlusion rims will avoid displacing occlusion rim in mouth due to patient closure or other uneven force. Polyvinyl Siloxane material has been evenly distributed around the face-bow fork, and care is exercised to position the fork to be centered at the mid-incisal position without any fork extension posterior to the record base, which could cause discomfort.

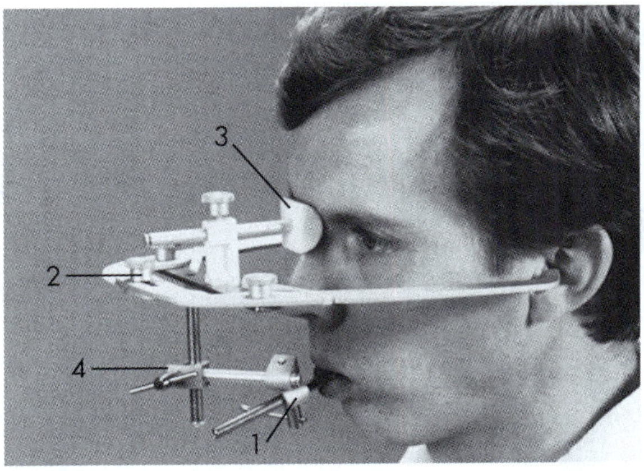

Figure 12-9 Horizontal toggle clamp of Whip-Mix earpiece face-bow *(1)* is slid onto shaft of face-bow fork protruding from patient's mouth. Patient then helps guide plastic earpieces into external auditory meatus and holds them in place while operator tightens three thumb screws *(2)* and centers plastic nosepiece *(3)* securely on nasion. Horizontal toggle clamp is positioned and secured near (but not touching) lip. T screw *(4)* on vertical bar is tightened. Note: Extreme care should be exercised not to tilt face-bow out of position when tightening.

noise. With the face-bow fork in position, the face-bow toggle is slipped over the anterior projection of the face-bow fork (Figure 12-9). The patient can assist in guiding the plastic earpieces into the external auditory meatus. The patient can then hold the arms of the face-bow in place with firm pressure while the operator secures the bitefork to the face-bow. This accomplishes the radius aspect of the face-bow transfer.

If an infraorbital pointer is used, it is placed on the extreme right side of the face-bow and angled toward the infraorbital point previously identified with an ink dot. It is then locked into position with its tip lightly touching the skin at the identified location marked by the dot. This establishes the elevation of the face-bow in relation to the axis-orbital plane. Extreme care must be taken to avoid any slip that might injure the patient's eye.

With all elements tightened securely, the patient is asked to open, and the entire assembly is removed intact, rinsed with cold water, and set aside. The face-bow records not only the radius from the condyles to the incisal contacts of the upper central incisors but also the angular relationship of the occlusal plane to the axis-orbital plane.

The face-bow must be positioned on the articulator in the same axis-orbital relationship as on the patient (Figure 12-10). If an arbitrary-type face-bow is used, the calibrated condyle rods of the face-bow ordinarily will not fit the condyle shafts of the articulator unless the width between the condyles just happens to be the same. With a Hanau model 132-25M face-bow, the calibrations must be made equal again when in position on the articulator. For example, they read 74 (mm) on each side of the patient but must be adjusted to read 69 (mm) on each side of the articulator. Some later model articulators have adjustable condyle rods and may be adjusted to fit the face-bow. It is necessary that the face-bow be centered in either case. Some face-bows are self-centering, such as the Hanau Spring-Bow.

The third point of reference is the orbital plane indicator, which must be swung to the right so that it will be above the tip of the infraorbital pointer. The entire face-bow, with maxillary cast in place, must be raised until the tip of the pointer contacts the orbital plane indicator. The elevation having been established, for all practical purposes the orbital plane indicator and pointer may now be removed because they may interfere with placing the mounting stone.

An auxiliary device called a **cast support** is available; it is used to support the face-bow fork and the maxillary cast during the mounting operation (Figure 12-11). With this device, the weight of the cast and the mounting stone is supported separately from the face-bow, thus preventing possible downward movement resulting from their combined weight. The cast support is raised to supporting contact with the face-bow fork after the face-bow height has been adjusted to the level of

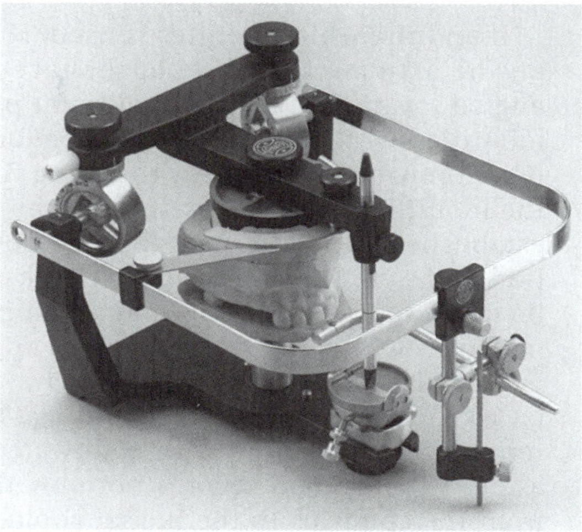

A

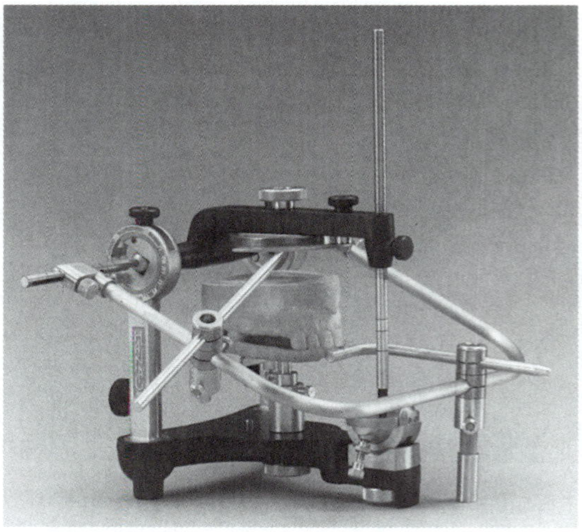

B

Figure 12-10 **A,** Hanau Wide-Vue articulator (model 183-2) with Spring-Bow (model 182-1) attached. Maxillary cast is secured to upper member of articulator by a split cast plate. Cast support is attached to lower member of articulator to support maxillary cast for mounting with stone. Orbitale indicator or articulator and pointer on bow are aligned as third point of reference during earpiece face-bow application and transfer. **B,** Facia-type Hanau face-bow (model 132-2SM) attached on Hanau model 96H2-0 articulator for mounting related maxillary cast. Bow is elevated to level orbitale pointer with underside of crescent-shaped orbitale indicator. Bitefork index is supported by cast support to preserve adjusted position under weight of stone.

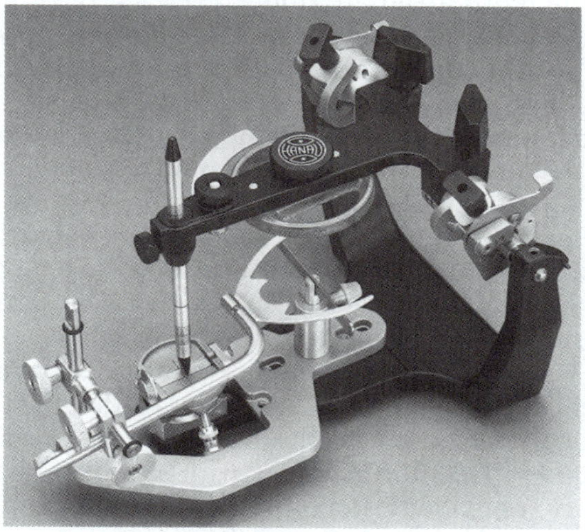

Figure 12-11 Mounting platform attached to lower member of Hanau modular articulator. Such platforms are helpful to prevent movement of the maxillary cast/bitefork assembly during mounting of the cast. This illustration shows the use of an indirect mounting technique that allows the face-bow to remain in the clinical area (to be used with another bitefork) while the bitefork adapts to a mounting jig designed to preserve the spatial relationship recorded on the patient for transfer to the articulator.

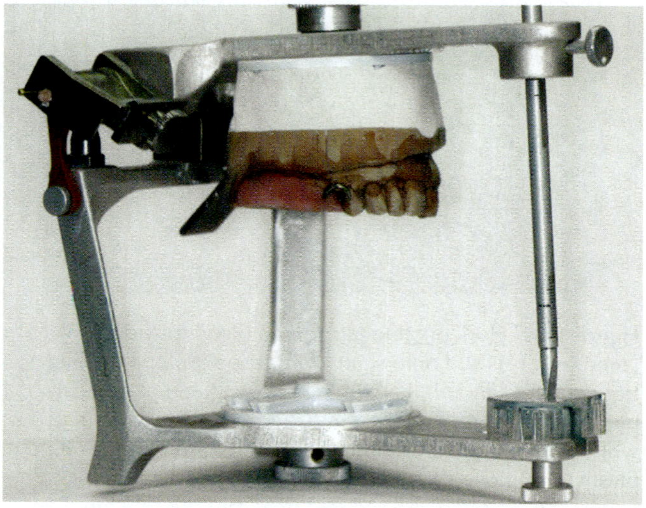

Figure 12-12 Face-bow mounting complete. Relationship of the maxillary cast to the articulator condylar components is anatomically similar to the patient's maxilla and the bilateral TMJ complex. Any subsequent tooth arrangement and occlusal contact development will more accurately represent the mouth than more arbitrary mountings. The benefits of the anatomic similarity are seen in more accurate occlusion for the finalized prosthesis (i.e., less intraoral adjustment required).

the orbital plane. Use of some type of cast support is highly recommended as an adjunct to face-bow mounting.

The keyed and lubricated maxillary cast is now attached to the upper arm of the articulator with the mounting stone, thus completing the face-bow transfer (Figure 12-12). Not only will the face-bow have permitted the upper cast to be mounted with reasonable accuracy, but it also will have served as a convenient means of supporting the cast during mounting. Once mastered, its use becomes a great convenience rather than a time-consuming nuisance.

It is preferable that the maxillary cast be mounted while the patient is still present, thus eliminating a possible reappointment if the face-bow record is unacceptable for some reason. Not too infrequently, the face-bow record has to be redone with the offset type face-bow fork repositioned to prevent interference with some part of the articulator.

Jaw Relationship Records for Diagnostic Casts

One of the first critical decisions that must be made in a removable partial denture service involves the selection of the horizontal jaw relationship to which the removable partial denture will be fabricated (centric relation or the maximum intercuspal position). All mouth-preparation procedures depend on this analysis. Failure to make this decision correctly may result in poor prosthesis stability, discomfort, and the deterioration of both the residual ridges and the supporting teeth.

It is recommended that deflective occlusal contacts in the maximum intercuspal and eccentric positions be corrected as a preventive measure. Not all dentists agree that centric relation and the maximum intercuspal position must be harmonious in the natural dentition. Many dentitions function satisfactorily with the opposing teeth maximally intercusping in an eccentric position without either diagnosable or subjective indications of TMJ dysfunction, muscle dysfunction, or disease of the supporting structures of the teeth. In many such situations, no attempt should be made to alter the occlusion. It is not a requirement to interfere with an occlusion simply because it does not completely conform to a relationship that is considered ideal.

If most natural posterior teeth remain—and if no evidence of TMJ disturbances, neuromuscular dysfunction, or periodontal disturbances related to occlusal factors exists—the proposed restorations may safely be fabricated with maximum intercuspation of the remaining teeth. However, when most natural centric stops are missing, the proposed prosthesis should be fabricated so that the maximum intercuspal position is in harmony with centric relation. By far the greater majority of removable partial dentures should be fabricated in the horizontal jaw relationship of centric relation. In most instances in which edentulous spaces have not been restored, the remaining posterior teeth will have assumed malaligned positions through drifting, tipping, or extrusion. Correction of the remaining natural occlusion to create a coincidence of centric relation and the maximum intercuspal position is indicated in such situations.

Regardless of the method used in creating a harmonious functional occlusion, an evaluation of the existing relationships of the opposing natural teeth must be made and is accomplished with a diagnostic mounting. This evaluation is in addition to, and in conjunction with, other diagnostic procedures that contribute to an adequate diagnosis and treatment plan.

Diagnostic casts provide an opportunity to evaluate the relationship of remaining oral structures when correctly mounted on a semiadjustable articulator by use of a face-bow transfer and interocclusal records. Diagnostic casts are mounted in centric relation (most retruded relation of the mandible to the maxillae) so that deflective occlusal contacts can be correlated with those observed in the mouth. Deflective contacts of opposing teeth are usually destructive to the supporting structures involved and should be eliminated. Diagnostic casts demonstrate the presence and location of such interfering tooth contacts and permit visualization of the treatment that would be necessary for their correction. Necessary alteration of teeth to harmonize the occlusion can be performed initially on duplicates of the mounted diagnostic casts to act as guides for similar necessary corrections in the mouth. In many instances the degree of alteration required will indicate the need for crowns or onlays to be fabricated or for the recontouring, repositioning, or elimination of extruded teeth.

As previously mentioned, the maxillary cast is correctly oriented to the opening axis of the articulator by means of the face-bow transfer and becomes spatially related to the upper member of the articulator in the same relationship that the maxilla are related to the hinge axis and the Frankfort plane. Similarly, when a centric relation record is made at an established vertical dimension, the mandible is in its most retruded relation to the maxilla. Therefore when the maxillary cast is correctly oriented to the axis of the articulator, the mandibular cast automatically becomes correctly oriented to the opening axis, when attached to and mounted with an accurate centric relation record.

Unlike recording the fixed relationship of the maxilla to the mandibular opening axis (using the face-bow transfer record), the mandibular position is recorded in space and is not a fixed point. Consequently, it is necessary to prove that the relationship of the mounted casts is correct. This can be done simply by making another interocclusal record at the centric relation, fitting the casts into the record, and checking to see that the condylar elements of the articulator are snug against the condylar housings. If this is not seen, another record is made until duplicate records are produced. Because centric relation is the only jaw position that can be repeated by the patient, mountings can be replicated and verified for correctness in this position.

A straightforward protrusive record is made to adjust the horizontal condylar inclines on the articulator. Lateral eccentric records are made so that the lateral condylar inclinations can be properly adjusted. All interocclusal records should be made as near the vertical relation of occlusion as possible. Opposing teeth or occlusion rims must not be allowed to make contact when the records are made. A contact of the inclined planes of opposing teeth will invalidate an interocclusal record.

In some instances a mounting of a duplicate diagnostic cast in the maximum intercuspal position may also be desirable to definitively study this relationship on the articulator. Because articulators only simulate jaw movements, it is not unreasonable to assume that the relationship of the casts mounted in centric relation may differ minutely from the maximum intercuspal position seen on the articulator and observed in the mouth. When diagnostic casts are hand related by maximum intercuspation for purposes of mounting on an articulator, it is essential that three (preferably four) positive contacts of opposing posterior teeth are present, having wide spread molar contacts on each side of the arch. If occlusion rims are necessary to correctly orient casts on an articulator, centric relation should usually be the horizontal jaw relationship to which the removable partial denture will be constructed.

Materials and Methods for Recording Centric Relation

Materials available for recording centric relation are (1) wax; (2) modeling plastic; (3) quick-setting impression plaster; (4) metallic oxide bite registration paste; (5) polyether impression materials; and (6) silicone impression materials. Of these, wax is likely to be least satisfactory unless carefully handled. If not uniformly softened when introduced into the mouth, it can record a position with unequal tissue placement. Also, it does not remain rigid and dimensionally stable unless carefully chilled and handled upon removal (Figure 12-13).

Modeling plastic is a satisfactory record medium because it can be flamed and tempered until uniformly soft before it is placed into the mouth. After modeling plastic is chilled, it is sufficiently stable to permit the mounting of casts with accuracy. For these reasons, it is a satisfactory medium for recording occlusal relations for either complete or partial dentures. It also can be used with opposing natural teeth.

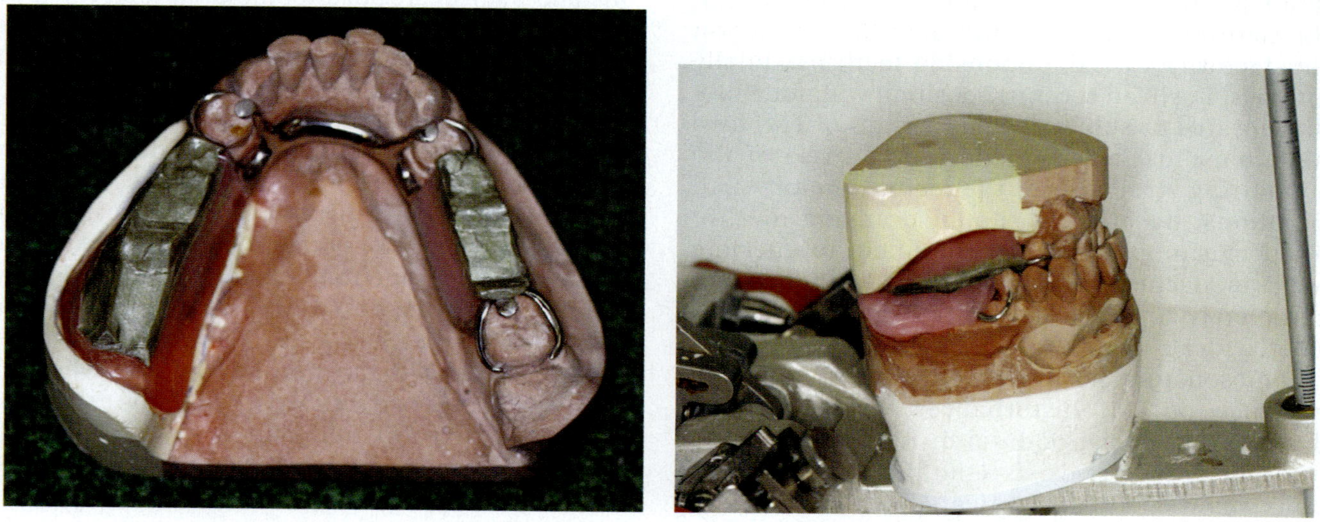

A B

Figure 12-13 **A,** A wax interocclusal record made on a cast framework. The modification spaces first had baseplate wax added, these were adjusted intraorally to provide space at the occlusal vertical dimension for recording wax, the wax was softened using a wax spatula and hot water bath, the framework was placed in the mouth, and care was exercised to guide the patient to close into a previously verified (and practiced) interocclusal position deemed appropriate (in this instance, centric relation position). The record was recovered from the mouth, excess wax was removed using a warm scalpel, and the wax was chilled and replaced in the mouth to verify the record. If not verified, the wax was re-softened (with additional wax added as needed) and the procedure was repeated. **B,** Immediately after verification, the framework with interocclusal registration was replaced on the mandibular cast and inverted on the maxillary cast for mounting.

Impression plaster has advantages of softness when introduced and rigidity when set, which make it a satisfactory material for recording jaw relations. Its use is highly recommended when occlusion rims are used to mount casts correctly or to adjust articulators with interocclusal eccentric records.

Metallic oxide bite registration paste offers many of the advantages of plaster, with less friability. Although not strong enough to be used alone, when supported by a gauze mesh attached to a metal frame, it is a satisfactory recording medium. Also it may be used with occlusion rims. After the paste sets, the frame is removed from the mouth and the buccal side of the gauze released where it was secured with sticky wax. The tube on the lingual side may then be slid off the lingual extension of the frame. The frame is not needed when mounting casts with this type of registration, because the tube alone lends sufficient support to the interocclusal record.

Elastomeric materials are excellent for recording interocclusal relationships (Figure 12-14). Some are specially formulated for this purpose and have the qualities of extremely low viscosity, minimal resistance to closure, rapid set, low rebound, lack of distortion, and stability after removal from the mouth. Care should be exercised to ensure that no elastic rebound results when the record is related to the cast during the mounting procedure.

The mandibular cast should be mounted on the lower arm of the articulator, with the articulator inverted (Figure 12-15, *A*). The articulator is first locked in centric position, and the incisal pin is adjusted so that the anterior distance between the upper and lower arms of the articulator will be increased 2 to 3 mm greater than the normal parallel relationship of the arms. This is done to compensate for the thickness of the interocclusal record so that the arms of the articulator will again be nearly parallel when the interocclusal record is removed and the opposing casts make contact.

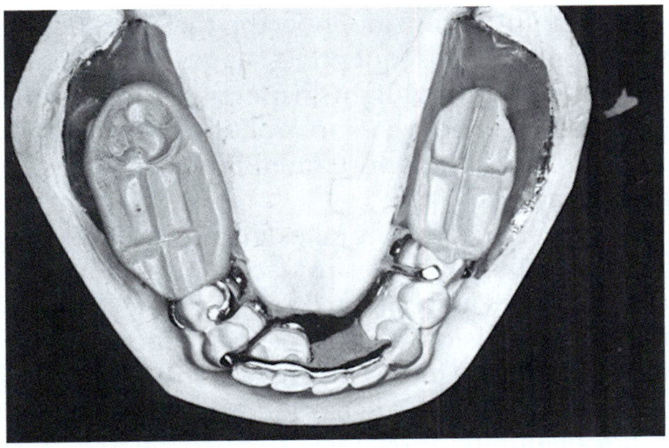

Figure 12-14 Elastomeric interocclusal registration material used to record mandibular position.

The base of the cast should be keyed and lightly lubricated for future removal. With the diagnostic casts accurately seated and secured in the occlusal record, the mandibular cast is affixed with stone to the lower member of the inverted articulator.

An articulator mounting thus made will have related the casts in centric relation (Figure 12-15, *B*). The dentist then can proceed to make an occlusal analysis by observing the influence of cusps in relation to one another after the articulator has been adjusted by using eccentric interocclusal records.

After an occlusal analysis has been made, the casts may be removed from their mounting for the purpose of surveying them individually and for other purposes as outlined previously. The indexed mounting ring record also should be retained throughout the course of treatment should the need arise for further study. It is advisable that the mounting be identified with the articulator that is used so that it may always be placed back onto the same articulator.

DIAGNOSTIC FINDINGS

The information gathered in the patient interview and clinical examination provides the basis for establishing whether treatment is indicated, and if so, what specific treatment should be considered. More than one treatment option can be considered, and financial implications need to be considered against long-term expectations to come to the best decision. Provision of a removable partial denture does not often preclude future considerations for other treatments, a fact that is not often the case for alternative treatments.

The patient interview can reveal medical considerations that impact the decision to provide any prosthesis. When it is felt that general medical health is being neglected, patients should be strongly encouraged to seek a general medical examination. Alternatively, patients who regularly see their physician may be found to take multiple medications that can contribute to a dry mouth and, potentially, an altered oral microflora with some increased risk for plaque-induced disease. Although such a condition can influence any prosthodontic care, given the unique features of removable partial denture service relative to the need for increased hygiene awareness and care, any factor that places an additional risk for plaque-induced disease should be pointed out to the patient and corrected if possible. Health conditions that negatively affect oral mucosa health (i.e., diabetes mellitus, Sjögren's syndrome, lupus, atrophic changes) may pose a risk for patient comfort for a tissue-supported prosthesis and factor into a treatment decision.

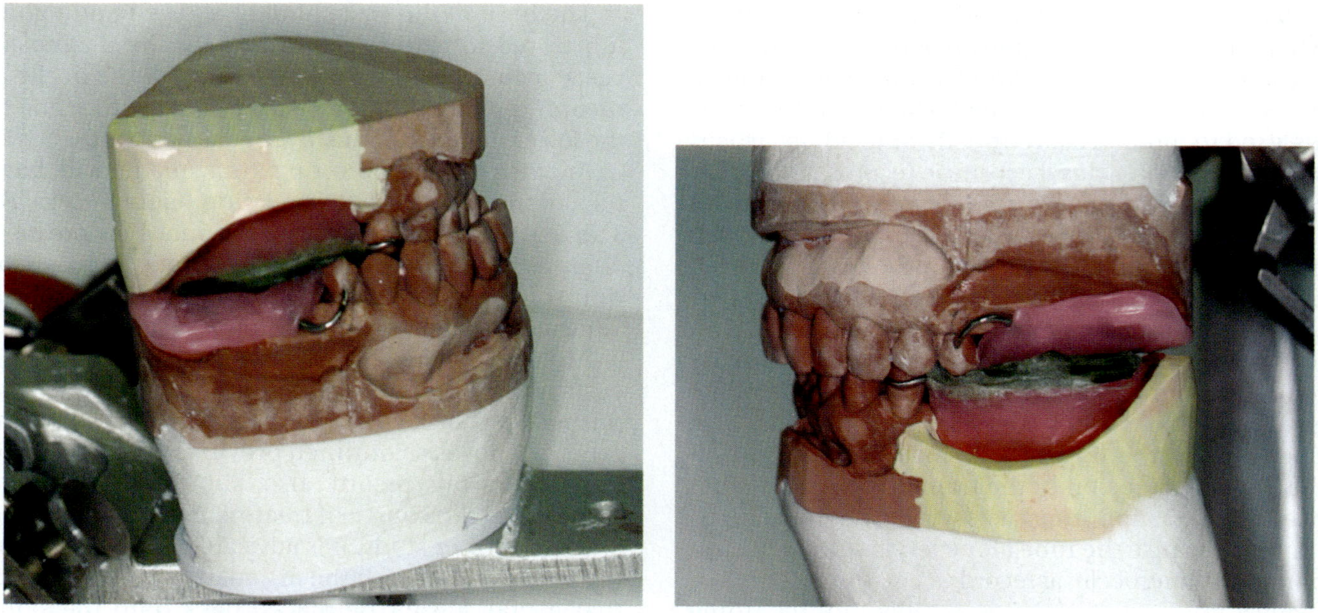

A B

Figure 12-15 **A,** Mandibular cast inverted on the mounted maxillary cast making sure that cast is fully seated into interocclusal record and stabilized to the opposing cast. It is important to check the posterior occlusion rim contact to be assured that no interfering contact has altered the record. Space should be observed between the opposing record bases (or record base and opposing occlusion). **B,** Mounted casts demonstrating occlusal plane as found in the mouth. Frankfort plane of the patient is oriented parallel to the articulator base and the floor. Also, inspection of the posterior rims demonstrates space between rims, which assures that the recorded position was registered without influence from rigid contacting components, only softened wax.

For the patient that has had previous experience with some form of prosthesis, the patient interview provides additional information that can impact treatment decisions. Identifying possible reasons (or more importantly a lack of any reasons) for both positive and negative past prosthesis experiences is important for determining whether a patient can predictably be helped. Although the clinical examination will point out the oral tissue responses to such therapy, the interview will highlight the subjective patient response to therapy and provides significant information that should be pursued. As mentioned previously, a patient complaint regarding a prosthesis needs to be confirmed through evaluation. The patient generally expresses concern about a symptom that can be related to support, stability, retention, and/or appearance. Confirmation of a design feature or oral condition that can explain the symptom is required to have a chance to correct it with a similar prosthesis. If examination does not confirm any such relationship, it would be difficult to proceed without some concern for repeating the patient response to therapy unless a different form of therapy is selected (i.e., replacing a problematic removable partial denture with an implant-supported prosthesis).

INTERPRETATION OF EXAMINATION DATA

As a result of the oral examination, several diagnoses are made related to the various tissue, conditions, and clinical information gathered. The integration of these diagnoses is the basis for the decisions that will ultimately form the suggested treatment. The treatment decision reflects a confluence of several aspects of the patient's past, present, and potential oral health status.

It is helpful to consider how the various diagnoses are integrated; consequently a suggested framework is provided that highlights aspects of disease management, followed by reconstruction considerations for (1) prosthesis support and (2) prosthesis design-specific aspects.

Disease management takes into account findings from the radiographic examination, periodontal disease and caries assessments, and pathology requiring endodontic considerations. Reconstruction considerations include diagnoses relative to prosthesis support (teeth and residual ridges) and prosthesis-specific design elements. Prosthesis support related to the remaining teeth requires radiographic examination of alveolar support and root morphology, endodontic evaluation, analysis of occlusal factors, assessment of the benefit for fixed prostheses or orthodontics, and evaluation for the need for extraction. Residual ridge support involves radiographic examination of the ridge contours and height, and evaluation of the need for preprosthetic surgical intervention. Prosthesis-specific design considerations include determination of anatomic relationships related to mandibular major connector design, the need for tooth modification to facilitate prosthesis function, and analysis of the occlusion. Each of these is considered as follows.

Radiographic Interpretation

Many of the reasons for radiographic interpretation during oral examination are outlined herein and are considered in greater detail in other texts. The aspects of such interpretation that are the most pertinent to removable partial denture construction are those relative to the prognosis of remaining teeth that may be used as abutments.

Disease Validation

It is important to verify disease found through radiographic interpretation by clinical evaluation. Also, if the clinical evaluation reveals dental caries and/or periodontal disease its severity can be confirmed by radiographic interpretation. It would be important to delineate the severity of caries, both in numbers of lesions and dentin and/or pulpal involvement, to gain insight as to the level of disease risk associated with the patient and to identify what therapy is required to maintain the teeth. The same is true for periodontal disease risk and severity, as such a diagnosis impacts both current and future tooth prognoses for prosthesis support.

The radiographic interpretation allows diagnosis of bone lesions associated with both the jaws and teeth. The implications for tooth stability and ridge support are important to factor into prosthesis prognosis. Surgical and postoperative management of such lesions can vary significantly with diagnosis (benign versus malignant), and definitive prosthesis treatment is often complicated by resection.

Tooth Support

The quality of the alveolar support of an abutment tooth is of primary importance, because the tooth will have to withstand greater stress loads when supporting a dental prosthesis. Abutment teeth providing total abutment support to the prosthesis, be it either fixed or removable, will have to withstand a greater load and especially greater horizontal forces. The latter may be minimized by establishing a harmonious occlusion and by distributing the horizontal forces among several teeth through the use of rigid connectors. Bilateral stabilization against horizontal forces is one of the attributes of a properly designed tooth-supported removable prosthesis. In many instances abutment teeth may be aided more than weakened by the presence of a bilaterally rigid removable partial denture.

In contrast, abutment teeth adjacent to distal extension bases are subjected not only to vertical and horizontal forces but to torque as well because of the movement of the tissue-supported base. Vertical support and stabilization against horizontal movement with rigid connectors are just as important as they are with a tooth-supported prosthesis, and the removable partial denture must be designed accordingly. In addition, the abutment tooth adjacent to the extension base will be subjected to torque in proportion to the design of the retainers, the size of the denture base, the tissue support received by the base, and the total occlusal load applied. With this in mind, each abutment tooth must be evaluated carefully as to the alveolar bone support present and the past reaction of that bone to occlusal stress.

It is important to judge whether the teeth and their respective periodontium can favorably respond to the demands of a prosthesis. Can the radiographic interpretation provide clues to predicting tooth response to increased loading from prostheses? Assessment of regions within the mouth that have been subjected to increased loading can provide some clues as to the predictability of future similar response. An understanding of bone density, index areas, and lamina dura response is helpful for these judgments.

Bone Density

The quality and quantity of bone in any part of the body are often evaluated by radiographic means. A detailed treatise concerning the bone support of the abutment tooth should include many considerations not possible to include in this text because of space limitations. The reader should realize that subclinical variations in bone may exist but may not be observed because of the limitations inherent in technical methods and equipment.

Of importance to the dentist when evaluating the quality and quantity of the alveolar bone are the height and the quality of the remaining bone. In estimating bone height, care must be taken to avoid interpretive errors resulting from angulation factors. Technically, when a radiographic exposure is made, the central ray should be directed at right angles to both the tooth and the film. The short-cone technique does not follow this principle; instead the ray is directed through the root of the tooth at a predetermined angle. This technique invariably causes the buccal bone to be projected higher on the crown than the lingual or palatal bone. Therefore in interpreting bone height, it is imperative to follow the line of the lamina dura from the apex toward the crown of the tooth until the opacity of the lamina materially decreases. At this point of opacity change, a less dense bone extends farther toward the tooth crown. This additional amount of bone represents false bone height. Thus the true height of the bone is ordinarily where the lamina shows a marked decrease in opacity. At this point, the trabecular pattern of bone superimposed on the tooth root is lost. The portion of the root between the cementoenamel junction and the true bone height has the appearance of being bare or devoid of covering.

Radiographic evaluation of bone quality is hazardous but is often necessary. It is essential to emphasize that changes in bone mineralization up to 25% often cannot be recognized by ordinary radiographic means. Optimum bone qualities are ordinarily expressed by normal-sized interdental trabecular spaces that tend to decrease slightly in size as examination of the bone proceeds from the root apex toward the coronal portion. The normal, interproximal crest is ordinarily shown by a relatively thin white line crossing from the lamina dura of one tooth to the lamina dura of the adjacent tooth. Considerable variation in the size of trabecular spaces may exist within normal limits, and the radiographic appearance of crestal alveolar bone may vary considerably, depending on its shape and the direction that the ray takes as it passes through the bone.

Normal bone usually responds favorably to ordinary stresses. Abnormal stresses, however, may create a reduction in the size of the trabecular pattern, particularly in that area of bone directly adjacent to the lamina dura of the affected tooth. This decrease in size of the trabecular pattern (so-called **bone condensation**) is often regarded as a favorable bone response, indicative of an improvement in bone quality. This is not necessarily an accurate interpretation. Such bone changes usually indicate stresses that should be relieved because if the resistance of the patient decreases, the bone may exhibit a progressively less favorable response in future radiographs.

An increased thickness of the periodontal space ordinarily suggests varying degrees of tooth mobility. This should be evaluated clinically. Radiographic evidence coupled with clinical findings may suggest to the dentist the inadvisability of using such a tooth as an abutment. Furthermore, an irregular intercrestal bone surface should make the dentist suspicious of active bone deterioration.

It is essential that the dentist realize that radiographic evidence shows the result of changes that have taken place and may not necessarily represent the present condition. For example, periodontal disease may have progressed beyond the stage visibly demonstrated in the radiograph. As was pointed out earlier, radiographic changes are not observed until approximately 25% of the mineral content has been depleted. On the other hand, bone condensation probably does represent the current situation.

Radiographic findings should serve the dentist as an adjunct to clinical observations. Too often the radiographic appearance alone is used to arrive at a diagnosis, therefore radiographic findings should always be confirmed by clinical examination. Radiographic interpretation will also serve an important function if used periodically after the prosthesis has been placed. Future bone changes of any type suggest traumatic interference from some source. The nature of such interference should be determined and corrective measures taken.

Index Areas

Index areas are those areas of alveolar support that disclose the reaction of bone to additional stress. Favorable reaction to such stress may be taken as an indication of future reaction to an added stress load. Teeth that have been subjected to abnormal loading because of the loss of adjacent teeth or that have withstood tipping forces, in addition to occlusal loading, may be better risks as abutment teeth than those that have not been called on to carry an extra occlusal load (Figures 12-16 and 12-17). If occlusal harmony can be improved and unfavorable forces minimized by the reshaping of occlusal surfaces and the favorable distribution of occlusal loading, such teeth may be expected to support the prosthesis without difficulty. At the same time, other teeth—although not at present carrying an extra load—may be expected to react favorably because of the favorable reaction of alveolar bone to abnormal loading elsewhere in the same arch.

Other index areas are those around teeth that have been subjected to abnormal occlusal loading; that have been subjected to diagonal occlusal loading caused by tooth migration; and that have reacted to additional loading, such as around existing fixed partial denture abutments. The reaction of the bone to additional stresses in these areas may be either positive or negative, with evidence of a supporting trabecular pattern, a heavy cortical layer, and a dense lamina dura, or the reverse response. With the former, the patient is said to have a positive bone factor, which means the ability to build additional support wherever needed. With the latter, the patient is said to have a negative bone factor, which means the inability to respond favorably to stress.

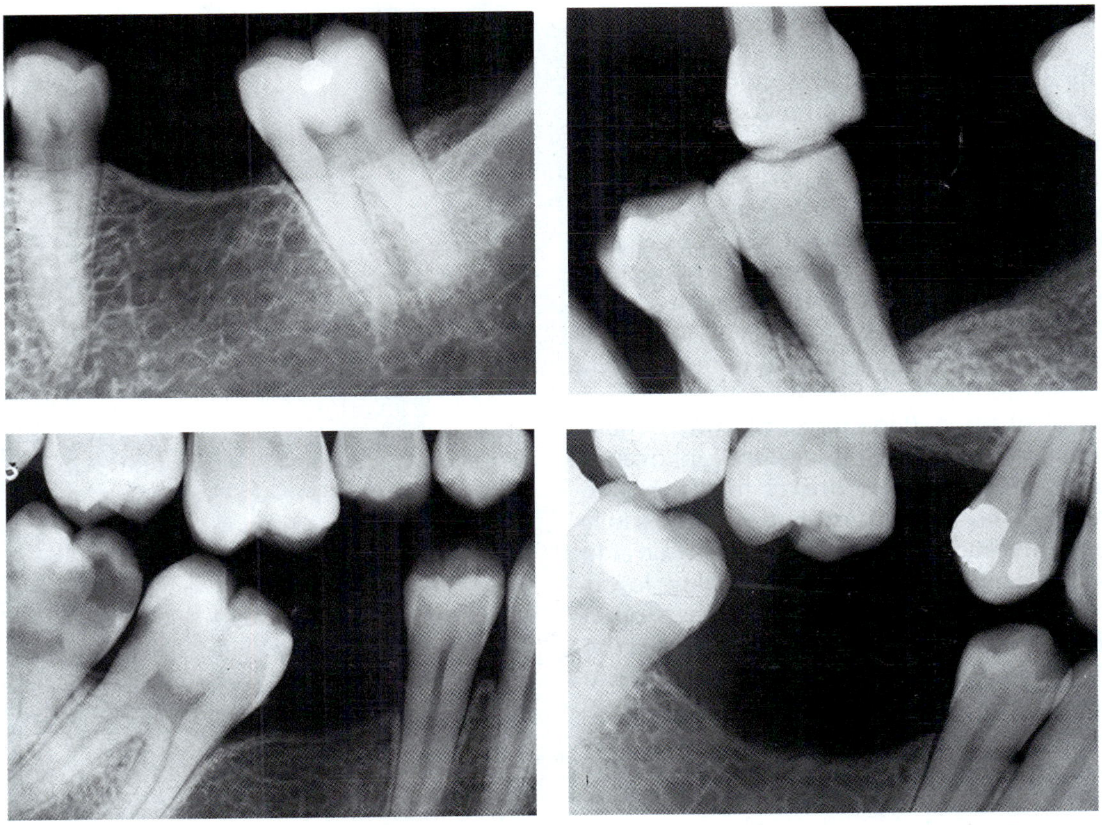

Figure 12-16 Reaction of bone adjacent to teeth that have been subjected to abnormal stress serves as indication of probable reactions of that bone when such teeth are used as abutments for fixed or removable restorations. Such areas are called *index areas*.

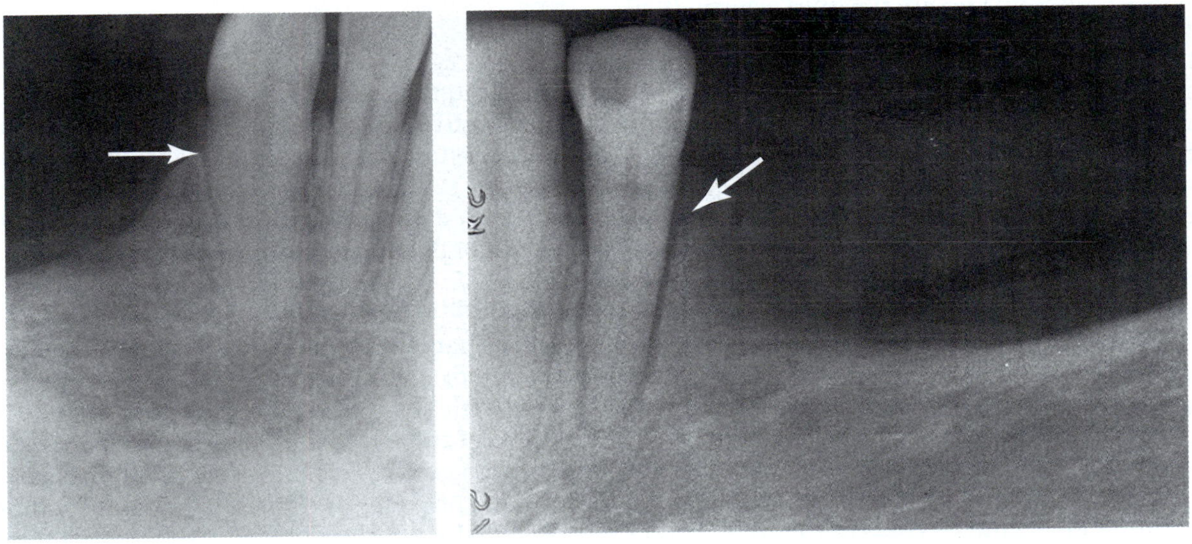

A B

Figure 12-17 **A,** Canine has provided support for distal extension removable partial denture for 10 years. There has obviously been positive bone response *(arrow)* to increased stress generated by removable partial denture. **B,** Mandibular first premolar has provided support for distal extension denture for 3 years. Bone response *(arrow)* to past additional stress has been unfavorable.

Alveolar Lamina Dura

The alveolar lamina dura is also considered in a radiographic interpretation of abutment teeth. The lamina dura is the thin layer of hard cortical bone that normally lines the sockets of all teeth. It affords attachment for the fibers of the periodontal membrane, and—as with all cortical bone—its function is to withstand mechanical strain. In a roentgenogram, the lamina dura is shown as a radiopaque white line around the radiolucent dark line that represents the periodontal membrane.

When a tooth is in the process of being tipped, the center of rotation is not at the apex of the root but in the apical third. Resorption of bone occurs where there is pressure, and apposition occurs where there is tension. Therefore during the active tipping process, the lamina dura is uneven, with evidence of both pressure and tension on the same side of the root. For example, in a mesially tipping lower molar the lamina dura will be thinner on the coronal mesial and apicodistal aspects and thicker on the apicomesial and coronal distal aspects because the axis of rotation is not at the root apex but is above it. When the tooth has been tipped into an edentulous space by some change in the occlusion and becomes set in its new position, the effects of leverage are discontinued. The lamina dura on the side to which the tooth is sloping becomes uniformly heavier, which is nature's reinforcement against abnormal stresses. The bone trabeculations are most often arranged at right angles to the heavier lamina dura.

Thus it is possible to say that for a given individual, nature is able to build support where it is needed and on this basis to predict future reaction elsewhere in the arch to additional loading of teeth used as abutments. However, because bone is approximately 30% organic, and this mostly protein, and because the body is not able to store a protein reserve in large amounts, any change in body health may be reflected in the patient's ability to maintain this support permanently. When systemic disease is associated with faulty protein metabolism and when the ability to repair is diminished, bone is resorbed and the lamina dura is disturbed. Therefore the loading of any abutment tooth must be kept to a minimum inasmuch as the patient's future health status and the eventualities of aging are unpredictable.

Root Morphology

The morphologic characteristics of the roots determine to a great extent the ability of prospective abutment teeth to resist successfully additional rotational forces that may be placed on them. Teeth with multiple and divergent roots will resist stresses better than teeth with fused and conical roots, because the resultant forces are distributed through a greater number of periodontal fibers to a larger amount of supporting bone (Figure 12-18).

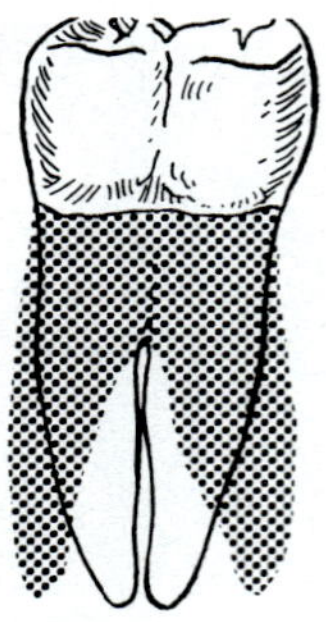

A

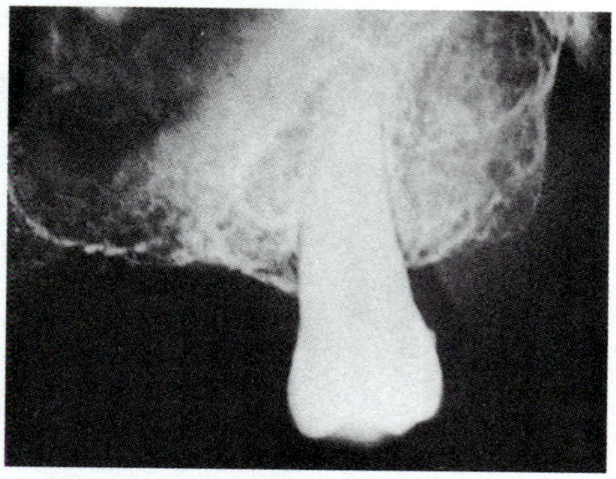

B

Figure 12-18 **A,** Prognosis for abutment service is more favorable for molar with divergent roots *(shaded)* than for same tooth if its roots were fused and conical. **B,** Evidence that prospective abutment has conical and fused roots indicates necessity for formulating framework design that will minimize additional stresses placed on tooth by abutment service.

Third Molars

Unerupted third molars should be considered as prospective future abutments to eliminate the need for a distal extension removable partial denture (Figure 12-19). The increased stability of a tooth-supported denture is most desirable to enhance the health of the oral environment.

Periodontal Considerations

An assessment of the periodontium in general and abutment teeth in particular must be made before prosthetic restoration. One must evaluate the condition of the gingiva, looking for adequate zones of attached gingiva and the presence or absence of periodontal pockets. The ideal periodontal condition is a disease-free periodontium with adequate attached mucosa in regions at or adjacent to removable partial denture component parts that cross the gingival margins to best resist the mechanical challenges posed because of function and use. The condition of the supporting bone must be evaluated, with specific attention to reduced bone support and mobility patterns

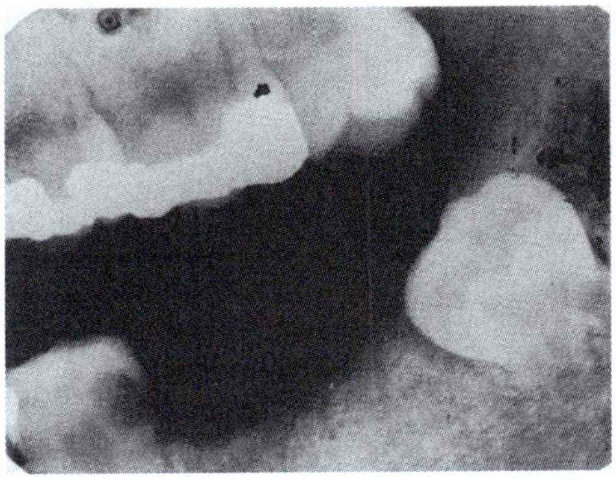

Figure 12-19 First and second molars have been lost by this 18-year-old patient. Distal extension removable partial denture may be constructed until third molar erupts and is fully formed. Tooth-supported restoration may then be considered.

recorded. If mucogingival involvement, osseous defects, or mobility patterns are recorded, the causes and potential treatment must be determined.

Oral hygiene habits of the patient must be determined and efforts made to educate the patient relative to plaque control. The most decisive evidence of oral hygiene habits is the condition of the mouth before the initial prophylaxis. Good or bad oral hygiene is basic to the patient's nature, and although it may be influenced somewhat by patient education, the long-range view must be taken. It is reasonably fair to assume that the patient will do little more in the long term than he or she has done in the past. In making decisions as to the method of treatment based on oral hygiene, the future in years, rather than in weeks and months, must be considered. It is probably best not to give the patient the benefit of any doubt as to future oral hygiene habits. Rather the benefit should come from protective measures when any doubt exists about future oral hygiene habits. Therefore for patients at greatest risk, an oral prophylaxis with continued oral hygiene instructions should be scheduled for 3- to 4-month intervals. In addition, the patient must be advised of the importance of regular maintenance appointments for tissue-supported prostheses to maintain occlusal relationships. In describing these on-going observation and prophylactic requirements, the patient is faced with the realization that they must be willing to share responsibility for maintaining the health of the mouth after restorative and prosthodontic treatment.

The remaining teeth and prosthesis will require meticulous plaque control after placement of a removable partial denture. Because of the nature of material coverage of oral tissue, the oral microflora can change with use of a removable prosthesis. Coupled with this microbial change is the potential for a mechanical challenge to tissue integrity if the appropriate relationship is not maintained for the prosthesis and soft tissue of the residual ridge and the marginal gingiva.

Caries Activity

Caries activity in the mouth, past and present, and the need for protective restorations must be considered. The decision to use full coverage is based on the need to reshape abutment teeth to accommodate the components of the removable partial denture, to prevent restoration breakdown when abutments have large direct restorations, evidence of caries activity, the patient's oral hygiene habits, and the age of the patient. Occasionally, three-quarter crowns may be used where buccal or lingual surfaces are completely sound, but intracoronal restorations (inlays) are seldom indicated in any mouth with evidence of past extensive caries or precarious areas of decalcification, erosion, or exposed cementum.

Frequent consumption of sugars can lead to carious involvement of roots, caries around restorations, or caries associated with clasps of removable partial dentures. Intelligent consumption of sweets (smaller amounts and less frequent consumption) and frequent plaque removal are the recommended countermeasures. Excellent protection from caries can be provided by fluoride applications via toothpastes and mouth rinses, or in extreme cases, such as postradiation xerostomia, by applying 1% NaF gels daily using plastic trays.

Xerostomia, caused by either degeneration of salivary glands (Sjögren's syndrome) or various medications, will enhance the occurrence and severity of caries and contribute to irritation of the oral mucosa. A possible way to alleviate xerostomia is the use of synthetic saliva, with a carboxymethylcellulose base, which can be enriched with fluoride in an effort to counteract caries. Frequent use provides an excellent means of maintaining high fluoride intraorally for long periods of time, thus enhancing the remineralization of incipient caries. Although the instructions for improvement of oral hygiene are a duty of the dental team, suspected problems of dietary deficiencies should be referred to a nutritionist.

Evaluation of the Prosthesis Foundation—Teeth and Residual Ridge

An evaluation of the prosthesis foundation is required to ensure that an appropriately stable base of sound teeth and/or residual ridge(s) is provided to maximize prosthesis function and patient comfort. To that end, the evaluation focuses on the identification of conditions that are inconsistent with sound support and predictably stable function.

Surgical Preparation

Need for preprosthetic surgery or extractions must be evaluated. The same criteria apply to surgical intervention in the partially edentulous arch as in the completely edentulous arch. Grossly displaceable soft tissue covering basal seat areas and hyperplastic tissue should be removed to provide a firm denture foundation. Mandibular tori should be removed if they will interfere with the optimum location of a lingual bar connector or a favorable path of placement. Any other areas of bone prominence that will interfere with the path of placement should be removed also. Primarily the guiding plane of the abutment teeth will dictate the path of placement. Therefore some areas may present interference to the path of placement of the removable partial denture by reason of the fact that other unalterable factors, such as retention and esthetics, must take precedence in selecting the path.

Clinical research in preprosthetic surgical concepts has contributed significantly to management of the compromised partially edentulous patient. Bone augmentation and guided bone regeneration procedures have been used with varying degrees of success as an alternative method of improving ridge support for the denture base areas. Skill and judgment must be exercised in patient selection, procedural planning, and surgical and prosthetic management to optimize clinical results. Use of osseointegrated implants can provide a foundation for developing suitable abutment support for removable partial dentures. As in any surgical procedure, results depend on careful treatment planning and cautious surgical management.

Extraction of teeth may be indicated for one of the following three reasons:

1. If the tooth cannot be restored to a state of health, extraction may be unavoidable. Modern advancements in the treatment of periodontal disease and in restorative procedures, including endodontic therapy, have resulted in the saving of teeth that were once considered untreatable. All reasonable avenues of treatment should be considered both from prognostic and economic standpoints before recommending extraction.
2. A tooth may be removed if its absence will permit a more serviceable and less complicated removable partial denture design. Teeth in extreme malposition (lingually inclined mandibular teeth, buccally inclined maxillary teeth, and mesially inclined teeth posterior to an edentulous space) may be removed if an adjacent tooth is in good alignment and if good support is available for use as an abutment. Justification for extraction lies in the decision that a suitable restoration, which will provide satisfactory contour and support, cannot be fabricated or that orthodontic treatment to realign the tooth is not feasible. An exception to the arbitrary removal of a malposed tooth is when a distal extension removable partial denture base would have to be made rather than using the more desirable tooth-supported base of the tooth in question. If alveolar support is adequate, a posterior abutment should be retained if at all possible in preference to a tissue-supported extension base. Teeth deemed to have insufficient alveolar support may be extracted if their prognosis is poor and if other adjacent teeth may be used to better advantage as abutments. The decision to extract such a tooth should be based on the degree of mobility and other periodontal considerations and on the number, length, and shape of the roots contributing to its support.
3. A tooth may be extracted if it is so unesthetic as to justify its removal to improve appearance. In this situation, a veneer crown should be considered in preference to removal if the crown can satisfy the esthetic needs. If removal is advisable because of unesthetic tooth position, the biomechanical problems involved in replacing anterior teeth with a removable partial denture must be weighed against the problems involved in making an esthetically acceptable fixed restoration. Admittedly the removable replacement is commonly the more esthetic of the two, despite modern advancements in retainers and pontics. However, the mechanical disadvantage of the removable restoration often makes the fixed replacement of missing anterior teeth preferable.

Another consideration for preprosthetic surgery involves the decision between use of a removable partial denture and an implant-supported prosthesis. The following categories of tooth loss are presented with comparative comments germane to such decisions.

Short Modification Spaces

For short spans (≤3 missing teeth), natural tooth, implant-supported fixed prostheses, and removable partial dentures can generally be considered. Implant placement requires the decision that ample bone volume exists, or can be provided with minimal morbidity, to adequately house sufficient implants to support prosthetic teeth. Implant prostheses have the advantage of not requiring the use of teeth for support, stability, and retention requirements, and consequently do not increase the functional burden on the natural dentition. Although the predictability of contemporary implant procedures (surgery and prosthodontics) makes them a consideration for short span prostheses, the main advantage is the opportunity to provide replacement teeth without involving adjacent teeth in the reconstruction. Therefore, when the adjacent teeth are in need of restoration, a conventional prosthesis should be considered.

Longer Modification Spaces

Longer span modification spaces (≥4 missing teeth) present a greater challenge for natural tooth-supported fixed prostheses. Consequently, the options for treatment are the removable partial denture or the implant-supported prosthesis. An implant prosthesis has the same bone volume requirements as stated above, and for an increased span will likely require more implants. Since residual ridge resorption can be greater with longer spans, the need for augmentation may also be greater. Both of these characteristics of longer spans cause implant use to be more costly and can significantly increase the cost difference between treatment options. The increased morbidity associated with augmentation procedures can also limit universal application. Because the removable partial denture remains largely tooth-supported (unless the span includes anterior and posterior segments that may cause it to function similar to a distal extension), the functional stability requirements should be efficiently met through the tooth support.

Distal Extension Spaces

Without tooth support at each end of the missing teeth, the removable partial denture and implant-supported prosthesis are the primary treatment considerations (double-abutted cantilevered fixed prostheses opposing maxillary complete dentures have been suggested to be a reasonable option for some patients). It then becomes obvious that when anatomic limitations to implant placement exist and surgical measures cannot be taken to correct this, the removable partial denture is the only option (unless no treatment is elected). Current surgical options are available to correct most anatomic limitations, yet frequently implant therapy is not elected because of patient medical factors, concerns for the risk of surgical morbidity, increased time required for treatment, or costs. It is important to note that a comparison of long-term maintenance requirements between these two options may demonstrate few cost differences over time. This is related to the effects of continued residual ridge resorption acting on the removable prosthesis and not the implant prosthesis.

Endodontic Treatment

Abutments for removable partial dentures are required to withstand various forces depending on the classification. The requirement for a distal extension abutment is different from that of a tooth-supported prosthesis in that torsional forces exist in the distal extension situation. For this reason, an abutment for a distal extension that is endodontically treated carries a greater risk for complications than a similar tooth not involved in removable partial denture function.

Because tooth support helps control prosthesis movement, the need for endodontic treatment should include assessment of overdenture abutments for removable partial dentures, especially to control movement of distal extensions.

Analysis of Occlusal Factors

From the occlusal analysis made by evaluating the mounted diagnostic casts the dentist must decide whether it is best to accept and maintain the existing occlusion or to attempt to improve on it by means of occlusal adjustment and/or restoration of occlusal surfaces. It must be remembered that the removable partial denture can only supplement the existing occlusion at the time the prosthesis is constructed. The dominant force that dictates the occlusal pattern will be the cuspal harmony or disharmony of the remaining teeth and their proprioceptive influence on mandibular movement. At best the artificial teeth can only be made to harmonize with the functional parameters of the existing occlusion.

Chapter 17 identifies schemes of occlusion recommended for partially edentulous configurations. A review of these recommendations will provide a guide for modifying the existing occlusion or developing the appropriate occlusal scheme for each partially edentulous configuration.

Improvements in the natural occlusion must be accomplished before the fabrication of the prosthesis, not subsequent to it. The objective of occlusal reconstruction by any means should be occlusal harmony of the restored dentition in relation to the natural forces already present or established. Therefore one of the earliest decisions in planning reconstructive treatment must be whether to accept or reject the existing vertical dimension of occlusion and the occlusal contact relationships in centric and eccentric positions. If occlusal adjustment is indicated, cuspal analysis always should precede any corrective procedures in the mouth by selective grinding. On the other hand, if reconstruction is to be the means of correction, the manner and sequence should be outlined as part of the overall treatment plan.

Fixed Restorations

There may be a need to restore modification spaces with fixed restorations rather than include them in the removable partial denture, especially when dealing with isolated abutment teeth. The advantage of splinting must be weighed against the total cost, with the weight of experience always in favor of using fixed restorations for tooth-bounded spaces unless the space will facilitate simplification of the removable partial denture design without jeopardizing the abutment teeth. One of the least successful removable partial denture designs is where multiple tooth-bounded areas are replaced with the removable partial dentures in conjunction with isolated abutment teeth and distal extension bases. Biomechanical considerations and the future health of the remaining teeth should be given preference over economic considerations when such a choice is possible.

Orthodontic Treatment

Occasionally, orthodontic movement of malposed teeth followed by retention through the use of fixed partial dentures makes it possible for a better removable partial denture design mechanically and esthetically than could otherwise be used. Although adequate anchorage for tooth movement can be a major limitation in partially edentulous arches, carefully placed implants, which subsequently can be used for prosthesis support, have been used to expand orthodontic applications for this patient group.

Need for Determining Type of Mandibular Major Connector

As discussed in Chapter 5, one of the criteria to determine the use of the lingual bar or linguoplate is the height of the floor of the patient's mouth when the tongue is elevated. Because the inferior border of both the lingual bar and linguoplate are placed at the same vertical level, and because subsequent mouth preparations depend in part on the design of the mandibular major connector, determination of the type of major connector must be made during the oral examination. This determination is facilitated by measuring the height of the elevated floor of the patient's mouth in relation to lingual gingiva with a periodontal probe and recording the measurement for later transfer to diagnostic and master casts. It is most difficult to make a determination of the type of mandibular major connector to be used solely from a stone cast that may or may not accurately indicate the active range of movement of the floor of the patient's mouth. Too many mandibular major connectors are ruined or made flexible because subsequent grinding of the inferior border is necessary to relieve impingement of the sensitive tissue of the floor of the mouth.

Need for Reshaping Remaining Teeth

The clinical crown shapes of anterior and posterior teeth are not capable of supporting a removable partial denture framework without appropriate modification. Without the required modifications, the prosthesis does not adequately benefit from the support and stability offered by the teeth and consequently will not be comfortable to the patient. Many failures of removable partial dentures can be attributed to the fact that the teeth were not reshaped properly to establish guiding planes or to receive clasp arms and occlusal rests before the impression for the master cast was made. Of particular importance are the paralleling of proximal tooth surfaces to act as guiding planes, the preparation of adequate rest areas, and the reduction of unfavorable tooth contours (Figure 12-20). To neglect planning such mouth preparations in advance is inexcusable and leads to unsuccessful removable prosthesis service.

The design of clasps is dependent on the location of the retentive, stabilizing, reciprocal, and supporting areas in relation to a definite path of placement and removal. Failure to reshape unfavorably inclined tooth surfaces and, if necessary, to place restorations with suitable contours not only complicates the design and location of clasp retainers but also often leads to failure of the removable partial denture because of poor clasp design.

A malaligned tooth or one that is inclined unfavorably may make it necessary to place certain parts of the clasp so that they interfere with the opposing teeth. Unparallel proximal tooth surfaces not only will fail to provide needed guiding planes during placement and removal but also will result in excessive blockout. This inevitably results in the connectors being placed so far out of contact with tooth surfaces that food traps are created. In order to pass lingually inclined lower teeth, clearance for a lingual bar major connector may have to be so great that a food trap will result when the restoration is fully seated. Such a lingual bar will be located so that it will interfere with tongue comfort and function. These are only some of the objectionable consequences of inadequate mouth preparations.

The amount of reduction of tooth contours should be kept to a minimum, and all modified tooth surfaces should not only be repolished after reduction but also should be subjected to fluoride treatment to lessen the incidence of caries. If it is not possible to produce the contour desired without perforating the enamel, then the teeth should be recontoured with an acceptable restorative material. The age of the patient, caries activity evidenced elsewhere in the mouth, and apparent oral hygiene habits must be taken into consideration when deciding between reducing the enamel or modifying tooth contours with protective restorations.

Some of the areas that frequently need correction are the lingual surfaces of mandibular premolars, the mesial and lingual surfaces of mandibular molars, the distobuccal line angle of maxillary premolars, and the mesiobuccal line angle of maxillary molars. The actual degree of inclination of teeth in relation to the path of placement and the location of retentive and supportive areas are not readily interpretable during visual examination. These are established during a comprehensive analysis of the diagnostic cast with a surveyor, which should follow the visual examination.

DIFFERENTIAL DIAGNOSIS: FIXED OR REMOVABLE PARTIAL DENTURES

Total oral rehabilitation (disease management, defective tooth restoration, and tooth replacement) is an objective in treating the partially edentulous patient.

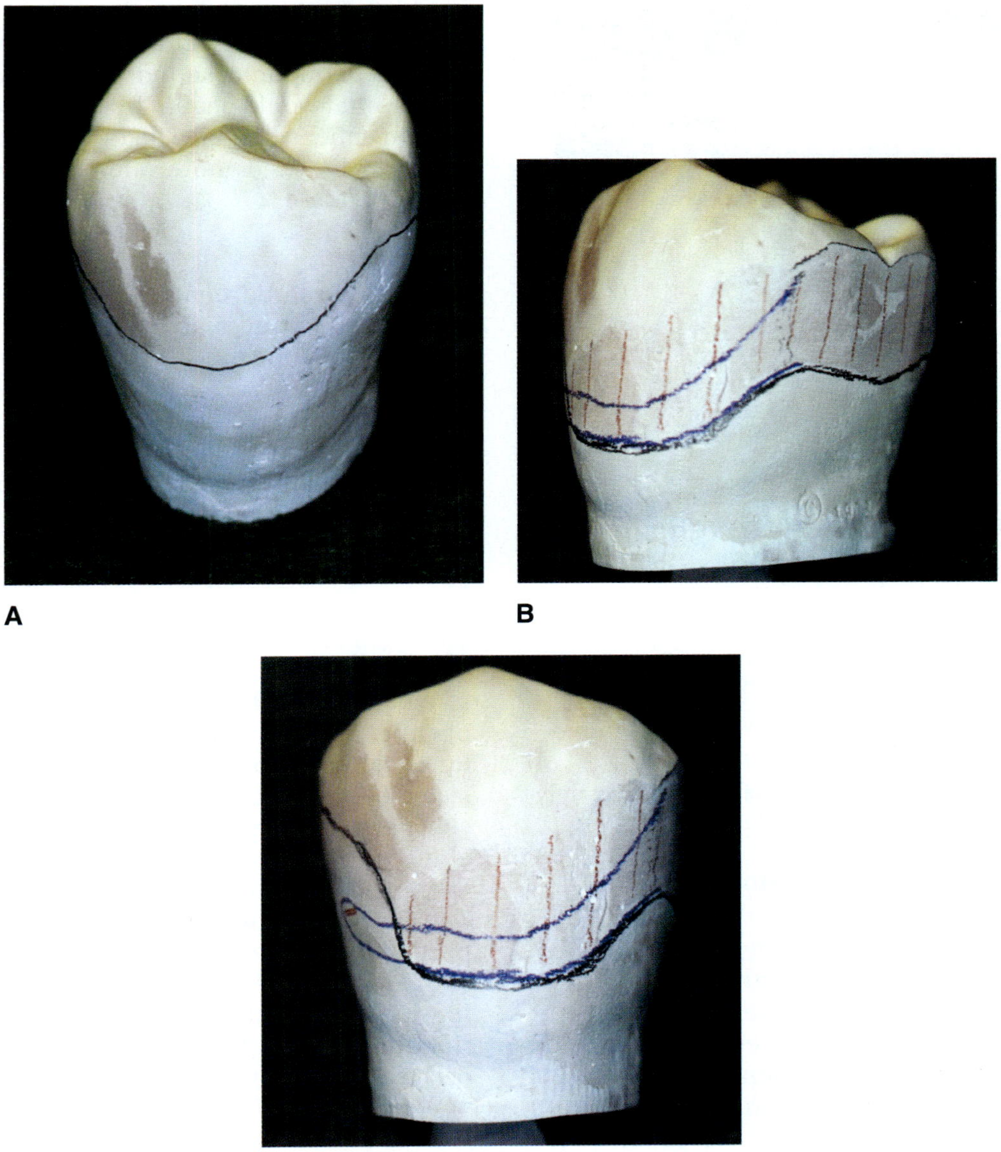

A B C

Figure 12-20 **A,** Unmodified buccal surface of mandibular premolar illustrating typical height of contour location natural for this tooth (middle and occlusal thirds of the tooth). **B,** Proximal surface modification required *(hatched region)* to produce guide plane surface. **C,** Buccal surface modification needed to position height of contour for favorable clasp location. The tooth modification is a continuation of the proximal surface modification onto the buccal surface, and generally requires less than 0.5 mm of tooth removal.

Although replacement of missing teeth by means of fixed partial dentures, either tooth- or implant-supported, is generally the method of choice, there are many reasons why a removable partial denture is the better method of treatment for a specific patient.

The dentist must follow the best procedure for the welfare of the patient, who is always free to seek more than one opinion. Ultimately, the choice of treatment must meet the economic limitations and personal desires of the patient. The exception to this guideline is the Class III arch with a modification space on the opposite side of the arch, which will provide better cross-arch stabilization and a simpler design for the removable partial denture (Figure 12-21).

Though uncommon, unilateral tooth loss is sometimes inappropriately treated using a unilateral removable partial denture in place of a fixed partial denture. This type of prosthesis does not benefit from cross-arch stabilization and places excessive stress on abutment teeth. Possibly more importantly, there is a significant risk for aspiration if such a prosthesis is dislodged during use. For these reasons, use

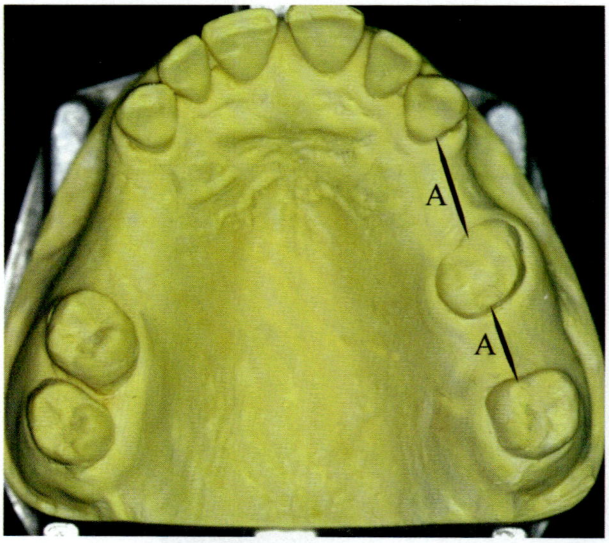

Figure 12-21 Class III, mod 2 arch in which modification spaces on the patient's left (spaces designated at *A*) will be included in design of removable partial denture rather than restored with a long-span fixed partial denture. Design for removable restoration is greatly simplified, resulting in significantly enhanced stability.

of the unilateral removable partial denture is strongly discouraged.

Indications for Use of Fixed Restorations

Tooth-Bounded Edentulous Regions

Generally, any unilateral edentulous space bounded by teeth suitable for use as abutments should be restored with a fixed partial denture cemented to one or more abutment teeth at either end. The length of the span and the periodontal support of the abutment teeth will determine the required number of abutments. As mentioned earlier, such a span could also be managed using dental implants if deemed feasible and elected by the patient. The fact that implant support does not place additional functional demands on adjacent teeth likely contributes to their preservation, though this has not been universally demonstrated.

For conventional fixed prostheses, a lack of parallelism of the abutment teeth may be counteracted with copings or locking connectors to provide parallel sectional placement. Sound abutment teeth make possible the use of more conservative retainers, such as partial veneer crowns, or resin bonded to metal restorations, rather than full crowns. The age of the patient, evidence of caries activity, oral hygiene habits, and soundness of remaining tooth structure must be considered in any decision to use less than full coverage for abutment teeth.

There are two specific contraindications for the use of unilateral fixed restorations. One is a long, edentulous span with abutment teeth that would not be able to withstand the trauma of nonaxial occlusal forces. The other is abutment teeth that exhibit reduced periodontal support because of periodontal disease that would benefit from cross-arch stabilization. In either situation a bilateral removable restoration can be used more effectively to replace the missing teeth.

Modification Spaces

A removable partial denture for a Class III arch is better supported and stabilized when a modification area on the opposite side of the arch is present. A fixed partial denture need not be used to restore such an edentulous area because its inclusion may simplify the design of the removable partial denture. However, when a lone-standing, single-rooted abutment binds a modification space, it is better restored by means of a fixed partial denture. This acts to stabilize the at-risk tooth, and the denture is made less complicated by not having to include other abutment teeth for the support and retention of an additional edentulous space or spaces.

When an edentulous space that is a modification of either a Class I or Class II arch exists anterior to a lone-standing abutment tooth, this tooth is subjected to trauma by the movements of a distal extension removable partial denture far in excess of its ability to withstand such stresses. The splinting of the lone abutment to the nearest tooth is mandatory. The abutment crowns should be contoured for support and retention of the removable partial denture and, in addition, a means usually should be provided for supporting a stabilizing component on the anterior abutment of the fixed partial denture or on the occlusal surface of the pontic.

Anterior Modification Spaces

Usually, any missing anterior teeth in a partially edentulous arch, except in a Kennedy Class IV arch in which only anterior teeth are missing, are best replaced by means of a fixed restoration. There are exceptions. Sometimes a better esthetic result is obtainable when the anterior replacements are supplied by the removable partial denture, at other times treatment is simplified by inclusion of an anterior modification space into the removable partial denture (Figure 12-22). This is also true when excessive tissue and bone resorption necessitates the placement of the pontics in a fixed partial denture too far palatally for good esthetics or for an acceptable relation with the opposing teeth. However, in most instances, from mechanical and biological standpoints, anterior replacements are best accomplished with fixed restorations. The replacement of missing posterior teeth with a removable partial denture is then made much less complicated and gives more satisfactory results.

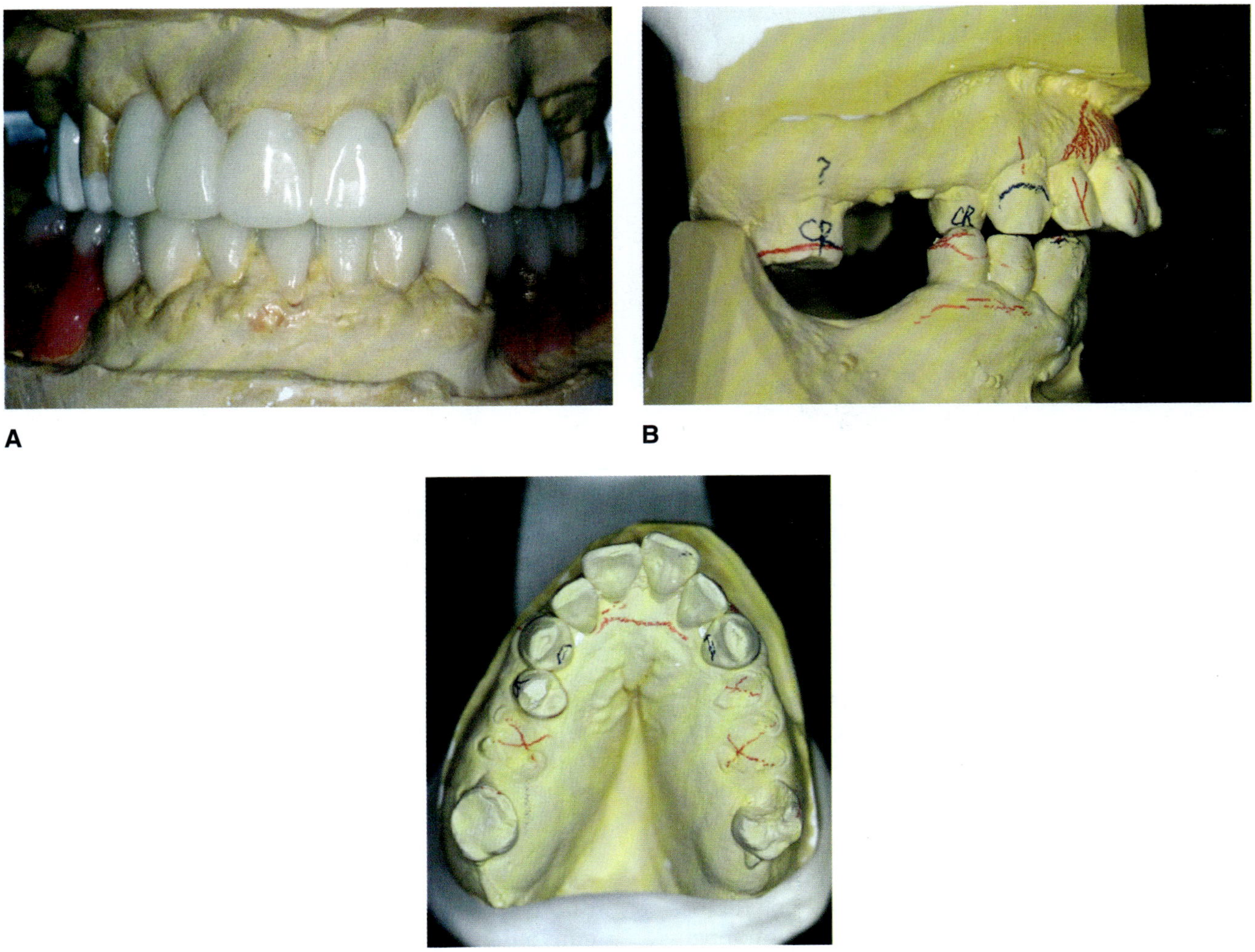

A B C

Figure 12-22 **A,** Diagnostic waxing of this complex case revealed the best means to manage replacement of teeth #s 6 and 7 was with a fixed prosthesis, especially since the ridge defect was not severe and the adjacent teeth offered good retainer support. **B,** In contrast, this complex situation requires the maxillary anterior to be re-positioned palatally to address an esthetic concern. **C,** Because of the condition of the maxillary canines and need to replace posterior teeth as well, the anterior teeth will be more easily managed as part of the removable partial denture. *(**A** Courtesy Dr. M. Alfaro.)*

Replacement of Unilaterally Missing Molars (Shortened Dental Arch)

Often the decision to replace unilaterally missing molars must be made (Figure 12-23). The decision must balance the impact of the treatment on the remaining oral structures with the potential benefit to the patient long term. To restore the missing molars with a fixed partial denture would require either a cantilever prosthesis or the use of dental implants. A cantilever fixed prosthesis is most applicable if the second molar is to be ignored, then only first molar occlusion need be supplied by using a cantilever-type fixed partial denture. Occlusion need be only minimal to maintain occlusal relations between the natural first molar in the one arch and the prosthetic molar in the opposite arch. The cantilevered pontic should be narrow buccolingually and need not occlude with more than one half to two thirds of the opposing tooth. Often, such a restoration is the preferred method of treatment. However, at least two abutments should be used to support a cantilevered molar opposed by a natural molar.

To replace unilaterally missing molars with a removable partial denture necessitates use of a distal extension prosthesis. This involves the major connector joining the edentulous side to retentive and stabilizing components located on the nonedentulous side of the arch. Leverage factors are frequently unfavorable, and the retainers used on the nonedentulous side are often unsatisfactory. Two

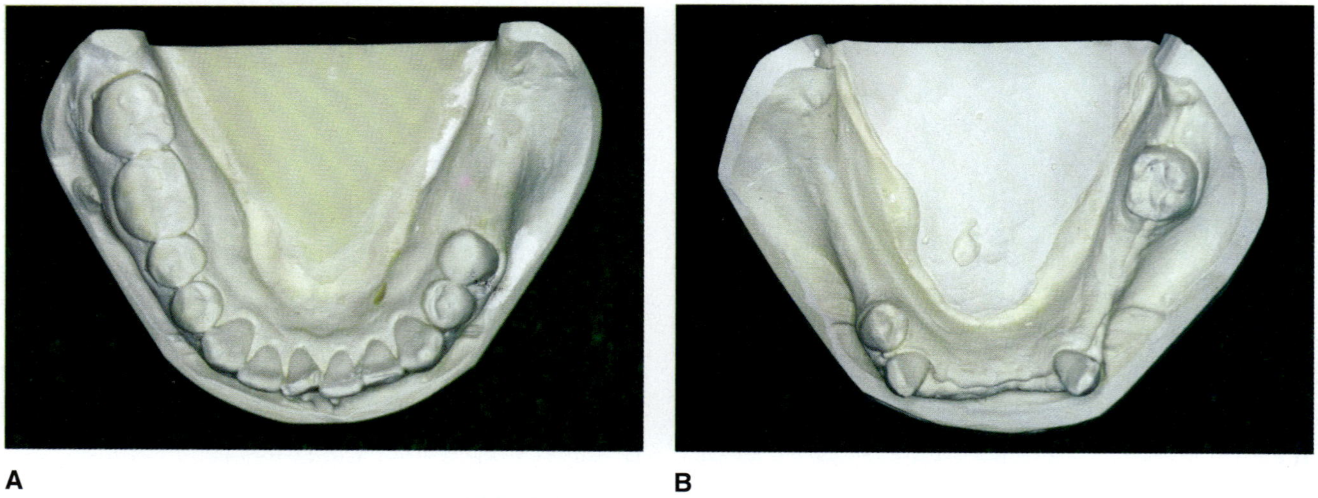

Figure 12-23 **A,** Unilaterally missing molars. If the patient exhibits opposing contacts to the remaining 6 posterior teeth (bilateral premolars, right first and second molars), there may be minimal functional gain from replacing the left molars. **B,** By contrast, the functional gain from replacement of the posterior occlusion in this patient is likely significant.

factors important to consider in making the decision to provide a unilateral, distal extension removable partial denture include the opposing teeth and the future effect of the maxillary tuberosity.

First the opposing teeth must be considered if it is considered important to prevent extrusion and migration. This influences the replacement of the missing molars far more than any improvement in masticating efficiency that might result. The replacement of missing molars on one side is seldom necessary for reasons of mastication alone.

Second the future effect of a maxillary tuberosity must be considered if concern exists for tuberosity enlargement. Often when left uncovered, the tuberosity increases in size, making future occlusal treatment difficult. However, covering the tuberosity with a removable partial denture base, in combination with the stimulating effect of the intermittent occlusion, helps maintain tuberosity size and position. In such an instance, it may be better to make a removable partial denture with cross-arch stabilization and retention than to leave a maxillary tuberosity uncovered.

Indications for Removable Partial Dentures

Although a removable partial denture should be considered only when a fixed restoration is contraindicated, there are several specific indications for the use of a removable restoration.

Distal Extension Situations

Replacement of missing posterior teeth is often best accomplished with a removable partial denture (see Figure 12-23, *B*), especially when implant treatment is not feasible for the patient. The exception to this includes situations in which the replacement of missing second (and third) molars is either inadvisable or unnecessary or in which unilateral replacement of a missing first molar can be accomplished by means of a multiple-abutment cantilevered fixed restoration or an implant-supported prosthesis. The most common partially edentulous situations are the Kennedy Class I and Class II. With the latter, an edentulous space on the opposite side of the arch is often conveniently present to aid in the required retention and stabilization of the removable partial denture. If no space is present, selected abutment teeth can be modified to accommodate appropriate clasp assemblies, or intracoronal retainers can be used. As previously stated, all other edentulous areas are best replaced with fixed partial dentures.

After Recent Extractions

The replacement of teeth after recent extractions often cannot be accomplished satisfactorily with a fixed restoration. When relining will be required later or when a fixed restoration using natural teeth or implants will be constructed later, a temporary removable partial denture can be used. If an all-resin denture is used rather than a cast framework removable partial denture, the immediate cost to the patient is much less, and the resin denture lends itself best to future temporary modifications—including those required after implant placement and before restoration.

Tissue changes are inevitable following extractions. Tooth-bounded edentulous areas (as a result of extractions) are best initially restored with removable partial dentures. Relining of a tooth-supported resin denture base is then possible. It is usually done to improve esthetics, oral cleanliness, or patient comfort. Support for such a restoration is supplied by occlusal rests on the abutment teeth at each end of the edentulous space.

Long Span

A long span may be totally tooth supported if the abutments and the means of transferring the support to the denture are adequate, and if the denture framework is rigid. There is little if any difference between the support afforded a removable partial denture and that afforded a fixed restoration by the adjacent abutment teeth. However, in the absence of cross-arch stabilization, the torque and leverage would be excessive on the two abutment teeth. Instead, a removable denture that derives retention, support, and stabilization from abutment teeth on the opposite side of the arch is indicated as the logical means of replacing the missing teeth.

Need for Effect of Bilateral Stabilization

In a mouth weakened by periodontal disease, a fixed restoration may jeopardize the future of the involved abutment teeth unless the multiple-abutment splinting effect is used. The removable partial denture, on the other hand, may act as a periodontal splint through its effective cross-arch stabilizing of teeth weakened by periodontal disease. When abutment teeth throughout the arch are properly prepared and restored, the beneficial effect of a removable partial denture can be far greater than that of a unilateral fixed partial denture.

Excessive Loss of Residual Bone

The pontic of a fixed partial denture must be correctly related to the residual ridge and in such a manner that the contact with the mucosa is minimal. Whenever excessive resorption has occurred, teeth supported by a denture base may be arranged in a more acceptable buccolingual position than is possible with a fixed partial denture (Figure 12-24).

Unlike a fixed partial denture, the artificial teeth supported by a denture base can be located without regard to the crest of the residual ridge and more nearly in the position of the natural dentition for normal tongue and cheek contacts. This is particularly true of a maxillary denture.

Anteriorly, loss of residual bone occurs from the labial aspect. Often the incisive papilla lies at the crest of the residual ridge. Because the central incisors are normally located anterior to this landmark, any other location of artificial central incisors is unnatural. An anterior fixed partial denture made for such a mouth will have pontics resting on the labial aspect of this resorbed ridge and will be too far lingual to provide desirable lip support. Often the only way the incisal edges of the pontics can be made to occlude with the opposing lower anterior teeth is to use a labial inclination that is excessive and unnatural, and both esthetics and lip support suffer. Because the same condition exists with a removable partial denture in which the anterior teeth are abutted on the residual ridge, a labial flange must be used to permit the teeth to be located closer to their natural position.

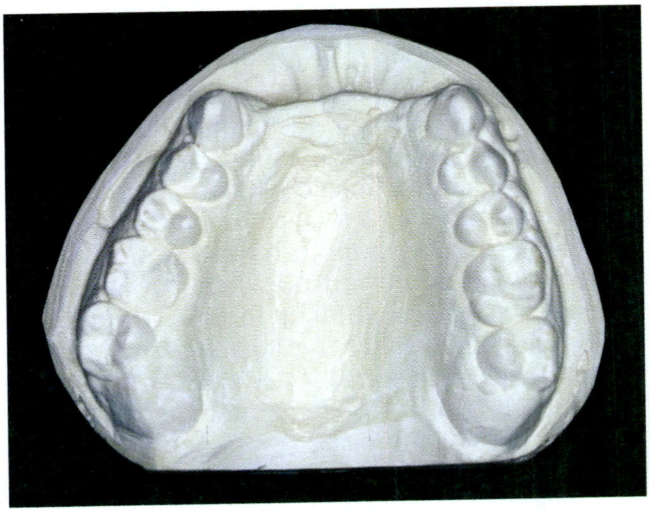

A

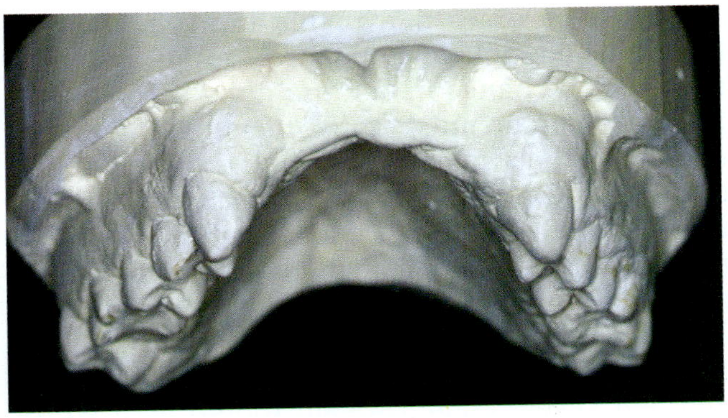

B

Figure 12-24 **A,** Occlusal view of anterior ridge defect (Kennedy Class IV) showing palatal position of the ridge crest. Incisal edge position of opposing dentition requires a more labial position of the prosthetic teeth, which would create difficult pontic form if a fixed partial denture were provided. **B,** View of the same cast from the labial showing significance of the vertical bone loss. Replacement of teeth and ridge anatomy is best accomplished by a removable partial denture.

The same method of treatment applies to the replacement of missing mandibular anterior teeth. Sometimes a mandibular anterior fixed partial denture is made six or more units in length, in which the remaining space necessitates either leaving out one anterior tooth or using the original number of teeth but with all of them too narrow for esthetics. In either instance the denture is nearly in a straight line because the pontics follow the form of the resorbed ridge. A removable partial denture will permit the location of the replaced teeth in a favorable relation to the lip and opposing dentition regardless of the shape of the residual ridge. When such a removable prosthesis is made, however, positive support must be obtained from the adjacent abutments.

Unusually Sound Abutment Teeth

Sometimes the reasoning for making a removable restoration is the desire to see sound teeth preserved in their natural state and not prepared for restorations. As mentioned previously, if this decision is made because it is felt that no tooth modification is necessary for removable partial dentures, then the prosthesis will lack tooth-derived stability and support.

When this condition exists, the dentist should not hesitate to reshape and modify existing enamel surfaces to provide proximal guiding planes, occlusal rest areas, optimum retentive areas, and surfaces on which nonretentive stabilizing components may be placed. The continued durability of the natural teeth is best ensured if the modifications that are provided optimize prosthesis function. This is because such modifications also ensure the most harmonious use of the natural dentition.

Abutments With Guarded Prognoses

If the prognosis of an abutment tooth is questionable, or if it becomes unfavorable during treatment, it might be possible to compensate for its impending loss by a change in denture design. The questionable or condemned tooth or teeth may then be included in the original design, and if subsequently lost, the removable partial denture can be modified or remade (Figure 12-25). Most removable partial denture designs do not lend themselves well to later additions, although this eventuality should be considered in the design of the denture.

When the tooth in question will be used as an abutment, every diagnostic aid should be used to determine its prognosis as a prospective abutment. It is usually not as difficult to add a tooth or teeth to a removable partial denture as it is to add a retaining unit when the original abutment is lost and the next adjacent tooth must be used for that purpose.

It is sometimes possible to design a removable partial denture so that a single posterior abutment, about which there is some doubt, can be retained and used at one end of the tooth-supported base. Then if the posterior abutment is lost, it could be replaced by adding an extension base to the existing denture framework. Such an original design must include provisions for future indirect retention, flexible clasping of the future abutment, and provision for establishing tissue support. Anterior abutments that are considered poor risks may not be so freely used because of the problems involved in adding a new abutment retainer when the original one is lost. It is rational that such questionable teeth be condemned in favor of more suitable abutments, even though the original treatment plan must be modified accordingly.

Economic Considerations

Economics should not be the sole criterion in arriving at a method of treatment. When for economic reasons, complete treatment is out of the question and yet replacement of missing teeth is indicated, the restorative procedures dictated by these considerations must be described clearly to the patient as a compromise and not representative of the best that modern dentistry has to offer. A prosthesis that is made to satisfy economic considerations alone may provide only limited success and result in more costly treatment in the future.

CHOICE BETWEEN COMPLETE DENTURES AND REMOVABLE PARTIAL DENTURES

One of the more difficult decisions to make for the partially edentulous patient involves making the choice of a complete denture over a removable partial denture. Many factors need to be considered when making such a decision and these generally fall under the categories of tooth-related factors, factors of comparative functional expectations between prostheses, and patient-specific factors. Because the difference between a tooth-tissue-borne prosthesis and a tissue-borne prosthesis can be important, especially since it is difficult for the partially edentulous patient to conceptualize the tissue-borne situation, such an irreversible decision is not trivial.

An evaluation of the remaining teeth will determine whether any caries or periodontal disease exists. The decision as to whether a tooth is useful for inclusion in a prosthetic treatment plan can be made based on an understanding that with appropriate disease management the tooth provides a reasonable 5-year prognosis for survival. This takes into account the added functional demand by the prosthesis and a risk assessment for recurrent disease. Since this scenario concerns teeth with disease, the expectation is that tooth structure and/or support

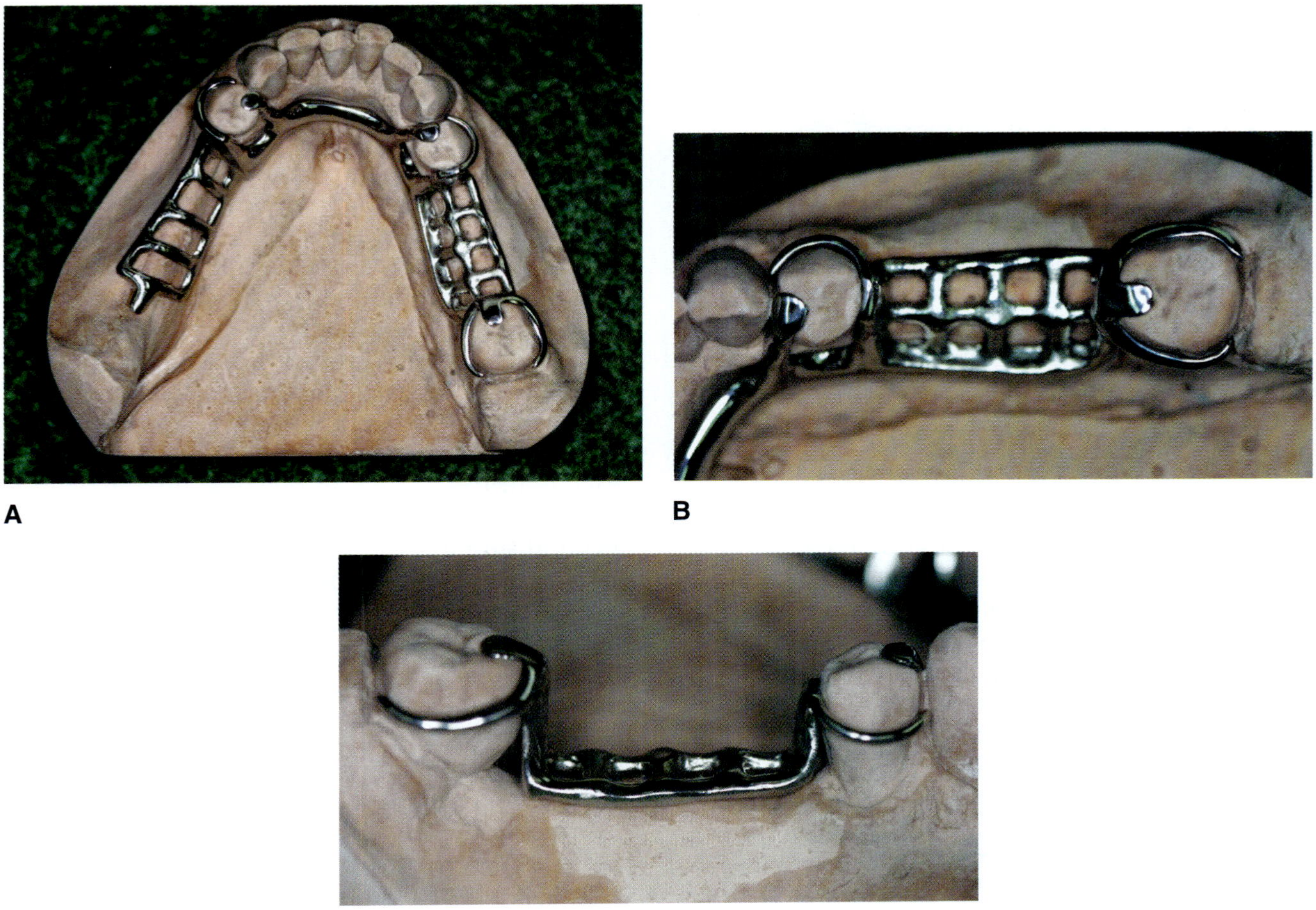

A B C

Figure 12-25 Kennedy Class II, mod 1 in which molar abutment has a guarded prognosis. **A,** Anterior abutment of modification space has a clasp assembly that accommodates for potential future loss of distal molar while currently providing adequate support, stability, and retention. **B,** Premolar clasp assembly is a mesial rest, distal guide plane, and wrought wire retainer design that will accommodate future distal extension movement. **C,** Buccal view showing guide plane contact and wrought wire location that is appropriate for a distal extension.

are compromised. The added functional burden along with a potentially increased risk for disease are important concerns when determining the long-term benefit for retaining teeth with a removable partial denture.

If the teeth can be maintained with a reasonable prognosis, the next questions to ask are "Do they require restoration with surveyed crowns?" and "How much improvement to the prosthesis support, stability, and retention do they provide?" If the expected prognosis for a given tooth is questionable, the costs associated with restoration high, and the added benefit to the prosthesis low, the tooth should likely not be maintained unless the patient strongly desires to maintain all teeth. However, if the same scenario exists and the long-term impact on the support, stability, and retention of the prosthesis is great, the decision strongly favors keeping the tooth.

The question of whether retained teeth offer a significant advantage to the prosthesis from a support, stability, and retention standpoint requires comparative evaluation of the potential denture-bearing foundations. If the expectation is that an edentulous arch would have unfavorable physical features (poor ridge form, poor arch configuration, displaceable mucosa, high frena attachments, minimal denture-bearing area, and/or an unfavorable jaw relationship) then retention of teeth is likely to provide a more significant benefit. If the retention of teeth can help prevent or delay age-related denture-bearing foundation changes seen with complete denture use, then retention of teeth can be of significant benefit.

When evaluation demonstrates that the remaining teeth have no active disease, then the often negative impact of disease management on the prognosis is not a concern. The decision to maintain teeth is again based on risk assessment, the costs for use of the teeth, the added benefit to the prosthesis functional stability, and the comparative functional expectations between a mucosal-borne denture and a removable partial denture, which uses teeth for some support, stability, and retention.

The remaining tooth location and distribution can also impact the decision to maintain teeth. It makes a difference if the remaining teeth are located only on one side of the arch. Having bilateral teeth remaining, especially if they are in similar locations (canines-canines, canines/premolars-canines/premolars), offers advantages to prosthesis design and occlusal development compared with asymmetrical tooth locations. Some teeth may not serve well as a stabilizing component to a removable partial denture and should not be maintained. If the remaining terminal tooth adjacent to a distal extension base is an incisor, the likelihood for long-term support, stability, and retention is poor.

An additional factor to consider when deciding between a complete denture and a removable partial denture is whether there is strong patient desire to maintain teeth. As mentioned previously, because the change to a complete denture is a significant transformation, there must be sufficient discussion before making this decision. The dentist must be very clear that the patient understands the functional difference between a mucosal-borne prosthesis for all aspects of function (i.e., chewing, talking, etc.) compared with the natural dentition or a removable partial denture.

The uniqueness of the patient is again appreciated when discussing these issues with various patients. One patient may prefer complete dentures rather than complete oral rehabilitation, regardless of ability to pay. Another may be so determined to keep their own teeth that they will make great financial sacrifices if given a reasonable assurance of success of oral rehabilitation. The value of listening to the patient during the examination and the diagnostic procedures pays off significantly when the treatment options differ so vastly as the complete and removable partial denture often do. During the presentation of pertinent facts, time should be allowed for patients to express themselves freely as to their desires in retaining and restoring their natural teeth. At this time a treatment plan may be influenced or even drastically changed to conform to the expressed and implied wishes of the patient. For example, there may be a reasonable possibility of saving teeth in both arches through the use of removable partial dentures. With only anterior teeth remaining, a removable partial denture can be made to replace the posterior teeth by use of good abutment support and, in the maxillary arch, use of full palatal coverage for retention and stability. If patients express a desire to retain their anterior teeth at any cost and if the remaining teeth are esthetically acceptable and functionally sound, the dentist should make every effort to provide successful treatment. If patients prefer a mandibular removable partial denture because of fear of difficulty in wearing a mandibular complete denture, then, all factors being acceptable, their wishes should be respected and treatment should be planned accordingly. The professional obligation to present the facts and then do the best in accordance with the patients' expressed desires still applies.

Other patients may wish to retain remaining teeth for an indefinite but relatively short period of time, with eventual complete dentures a foregone conclusion. In this instance the professional obligation may be to recommend interim removable partial dentures without extensive mouth preparations. Such dentures will aid in mastication and will provide esthetic replacements, at the same time serving as conditioning restorations, which will make the later transition to complete dentures somewhat easier. Such removable partial dentures should be designed and fabricated with care, but the total cost of removable partial denture service should be considerably less.

An expressed desire on the part of patients to retain only six mandibular anterior teeth must be considered carefully before being agreed to as the planned treatment. The advantages to the patients are obvious: they may retain six esthetically acceptable teeth, they do not become totally edentulous, and they have the advantage of direct retention for the removable partial denture that would not be possible if they were completely edentulous. Retaining even the mandibular canine teeth would accomplish the latter two objectives. The potential disadvantages relate directly to the patient keeping up with prosthesis maintenance procedures. The disadvantages relate to the poor response of the anterior maxilla to functional stress concentrated from the opposing natural dentition. If the functional forces of occlusion are not well distributed, the natural anterior can concentrate stress to the anterior maxillary arch. The possible result of such poorly distributed functional force is the loss of residual maxillary bone, loosening of the maxillary denture because of the tripping influence of the natural mandibular teeth, and the loss of basal foundation for the support of future prostheses. However, if the maxillary anterior teeth are arranged to contact in balanced eccentric positions and patients comply with periodic recall to maintain these relationships, these problems are minimized. The prevention of this sequence of events lies in the maintenance of positive occlusal support posteriorly and the continual elimination of traumatic influence from the remaining anterior teeth. Such support is sometimes impossible to maintain without frequent relining or remaking of the lower removable partial denture base. The presence of inflamed hyperplastic tissue is a frequent sequela to continued loss of support and denture movement.

Although some patients are able to successfully function with a lower removable partial denture supported only by anterior teeth against a complete maxillary denture, it is likely that undesirable consequences will result unless the patient faithfully follows the instructions of the dentist. In no other situation in treatment planning are the general health of the patient and the quality of residual alveolar bone as critical as they are in this situation.

CLINICAL FACTORS RELATED TO METAL ALLOYS USED FOR REMOVABLE PARTIAL DENTURE FRAMEWORKS

The cast framework offers significant advantages over the all acrylic-resin removable partial denture. In general, the ability to predictably use the remaining teeth for support, stability, and retention over time is best ensured with the interface between prosthesis and teeth consisting of a cast structure and not a polymer. Although the utility of all acrylic-resin prostheses can be extended if wire "rests" are provided, typical polymer properties do not allow for a durable interface, which is required to take advantage of the stabilizing effect of tooth contact. The expectations of how the metal framework improves functional performance are related to the properties of the metal alloy. Various alloys can be considered for use, and the following is a discussion of the most common framework alloys in use today.

Practically all cast frameworks for removable partial dentures are made from a chromium-cobalt alloy. The choice of the alloy from which the framework of a removable partial denture will be constructed is logically made during the treatment-planning phase. Inherent differences in the physical properties of alloys presently available to the dental profession must be considered when making this choice. For example, mouth preparation procedures, especially the recontouring of abutment teeth for the optimum placement of retentive elements, depend to a large extent on the modulus of elasticity (stiffness) of a particular alloy.

Chromium-Cobalt Alloys

The popularity of the chromium-cobalt alloys has been attributed to their low density (weight), high modulus of elasticity (stiffness), low material cost, and resistance to tarnish. Each of the alloys has advantages under certain conditions. The material considered capable of rendering the best overall service to the patient over a period of years is the one that should be used (Table 12-1). The choice of alloy is based on several factors: (1) weighed advantages or disadvantages of the physical properties of the alloy; (2) the dimensional accuracy with which the alloy can be cast and finished; (3) the availability of the alloy; (4) the versatility of the alloy; and (5) the individual clinical observation and experiences with alloys in respect to quality control and service to the patient.

The following are comparable characteristics of gold alloys and chromium-cobalt alloys: (1) each is well tolerated by oral tissues; (2) they are equally acceptable esthetically; (3) enamel abrasion by either alloy is insignificant on vertical tooth surfaces; (4) a low-fusing, chrome-cobalt alloy or gold alloy can be cast to wrought wire, and wrought-wire components may be soldered to either gold or chrome-cobalt alloys (these characteristics are important in overcoming the objection by some dentists to the increased stiffness of chromium-cobalt alloys for the portions of direct retainers that must engage an undercut of the abutment tooth); (5) the accuracy obtainable in casting either alloy is clinically acceptable under strictly controlled investing and casting procedures; and (6) soldering procedures for the repair of frameworks can be performed on each alloy.

Comparative Physical Properties

Chromium-cobalt alloys generally have lower yield strength than the gold alloys used for removable partial dentures (Table 12-2). Yield strength is the greatest amount of stress an alloy will withstand and still return to its original shape in an unweakened condition. Possessing a lower proportional limit, the chromium-cobalt alloys will deform permanently at lower loads than gold alloys. Therefore the dentist must design the chromium-cobalt framework so

TABLE 12-1. Comparative Physical Properties of Alloys

	Density	Modulus of Elasticity	Yield Strength	Tarnish Resistance	Cost	Hardness
Chromium-Cobalt	Low	High	Low	Good	Low	High
Gold	High	Low	High	Good	High	Mod
Titanium	Low	Low	Low	Good	Mod-high	High

TABLE 12-2. Mechanical Properties of Representative Stellite Alloys

	Stellite Alloys*					Hardened Partial Denture
Properties	**A**	**B**	**D**	**E**	**21**	**Gold Alloys**
Yield strength (psi)	64,500	61,000	56,000	62,400	82,300	65,000–90,000
Tensile strength (psi)	180,500	107,500	84,500	102,500	101,300	107,000–120,000
Elongation (%)	3.4	3.2	6.0	1.9	8.2	1.5–8.0
Modulus of elasticity (psi × 10^6)	28.0	29.5	27.5	28.5	36.0	13–15
Hardness (R[30N])†	53.0	60.0	51.0	55.0	—	—

From Peyton FA: Dent Clin North Am 759–771, 1958.

*Data for lettered alloys from Taylor DF, Liebfritz WA, Adler AG: J Am Dent Assoc 56:343–351, 1958; for Stellite No. 21 from Metals Handbook, 1948 ed, p. 579, for gold alloys from manufacturers' property charts.

†Rockwell 30N hardness scale.

that the degree of deformation expected in a direct retainer is less than a comparable degree of deformation for a gold component. The modulus of elasticity refers to stiffness of an alloy. Gold alloys have a modulus of elasticity approximately one half of that for chromium-cobalt alloys for similar uses. The greater stiffness of chromium-cobalt alloy is advantageous but at the same time offers disadvantages. Greater rigidity can be obtained with the chromium-cobalt alloy in reduced sections in which cross-arch stabilization is required, thereby eliminating an appreciable bulk of the framework. Its greater rigidity is also an advantage when the greatest undercut that can be found on an abutment tooth is in the nature of 0.05 inch. A gold retentive element would not be as efficient in retaining the restoration under such conditions as would the chromium-cobalt clasp arm.

A high yield strength and a low modulus of elasticity produce higher flexibility. The gold alloys are approximately twice as flexible as the chromium-cobalt alloys, which is a distinct advantage in the optimum location of retentive elements of the framework in many instances. The greater flexibility of the gold alloys usually permits location of the tips of retainer arms in the gingival third of the abutment tooth. The stiffness of the chromium-cobalt alloys can be overcome by including wrought-wire retentive elements in the framework.

The bulk of a retentive clasp arm for a removable partial denture is often reduced for greater flexibility when chromium-cobalt alloys are used as opposed to gold alloys. This, however, is inadvisable because the grain size of the chromium-cobalt alloys is usually larger and is associated with a lower proportional limit, and so a decrease in the bulk of chromium-cobalt cast clasps increases the likelihood of fracture or permanent deformation. The retentive clasp arms for both alloys should be approximately the same size, but the depth of undercut used for retention must be reduced by one half when chromium-cobalt is the choice of alloys. Chromium-cobalt alloys are reported to work-harden more rapidly than gold alloys, and this, associated with coarse grain size, may lead to failure in service. When adjustments by bending are necessary, they must be executed with extreme caution and limited optimism.

Chromium-cobalt alloys have a lower density *(weight)* than gold alloys in comparable sections and are therefore about one half as heavy as the gold alloys. Weight of the alloy in most instances is not a valid criterion for selection of one metal over another, because after placement of a removable partial denture the patient seldom notices the weight of the restoration. The comparable lightness of the chromium-cobalt alloys, however, is an advantage when full palatal coverage is indicated for the bilateral distal extension removable partial denture. Weight is a factor that must be considered when the force of gravity must be overcome so that usually passive direct retainers will not be activated constantly to the detriment of abutment teeth.

The hardness of chromium-cobalt alloys presents a disadvantage when a component of the framework, such as a rest, is opposed by a natural tooth or by one that has been restored. We have observed more wear of natural teeth opposed by some of the various chromium-cobalt alloys as contrasted to the Type IV gold alloys.

It has been observed that gold frameworks for removable partial dentures are more prone to produce

TABLE 12-3. Comparative Specifications Contained in ADA Specification No. 7

	Type I	Type II
Content of metals of the gold, platinum group (minimum)	75%	65%
Minimum fusion temperature	1742° F	1898° F
Minimum yield point value (hardened or oven cooled)	125,000 psi	95,000 psi
Minimum elongation (hardened)	4%	2%
Minimum elongation (softened)	15%	15%

uncomfortable galvanic shocks to abutment teeth restored with silver amalgam than frameworks made of chromium-cobalt alloy. This may not be a valid criterion for the selection of a particular alloy when the dentist has complete control over the choice of restorative materials.

Commercially pure (CP) titanium and titanium in alloys containing aluminum and vanadium, or palladium (Ti-O Pd), should be considered potential future materials for removable partial denture frameworks. Their versatility and well-known biocompatibility are promising; however, long-term clinical trials are needed to validate their potential usefulness. Currently, when CP titanium is cast under dental conditions, the material properties change dramatically. During the casting procedure, the high affinity of the liquid metal for elements such as oxygen, nitrogen, and hydrogen results in their incorporation from the atmosphere. As interstitial alloying elements, their deleterious effect on mechanical properties is a problem. Also, reactions between molten titanium metal and the investment refractory produce gases, which cause porosity. In alpha-beta alloys, such as Ti-6Al-4V, a surface skin of alpha titanium can form (alpha-case zone), which has a tremendous effect on the electrochemical behavior and mechanical properties. This could be important for small thin structures, such as clasp assemblies and major and minor connectors. Table 12-3 shows selected mechanical properties of commercially pure titanium and Ti-6Al-4V alloys. The CP grades of titanium have yield strengths that are too low for clinical use as clasps (450 MPa minimum), although the ductility is high. The much higher yield strengths of the Ti-6Al-4V alloys are the same as that of a typical bench-cooled, chromium-cobalt alloy but with far superior ductility. The typical Young's modulus of elasticity of titanium alloy is half that of chromium-cobalt and just slightly higher than type IV gold alloys. This would require a different approach to clasp design than with chromium-cobalt alloys and present some advantages. Wrought titanium alloy wires are also flexible because of the same low elastic modulus. Beta alloys, which are used in orthodontics, have two thirds the elastic modulus of CP titanium and Ti-6Al-4V. The joining of titanium by brazing is a problem because, like casting, inert atmospheres must be used. The corrosion and fatigue behavior of brazed joints has yet to be tested for long-term corrosion resistance and clinical efficacy. Clinical use has demonstrated reasonable short-term results, but laboratory fabrication difficulties need to be addressed, and long-term advantages over existing alloys need to be demonstrated before titanium will gain broad clinical use.

Wrought Wire: Selection and Quality Control

Wrought-wire direct retainer arms may be attached to the restoration by embedding a portion of the wire in a resin denture base, by soldering to the fabricated framework, or by casting the framework to a wire embedded in the wax pattern (Figure 12-26). The

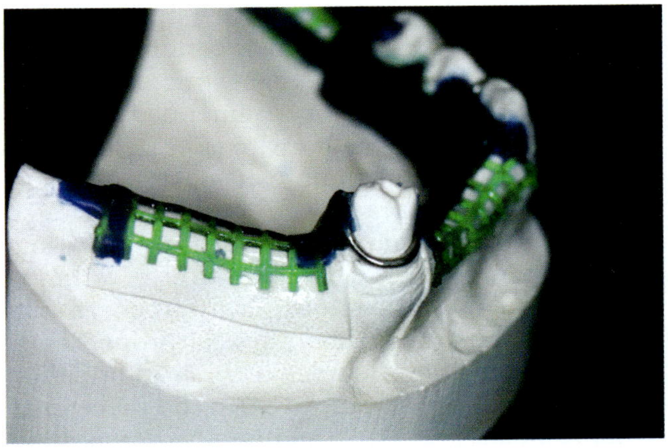

Figure 12-26 Wrought-wire retainer arm has been contoured to follow the design and is incorporated into the wax pattern of this frame where it will become an integral part of framework. Wire is contoured in two planes and will be mechanically retained in casting.

NEY WIRE PROPERTIES

ALLOY	Condition	Ultimate Tensile Strength Lbs/in.²	Ultimate Tensile Strength Kg/cm²	Proportional Limit Lbs/in.²	Proportional Limit Kg/cm²	Elongation Percent 2 in. or 5.1 cm	Hardness BHN	Hardness HV	Fusion Temp. °F	Fusion Temp. °C	Density dwt./in.³	Density gm/cm³	Nobility Gold & Platinum Group Metals
ELASTIC #4*	S	117,500	8,260	86,500	6,080	15	190	215					
	H	173,000	12,160	131,000	9,170	7	270	305	1925	1050	164	15.6	79.5%
ELASTIC #12	S	125,000	8,790	88,000	6,190	20	175	200					
	H	178,000	12,510	135,000	9,490	15	275	310	2010	1150	127	12.1	61.0%
PALINEY #7**	S	120,000	8,440	89,000	6,260	24	180	205					
	H	180,000	12,650	148,000	10,400	9	280	315	1985	1085	125	11.9	55.0%
PALINEY #6**	S	110,000	7,730	63,500	4,460	24	150	170					
	H	170,000	11,950	127,000	8,930	15	270	305	1970	1075	115	10.9	45.0%
NEYLASTIC H.F.**	S	110,000	7,730	75,000	5,270	20	215	245					
	H	145,000	10,190	85,000	5,980	6	260	295	1830	1000	183	17.4	76.0%
GOLD COLOR ELASTIC*	S	120,000	8,440	73,000	5,130	14	200	225					
	H	165,000	11,600	135,000	9,490	1	290	330	1675	915	160	15.2	73.0%
DENTURE CLASP (GOLD COLOR)	S	100,000	7,030	52,000	3,660	22	160	180					
	H	157,000	11,040	122,000	8,580	1	265	300	1650	900	145	13.8	61.5%
PGP***		125,000	8,790	80,000	5,620	15	200	225	2790	1535	185	17.6	100%
P & I***		120,000	8,440	115,000	8,080	2	180	200	3250	1790	226	21.5	100%

* This product appears on The American Dental Association List of Certified Dental Material.
** This wire recommended for Crozat Technic.
*** This wire recommended for cast-to applications.

A

Figure 12-27 Physical properties and nobility (gold and platinum group metal content of various wires) are furnished in manufacturers' charts **A** and **B**. Such information is necessary to select wrought wire for particular purpose and attachment method. *(**A** Courtesy JM Ney Company, Bloomfield, Conn.; **B** Courtesy JF Jelenko & Company, New Rochelle, NY.)*

Continued

physical (mechanical) properties of available wrought wires are most important considerations in selecting a proper wire for the desired method of attachment. These properties are yield strength or proportional limit, percentage elongation, tensile strength, and fusion temperature. After selection of the wire, the procedures to which the wire is subjected in fabricating the restoration become critical. Improper laboratory procedures can diminish certain desirable physical properties of the wrought structure, rendering it relatively useless for its intended purpose. For example, when wrought wire is heated, as in a cast-to or soldering procedure, its physical properties and microstructure may be considerably altered depending on the temperature, heating time, and cooling operation. Each manufacturer of wrought forms for dental applications furnishes charts listing their products and the physical properties of each product. Two examples of such information are demonstrated in Figure 12-27. The percentage of noble metals is given. In addition, most manufacturers designate wires that may be used in a cast-to procedure. American Dental Association (ADA) specification No. 7 addresses itself to wrought gold wire both as to content and minimum physical properties (Table 12-4).

Craig* has suggested that the tensile strength of the wrought structure is approximately 25% greater than that of the cast alloy from which it was made. The wrought structure's hardness and strength are also greater. This means that a wrought structure having a smaller cross-section than a cast structure may be used as a retainer arm (retentive) to perform the same function. Craig has also suggested that a minimum yield strength of 60,000 psi is required for the retentive element of a direct retainer. A percentage elongation of less than 6% is indicative that a wrought wire may not be amenable to contouring without attendant undesirable changes in microstructure.

Regardless of the method of attaching the wrought wire retainer, either by embedding, soldering, or cast-to, tapering the wrought arm seems most rational. A retainer arm is in essence a cantilever and can be made more serviceable and efficient by tapering. Tapering to 0.8 mm permits more uniform distribution of service stresses throughout the length of the arm, being readily demonstrated by photoelastic stress analysis. Uniform tapering of an 18-gauge,

*From Craig RG: Restorative dental materials, ed 11, St. Louis, 2002, Mosby.

JELENKO GOLD WIRES		Solders Recommended	Hardness: Brinell D.P.H.	U. T. S. lbs./sq. in. (kg./cm.²)	% Elong. in 2 in. (5 cm.)	Yield Strength lbs./sq. in. (kg./cm.²)	No. of Cold Bends	Fusion Temperature (Approx.)
EXTRA HIGH FUSING **(All Gold Alloys Can Be Cast To It, Including Jelenko "O")**	**† NO. 12 WIRE** (Plat. Color)	Jelenko "O" Ortho Solder Can Be Used With All Others	Q 183 Q 200 H 204 H 225	88,500 (6,220) 103,000 (7,240)	11 9	66,500 (4,675) 70,000 (4,920)	6 5	2225°F. 1218°C.
HIGH FUSING **(Can be Cast Against)** **For** **Clasps, Bars, Pins** **Including Jelenko "O"**	**SUPER WIRE*** (Plat. Color)	Orthoflex H.F.	Q 200 Q 220 H 255 H 280	132,000 (9,280) 175,000 (12,303)	20 12	89,000 (6,260) 127,000 (8,930)	6.5 3.5	1845°F. 1007°C.
	THRIFT WIRE (Plat. Color)	Alboro H.F.	Q 200 Q 220 H 250 H 275	126,000 (8,860) 170,000 (11,950)	20 4	78,000 (5,485) 118,000 (8,295)	6.0 3.5	1890°F. 1032°C.
MEDIUM HIGH FUSING **(Can Be Cast Against) For Clasps, Bars and Wrought Structures**	**STANDARD WIRE** (Gold Color)	708 650 615	Q 165 Q 180 H 260 H 285	110,400 (7,760) 165,000 (11,600)	22 8	54,000 (3,795) 112,000 (7,875)	6.0 3.5	1735°F. 946°C.
MEDIUM FUSING **(Not to be Cast Against)** **For Clasps, Bars and Dowels**	**NO. 25 WIRE** (Gold Color)	650 615 585	Q 145 Q 160 H 230 H 250	93,200 (6,550) 147,000 (10,330)	26 9	53,000 (3,725) 112,000 (7,875)	6.0 3.5	1615°F. 879°C.
	NO. 2 WIRE (Gold Color)	650 615 585	Q 140 Q 155 H 250 H 275	95,000 (6,680) 155,000 (10,900)	27 5	48,000 (3,375) 110,000 (7,735)	5.0 1.5	1620°F. 882°C.
For PARALLEL PIN WORK	**PONTO WIRE** (Plat. Color)		230 250	136,000 (9,560)	20	105,000 (7,380)	5.5	2732°F. 1500°C.

† Hardens in a manner similar to Jelenko "O" Cast Gold. (After casting, slow cool from approximately 1800°F. (982°C.) in flask.)

NOTE: Ponto wire is knurled. "Q" is quenched or softened and H is hardened.

Heat treatment instructions included with each wire.

Jelenko Wires are immunized, Calor-Ohmically Heat Hardened, and furnished in straight 1 ft. (0.3m) lengths unless otherwise specified.

MADE IN THESE GAUGES

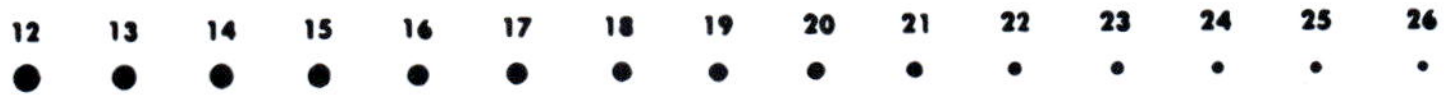

AVAILABLE IN THESE STYLES

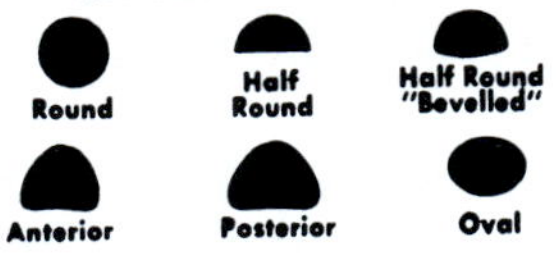

B

Figure 12-27 Cont'd

round-wire arm can be accomplished by rapidly rotating the wire in angled contact with an abrasive disk in dental lathe. It is then polished by rotating the wire in angled contact with a mildly abrasive rubber disk in dental lathe. The appropriate taper is shown in Figure 12-28.

SUMMARY

In making a selection of materials, it must be remembered that fundamentals do not change. These are inviolable. It is only methods, procedures, and substances—by which the dentist effects the best possible end result—that change. The responsibility of decision still rests with the dentist, who must evaluate all factors in relation to the desired results. In any instance, therefore, the dentist must weigh the problems involved, compare and evaluate the characteristics of different potential materials, and then make a decision that leads to the greatest possible service to the patient.

TABLE 12-4. Mechanical Properties of Titanium*

Properties	Commercially Pure Titanium				
	G1	G2	G3	G4	Ti-6A1-4V
Yield strength *MPa (minimum)*	170	280	380	480	825
Tensile strength	240	340	450	550	895
Elongation (%)	24	20	18	15	10
Elasticity *MPa (minimum)*	103	103	107	107	110
Hardness	120 HB	200 HB	225 HB	245 HB	37 HRC

*Annealed bar.
HB, Brinell hardness; *HRC*, Rockwell C.
NOTE: Little difference except for hardness.

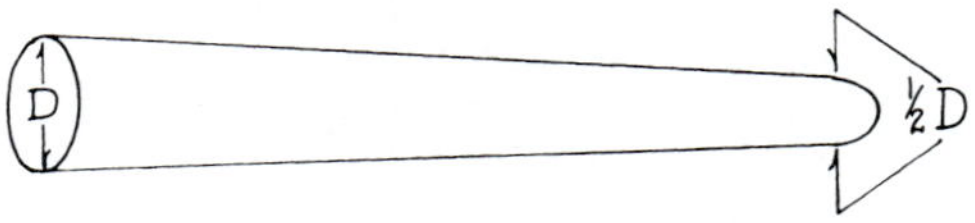

Figure 12-28 Round, 18-gauge wrought wire for retentive component of direct retainer assembly (clasp) is uniformly tapered to 0.8 mm from its full diameter to its terminus. Tapering should precede contouring wire for retainer arm.

SELF-ASSESSMENT AIDS

1. State the purpose of dental treatment.
2. Meaningful treatment of a patient embodies four fundamentally different processes. Please name these processes in chronological order of accomplishment.
3. What are the objectives of prosthodontic treatment for a partially edentulous patient?
4. In what ways would ascertaining the past dental experiences of a patient that one is treating for the first time contribute to patient management?
5. Why should one review the present health status of the patient before conducting an oral examination?
6. Diagnostic casts should be made before definitive treatment is undertaken. What two specific purposes would they serve?
7. It is not unusual for a patient to be primarily concerned with the cosmetic implications of a missing tooth. What are the obligations of the dentist to broaden the concern of total treatment?
8. A logical sequence of a thorough oral examination includes at least eight different procedures accomplished in order. Two of the eight procedures are a thorough prophylaxis and the placement of individual temporary restorations. What are the other six factors?
9. For what reason should the definitive location of the inferior border of a mandibular major connector be ascertained as a part of an oral examination?
10. Rationalize the importance of the following areas that must be ascertained by radiographic interpretation:
    a. Quality of alveolar support of prospective abutment teeth
    b. Interpretation of relative bone density
    c. Increased width of the periodontal space
    d. Index areas
    e. Lamina dura
    f. Root morphology
    g. Unerupted third molars
11. What is a diagnostic cast?
12. Describe the characteristic of a diagnostic cast of a partially edentulous arch that may be considered a quality cast.
13. Diagnostic casts serve several purposes as aids in diagnosis and treatment planning. What are six different uses for them?
14. Two sets of diagnostic casts (one a duplicate set) should be made for a patient requiring treatment. Why?
15. What can be gained from a study of accurately mounted diagnostic casts on a programmed, semiadjustable articulator?
16. The base of a diagnostic cast should be prepared in a certain way before any mounting on the articulator. Describe the preparation and state its importance.
17. What is a record base? An occlusion rim?

18. Are record bases usually necessary to correctly orient diagnostic casts of partially edentulous arches to an articulator? Why?
19. What four maxillomandibular records are necessary to orient casts to an arcon type of articulator and to program the articulator?
20. What is meant by proving the articulator, and how is it accomplished?
21. Name and describe the use of at least six different materials used for recording maxillomandibular relations.
22. In relation to occlusion, one of the earliest decisions to be made in diagnosis is whether to accept or reject the existing occlusion as demonstrated by the correctly oriented and articulated diagnostic casts. True or false?
23. Improvements in the natural occlusion must be accomplished before fabrication of the denture, not subsequent to it. True or false?
24. The decision-making process in planning the restoration of a partially edentulous mouth must include a differential diagnosis of fixed or removable restorations or a combination of both as a means of restoration. Usually, where indicated, a fixed restoration is preferable to a removable restoration. True or false?
25. What are the indications for the use of fixed restorations in (1) tooth-bounded edentulous regions; (2) posterior modification spaces; and (3) anterior modification spaces?
26. Although a removable partial denture should be considered as the means of treatment only when a fixed partial denture is contraindicated, there are several specific indications for the use of a removable restoration. Briefly discuss these indications related to (1) distal extension situations; (2) postextraction periods; (3) long tooth-bounded edentulous spans; (4) need for bilateral stabilization; (5) excessive loss of residual bone; (6) esthetics in the anterior region of the mouth; (7) abutments with guarded prognoses; and (8) economic considerations.
27. In many instances the dentist is confronted with the decision of treating the partially edentulous patient with removable partial dentures or complete dentures. Discuss the following factors that have a bearing on the decision-making process: (1) economics; (2) patient preference or desires of patient; (3) age; (4) health; (5) present periodontal status; and (6) dental IQ or prospective IQ.
28. As a result of oral examination and diagnosis, certain data should be recorded, many of which are based on decisions that are the result of diagnosis, patient attitude, and economics. Some of these data are present and predictable health status, periodontal conditions present, oral hygiene habits, caries activity, need for extractions or surgery, need for fixed restorations, and need for orthodontic treatment. There are at least five more areas of treatment that should be recorded at this time. What are they?
29. Most frameworks for removable partial dentures today are made of some type of chromium-cobalt alloy rather than with an extra hard gold alloy. Four reasons are usually projected for this wide variation. What are they?
30. The choice of an alloy(s) is based on what factors?
31. Compare the physical properties of yield strength (proportional limit) and percentage elongation of chromium-cobalt alloy and removable partial denture gold alloy.
32. Which alloy is the stiffest in comparable sections—gold, titanium, or chromium-cobalt? What are the advantages and disadvantages of comparable stiffness?
33. The retentive clasp arms for chromium-cobalt, titanium, and gold alloys should be dimensionally the same. Why or why not?
34. Many dentists prefer to use wrought-wire retentive arms in certain instances. Wrought wire may be attached to the denture by being cast-to, soldered, or embedded in the resin base. Does the method of attachment have a bearing on the selection of framework alloy and wrought wire? Why?
35. How would you go about selecting a wrought wire for a specific application of the wire?
36. There are inherent risks in the use of unilateral removable partial dentures. One is the risk of aspiration. What are some other risks?
37. Recent clinical research has contributed several significant developments to the management of compromised partially edentulous patients. Two of these developments are related to the field of implant prosthodontics. Name them.

13

PREPARATION OF MOUTH FOR REMOVABLE PARTIAL DENTURES

The preparation of the mouth is fundamental to a successful removable partial denture service. Mouth preparation, perhaps more than any other single factor, contributes to the philosophy that the prescribed prosthesis must not only replace what is missing but also preserve the remaining tissue and structures that will enhance the removable partial denture.

Mouth preparation follows the preliminary diagnosis and the development of a tentative treatment plan. Final treatment planning may be deferred until the response to the preparatory procedures can be ascertained. In general, mouth preparation includes procedures in four categories: oral surgical preparation, conditioning of abused and irritated tissue, periodontal preparation, and preparation of abutment teeth. The objectives of the procedures involved in all four areas are to return the mouth to optimum health and to eliminate any condition that would be detrimental to the success of the removable partial denture.

Naturally, mouth preparation must be accomplished before the impression procedures that will produce the master cast on which the removable partial denture will be fabricated. Oral surgical and periodontal procedures should precede abutment tooth preparation and should be completed far enough in advance to allow the necessary healing period. If at all possible, at least 6 weeks, but preferably 3 to 6 months, should be provided between surgical and restorative dentistry procedures. This depends on the extent of the surgery and its impact on the overall support, stability, and retention of the proposed prosthesis.

ORAL SURGICAL PREPARATION

As a rule, all preprosthetic surgical treatment for the removable partial denture patient should be completed as early as possible. When possible, necessary endodontic surgery, periodontal surgery, and oral surgery should be planned so that they can be completed during the same time frame. The longer the interval between the surgery and the impression procedure, the more complete the healing and consequently the more stable the denture-bearing areas.

A variety of oral surgical techniques can prove beneficial to the clinician in preparing the patient for prosthetic replacements. However, it is not the purpose of this section to present the details of surgical correction. Rather, attention is called to some of the more common oral conditions or changes in which surgical intervention is indicated as an aid to removable partial denture design and fabrication, and as an aid to the restoration's successful function. Additional information concerning the techniques used is available in oral surgery texts and journal publications. It is important to emphasize, however, that the dentist providing the removable partial denture treatment bears the responsibility for ensuring that the necessary surgical procedures are accomplished in accordance with the treatment plan. Measures to control apprehension, including the use of intravenous and inhalation agents, have made the most extensive surgery acceptable to patients. Whether the dentist chooses to perform these procedures or elects to refer the patient to someone more qualified is immaterial. The important consideration is that the patient not be deprived of any treatment that would enhance the success of the removable partial denture.

Extractions

Planned extractions should occur early in the treatment regimen but not before completion of a careful and thorough evaluation of each remaining tooth in the dental arch (Figure 13-1). Regardless of its condition, each tooth must be evaluated concerning its strategic importance and its potential contribution to the success of the removable partial denture. With the knowledge and technical capability available in dentistry today, almost any tooth may be salvaged if its retention is sufficiently important to warrant the procedures necessary. On the other hand, heroic attempts to salvage seriously involved teeth or those with doubtful prognoses, for which retention would contribute little if anything—even if successfully treated and maintained—are contraindicated. The extraction of nonstrategic teeth that would present complications or those that may be detrimental to the design of the removable partial denture is a necessary part of the overall treatment plan.

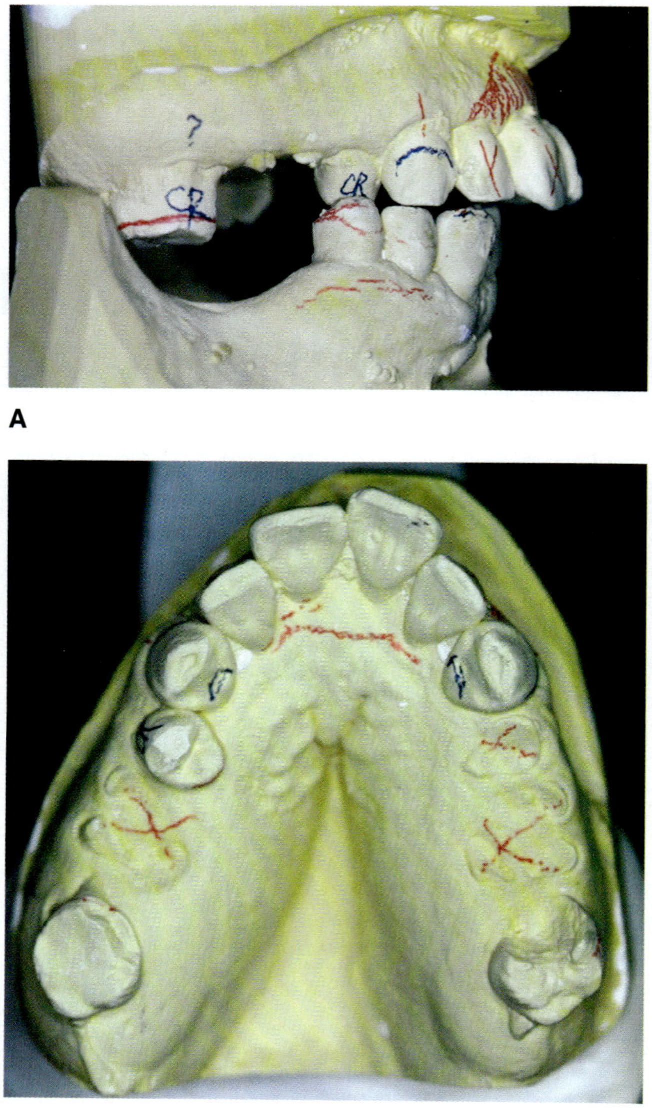

A

B

Figure 13-1 Diagnostic mounting allows confirmation of need for extraction after clinical examination. **A,** Anterior tooth position and chronic periodontal disease status require extraction to address patient's concern of malpositioned and painful teeth. **B,** Root tips require immediate extraction to allow ridge healing to begin. The status of molar (#15) requires additional workup determine pulpal involvement of carious lesion and extent of occlusal reduction required to optimize occlusal plane. The decision to maintain this tooth, though potentially costly, must consider the stabilizing effect it will have on the posterior left functional occlusion.

Removal of Residual Roots

Generally, all retained roots or root fragments should be removed. This is particularly true if they are in close proximity to the tissue surface or if there is evidence of associated pathological findings. Residual roots adjacent to abutment teeth may contribute to the progression of periodontal pockets and compromise the results from subsequent periodontal therapy. The removal of root tips can be accomplished from the facial or palatal surfaces without resulting in a reduction of alveolar ridge height or endangering adjacent teeth (Figure 13-2).

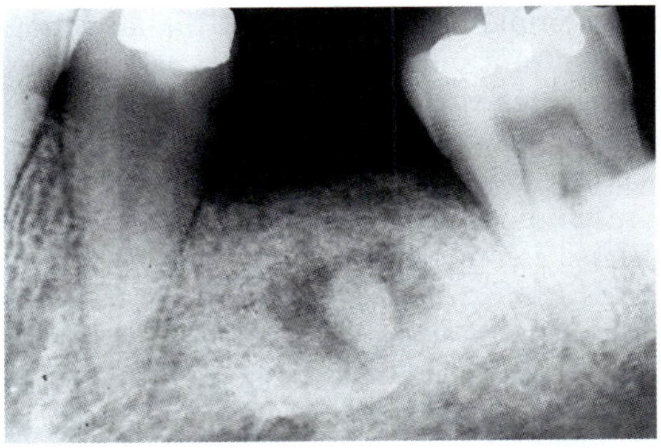

Figure 13-2 Retained root with associated bone resorption. *(From Costich ER, White RP Jr: Fundamentals of oral surgery, Philadelphia, 1971, Saunders.)*

Impacted Teeth

All impacted teeth, including those in edentulous areas and those adjacent to abutment teeth, should be considered for removal. The periodontal implications of impacted teeth adjacent to abutments are similar to those for retained roots. These teeth are often neglected until serious periodontal implications arise.

The skeletal structure of the body changes with age. Asymptomatic impacted teeth in the elderly that are covered with bone, with no evidence of a pathological condition, should be left to preserve the arch morphology. If an impacted tooth is left, it should be recorded in the patient's record and the patient should be informed of its presence. Roentgenograms should be taken at reasonable intervals to be sure that no adverse changes occur.

Alterations that affect the jaws can result in minute exposures of impacted teeth to the oral cavity via sinus tracts. Resultant infections can cause considerable bone destruction and serious illness for persons who are elderly and not physically able to tolerate the debilitation. Early elective removal of impactions prevents later serious acute and chronic infection with extensive bone loss. Any impacted teeth that can be reached with a periodontal probe must be removed to treat the periodontal pocket and prevent more extensive damage (Figure 13-3).

Malposed Teeth

The loss of individual teeth or groups of teeth may lead to extrusion, drifting, or combinations of malpositioning of the remaining teeth (Figure 13-4). In most instances the alveolar bone supporting extruded teeth will be carried occlusally as the teeth continue to erupt. Orthodontics may be useful in correcting many occlusal discrepancies, but for some patients, such treatment may not be practical because of a lack of teeth for anchoring orthodontic appliances or for other reasons. In such situations individual teeth or groups of teeth and their supporting alveolar bone can be surgically repositioned. This type of surgery can be accomplished in an outpatient setting and should be given serious consideration before condemning additional teeth or compromising the design of removable partial dentures.

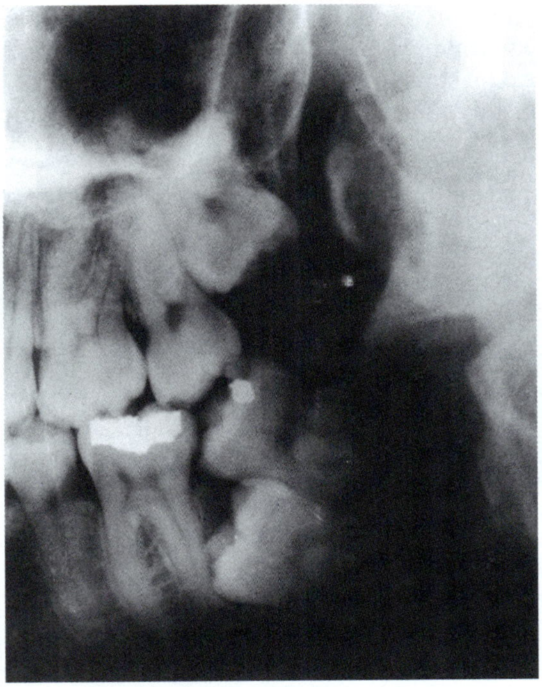

Figure 13-3 Lateral oblique roentgenogram showing unerupted maxillary third molar and impacted mandibular second and third molars. Maxillary third molar and mandibular second molar could be contacted by periodontal probe. *(From Costich ER, White RP Jr: Fundamentals of oral surgery, Philadelphia, 1971, Saunders.)*

Cysts and Odontogenic Tumors

Panoramic roentgenograms of the jaws are recommended to survey for unsuspected pathological conditions. When a suspicious area appears on the survey film, a periapical roentgenogram should be taken to confirm or deny the presence of a lesion. All radiolucencies or radiopacities observed in the jaws should be investigated. Although the diagnosis may appear obvious from clinical and roentgenographic examinations, the dentist should confirm that diagnosis through appropriate consultation and if necessary perform a biopsy of the area and submit the specimens to a pathologist for microscopic study. The patient should be informed of the diagnosis and provided with various options for resolution of the abnormality as confirmed by the pathologist's report.

Exostoses and Tori

The existence of abnormal bony enlargements should not be allowed to compromise the design of the removable partial denture (Figure 13-5). Although modification of denture design can at times accommodate for exostoses, more frequently this results in additional stress to the supporting elements and compromised function. The removal of exostoses and tori is not a complex procedure, and the advantages to be realized from such removal are great in contrast to the deleterious effects their continued presence can create. Ordinarily the mucosa covering bony protuberances is extremely thin and friable. Removable partial denture components in proximity to this type of tissue may cause irritation and chronic ulceration. Also, exostoses approximating gingival margins may complicate the maintenance of periodontal health and lead to the eventual loss of strategic abutment teeth.

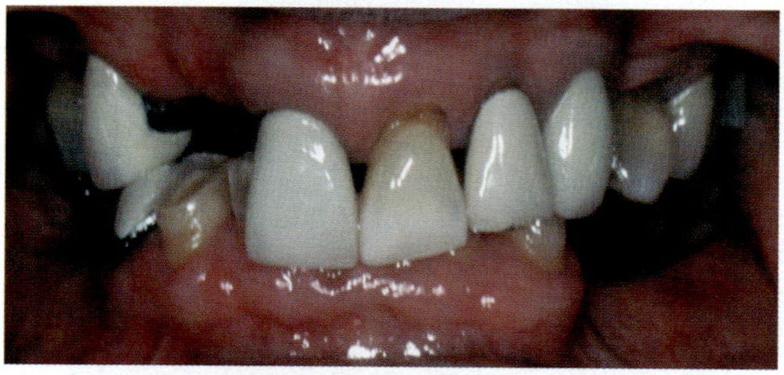

A

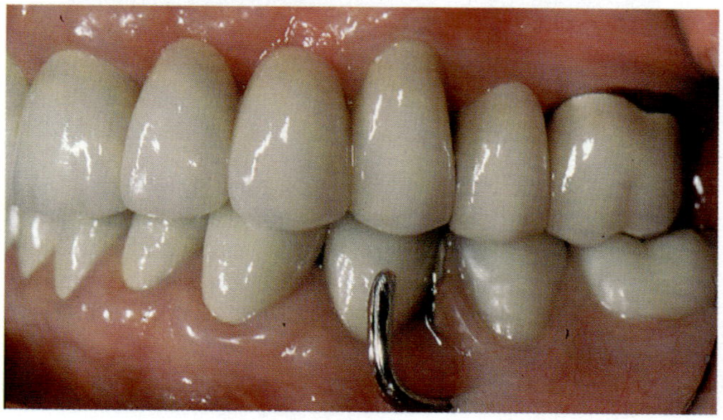

B

Figure 13-4 **A,** Malpositioned maxillary dentition due to loss of posterior occlusion and excessive wear of opposing mandibular anterior teeth. **B,** Restored dentition made possible by a combination of endodontics, periodontics, and fixed and removable partial prosthodontics. *(Courtesy Dr. M. Alfaro, Columbus, OH.)*

Hyperplastic Tissue

Hyperplastic tissue is seen in the form of fibrous tuberosities, soft flabby ridges, folds of redundant tissue in the vestibule or floor of the mouth, and palatal papillomatosis (Figure 13-6). All these forms of excess tissue should be removed to provide a firm base for the denture. This removal will produce a more stable denture, reduce stress and strain on the supporting teeth and tissue, and in many instances will provide a more favorable orientation of the occlusal plane and arch form for the arrangement of the artificial teeth. The appropriate surgical approaches should not reduce vestibular depth. Hyperplastic tissue can be removed with any preferred combination of scalpel, curette, electrosurgery, or laser. Some form of surgical stent should always be considered for these patients so that the period of healing is more comfortable. An old removable partial denture properly modified can serve as a surgical stent. Although hyperplastic tissue has no great malignant propensity, all such excised tissue should be sent to an oral pathologist for microscopic study.

Muscle Attachments and Frena

As a result of the loss of bone height, muscle attachments may insert on or near the residual ridge crest.

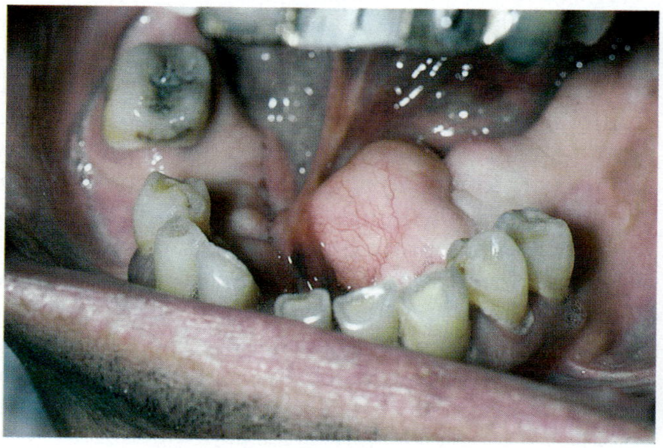

A

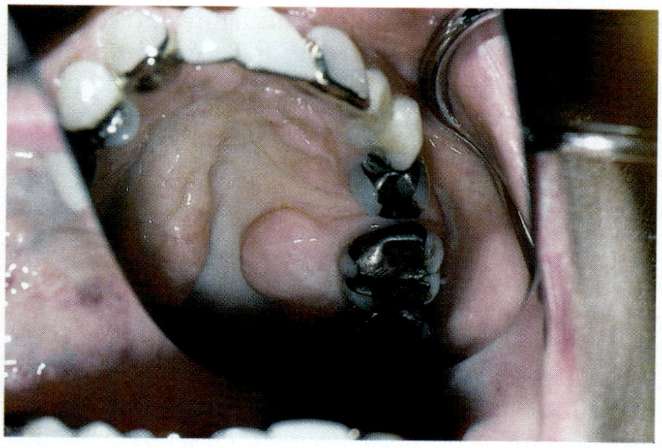

B

Figure 13-5 **A,** Bilateral mandibular removable partial denture without surgical removal. **B,** Maxillary mid-palatal torus and exostosis palatal to maxillary molar. Without removal any contact with the overlying mucosa would be quite painful.

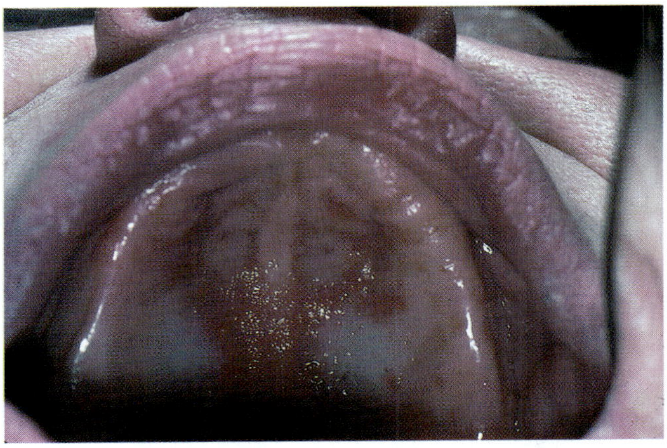

Figure 13-6 Palatal papillomatosis likely the result of continual use of an ill-fitting prosthesis. If longstanding, corrective procedures may require surgical removal.

The mylohyoid, buccinator, mentalis, and genioglossus muscles are those most likely to introduce problems of this nature. In addition to the problem of the attachments of the muscles themselves, the mentalis and genioglossus muscles occasionally produce bony protuberances at their attachments, which may also interfere with removable partial denture design. Appropriate ridge extension procedures can reposition attachments and remove bony spines, which will enhance the comfort and function of the removable partial denture.

Repositioning of the mylohyoid is successfully achieved by several methods. The genioglossus is more difficult to reposition, but careful surgery can reduce the prominence of the genial tubercles and provide some sulcus depth in the anterior lingual area.

Surgical procedures that use skin or mucosal grafts have largely replaced secondary epithelialization procedures for the facial aspect of the mandible. Mucosal grafts using the palate as a donor site offer the best possibility for success. Transplanted skin can be used when large areas must be grafted.

The maxillary labial and mandibular lingual frena are the most common sources of frenum interference with denture design. These can be modified easily with any of several surgical procedures. Under no circumstances should a frenum be allowed to compromise the design or comfort of a removable partial denture.

Bony Spines and Knife-Edge Ridges

Sharp bony spicules should be removed and knifelike crests gently rounded. These procedures should be carried out with minimum bone loss. If, however, the correction of a knife-edge residual crest results in insufficient ridge support for the denture base, the dentist should resort to vestibular deepening for correction of the deficiency or insertion of the various bone grafting materials that have demonstrated successful clinical trials.

Polyps, Papillomas, and Traumatic Hemangiomas

All abnormal soft tissue lesions should be excised and submitted for pathological examination before the fabrication of a removable partial denture. Even though the patient may relate a history of the condition having been present for an indefinite period, its removal is indicated. New or additional stimulation to the area introduced by the prosthesis may produce discomfort or even malignant changes in the tumor.

Hyperkeratoses, Erythroplasia, and Ulcerations

All abnormal, white, red, or ulcerative lesions should be investigated regardless of their relationship to the proposed denture base or framework. A biopsy of areas larger than 5 mm should be completed, and if the lesions are large (more than 2 cm in diameter), multiple biopsies should be taken. The biopsy report will determine whether the margins of the tissue to be excised can be wide or narrow. The lesions should be removed and healing accomplished before fabrication of the removable partial denture. On occasion the removable partial denture design will have to be radically modified to prevent areas of possible sensitivity, such as after irradiation treatments or the excoriation of erosive lichen planus.

Dentofacial Deformity

Patients with a dentofacial deformity often have multiple missing teeth as part of their problem. Correction of the jaw deformity can simplify the dental rehabilitation. Before specific problems with the dentition can be corrected, the patient's overall problem must be evaluated thoroughly. Several dental professionals (prosthodontist, oral surgeon, periodontist, orthodontist, and general dentist) may play a role in the patient's treatment. These individuals must be involved in producing the diagnostic database and in planning treatment for the patient. Information obtained from a general patient evaluation to determine the patient's health status, a clinical evaluation directed toward facial esthetics and the status of the teeth and oral soft tissue, and an analysis of appropriate diagnostic records produces a database. From this database, the patient's problems can be enumerated, with the most severe problem being placed at the top of the list. Other identified problems would follow in the order of their severity. It is only after this step that input from several dentists can provide a correctly sequenced final treatment plan for the patient.

Surgical correction of a jaw deformity can be made in horizontal, sagittal, or frontal planes. Mandibles and maxillae may be positioned anteriorly or posteriorly, and their relationship to the facial planes may be surgically altered to achieve improved appearance. Replacement of missing teeth and development of a harmonious occlusion are almost always major problems in treating these patients.

Osseointegrated Devices

A number of implant devices to support the replacement of teeth have been introduced to the dental profession. These devices offer a significant stabilizing effect on dental prostheses through a rigid connection to living bone. The system that pioneered clinical prosthodontic applications with the use of commercially pure (CP) titanium endosseous implants is that of Brånemark and co-workers (Figure 13-7). This titanium implant was designed to provide a direct

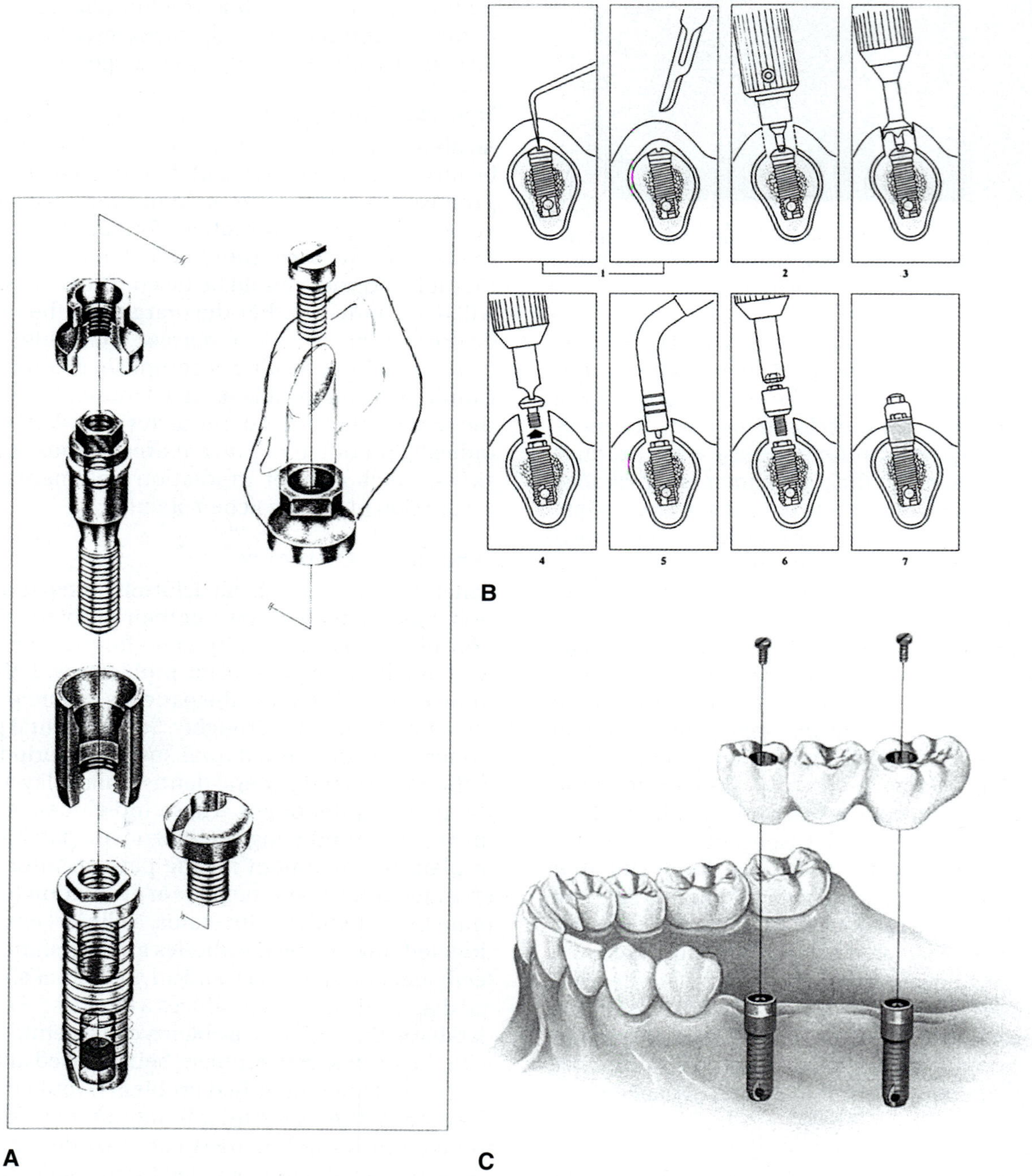

Figure 13-7 **A,** Brånemark System components. From lower to upper: implant, cover screws, abutment, abutment screw, gold cylinder, gold screw. **B,** Basic procedures in second-stage surgery: (1) exploration to locate cover screw; (2) removal of soft tissue; (3) removal of bony tissue; (4) removal of cover screw; (5) use of depth gauge to measure the amount of soft tissue; (6) abutment connection; (7) placement of healing cap. **C,** Freestanding three-unit fixed partial denture supported by two osseointegrated implants that restore the extension base area, which would have been restored with a Class II removable partial denture if implants had not been used. *(**A** and **C**, From Hobo S, Ichida E, Garcia L: Osseointegration and occlusal rehabilitation, Carol Stream, IL, Quintessence Co., Inc.,1989. **B**, Courtesy Nobel Biocare, Göteborg, Sweden.)*

titanium-to-bone interface (osseointegrated), with the basic laboratory and clinical results supporting the value of this procedure.

Implants are carefully placed using controlled surgical procedures, and in general bone healing to the device is allowed to occur before fabrication of a dental prosthesis. Long-term clinical research has demonstrated good results for the treatment of complete and partially edentulous patients using dental implants. Although there has been very limited research on implant applications with removable partial dentures, the inclusion of strategically placed implants can significantly control prosthesis movement (Figures 13-8 through 13-10).

Augmentation of Alveolar Bone

Considerable attention has been devoted to ridge augmentation with the use of autogenous and alloplastic materials, especially in preparation for implant placement. Larger ridge volume gains necessitate consideration of autogenous grafts; however, these procedures are accompanied with concerns for surgical morbidity. Although alloplastic materials have displayed short-term success, no randomized controlled trials have been conducted to provide evidence of long-term increases in ridge width and height for removable prostheses.

Clinical results depend on careful evaluation of the need for augmentation, the projected volume of required material, and the site and method of placement. Considerable emphasis must be placed on sound clinical understanding that some of the alloplastic materials can migrate or be displaced under occlusal loads if not appropriately supported by underlying bone and contained by buttressing soft tissue. Careful clinical judgment, with

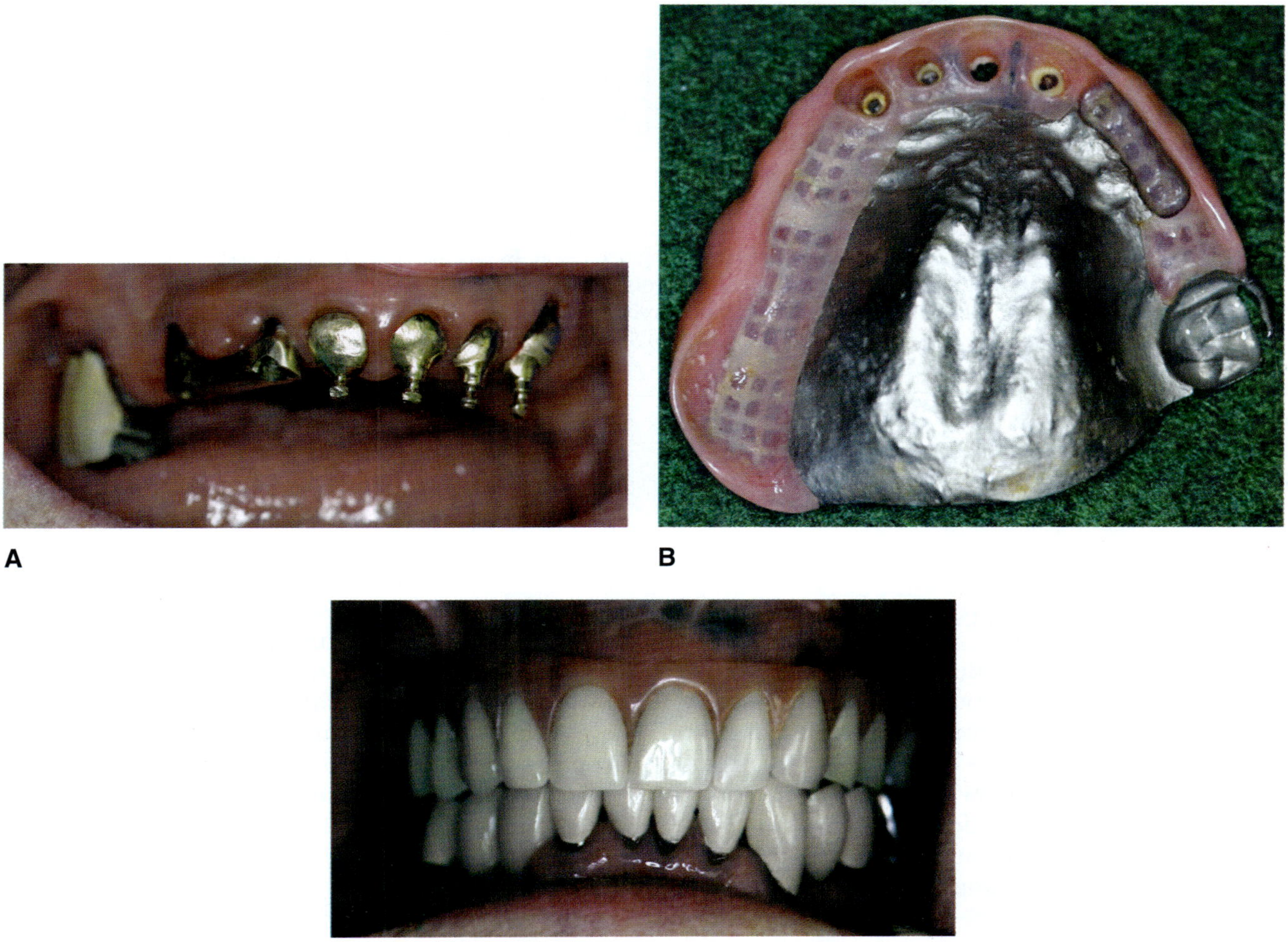

A B C

Figure 13-8 **A,** Implant bar and natural tooth copings used to support and retain this maxillary prosthesis. **B,** Tissue side of prosthesis showing the implant bar space, which when fitted will derive both support and stability from the implants while retention is gained through resilient O-rings on the natural tooth copings. **C,** Maxillary prosthesis seated and in occlusion. *(Courtesy Dr. N. Van Roekel, Palm Springs, CA.)*

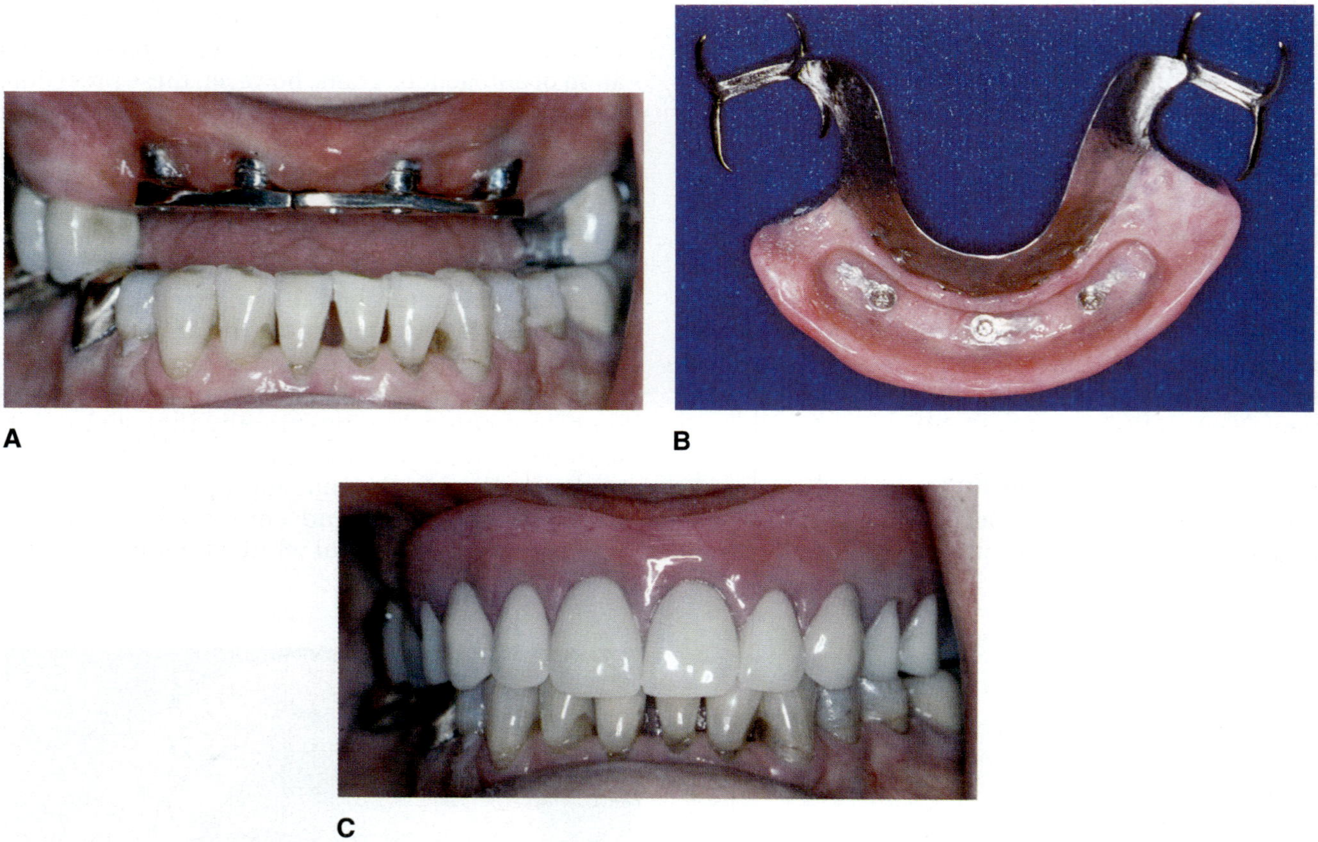

Figure 13-9 **A,** An anterior implant-supported bar demonstrating excellent access for hygiene and a parallel relationship to opposing occlusion. **B,** Prosthesis with implant bar space (housing three retentive male components for retention and a flat surface for bar contact and support) and bilateral posterior embrasure clasps. **C,** Prosthesis seated and in occlusion. *(Courtesy Dr. N. Van Roekel, Palm Springs, CA.)*

sound surgical and prosthetic principles, must be exercised.

CONDITIONING OF ABUSED AND IRRITATED TISSUE

Many removable partial denture patients require some conditioning of supporting tissue in edentulous areas before the final impression phase of treatment. Patients who require conditioning treatment often demonstrate the following symptoms:

1. Inflammation and irritation of the mucosa covering the denture-bearing areas (Figure 13-11)
2. Distortion of normal anatomic structures, such as incisive papillae, the rugae, and the retromolar pads
3. A burning sensation in residual ridge areas, the tongue, and the cheeks and lips

These conditions are usually associated with ill-fitting or poorly occluding removable partial dentures. However, nutritional deficiencies, endocrine imbalances, severe health problems (diabetes or blood dyscrasias), and bruxism must be considered in a differential diagnosis.

If a new removable partial denture or the relining of a present denture is attempted without first correcting these conditions, the chances for successful treatment will be compromised because the same old problems will be perpetuated. The patient must be made to realize that fabrication of a new prosthesis should be delayed until the oral tissue can be returned to a healthy state. If there are unresolved systemic problems, removable partial denture treatment will usually result in either failure or limited success.

The first treatment procedure should be an immediate institution of a good home care program. A suggested home care program includes rinsing the mouth three times a day with a prescribed saline solution; massaging the residual ridge areas, palate, and tongue with a soft toothbrush; removing the prosthesis at night; and using a prescribed therapeutic multiple vitamin along with a prescribed

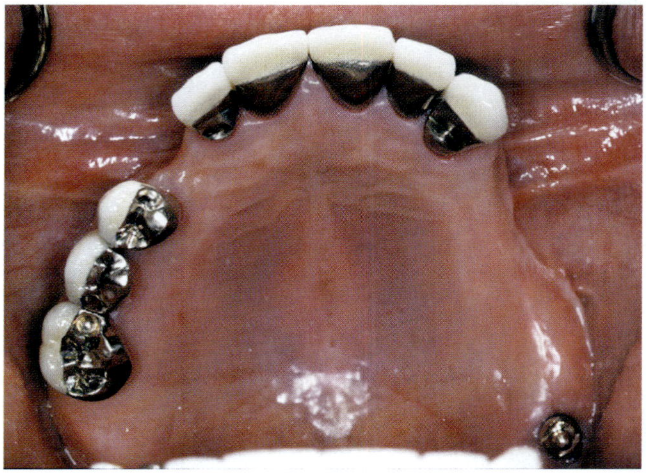

A

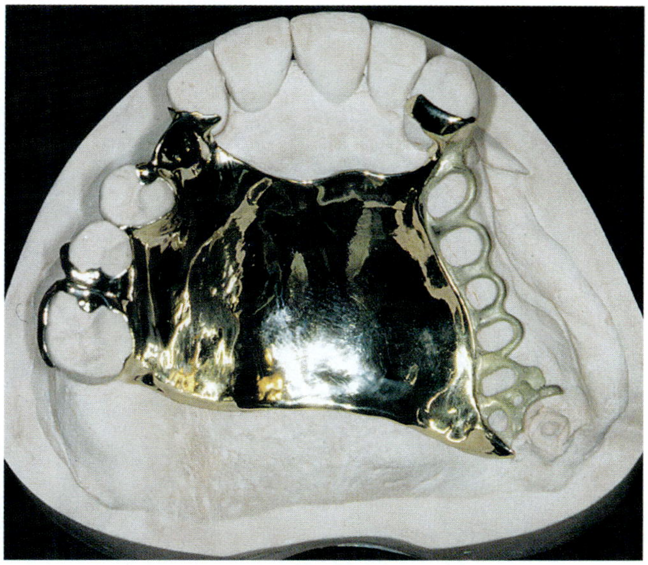

B

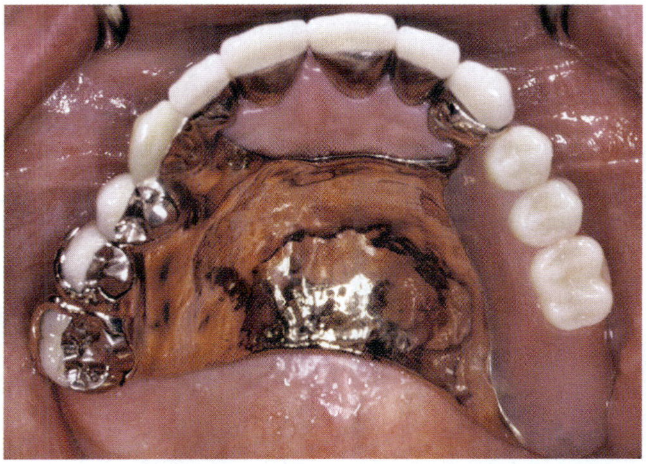

C

Figure 13-10 **A,** A Class II, mod 1 maxillary arch with posterior implant at distal location of extension base. **B,** Maxillary gold framework with broad palatal coverage, maximum stabilization through palatal contacts of multiple maxillary teeth, and implant position at the distal of extension base. Single implant should be protected from excessive occlusal forces, consequently the broad palatal coverage and maximum bracing are important features of the overall design. Ball attachment abutment was used for retentive purposes. **C,** Occlusal view of prosthesis with implant (see **A**) providing improved retention to distal extension base. *(Courtesy Dr. James Taylor, Toronto, Ontario, Canada.)*

high-protein, low-carbohydrate diet. Some inflammatory oral conditions caused by ill-fitting dentures can be resolved by removing the dentures for extended periods. However, few patients are willing to undergo such inconveniences.

Use of Tissue Conditioning Materials

The tissue conditioning materials are elastopolymers that continue to flow for an extended period, permitting distorted tissue to rebound and assume its normal form. These soft materials apparently have a massaging effect on irritated mucosa, and because they are soft, occlusal forces are probably more evenly distributed.

Maximum benefit from using tissue conditioning materials may be obtained by (1) eliminating deflective or interfering occlusal contacts of old dentures (by remounting in an articulator if necessary); (2) extending denture bases to proper form to enhance support, retention, and stability (Figure 13-12);

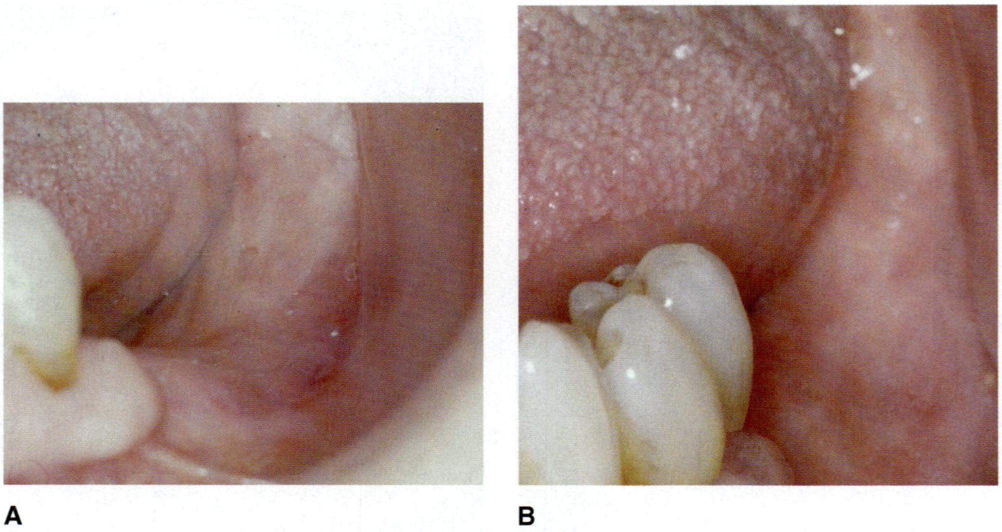

Figure 13-11 A, Inflamed and distorted denture-bearing mucosa due to an ill-fitting prosthesis that is worn 24 hours a day. B, After treating the tissue abuse using a modification of the denture base with a tissue conditioning material, removal of the prosthesis for portions of the day, and massaging the abused tissue, the denture-bearing foundation is healthy again.

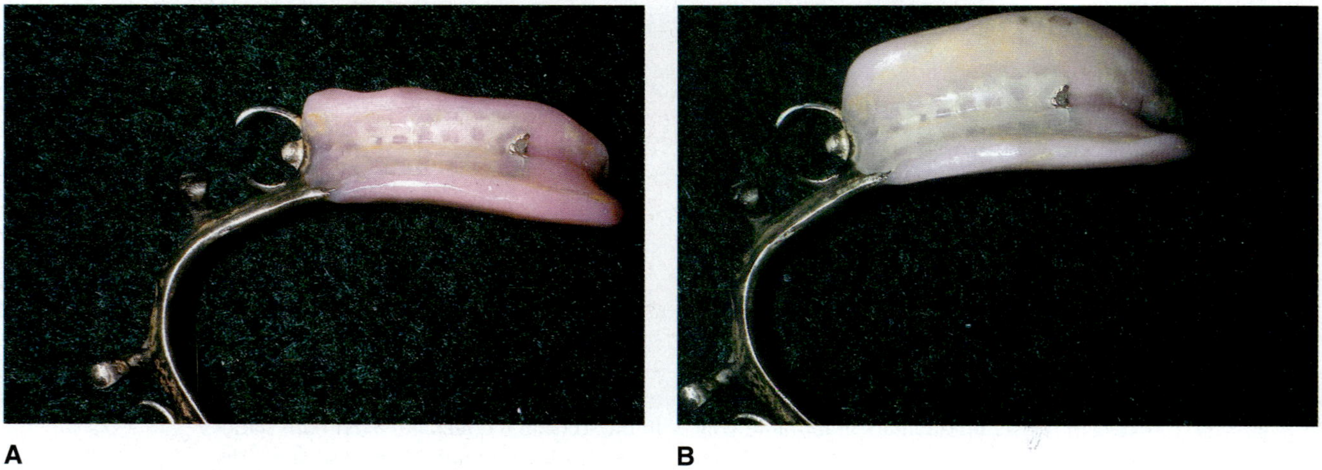

Figure 13-12 A, Mandibular removable partial denture distal extension base exhibiting an underextended form. Such a reduced area of residual ridge coverage can contribute to tissue irritation. B, Denture base properly extended to enhance support, stability, and retention.

(3) relieving the tissue side of denture bases sufficiently (2 mm) to provide space for even thickness and distribution of conditioning material; (4) applying the material in amounts sufficient to provide support and a cushioning effect (Figure 13-13); and (5) following the manufacturer's directions for manipulation and placement of the conditioning material.

The conditioning procedure should be repeated until the supporting tissues display an undistorted and healthy appearance. Many dentists find that intervals of 4 to 7 days between changes of the conditioning material are clinically acceptable. An improvement in irritated and distorted tissue is usually noted within a few visits, and in some patients a dramatic improvement will be seen. Usually three or four changes of the conditioning material are adequate, but in some instances more changes are required. If positive results are not seen within 3 to 4 weeks, one should suspect more serious health problems and request a consultation from a physician.

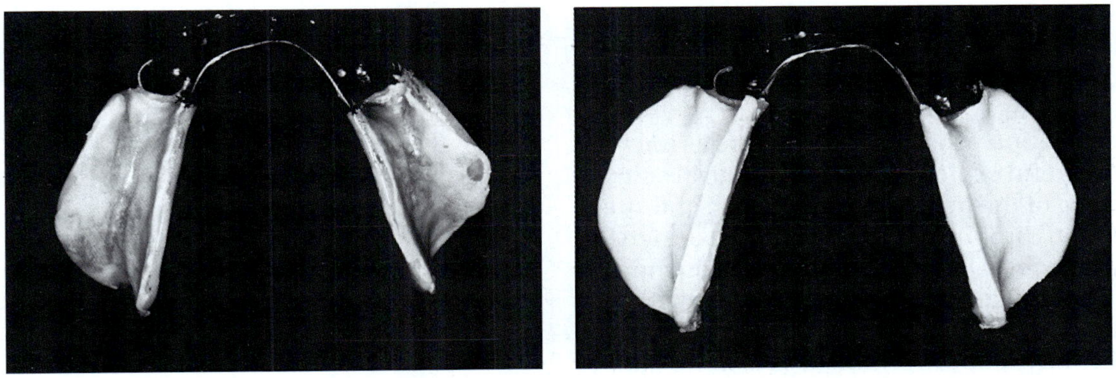

A B

Figure 13-13 A, Unsuccessful attempt to apply tissue conditioning material. Bases incorrectly relieved and conditioning material improperly applied. B, Tissue conditioning of sufficient thickness and distribution for effective treatment.

PERIODONTAL PREPARATION*

The periodontal preparation of the mouth usually follows any oral surgical procedure and is performed simultaneously with tissue conditioning procedures. Ordinarily, tooth extraction and removal of impacted teeth and retained roots or their fragments are accomplished before definitive periodontal therapy. However, it is strongly recommended that a gross debridement be performed before tooth extraction when patients have significant calculus accumulation. This helps limit the possibility of accidentally dislodging a piece of calculus into the extraction socket, which could lead to an infection. The elimination of exostoses, tori, hyperplastic tissue, muscle attachments, and frena, on the other hand, can be incorporated with periodontal surgical techniques. In any situation, periodontal therapy should be completed before restorative dentistry procedures are begun for any dental patient. This is particularly true when a removable partial denture is contemplated because the ultimate success of this restoration depends directly on the health and integrity of the supporting structures of the remaining teeth. The periodontal health of the remaining teeth, especially those to be used as abutments, must be evaluated carefully by the dentist and corrective measures instituted before removable partial denture fabrication. It has been demonstrated that following periodontal therapy and with a good recall and oral hygiene program, properly designed removable partial dentures will not adversely impact the progression of periodontal disease or carious lesions.

This discussion attempts to demonstrate how periodontal procedures affect diagnoses and treatment planning in a removable partial denture service rather than how the procedures are actually accomplished. For technical details, the reader is referred to any of several excellent textbooks on periodontics.

*This section edited by Vanchit John DDS, Assistant Professor, Department of Periodontics, Indiana University School of Dentistry, Indianapolis, Indiana.

Objectives of Periodontal Therapy

The objective of periodontal therapy is the return to health of the supporting structures of the teeth, creating an environment in which the periodontium may be maintained. The specific criteria for satisfying this objective are as follows:

1. Removal and control of all etiological factors contributing to periodontal disease, along with a reduction or elimination of bleeding on probing
2. Elimination of, or reduction in, pocket depths of all pockets, with the establishment of healthy gingival sulci whenever possible
3. Establishment of functional atraumatic occlusal relationships and tooth stability
4. Development of a personal plaque control program and definitive maintenance schedule

A complete periodontal charting should be performed that includes the recording of pocket depths, assessment of attachment levels, recording furcation involvements, mucogingival problems, and tooth mobility. Determining the severity of periodontal disease should also include the use of appropriate radiographs. The dentist considering removable partial denture fabrication must be certain that these criteria have been satisfied before continuing with impression procedures for the master cast.

Periodontal Diagnosis and Treatment Planning

Diagnosis

The diagnosis of periodontal diseases is based on a systematic and carefully accomplished examination of the periodontium. It follows the procurement of the health history of the patient and is performed using direct vision, palpation, periodontal probe, mouth mirror, and other auxiliary aids, such as curved explorers, furcation probes, diagnostic casts, and appropriate radiographs.

In the evaluation procedure, nothing is as important as the careful exploration of the gingival sulcus and recording of the probing pocket depth and sites that bleed on probing with a suitably designed periodontal probe. Under no circumstances should removable partial denture fabrication begin without an accurate appraisal of sulcus and/or pocket depth and health. The probe is positioned as close to parallel with the long axis of the tooth as possible and is inserted gently between the gingival margin and the tooth surface, and the depth of the sulcus/pocket is determined circumferentially around each tooth. At least six probing depth readings are recorded on the patient's chart for each tooth. Usually depths are recorded for the distobuccal, buccal, mesiobuccal, distolingual, lingual, and mesiolingual aspects of each tooth. An assessment of sulcular health can also be determined by the presence or absence of bleeding upon probing.

Dental radiographs can be used to supplement the clinical examination but should not be used as a substitute for it. A critical evaluation of the following factors should be made: (1) type, location, and severity of bone loss; (2) location, severity, and distribution of furcation involvements; (3) alterations of the periodontal ligament space; (4) alterations of the lamina dura; (5) presence of calcified deposits; (6) location and conformity of restorative margins; (7) evaluation of crown and root morphologies; (8) root proximity; (9) caries; and (10) evaluation of other associated anatomic features, such as the mandibular canal or sinus proximity. This information serves to substantiate the impression gained from the clinical examination.

Each tooth should be evaluated carefully for mobility. Unfortunately, there is no universally accepted standard for mobility. In general, mobility is graded according to the ease and extent of tooth movement. Normal mobility is in the order of 0.05 to 0.10 mm. Grade I mobility is present when there is less than 1 mm of movement in a buccolingual direction; grade II is present when mobility in the buccolingual direction is between 1 to 2 mm, and grade III is present when there is greater than 2 mm of mobility in the buccolingual direction and/or the tooth is vertically depressible.

Tooth mobility is an indication of the condition of the supporting structures, namely the periodontium, and is usually caused by inflammatory changes in the periodontal ligament, traumatic occlusion, loss of attachment, or a combination of the three factors (Figure 13-14). The degree of mobility present, coupled with a determination of the etiological factors responsible, provides additional information that is invaluable in planning for the removable partial denture. If the etiological factor can be removed, many grade I and grade II mobile teeth can become stable and may be used successfully to help support, stabilize, and retain the removable partial denture. Mobility is not in itself an indication for extraction unless the mobile tooth cannot aid in the support or stability of the removable partial denture or the mobility cannot be reduced. (Grade III usually cannot be reversed and will not provide support or stability.)

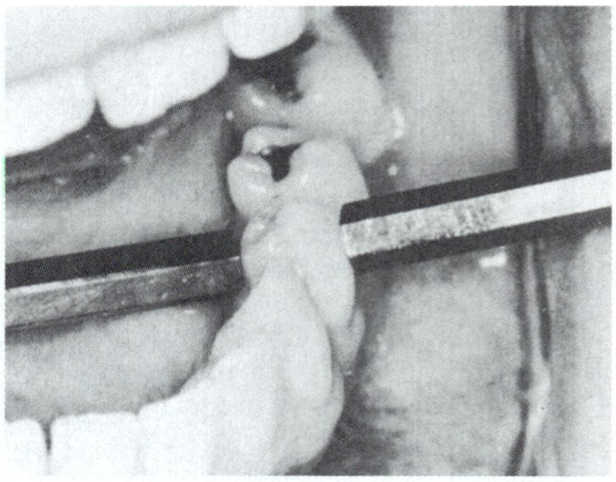

Figure 13-14 Mobility can be visualized best when pressure is exerted on tooth through instrument handles. If fingers are used for this purpose, movement of soft tissue may mask accurate determination of mobility. Mobility should also be evaluated by checking for fremitus. This is most important for more anterior teeth, which may serve as abutments. It is important for such teeth to have careful adjustment of frameworks so as to eliminate any potential framework interference, which could cause tooth mobility.

Treatment Planning

Depending on the extent and severity of the periodontal changes present, a variety of therapeutic procedures, ranging from simple to relatively complex, may be indicated. As was the situation with the previously discussed oral surgical procedures, it is the responsibility of the dentist rendering the removable partial denture treatment to see that the required periodontal care is accomplished for the patient. Periodontal treatment planning can usually be divided into three phases. The first phase is considered disease control or initial therapy because the objective is to essentially eliminate or reduce local etiological factors before any periodontal surgical procedures are accomplished. The procedures that are accomplished as part of the initial preparation phase include oral hygiene instruction, scaling, and root planing and polishing along with endodontics, occlusal adjustment, and temporary splinting, if indicated. In many instances, carefully performed scaling and root planing combined with excellent patient compliance may negate the need for periodontal surgery.

During the second—or periodontal—surgical phase, any needed periodontal surgery is accomplished, including free gingival grafts, osseous grafts, or pocket reduction. It is advisable to discuss the possible need for these treatment procedures with the patient either at the initial examination appointment or during the initial phase of therapy because this will likely involve the referral of the patient to a periodontist. The maintenance of periodontal health is accomplished in phase 3 and is always ongoing. A definitive recall schedule should be established with the patient and is usually kept at 3- to 4- month intervals.

Initial Disease Control Therapy (Phase 1)

Oral Hygiene Instruction

Ordinarily, dental treatment should be introduced to the patient through instruction in a carefully devised oral hygiene regimen. The cooperation witnessed by the patient's acceptance and compliance with the prescribed procedure, as evidenced by improved oral hygiene, will provide the dentist with a valuable means of evaluating the patient's interest and the long-term prognosis of treatment.

For the oral hygiene routine to be successful, the patient must be convinced to follow the prescribed procedure regularly and conscientiously. The most effective motivation techniques require a good understanding by the patient of his/her periodontal condition. Only then can the benefits of routine treatment become evident. Hence, an explanation of dental/periodontal disease, its causes, initiation, and progression, is an important component of oral hygiene instruction. After this discussion, the patient should be instructed in the use of disclosing wafers/tablets, a soft/medium bristle toothbrush, and unwaxed/waxed dental floss. At subsequent appointments, oral hygiene can be evaluated carefully and other oral hygiene aids—such as an interdental and or sulcular brushes—can be incorporated as needed. Further treatment should be withheld until achievement of a satisfactory level of plaque control. This is a particularly critical point for the patient who requires extensive restorative dentistry or a removable partial denture. Without good oral hygiene, any dental procedure—regardless of how well it is performed—is ultimately doomed to failure. The informed dentist insists that acceptable oral hygiene be demonstrated and maintained before embarking on an extensive restorative dentistry treatment plan.

Scaling and Root Planing

One of the most important services rendered to the patient is the removal of calculus and plaque deposits from the coronal and root surfaces of the teeth. Careful scaling and root planing are fundamental to the reestablishment of periodontal health. Without meticulous removal of calculus, plaque, and toxic material in the cementum, other forms of periodontal therapy cannot be successful.

The use of ultrasonic instrumentation is recommended for calculus removal followed by root planing with sharp periodontal curettes. The curette is designed specifically for root planing and, when used correctly in combination with ultrasonic instrumentation, results in calculus removal and root surface decontamination. Thorough scaling and root planing should precede definitive surgical periodontal procedures, which may be indicated before removable partial denture fabrication.

Elimination of Local Irritating Factors Other Than Calculus

Overhanging restoration margins and open contacts that allow food impaction should be corrected before beginning definitive prosthetic treatment. Although periodontal health predisposes to a much better environment for restorative procedures, it is not always possible or prudent to delay all restorative procedures until complete periodontal therapy and healing have occurred. This is especially true for patients with severe carious lesions where pulpal involvement is likely. Excavation of these areas and placement of adequate restorations must be incorporated early in treatment. The placement of temporary or treatment fillings must not, in itself, become a local etiological factor.

Elimination of Gross Occlusal Interferences

Bacterial plaque accumulations and calculus deposits are the primary factors involved in the initiation and progression of inflammatory periodontal disease. However, poor restorative dentistry can contribute to the damage of the periodontium, and poor occlusal relationships may act as another factor that contributes to more rapid loss of periodontal attachment. Although occlusal interferences may be eliminated by a variety of techniques, at this stage of treatment, selective grinding is the generally applied procedure. Particular attention is directed to the occlusal relationships of mobile teeth. Traumatic cuspal interferences are removed by a selective grinding procedure. An attempt is made to establish a positive planned intercuspal position that coincides with centric relation. Deflective contacts in the centric path of closure are removed, eliminating mandibular displacement from the closing pattern. After this, the relationship of the teeth in the various excursive movements of the mandible is observed, with special attention to cuspal contact, wear, mobility, and roentgenographic changes in the periodontium. The presence of working and nonworking interferences should be evaluated, and if present, they should be removed.

The mere presence of occlusal abnormalities in the absence of demonstrable pathological change associated with the occlusion does not necessarily constitute an indication for selective grinding. The indication for occlusal adjustment is based on the presence of a pathological condition rather than on a preconceived articulation pattern. In the natural dentition, the attempt to create bilateral balance in the prosthetic sense has no place in the occlusal adjustment procedure. Bilateral balanced occlusion not only is difficult to obtain in a natural dentition but also is apparently unnecessary in view of its absence in most normal healthy mouths. Occlusion on natural teeth needs to be perfected only to a point at which cuspal interference within the patient's functional range of contact is eliminated and normal physiologic function can occur.

Guide to Occlusal Adjustment

In the study or evaluation of occlusal disharmony of the natural dentition, accurately mounted diagnostic casts are extremely helpful—if not essential—in determining static cusp to fossa contacts of opposing teeth and as a guide in the correction of occlusal anomalies in both centric and eccentric functional relations. Occlusion can be coordinated only by selective spot grinding. Ground tooth surfaces should be subsequently smoothed and polished.

Schuyler has provided the following guide to occlusal adjustment by selective grinding*:

1. A static coordinated occlusal contact of the maximum number of teeth (maximum intercuspal position) when the mandible is in centric relation to the maxilla should be the first objective.
   a. A prematurely contacting cusp should be reduced only if the cusp point is in premature contact in both centric and eccentric relations. If a cusp point is in premature contact in centric relation only, the opposing sulcus should be deepened.
   b. When anterior teeth are in premature contact in centric relation, or in both centric and eccentric relations, corrections should be made by grinding the incisal edges of the mandibular teeth. If premature contact occurs only in the eccentric relation, correction must be made by grinding the lingual inclines of the maxillary teeth.
   c. Usually, premature contacts in centric relation are relieved by grinding the buccal cusps of the mandibular teeth, the lingual cusps of maxillary teeth, and the incisal edges of the mandibular anterior teeth. Deepening the fossa of a posterior tooth or the lingual contact area in centric relation of a maxillary anterior tooth changes and increases the steepness of the eccentric guiding inclines of the tooth. Although this relieves trauma in centric relation, it may predispose the tooth to trauma in eccentric relations.
2. After establishing a static, even distribution of stress over the maximum number of teeth in centric relation, the dentist is ready to evaluate opposing tooth contact or lack of contact in eccentric functional relations. The attention is directed first to balancing side contacts. In extreme cases of pathological condition balancing contacts, relief may be needed even before the corrective procedures in centric relation. Where balancing contacts exist, it is extremely difficult to differentiate the harmless from the destructive because we cannot visualize the influence of these fulcrum contacts on the functional movements of the condyle in the articular fossa. Subluxation, pain, lack of normal functional movement of the joint, or loss of alveolar support of the teeth involved may be evidence of excessive balancing contacts. Balancing-side contacts receive less frictional wear than working-side contacts, and premature contacts may develop progressively with wear. A reduction in the steepness of the guiding tooth incline on the working side will increase the proximity of the teeth on the balancing side and may contribute to destructive premature contact. In all corrective grinding to relieve premature or excessive contacts in eccentric relations, care must be exercised to prevent the loss of a static supporting contact in centric relation. This static support in centric relation may exist between the mandibular buccal cusp fitting into the central fossa of the maxillary tooth or between the maxillary lingual cusp fitting into the central fossa of the mandibular tooth or it may exist in both situations. Although both the maxillary lingual cusp and the mandibular buccal cusp may sometimes have a static centric contact in the sulcus of the opposing tooth, often only one of these cusps has this static contact. In such instances the contacting cusp must be left untouched to maintain this essential support in the planned intercuspal position, and all corrective grinding to relieve premature contacts in eccentric positions would be done on the opposing tooth inclines. The mandibular buccal cusp is in a static central contact in the maxillary sulcus more often than the maxillary lingual cusp is in a static contact in its opposing mandibular sulcus. Therefore corrective grinding to relieve premature balancing contacts is more often done on the maxillary lingual cusps.
3. To obtain maximum function and the distribution of functional stress in eccentric positions on the working side, necessary grinding must be done

*Courtesy Dr. C.H. Schuyler, Montclair, NJ.

on the lingual surfaces of the maxillary anterior teeth. Corrective grinding on the posterior teeth at this time should always be done on the buccal cusp of the maxillary premolars and molars and on the lingual cusp of the mandibular premolars and molars. The grinding of mandibular buccal cusps or maxillary lingual cusps at this time would rob these cusps of their static contact in the opposing central sulci in centric relation.

4. Corrective grinding to relieve premature protrusive contacts of one or more anterior teeth should be accomplished by grinding the lingual surface of the maxillary anterior teeth. Anterior teeth should never be ground to bring the posterior teeth into contact in either protrusive position or on the balancing side. In the elimination of premature protrusive contacts of posterior teeth, neither the maxillary lingual cusps nor the mandibular buccal cusps should be ground. Corrective grinding should be done in the eccentric position on the surface of the opposing teeth on which these cusps function, leaving the centric contact undisturbed.
5. Any sharp edges left by grinding should be rounded off.

Temporary Splinting

Teeth that are mobile at the time of the initial examination frequently present a diagnostic problem for the dentist. The cause of the mobility must be determined and then a decision made for elimination of the causal factors. The response of these teeth to temporary immobilization, followed by appropriate treatment, may be a helpful indicator in establishing a prognosis for them and may lead to a rational decision as to whether they should be retained or sacrificed. Secondary mobility resulting from the presence of an inflammatory lesion may be reversible if the disease process has not destroyed too much of the attachment apparatus. Primary mobility caused by occlusal interference also may disappear after selective grinding. In instances of angular types of osseous defects, one should consider guided tissue regeneration as a means of increasing attachment levels. In some situations, however, the teeth must be stabilized because of loss of supporting structure from the periodontal process.

Teeth may be immobilized during periodontal treatment by acid etching teeth with composite resin, with fiber reinforced resins, with cast removable splints, or with intracoronal attachments (Figure 13-15). The latter, an example of which is the A-splint, necessitates cutting tooth surfaces and embedding a ridge connector between adjacent teeth.

After periodontal treatment, splinting may be accomplished with cast removable restorations or cast cemented restorations. The preferred form of permanent splinting is with two or more cast restorations soldered or cast together. They may be cemented with either permanent (zinc oxyphosphate or resin) cements or temporary (zinc oxide–eugenol) cements. A properly designed removable partial denture can also stabilize mobile teeth if provision for such immobilization is planned as the denture is designed.

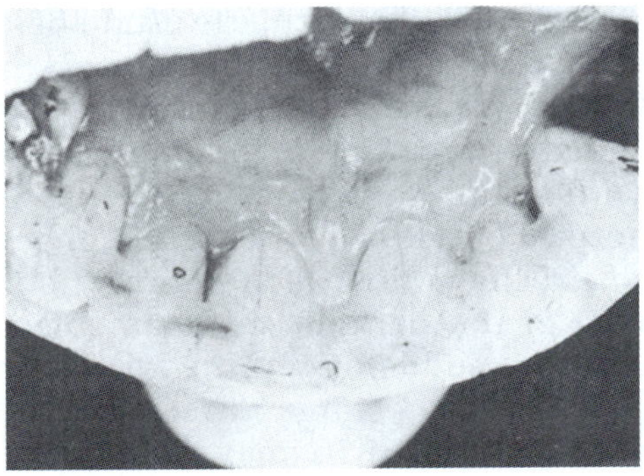

Figure 13-15 A splint used to stabilize mobile anterior segment. Markley pins embedded in plastic filling material in dovetail preparations on lingual surfaces. *(Courtesy Dr. Daniel R. Trinler, Lexington, KY.)*

Use of a Nightguard

The removable acrylic resin splint, originally designed as an aid in eliminating the deleterious effects of nocturnal clenching and grinding, has been used to advantage for the removable partial denture patient. The nightguard may be helpful as a form of temporary splinting if worn at night after the removal of the removable partial denture. The flat occlusal surface prevents the intercuspation of the teeth, which eliminates lateral occlusal forces (Figure 13-16).

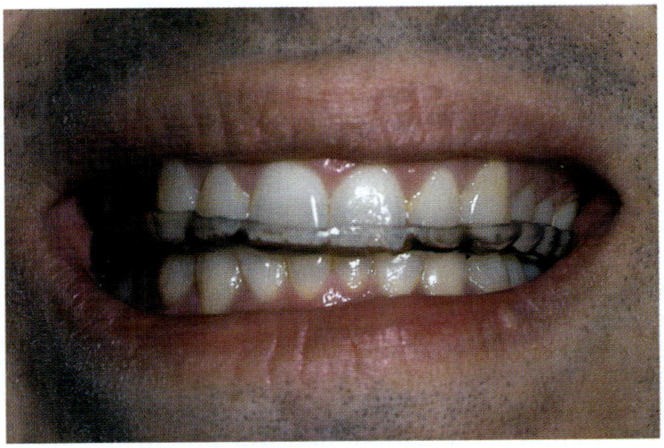

Figure 13-16 Removable acrylic resin splint with flat occlusal plane can be used effectively as a form of temporary stabilization and as means of eliminating excessive lateral forces created by clenching and grinding habits.

The nightguard is particularly useful before fabrication of a removable partial denture when one of the abutment teeth has been unopposed for an extended period. The periodontal ligament of a tooth without an antagonist undergoes changes characterized by a loss of orientation of periodontal ligament fibers, loss of supporting bone, and narrowing of the periodontal ligament space. If such a tooth is suddenly returned to full function when it is carrying an increased burden, pain and prolonged sensitivity may result. However, if a nightguard is used to return some functional stimulation to the tooth, the periodontal ligament changes are reversed and an uneventful course can be experienced when the tooth is returned to full function.

Minor Tooth Movement

The increased use of orthodontic procedures in conjunction with restorative and prosthetic dentistry has contributed to the success of many restorations by altering the periodontal environment in which they are placed. Malposed teeth that were once doomed to extraction now should be considered for repositioning and retention. The additional stability provided for a removable partial denture from uprighting a tilted or drifted tooth may mean much in terms of comfort to the patient. The techniques employed are not difficult to master, and the rewards in terms of a better restorative dentistry service are great (Figure 13-17).

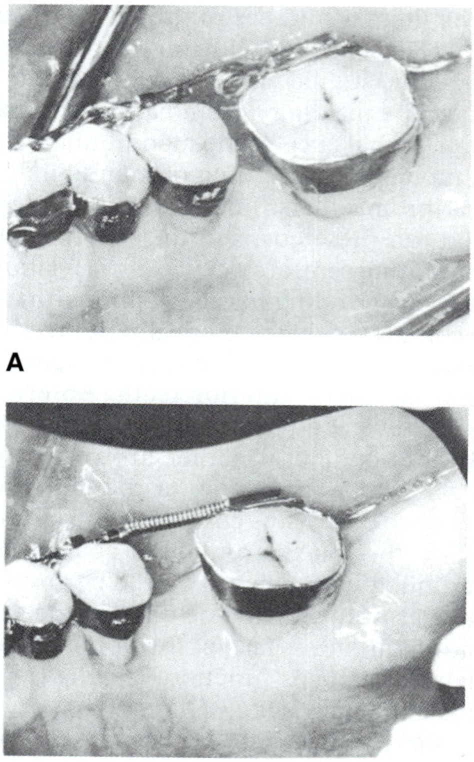

A

B

Figure 13-17 Tooth movement used to upright tilted molar to prepare the segment for receipt of pontic. **A,** Placement of orthodontic appliance. **B,** Space gained after 3 months' active movement.

Definitive Periodontal Surgery (Phase 2)

Periodontal Surgery

After initial therapy is completed, the patient is reevaluated for the surgical phase. If oral hygiene is at an optimum level, yet pockets with inflammation and osseous defects are still present, a variety of periodontal surgical techniques should be considered to improve periodontal health. The procedures selected should have the potential to enhance the results obtained during phase 1 therapy.

Pocket reduction or elimination may be achieved by root planing when the cause of pocket depth is edema caused by gingival inflammation. Apically positioned flap surgery or occasionally a gingivectomy may be considered for reduction of suprabony pockets. Osseous resection or regeneration using a flap approach is also a commonly employed form of surgical therapy to help with the treatment of the diseased periodontium. It must be noted that elimination of the inflammatory disease process and restoration of the periodontal attachment apparatus are the major objectives of periodontal therapy.

Periodontal flaps. Today the use of one of the various flap procedures is the surgical approach offering the greatest versatility. Periodontal flap surgery involves the elevation of either mucosa alone or both the mucosa and the periosteum. Although there are several indications for flap elevation, the most important goal of flap elevation is to allow access to the bone and the root surfaces for complete instrumentation. The other goals of the flap approach include access for pocket elimination, caries control, crown lengthening to allow for optimum restorative dental treatment, root amputation or hemisection as required, and access to the furcation of the tooth.

A decision is made prior to surgery if the aim is resection of osseous tissue to allow for a more physiological osseous anatomy and subsequently gingival contour or to regenerate some of the lost periodontal attachment apparatus. However, sometimes changes have to be made during surgery based on the anatomy of the defects following the removal of diseased granulation tissue. Osseous resection involves use of both osteoplasty and ostectomy procedures. Osteoplasty refers to reshaping the bone without removing tooth-supporting bone, whereas ostectomy includes the removal of tooth-supporting bone. Consequently, the flap is widely applied in the treatment of periodontal diseases.

Guided tissue regeneration. Guided tissue regeneration (GTR) has been defined as those procedures that attempt regeneration of lost periodontal structures through differing tissue responses. The rationale for GTR is based on the physiological healing response of the tissue after periodontal surgery. After periodontal surgery, a race to repopulate the root surface begins among the 4 tissue types of the periodontium, namely the epithelium, connective tissue, periodontal ligament (PDL), and bone. Epithelium, which migrates at a rate of 0.5 mm per day, typically migrates first along the root surface, preventing new attachment. Therefore to allow the undifferentiated mesenchymal cells from the PDL and the endosteum to repopulate the root against surfaces, the epithelial cells and the gingival connective tissue cells should be isolated. This isolation during initial healing enables periodontal structures to become reestablished and may lead to better long-term health of the tooth. The GTR procedure commonly involves the use of an osseous graft along with a resorbable membrane (Figure 13-18). This technique has the potential to lead to substantial

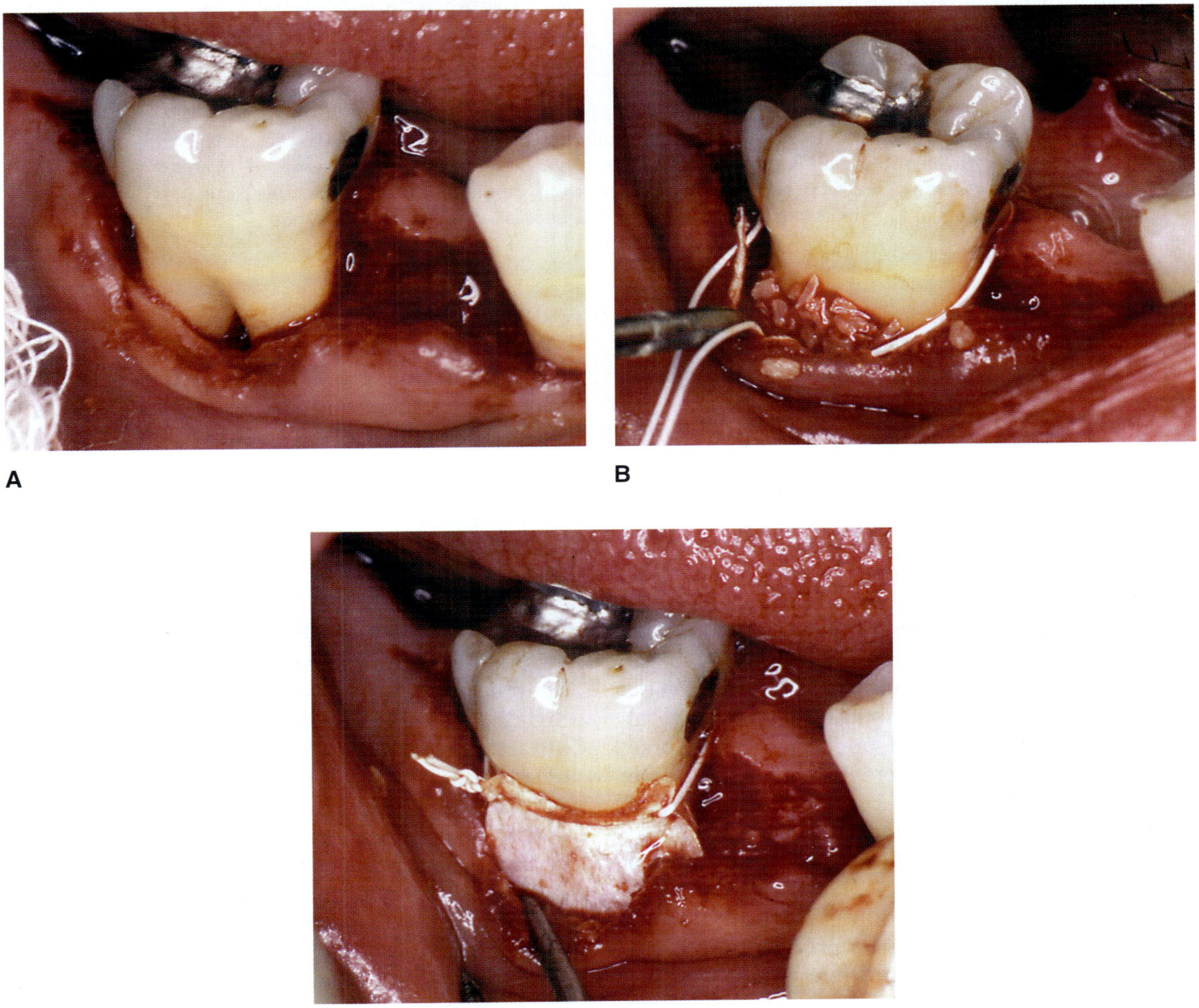

A

B

C

Figure 13-18 Guided tissue regeneration (GTR) procedure to address a furcation involvement. **A,** Tooth #30 presented with a grade 2 furcation involvement with the probe entering 3 mm in a horizontal direction. A GTR procedure using a combination of a bone graft and a nonresorbable membrane was planned. **B,** Following hand and ultrasonic instrumentation, decalcified freeze-dried bone allograft was grafted around the furcation. **C,** A nonresorbable membrane was placed over the bone graft.

Continued

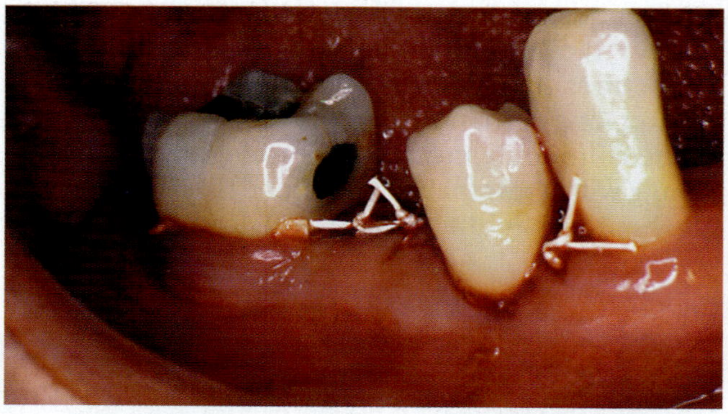

D

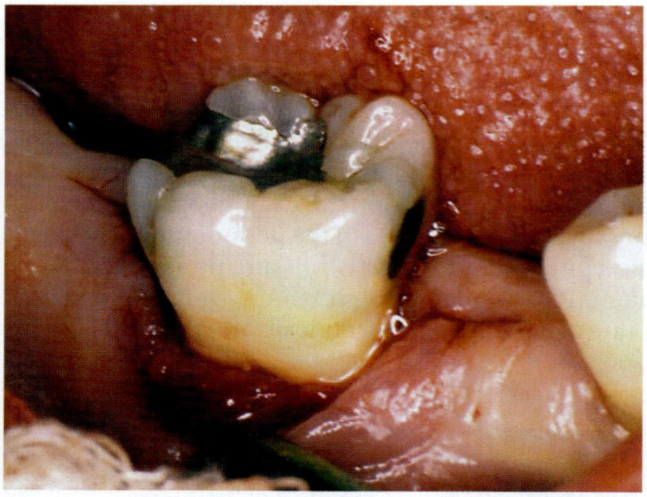

E

Figure 13-18 Cont'd D, The flap was then sutured with a nonresorbable expanded poly tetra ethylene suture. **E,** Two months following surgery, the membrane was removed. Note the presence of red rubbery tissue filling the previously exposed furcation site. This tissue has the potential to form osseous tissue and close the access to the furcation entrance.

improvement of the periodontal condition when used to treat carefully selected two- and three-walled osseous defects and mandibular furcation involvements.

Periodontal plastic surgery. The term *periodontal plastic surgery,* which was previously referred to as "mucogingival surgery," is applied to those procedures used to resolve problems involving the interrelationship between the gingiva and the alveolar mucosa. Mucogingival surgery consists of plastic surgical procedures that are used for the correction of the gingiva–mucous membrane relationships that complicate periodontal disease and may interfere with the success of periodontal treatment. The objectives of periodontal plastic surgery are several and include elimination of pockets that traverse the mucogingival junction, creation of an adequate zone of attached gingiva, and correction of gingival recession by root coverage techniques. In addition, the objectives include relief of the pull of frena and muscle attachments on the gingival margin, correction of deformities of edentulous ridges to permit access to the underlying alveolar process, correction of osseous deformities when there is sufficient or insufficient attached gingiva to deepen a shallow vestibule, and assistance in orthodontic therapy. Commonly used periodontal plastic surgical procedures include lateral sliding flaps, free gingival grafts, pedicle grafts, coronally positioned grafts, double papilla flaps, semilunar coronally positioned flaps, subepithelial connective tissue grafts and edentulous ridge augmentation using one of the above techniques. In addition, GTR has also been used for periodontal plastic surgical procedures. More recently, the use of the commercially available acellular dermal graft has gained popularity. However, the most commonly used procedure is the subepithelial connective tissue graft (Figure 13-19).

These plastic surgical procedures should be considered whenever an abutment tooth lacks adequate attached keratinized gingiva and requires root coverage to facilitate removable partial denture construction and maintenance.

Recall Maintenance (Phase 3)

Several longitudinal studies have now demonstrated the increasing importance of maintenance for all patients who have undergone any periodontal therapy. This includes not only reinforcement of plaque control measures but also thorough debridement of all root surfaces of supragingival and subgingival calculus and plaque by the dentist or an auxiliary.

The frequency of recall appointments should be customized for the patient depending on the susceptibility and severity of periodontal disease. It is now understood that patients with a history of moderate to severe periodontitis should be placed on a 3- to 4-month recall system to maintain results achieved by nonsurgical and surgical therapy.

Advantages of Periodontal Therapy

Periodontal therapy before the fabrication of a removable prosthesis has several advantages. First, the elimination of periodontal disease removes a primary etiological factor in tooth loss. The long-term

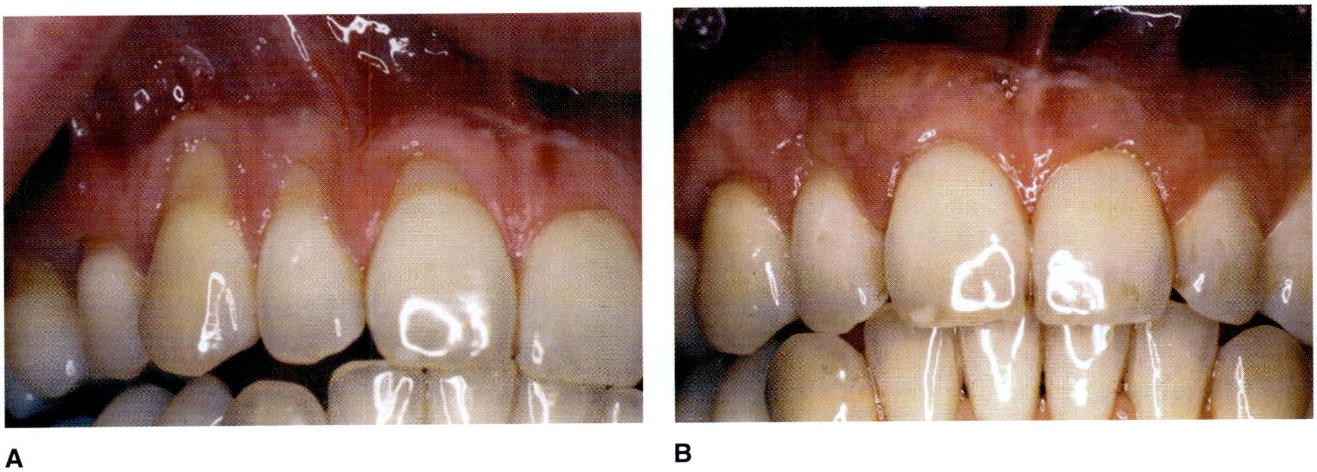

Figure 13-19 Gingival recession addressed with subepithelial connective tissue graft procedure. **A,** The patient presents with evidence of severe gingival recession associated with teeth #s 6, 7, and 8. It was an esthetic problem. The patient also complained of hypersensitivity associated with these teeth. A subepithelial connective tissue graft was planned to help correct the gingival recession. **B,** Clinical appearance 6 months following treatment with a subepithelial connective tissue graft on teeth #s 6, 7, and 8. The patient was very satisfied with the postoperative appearance and clinically the symptom of hypersensitivity was no longer significant.

success of dental treatment depends on the maintenance of the remaining oral structures, and periodontal health is mandatory if further loss is to be prevented. Second, a periodontium free of disease presents a much better environment for restorative correction. The elimination of periodontal pockets with the associated return of a physiological architectural pattern establishes a normal gingival contour at a stable position on the tooth surface. Thus the optimum position for gingival margins of individual restorations can be established with accuracy. The coronal contours of these restorations can also be developed in correct relationships to the gingival margin, ensuring the proper degree of protection and functional stimulation to the gingival tissue. Third, the response of strategic but questionable teeth to periodontal therapy provides an important opportunity for reevaluating their prognosis before the final decision is made to include (or exclude) them in the removable partial denture design. And last, the overall reaction of the patient to periodontal procedures provides the dentist with an excellent indication of the degree of cooperation to be expected in the future.

Even in the absence of periodontal disease, certain periodontal procedures may be an invaluable aid in removable partial denture construction. Through periodontal surgical techniques, the environment of potential abutment teeth may be altered to the point of making an otherwise unacceptable tooth a most satisfactory retainer for a removable partial denture.

ABUTMENT TEETH PREPARATION

Abutment Restorations

Equipped with the diagnostic casts, on which a tentative removable partial denture design has been drawn, the dentist is able to accomplish preparation of abutment teeth with accuracy. The information at hand should include the proposed path of placement, the areas of teeth to be altered and tooth contours to be changed, and the location of rest seats and guiding planes (see Figure 12-5).

During examination and subsequent treatment planning, in conjunction with a survey of diagnostic casts, each abutment tooth is considered individually as to what type of restoration is indicated. Abutment teeth presenting sound enamel surfaces in a mouth in which good oral hygiene habits are evident may be considered a fair risk for use as removable partial denture abutments. One should not be misled, however, by a patient's promise to do better as far as oral hygiene habits are concerned. Good or bad oral hygiene is a habit of long standing and is not likely to be changed appreciably because a removable partial denture is being worn. Therefore one must be conservative in evaluating the oral hygiene habits of the patient in the future. Remember that clasps as such do not cause teeth to decay, and if the individual will keep the teeth and the removable partial denture clean, one need not condemn clasps from a cariogenic standpoint. On the other hand, more removable partial dentures have been condemned as cariogenic because the dentist did not provide for the protection of abutment teeth rather than because of inadequate care on the part of the patient.

Esthetic veneer type of crowns should be used when a canine or premolar abutment is to be restored or protected. Less frequently does the molar have to be treated in such a manner, and except for maxillary first molars the full cast crown is usually acceptable.

When there is proximal caries on abutment teeth with sound buccal and lingual enamel surfaces, in a mouth exhibiting average oral hygiene and low caries activity, a gold inlay may be indicated. However, silver amalgam or composite for the restoration of those teeth with proximal caries should not be condemned, although one must admit that an inlay cast of a hard type of gold will provide the best possible support for occlusal rests, at the same time giving an esthetically pleasing restoration. However, an amalgam restoration, properly condensed, is capable of supporting an occlusal rest without appreciable flow over a long period.

The most vulnerable area on the abutment tooth is the proximal gingival area, which lies beneath the minor connector of the removable partial denture framework and is therefore subject to accumulation of debris in an area most susceptible to caries. Even when the removable partial denture is removed, these areas are often missed by the toothbrush, which allows bacterial plaque and debris to remain for long periods. Because of this unique removable partial denture concern, special attention should be paid to these areas during patient education and follow up. Even when a complete crown restoration is placed in this most vulnerable area, recurrent caries can occur. Caries risk is best managed through effective home care and professional follow-up procedures, rather than through the placement of restorations.

All proximal abutment surfaces that are to serve as guiding planes for the removable partial denture should be prepared so that they will be made as nearly parallel as possible to the path of placement. Preparations may include modifying the contour of existing ceramic restorations, if necessary. This may be accomplished with abrasive stones or diamond finishing stones. A polished surface for the altered ceramic restoration may be restored by using any of several polishing kits supplied by manufacturers.

When preparing abutments that will receive surveyed crowns, it is important to plan for the tooth reduction necessary to allow placement of sufficient restorative material for durability, contour, and esthetics, and the contours prescribed for the desired clasp assembly (Figure 13-20). This can be accomplished by first modifying the axial contours of the abutments to those required by the completed crown, then starting the controlled tooth reduction (preparation) to accommodate the thickness of the materials for durability, contour, and esthetics. This ensures that the wax patterns and resultant crowns can be restored to the desired form.

Contouring Wax Patterns

Modern indirect techniques permit the contouring of wax patterns on the master cast with the aid of the surveyor blade. All abutment teeth to be restored with castings can be prepared at one time and an impression made that will provide an accurate stone replica of the prepared arch. Wax patterns may then be refined on separated individual dies or removable dies. All abutment surfaces facing edentulous areas should be made parallel to the path of placement by the use of the surveyor blade (Figure 13-21). This technique will provide proximal surfaces that will be parallel without any further alteration in the mouth, will permit the most positive seating of the removable partial denture along the path of placement, and will provide the least amount of undesirable space beneath minor connectors for the lodgment of debris.

Rest Seats

After the proximal surfaces of the wax patterns have been made parallel, and buccal and lingual contours have been established to satisfy the requirements of stability and retention with the best possible esthetic placement of clasp arms, the occlusal rest seats should be prepared in the wax pattern rather than in the finished restoration. The placement of occlusal rests should be considered at the time the teeth are prepared to receive cast restorations so that there will be sufficient clearance beneath the floor of the occlusal rest seat. Too many times a completed cast restoration is cemented in the mouth for a removable partial denture abutment without any provision for the occlusal rest having been made in the wax pattern. The dentist then proceeds to prepare an occlusal rest seat in the cast restoration, being ever conscious of the fact that he or she may perforate the casting during the process of forming the rest seat. The unfortunate result is usually a poorly formed rest seat that is too shallow.

If tooth structure has been removed to provide placement of the occlusal rest seat, it may be ideally placed in the wax pattern by using a No. 8 round bur to lower the marginal ridge and establish the outline form of the rest, and then using a No. 6 round bur to slightly deepen the floor of the rest seat inside this lowered marginal ridge. This approach provides an occlusal rest that best satisfies the requirements that it be placed so that any occlusal force will be directed axially and that there will be the least possible interference to occlusion with the opposing teeth.

Perhaps the most important function of a rest is the division of stress loads from the removable partial

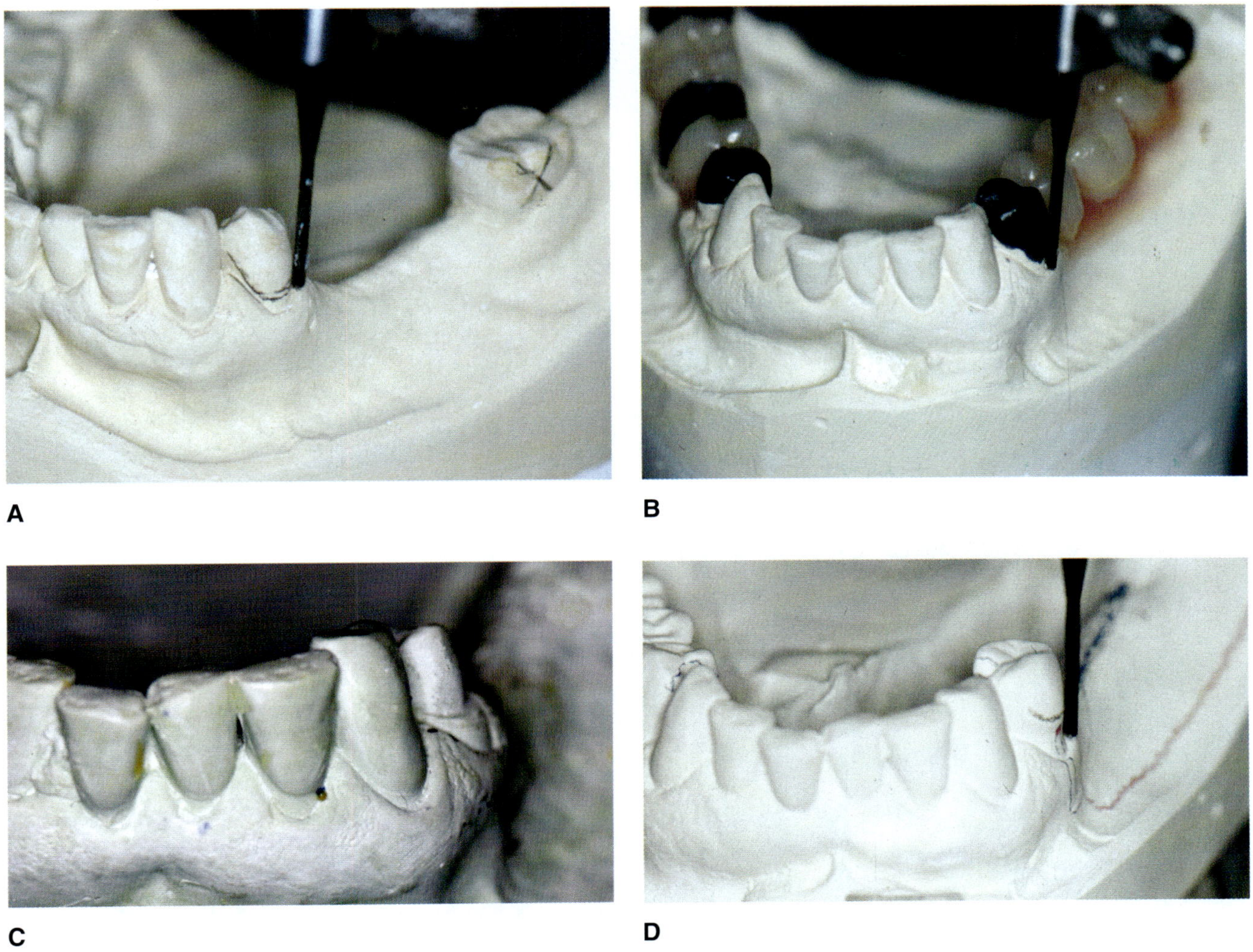

Figure 13-20 **A,** Diagnostic cast at an orientation best for all abutments considered. Buccal survey line is too close to the marginal gingival and the distal surface does not lend itself to guide plane preparation. A surveyed crown is indicated. **B,** Abutment contours, appropriate to clasp design (distal guide plane and mid-buccal 0.01 inch undercut), are produced in wax. The benefit of this procedure is to determine tooth preparation requirements necessary to produce the surveyed crown contours. Tooth reduction needs differ if the contours are excessive (high survey lines) versus under-contoured (low survey line, as in this example). **C,** Cast of abutment preparation providing buccal surface reduction adequate to replace with metal ceramic material at the required contour. Without careful consideration of survey line placement needs prior to and during preparation it is easy to reproduce incorrect contours in finished crowns. **D,** Cast of seated surveyed crown demonstrating desired contours for clasp design chosen.

denture to provide the greatest efficiency with the least damaging effect to the supporting abutment teeth. For a distal extension removable partial denture, the rest must be able to transmit occlusal forces to the abutment teeth in a vertical direction only, thereby permitting the least possible lateral stress to be transmitted to the abutment teeth.

For this reason, the floor of the rest seat should incline toward the center of the tooth so that the occlusal forces, insofar as possible, are centered over the root apex. Any form other than spoon shape can permit a locking of the occlusal rest and the transmission of tipping forces to the abutment tooth. A ball-and-socket type of relationship between occlusal rest and abutment tooth is the most desirable. At the same time, the marginal ridge must be lowered so that the angle formed by the occlusal rest with the minor connector will stand as little as possible above the occlusal surface of the abutment tooth, thus avoiding interference with the opposing teeth. Simultaneously, sufficient bulk must be provided to prevent a weakness in the occlusal rest at the marginal ridge.

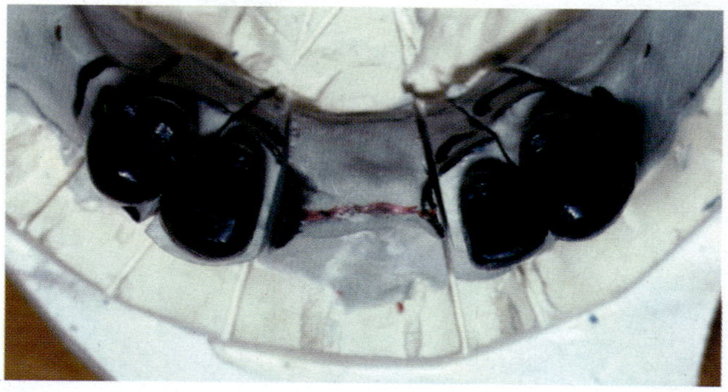

A

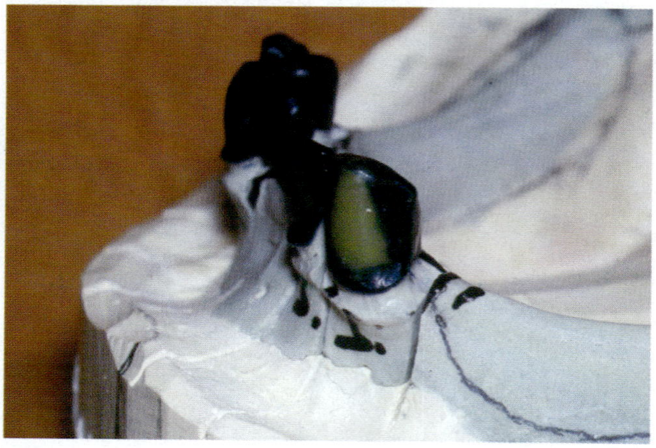

B

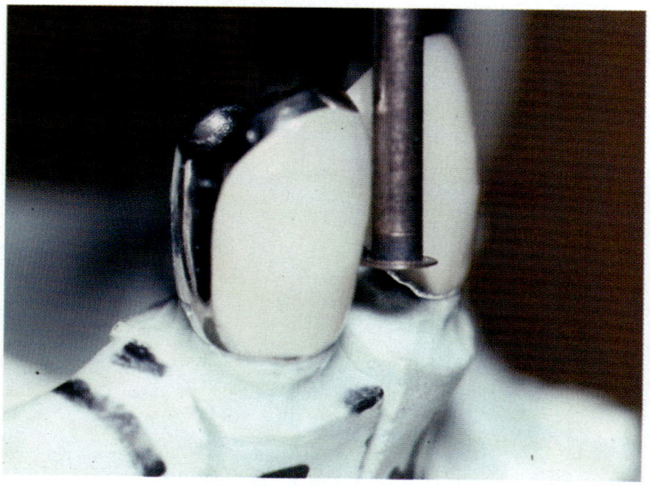

C

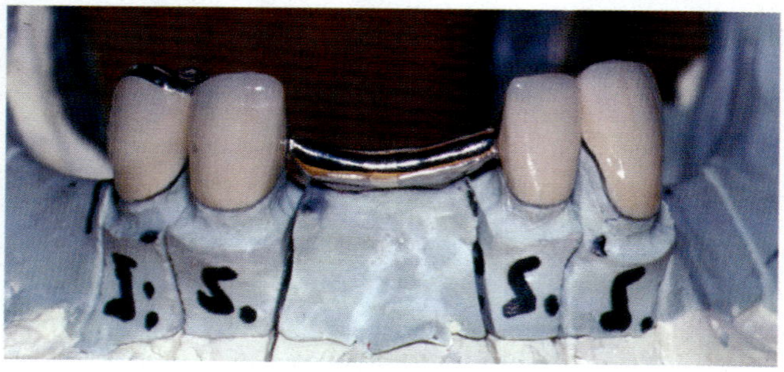

D

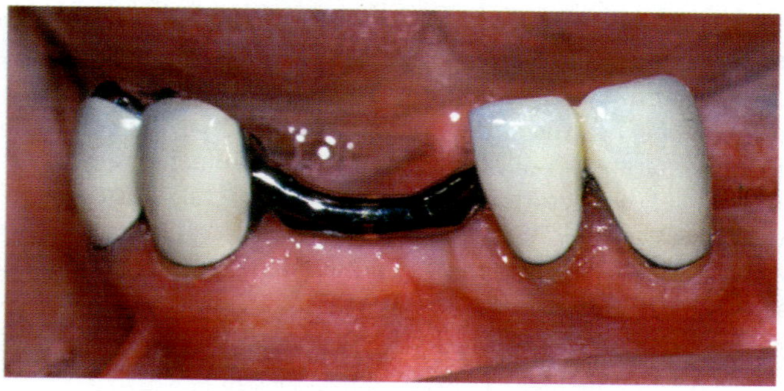

E

Figure 13-21 **A,** Occlusal view of full contour wax patterns. Crowns will be splinted together (#s 22-23, #s 27-28) and across the midline using a 13-gauge splint bar. Rests are evident on the lingual surfaces of the abutment wax patterns. **B,** Wax patterns showing labial cut-back for porcelain. Bilateral guide plane surfaces will be reproduced in metal and are parallel to the path of insertion. **C,** An abutment veneered crown with an appropriate height of contour and 0.02-inch undercut for the anticipated wrought wire retainer. **D,** Completed prosthesis splinted between retainer crowns and across the midline. Splint bar with added vertical support and provide indirect retention. **E,** Prosthesis inserted intraorally.

The marginal ridge must be lowered and yet not be the deepest part of the rest preparation. To permit occlusal stresses to be directed toward the center of the abutment tooth, the angle formed by the floor of the occlusal rest with the minor connector should be less than 90°. In other words, the floor of the occlusal rest should incline slightly from the lowered marginal ridge toward the center of the tooth.

This proper form can be readily accomplished in the wax pattern if care is taken during crown or inlay preparation to provide the location of the rest. If direct restorations are used, sufficient bulk must be present in this area to allow proper occlusal rest seat form without weakening the restoration. There is insufficient evidence to show that direct restorations used as rest seats perform equal to enamel. When the rest seat is placed in sound enamel, it is best accomplished by the use of round carbide burs (No. 4, 6, and 8 sizes) that leave a smooth enamel surface.

Rest seat preparations in sound enamel (or in existing restorations that are not to be replaced) should always follow the recontouring of proximal tooth surfaces. The preparation of proximal tooth surfaces should be done first because if the occlusal portion of the rest seat is placed first and the proximal tooth surface is altered later, the outline form of the rest seat is sometimes irreparably altered.

Following proximal surface recontouring (guide plane preparation), the larger round bur is used to lower the marginal ridge 1.5 to 2.0 mm while creating the relative outline form of the rest seat. The result is a rest seat preparation with the marginal ridge lowered and the gross outline form established, but without sufficient deepening of the rest seat preparation toward the center of the tooth. A smaller round bur (a No. 4 or 6) may then be used to deepen the floor of the rest seat to a gradual incline toward the center of the tooth. Enamel rods are then smoothed by the planing action of a round bur revolving with little pressure. Abrasive rubber points are sufficient to complete the polishing of the rest seat preparation.

The success or failure of a removable partial denture depends on how well the mouth preparations are accomplished. It is only through intelligent planning and competent execution of mouth preparations that the denture can satisfactorily restore lost dental functions and contribute to the health of the remaining oral tissue.

SELF-ASSESSMENT AIDS

1. A prescribed prosthesis not only must replace what is missing but also, of even greater importance, must ________ what is remaining.
2. Preparation of oral structures most often involves three categories. One of these categories is oral surgical preparation. What are the other two?
3. Which treatment should be accomplished first—oral surgery or preparation of abutment teeth? Why?
4. Generally, all retained roots or root fragments should be removed as a mouth preparation procedure. True or false?
5. All impacted teeth should be considered for removal. However, any impacted tooth that can be reached with a periodontal probe must be removed. True or false?
6. Unopposed posterior teeth quite often extrude, severely limiting space for a prosthesis and the opportunity to create a harmonious occlusion. Name different methods by which these discrepancies may be corrected, depending of course on the severity of the malpositions.
7. When a suspicious radiopaque area is seen while viewing a panoramic roentgenogram of a patient, what procedures—listed in chronological order—must be undertaken to resolve the possible problem?
8. Visual examination, carefully conducted, reveals undesirable bony exostoses or tori in some patients. Unless these are removed, the restoration design will be compromised. In what areas are these various protuberances likely to be found?
9. Why should hyperplastic tissue seen in the form of fibrous tuberosities, flabby ridges, folds of redundant tissue in vestibular regions, and palatal papillomatosis be surgically removed before the construction of a removable restoration?
10. Discuss the influence of muscle attachments and frena that are inserted on the crest of residual ridges in relation to denture stability.
11. Should all abnormal soft tissue lesions be excised and submitted for pathological examination before fabrication of a removable restoration? Why or why not?
12. Excessively resorbed residual ridges offer comparatively poor support for removable restorations. Augmentation of alveolar bone to increase ridge height and width may be a viable surgical procedure for certain patients. Name a material used for such a procedure.
13. What is an oral osseointegrated device? What role can be envisioned for such devices in removable prosthodontics?
14. What are elastopolymers used for in removable prosthodontics?
15. Should irritated and distorted oral tissues optimally be returned to a state of health before final impressions are made? Why or why not?
16. Examination of a patient having removable partial dentures discloses a palatal inflammation. What other factors must be considered in formulating a thorough differential diagnosis?

17. Abused and irritated oral tissues most often respond favorably to tissue-conditioning procedures. Describe an acceptable order of procedures to be undertaken to institute a good tissue conditioning program.
18. Periodontal therapy should be completed before restorative procedures are undertaken. True or false?
19. What are the overall objectives of periodontal therapy for the partially edentulous patient?
20. The indication for occlusal adjustment is based on the presence of a pathological condition rather than on a preconceived articular pattern. Support and explain this statement.
21. What procedure(s) are most often used to eliminate gross occlusal interferences initially as a phase of periodontal considerations?
22. What is a nightguard and what purpose does it serve?
23. Teeth that demonstrate mobility at the time of the initial examination may be temporarily splinted. How does this help to establish a prognosis?
24. Under what clinical circumstances should minor tooth movement by orthodontic means be considered to enhance treatment?
25. State five distinct advantages of performing periodontal therapy (when indicated) before fabricating a removable prosthesis.
26. Through intelligent planning and competent execution of mouth preparations, the denture can satisfactorily restore lost dental functions and contribute to the health of the remaining oral tissue. True or false?

14

PREPARATION OF ABUTMENT TEETH

After surgery, periodontal treatment, endodontic treatment, and tissue conditioning of the arch involved, the abutment teeth may be prepared to provide support, stabilization, reciprocation, and retention for the removable partial denture. Rarely if ever is the situation encountered in which alterations of the abutment are not indicated because teeth do not develop with guiding planes, rests, and contours to accommodate clasp assemblies.

A favorable response to any deep restorations, endodontic therapy, and the results of periodontal treatment should be established before fabrication of the removable partial denture. If the prognosis of a tooth under treatment becomes unfavorable, its loss can be compensated for by a change in the removable partial denture design. If teeth are lost after the removable partial denture is fabricated, then the removable partial denture must be added to or replaced. Most removable partial denture designs do not lend themselves well to later additions, although this possibility should be considered in the original design of a denture. Every diagnostic aid should be used to determine which teeth are to be used as abutments or are potential abutments for future designs. When an original abutment is lost, it is extremely difficult to effectively modify the removable partial denture to use the next adjacent tooth as a retaining unit.

It is sometimes possible to design a removable partial denture so that a single posterior abutment that is questionable can be retained and used to support one end of a tooth-supported base. Then, if that posterior abutment were to be lost, it can be replaced with a distal extension base (see Figure 12-25). Such a design must include provision for future indirect retention, flexible clasping on the remaining terminal abutment, and provision for establishing tissue support by a secondary impression. *Anterior abutments, which are considered poor risks, may not be so freely used because of the problems involved in adding a new abutment retainer when the original one is lost.* Such questionable teeth should be planned for extraction in favor of a better abutment.

CLASSIFICATION OF ABUTMENT TEETH

The subject of abutment preparations may be grouped as follows: (1) those abutment teeth that require only minor modifications to their coronal portions, (2) those that are to have restorations other than complete coverage crowns, and (3) those that are to have crowns (complete coverage).

Abutment teeth that require only minor modifications include teeth with sound enamel, those with small restorations not involved in the removable partial denture design, those with acceptable restorations that will be involved in the removable partial denture design, and those that have existing crown restorations requiring minor modification that will not jeopardize the integrity of the crown. The latter may exist either as an individual crown or as the abutment of a fixed partial denture.

The use of unprotected abutments has been discussed previously. Although complete coverage of all abutments may be desirable, it is not always possible or practical. The decision to use unprotected abutments involves certain risks of which the patient must be advised and includes responsibility for maintaining oral hygiene and caries control. Making crown restorations fit existing denture clasps is a difficult task; however, the fact that it is possible may influence the decision to use uncrowned but otherwise sound teeth as abutments.

Complete coverage restorations provide the best possible support for occlusal rests. If the patient's economic status or other factors beyond the control of the dentist prevent the use of complete coverage restorations, then an amalgam alloy restoration if properly condensed is capable of supporting an occlusal rest without appreciable flow for a long period. Any existing silver amalgam alloy restoration about which there is any doubt should be replaced with new amalgam restorations. This should be done before the preparation of guiding planes and occlusal rest seats to allow the restoration to reach maximum strength and to be polished.

Continued improvement in dimensional stability, strength, and wear resistance of composite resin restorations will add another dimension to the preparation and modification of abutment teeth for removable partial dentures that should be less invasive than placement of complete coverage restorations and more economical.

SEQUENCE OF ABUTMENT PREPARATIONS ON SOUND ENAMEL OR EXISTING RESTORATIONS

Abutment preparations on sound enamel or on existing restorations that have been judged as acceptable should be done in the following order:

1. Proximal surfaces parallel to the path of placement should be prepared to provide guiding planes (Figure 14-1, *A*).
2. Tooth contours should be modified (Figure 14-1, *B* and *C*), lowering the height of contour so that (a) the origin of the circumferential clasp arms may be placed well below the occlusal surface, preferably at the junction of the middle and gingival thirds; (b) retentive clasp terminals may be placed in the gingival third of the crown for better esthetics and better mechanical advantage; and (c) reciprocal clasp arms may be placed on and above a height of contour that is no higher than the cervical portion of the middle third of the crown of the abutment tooth.
3. After alterations of axial contours are accomplished and before rest seat preparations are instituted, an impression of the arch should be made in irreversible hydrocolloid and a cast formed in a fast-setting stone. This cast can be returned to the surveyor to determine the adequacy of axial alterations before proceeding with rest seat preparations. If axial surfaces require additional axial recontouring, it can be performed during the same appointment and without compromise.
4. Occlusal rest areas should be prepared that will direct occlusal forces along the long axis of the abutment tooth (Figure 14-1, *D*). Mouth preparation should follow the removable partial denture design that was outlined on the diagnostic cast at the time the cast was surveyed and the treatment plan confirmed. Proposed changes to abutment teeth should be made on the diagnostic cast and outlined in colored pencil to indicate the area, amount, and angulation of the modification to be done (see Chapter 12). Although occlusal rest seats may also be prepared on the diagnostic cast, indication of their location in colored pencil is usually sufficient for the experienced dentist because rest preparations follow a definite pattern (see Chapter 6).

ABUTMENT PREPARATIONS USING CONSERVATIVE RESTORATIONS

Conventional inlay preparations are permissible on the proximal surface of a tooth not to be contacted by a minor connector of the removable partial denture. On the other hand, proximal and occlusal surfaces that support minor connectors and occlusal rests require somewhat different treatment. The extent of occlusal coverage (i.e., whether cusps are covered) will be governed by the usual factors, such as the extent of caries, the presence of unsupported enamel walls, and the extent of occlusal abrasion and attrition.

When an inlay is the restoration of choice for an abutment tooth, certain modifications of the outline form are necessary. To prevent the buccal and lingual proximal margins from lying at or near the minor connector or the occlusal rest, these margins must be extended well beyond the line angles of the tooth. This additional extension may be accomplished by widening the conventional box preparation. However, the margin of a cast restoration produced for such a preparation may be quite thin and may be damaged by the clasp during placement or removal of the removable partial denture. This hazard may be prevented by extending the outline of the box beyond the line angle, thus producing a strong restoration-to-tooth junction.

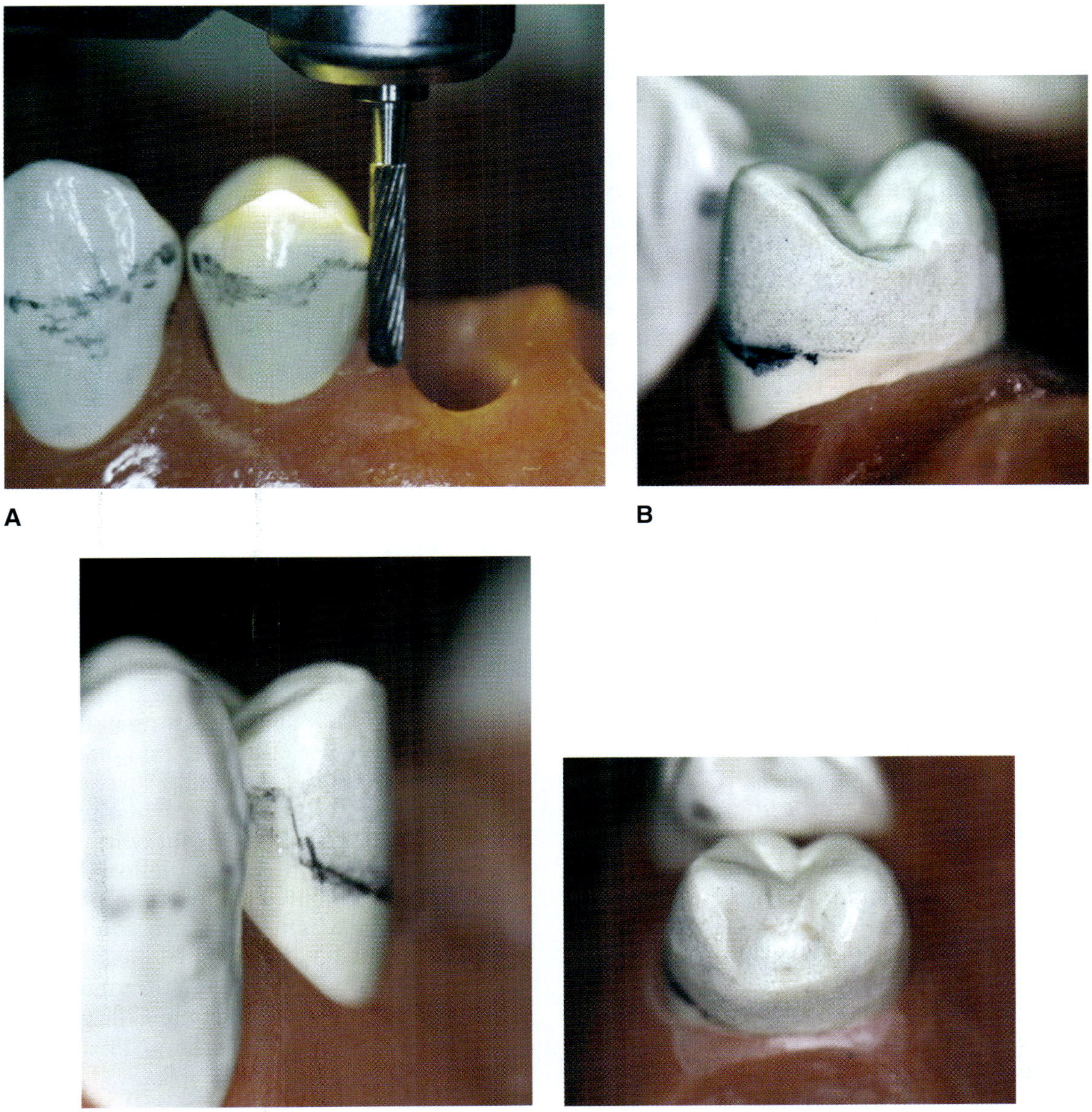

A B C D

Figure 14-1 Abutment contours should be altered during mouth preparations in the following sequence. **A,** Proximal surface is prepared parallel to path of insertion to create guiding plane. **B,** Height of contour on buccal (and lingual) is lowered when necessary to permit clasp placement to be located more favorably (i.e., middle-gingival third). Tooth reduction should be parallel to the guide plane reduction, followed by contouring the tooth occlusal to the new height of contour to allow a gradual convergence. **C,** Labial reduction demonstrating favorable location of height of contour and mesio-buccal undercut location. Occlusal convergence of height of contour is also evident. **D,** Spoon-shaped disto-occlusal rest preparation that will direct occlusal forces along long axis of tooth should be the final step in mouth preparations.

In this type of preparation, the pulp is particularly vulnerable unless the axial wall is curved to conform to the external proximal curvature of the tooth. When caries is of minimal depth, the gingival seat should have an axial depth at all points about the width of a No. 559 fissure bur. It is of utmost importance that the gingival seat be placed where it can be easily accessed to maintain good oral hygiene. The proximal contour necessary to produce the proper guiding plane surface and the close proximity of the minor connector render this area particularly vulnerable to future caries. Every effort should be made to provide the restoration with maximum resistance and retention, and with clinically imperceptible margins. The first requisite can be satisfied by preparing opposing cavity walls 5° or less from parallel and producing flat floors and sharp, clean line angles.

It is sometimes necessary to use an inlay on a mandibular first premolar for the support of an indirect retainer. The narrow occlusal width buccolingually and the lingual inclination of the occlusal surface of such a tooth often complicate the two-surface inlay preparation. Even the most exacting occlusal cavity preparation often leaves a thin and weak lingual cusp remaining.

ABUTMENT PREPARATIONS USING CROWNS

When multiple crowns are to be restored as removable partial denture abutments, it is best that all wax patterns be made at the same time. A cast of the arch with removable dies may be used if they are stable and sufficiently keyed for accuracy. If preferred, contouring wax patterns and making them parallel may be done on a solid cast of the arch (Figure 14-2), with individual dies to refine margins. Modern impression materials and indirect techniques make either method equally satisfactory.

The same sequence for preparing teeth in the mouth applies to the contouring of wax patterns. After the cast has been placed on the surveyor to conform to the selected path of placement and after the wax patterns have been preliminarily carved for occlusion and contact, proximal surfaces that are to act as guiding planes are carved parallel to the path of placement with a surveyor blade. Guiding planes are extended from the marginal ridge to the junction of the middle and gingival thirds of the involved tooth surface. One must be careful not to extend the guiding plane to the gingival margin, because the minor connector must be relieved when it crosses the gingiva. A guiding plane that includes the occlusal two thirds or even one third of the proximal area is usually adequate without endangering gingival tissue.

After the guiding planes are parallel and any other contouring is accomplished to accommodate the removable partial denture design, occlusal rest seats are carved in the wax pattern. This method has been outlined in Chapter 6.

It should be emphasized that critical areas prepared in wax should not be destroyed by careless spruing or polishing. The wax pattern should be sprued to preserve paralleled surfaces and rest areas. Polishing should consist of little more than burnishing. Rest seat areas should need only refining with round finishing burs. If some interference by spruing is unpreventable, the casting must be returned to the surveyor for proximal surface refinement. This can be done accurately with the aid of a handpiece holder attached to the vertical spindle of the surveyor or some similar machining device.

One of the advantages of making cast restorations for abutment teeth is that mouth preparations that would otherwise have to be done in the mouth may be done on the surveyor with far greater accuracy. It is generally impossible to make several proximal surfaces parallel to one another when preparing them intraorally. The opportunity for contouring wax patterns and making them parallel on the surveyor in relation to a path of placement should be used to its full advantage whenever cast restorations are being made (Figure 14-3).

The ideal crown restoration for a removable partial denture abutment is the complete coverage crown, which can be carved, cast, and finished to ideally

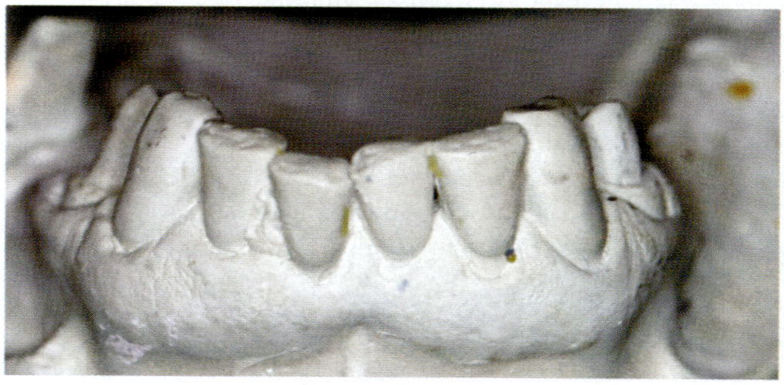

Figure 14-2 Solid cast of multiple abutment crowns for a removable partial denture. Wax patterns for crown #s 21, 28, 30, and 31 can be completed at the same time using the identical cast orientation. This allows control of the path of insertion features on all fitting surfaces of the removable prostheses.

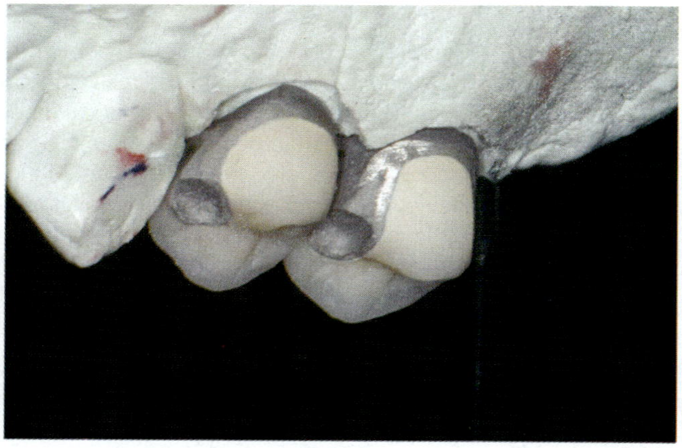

Figure 14-3 Metal ceramic crowns for teeth #s 4 and 5 demonstrating occlusal rests in metal and evidence of palatal finishing procedures. Distal surface of tooth #4 provides a guide plane surface that is continued on to a portion of the lingual surface for maximum stabilization.

satisfy all requirements for support, stabilization, and retention without compromise for cosmetic reasons. Porcelain veneer crowns can be made equally satisfactory but only by the added step of contouring the veneered surface on the surveyor before the final glaze. If this is not done, retentive contours may be excessive or inadequate.

The three-quarter crown does not permit creating retentive areas as does the complete coverage crown. However, if buccal or labial surfaces are sound and retentive areas are acceptable or can be made so by slight modification of tooth surfaces, the three-quarter crown is a conservative restoration of merit. The same criteria apply in the decision to leave a portion of an abutment unprotected as in the decision to leave any tooth unprotected that is to serve as a removable partial denture abutment.

Regardless of the type of crown used, the preparation should be made to provide the appropriate depth for the occlusal rest seat. This is best accomplished by altering the axial contours of the tooth to the ideal before preparing the tooth and creating a depression in the prepared tooth at the occlusal rest area (Figure 14-4). Because the location of occlusal rests is established during treatment planning, this information will be known in advance of any tooth preparations. If, for example, double occlusal rests are to be used, this will be known so that the tooth can be prepared to accommodate the depth of both rests. It is inexcusable when waxing a pattern to find that a rest seat has to be made more shallow than is desirable because of posttreatment planning. It can also create serious problems when having to make a rest seat shallow in an existing crown or inlay because its thickness is not known. The opportunity for creating an ideal rest seat (if it has been properly planned) depends only on the few seconds it takes to create a space for it.

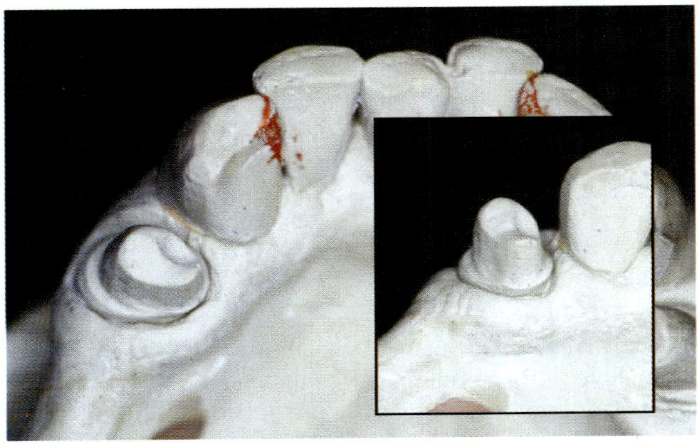

Figure 14-4 Metal-ceramic crown preparation on tooth #21 showing MO rest space provided in the crown preparation at the mesial. Inset shows perspective of the vertical height this provides for the rest to be prepared in the wax pattern.

Ledges on Abutment Crowns

In addition to providing abutment protection, more ideal retentive contours, definite guiding planes, and optimum occlusal rest support, complete coverage restorations on teeth used as removable partial denture abutments offer still another advantage not obtainable on natural teeth. This is the crown ledge or shoulder, which provides effective stabilization and reciprocation.

The functions of the reciprocal clasp arm have been stated in Chapter 6. Briefly, these are reciprocation, stabilization, and auxiliary indirect retention. Any rigid reciprocal arm may provide horizontal stabilization if it is located on axial surfaces parallel to the path of placement. To a large extent, because it is placed at the height of convexity, a rigid reciprocal arm may also act as an auxiliary indirect retainer. However, its function as a reciprocating arm against the action of the retentive clasp arm is limited only to stabilization against possible orthodontic movement when the denture framework is in its terminal position. Such reciprocation is needed when the retentive clasp produces an active orthodontic force because of accidental distortion or improper design. Reciprocation to prevent transient horizontal forces that may be detrimental to abutment stability is most needed when the restoration is placed or when a dislodging force is applied. Perhaps the term orthodontic force is incorrect, because the term signifies a slight but continuous influence that would logically reach equilibrium when the tooth is orthodontically moved. Instead the transient forces of placement and removal are intermittent but forceful, which can lead to periodontal destruction and eventual instability rather than to orthodontic movement.

True reciprocation is not possible with a clasp arm that is placed on an occlusally inclined tooth surface because it does not become effective until the prosthesis is fully seated. When a dislodging force is applied, the reciprocal clasp arm, along with the occlusal rest, breaks contact with the supporting tooth surfaces, and they are no longer effective. Thus as the retentive clasp flexes over the height of contour and exerts a horizontal force on the abutment, reciprocation is nonexistent just when it is needed most (Figure 14-5).

True reciprocation can be obtained only by creating a path of placement for the reciprocal clasp arm that is parallel to other guiding planes. In this manner the inferior border of the reciprocal clasp makes contact with its guiding surface before the retentive clasp on the other side of the tooth begins to flex (Figure 14-6). Thus reciprocation exists during the entire path of placement and removal. The presence of a ledge on the abutment crown acts as a terminal stop for the reciprocal clasp arm. It also augments the occlusal rest and provides indirect retention for a distal extension removable partial denture.

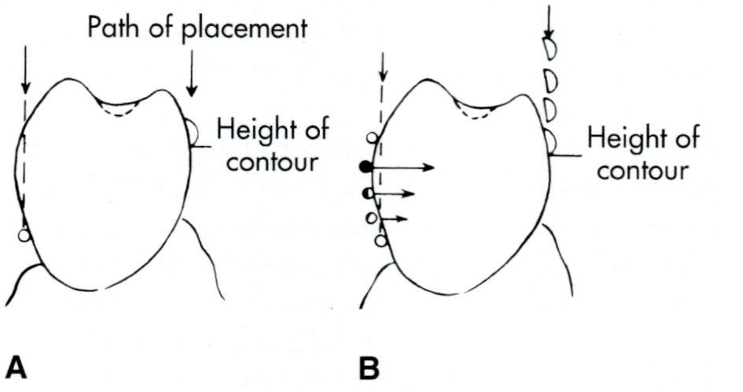

Figure 14-5 **A,** Incorrect relationship of retentive and reciprocal clasp arm to each other when removable partial denture framework is fully seated. As retentive clasp arm flexes over height of contour during placement and removal, reciprocal clasp arm cannot be effective because it is not in contact with tooth until denture framework is fully seated. **B,** Horizontal forces applied to abutment tooth as retentive clasp flexes over height of contour during placement and removal. Open circle at top and bottom illustrates that retentive clasp is only passive at its first contact with tooth during placement and when in its terminal position with denture fully seated. During placement and removal, rigid clasp arm placed on opposite side of tooth cannot provide resistance against these horizontal forces. See Figure 14-6 for a method to ensure true reciprocation.

A ledge on an abutment crown has still another advantage. The usual reciprocal clasp arm is half-round, and therefore convex, and is superimposed on and increases the bulk of an already convex surface. A reciprocal clasp arm built on a crown ledge is actually inlayed into the crown and reproduces more normal crown contours (see Figure 14-6). The patient's tongue then contacts a continuously convex surface rather than the projection of a clasp arm. Unfortunately the enamel is neither thick enough nor the tooth so shaped that an effective ledge can be created on an unrestored tooth. Narrow enamel shoulders are sometimes used as rest seats on anterior teeth, but these do not provide the parallelism that is essential to reciprocation during placement and removal.

The crown ledge may be used on any complete or three-quarter crown restored surface that is opposite the retentive side of an abutment tooth. It is used most frequently on premolars and molars but also may be used on canine restorations. It is not ordinarily used on buccal surfaces for reciprocation against lingual retention because of the excessive display of metal, but it may be used just as effectively on posterior abutments when esthetics is not a factor.

The fact that a crown ledge is to be used should be known in advance of crown preparation to ensure sufficient removal of tooth structure in

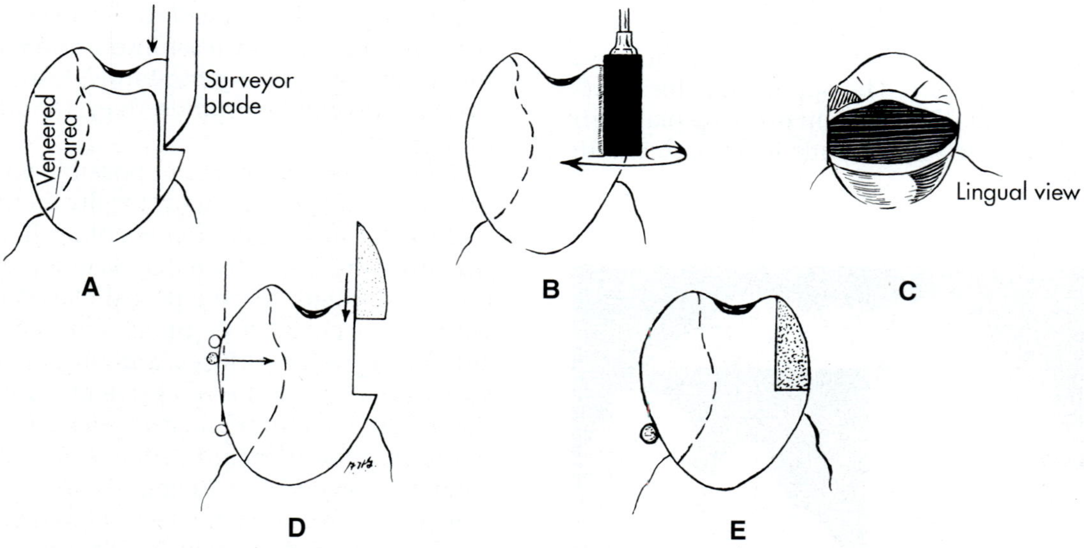

Figure 14-6 **A,** Preparation of ledge in wax pattern with surveyor blade parallel to path of placement. **B,** Refinement of ledge on casting, using suitable stone or milling device in handpiece attached to dental surveyor or specialized drill press for same purpose. **C,** Approximate width and depth of ledge formed on abutment crown, which will permit reciprocal clasp arm to be inlaid within normal contours of tooth. **D,** True reciprocation throughout full path of placement and removal is possible when reciprocal clasp arm is inlaid onto ledge on abutment crown. **E,** Direct retainer assembly is fully seated. Reciprocal arm restores lingual contour of abutment.

this area. Although a shoulder or ledge is not included in the preparation itself, adequate space must be provided so that the ledge may be made sufficiently wide and the surface above it made parallel to the path of placement. The ledge should be placed at the junction of the gingival and middle thirds of the tooth, curving slightly to follow the curvature of the gingival tissue. On the side of the tooth where the clasp arm will originate, the ledge must be kept low enough to allow the origin of the clasp arm to be wide enough for sufficient strength and rigidity.

In forming the crown ledge, which is usually located on the lingual surface, the wax pattern of the crown is completed—except for refinement of the margins—before the ledge is carved. After the proximal guiding planes and the occlusal rests and retentive contours are formed, the ledge is carved with the surveyor blade so that the surface above is parallel to the path of placement. Thus a continuous guiding plane surface will exist from the proximal surface around the lingual surface.

The full effectiveness of the crown ledge can only be achieved when the crown is returned to the surveyor for refinement after casting. To afford true reciprocation, the crown casting must have a surface above the ledge that is parallel to the path of placement. This can be accomplished with precision only by machining the casting parallel to the path of placement with a handpiece holder in the surveyor or some other suitable machining device (Figure 14-7). Similarly the parallelism of proximal guiding planes needs to be perfected after casting and polishing. Although it is possible to approximate parallelism and, at the same time, form the crown ledge on the wax pattern with a surveyor blade, some of its accuracy is lost in casting and polishing. The use of suitable burs, such as No. 557, 558, and 559 fissure burs and true cylindrical carborundum stones in the handpiece holder, permits the paralleling of all guiding planes on the finished casting with the accuracy necessary for the effectiveness of those guiding plane surfaces.

The reciprocal clasp arm is ultimately waxed on the investment cast so that it is continuous with the ledge inferiorly and contoured superiorly to restore the crown contour, including the tip of the cusp.

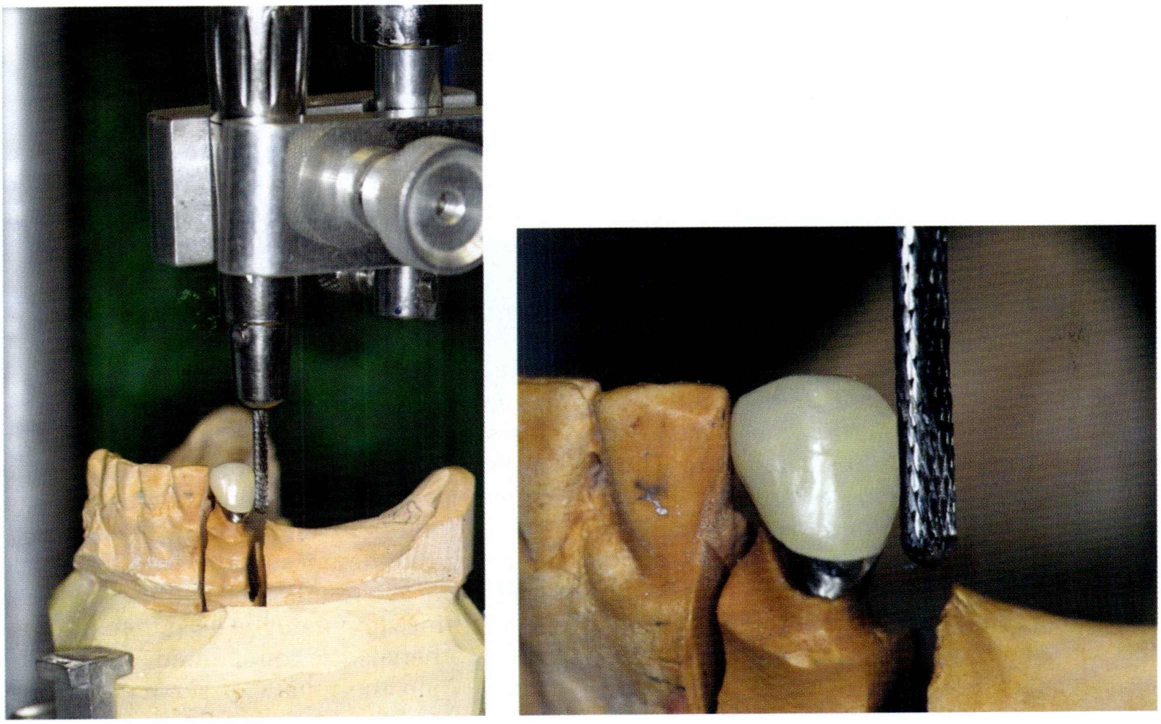

A B

Figure 14-7 Milling of surveyed crowns to prepare parallel surfaces, internal rest seats, lingual grooves, and ledges in cast restorations requires use of either a specialized milling machine, or a handpiece holder attached to a surveyor, as shown in **A**. This allows final adjustments to surveyed crowns before cementation, and assures maximum parallelism or ledge preparation. **B,** Close-up of proximal guide plane preparation with metal finishing bur.

It is obvious that polishing must be controlled so as not to destroy the form of the shoulder that was prepared in wax or the parallelism of the guiding plane surface. It is equally vital that the removable partial denture casting be finished with great care so that the accuracy of the counterpart is not destroyed. Modern investments, casting alloys, and polishing techniques make this degree of accuracy possible.

Spark Erosion

Spark erosion technology is a highly advanced system for producing the ultimate in precision fit of the reciprocal arm to the ledge on the casting. This technology uses a tool system that permits repositioning the casting with great accuracy and an electric discharge machine that is programmed to erode minute metal particles through periodic spark intervals.

Regardless of the method or technique used, it is imperative that the predetermined cast orientation be maintained to ensure that ledges and proximal guide planes remain parallel.

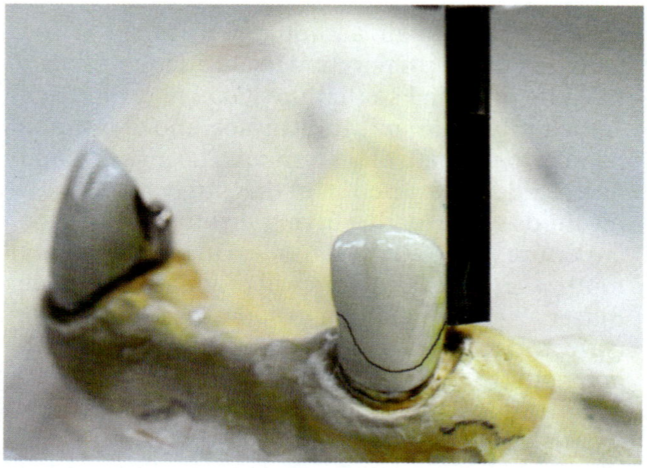

Figure 14-8 Porcelain veneer crown is resurveyed following adjustment, glazing, and polishing. It is important to survey crowns returned from the laboratory prior to cementation. The best means to ensure control of all abutment contours for a removable partial denture is when surveyed crowns are used and they are resurveyed prior to permanent placement.

Veneer Crowns for Support of Clasp Arms

For cosmetic reasons, resin and porcelain veneer crowns are used on abutment teeth that would otherwise display an objectionable amount of metal. They may be in the form of porcelain veneers retained by pins and cemented to the crown; porcelain fused directly to a cast metal substructure; porcelain fused to a machined coping; cast porcelain; pressed ceramic crowns; computer assisted designed and machined ceramic restorations; or acrylic resin processed directly to a cast crown. The development of abrasion-resistant composites offers materials suitable for veneering that can withstand clasp contact, thereby eliminating an undesirable display of metal.

Veneer crowns must be contoured to provide suitable retention. This means that the veneer must be slightly overcontoured and then shaped to provide the desired undercut for the location of the retentive clasp arm (Figure 14-8). If the veneer is of porcelain, this procedure must precede glazing; if it is of resin, it must precede final polishing. If this important step in making veneered abutments is neglected or omitted, excessive or inadequate retentive contours may result.

In limited clinical trials, porcelain laminates have demonstrated resistance to wear for the equivalent of 5 years. The porcelain, however, resulted in slight wear on the clasps.

The flat underside of the cast clasp makes sufficient contact with the surface of the veneer so that abrasion of the resin veneer may result. Although the underside of the clasp may be polished (with some loss in accuracy of fit), abrasion results from the trapping and holding of food debris against the tooth surface as the clasp moves during function. Therefore, unless the retentive clasp terminal rests on metal, glazed porcelain should be used to ensure the future retentiveness of the veneered surface. Present-day acrylic resins, being cross-linked copolymers, will withstand abrasion for considerable time but not nearly to the same degree as porcelain. Therefore acrylic resin veneers are best used in conjunction with metal that supports the half-round clasp terminal.

SPLINTING OF ABUTMENT TEETH

Often a tooth is considered too weak to use alone as a removable partial denture abutment because of the short length or excessive taper of a single root or because of bone loss resulting in an unfavorable crown-root ratio. In such instances, splinting to the adjacent tooth or teeth can be used as a means of improving abutment support. Thus two single-rooted teeth serve as a multirooted abutment.

Splinting should not be used to retain a tooth that would otherwise be condemned for periodontal reasons. When the length of service of a restoration depends on the serviceability of an abutment, any periodontally questionable tooth should be condemned in favor of using an adjacent healthy tooth as the abutment, even though the span is increased one tooth by doing so.

The most common application of the use of multiple abutments is the splinting of two premolars or a first premolar and a canine (Figure 14-9). Mandibular premolars generally have round and tapered roots, which are easily loosened by rotational and tipping forces. They are the weakest of the posterior abutments. Maxillary premolars also often have tapered roots, which may make them poor risks as abutments, particularly when they will be called on to resist the leverage of a distal extension base. Such teeth are best splinted by casting or soldering two crowns together. When a first premolar to be used as an abutment has poor root form or support, it is best that it be splinted to the stronger canine.

Anterior teeth on which lingual rests are to be placed often must be splinted together to prevent orthodontic movement of individual teeth. Mandibular anterior teeth are seldom used for support, but if they are, splinting of the teeth involved is advisable. When splinting is impossible, individual lingual rests on cast restorations may be slightly inclined apically to prevent possible tooth displacement, or lingual rests may be used in conjunction with incisal rests, slightly engaging the labial surface of the teeth.

Lingual rests should always be placed as low on the cingulum as possible, and single anterior teeth, other than canines, should not be used for occlusal support. Where lingual rests are used on central and lateral incisors, as many teeth as possible should be included to distribute the load, thereby minimizing the force on any one tooth. Even so, some movement of individual teeth is likely to occur, particularly when they are subjected to the forces of indirect retention or when bone support is compromised. This is best prevented by splinting several teeth with united cast restorations. The condition of the teeth and cosmetic considerations will dictate whether complete crowns, three-quarter crowns, pin ledge inlays, resin-bonded retainers, or composite restorations will be used for this purpose.

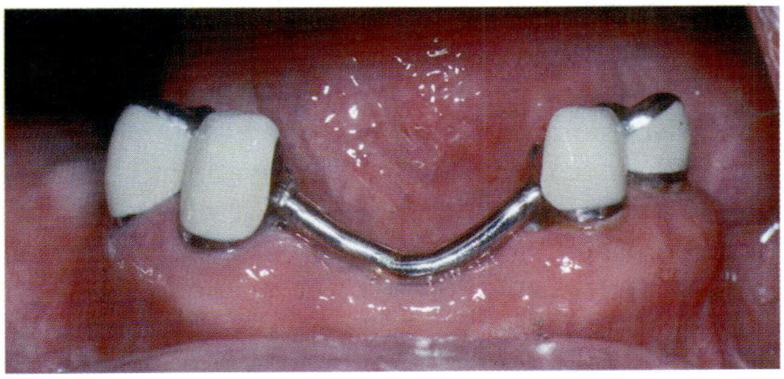

Figure 14-9 First premolars and canines have been splinted in this Class I, mod 1, partially edentulous arch. Splint bar was added to provide cross-arch stabilization for splinted abutments and to support and retain anterior segment of removable restoration. Prospective longevity of abutments has been enhanced.

Splinting of molar teeth for multiple abutment support is less frequently used because they are generally multirooted. A two- or three-rooted tooth that is not strong enough alone is probably a poor abutment risk. However, there may be notable exceptions when a molar abutment would benefit from the effect of splinting as in a hemisected molar root (Figure 14-10).

USE OF ISOLATED TEETH AS ABUTMENTS

The average abutment tooth is subjected to some distal tipping, rotation, torquing, and horizontal movement, all of which must be held to a minimum by the quality of tissue support and the design of the removable partial denture. The isolated abutment tooth, however, is subjected also to mesial tipping because of lack of proximal contact. Despite indirect retention, some lifting of the distal extension base is inevitable, causing torque to the abutment.

In a tooth-supported prosthesis, an isolated tooth may be used as an abutment by including a fifth abutment for additional support. Thus rotational and horizontal forces are resisted by the additional stabilization obtained from the fifth abutment. When two such isolated abutments exist, a sixth abutment should be included for the same reason. Thus the two canines, the two isolated premolars, and the two posterior teeth are used as abutments.

In contrast, an isolated anterior abutment adjacent to a distal extension base usually should be splinted to the nearest tooth by means of a fixed partial denture. The effect is twofold: (1) the anterior edentulous segment is eliminated, thereby creating an intact dental arch anterior to the edentulous space; and (2) the isolated tooth is splinted to the other abutment of the fixed partial denture, thereby providing multiple abutment support. Splinting should be used here only to gain multiple abutment support rather than to support an otherwise weak abutment tooth.

Although splinting is advocated for abutment teeth that are considered too weak to risk using alone, a single abutment standing alone in the dental arch anterior to a distal extension basal seat generally requires the splinting effect of a fixed partial denture (Figures 14-11 and 14-12). Even though the form and length of the root and the supporting bone seem to be adequate for an ordinary abutment, the fact that the tooth lacks proximal contact endangers the tooth when it is used to support a distal extension base removable partial denture.

A second factor that may influence the decision to use an isolated tooth as an abutment is an esthetic consideration. However, neither esthetics nor economics should deter the dentist from recommending

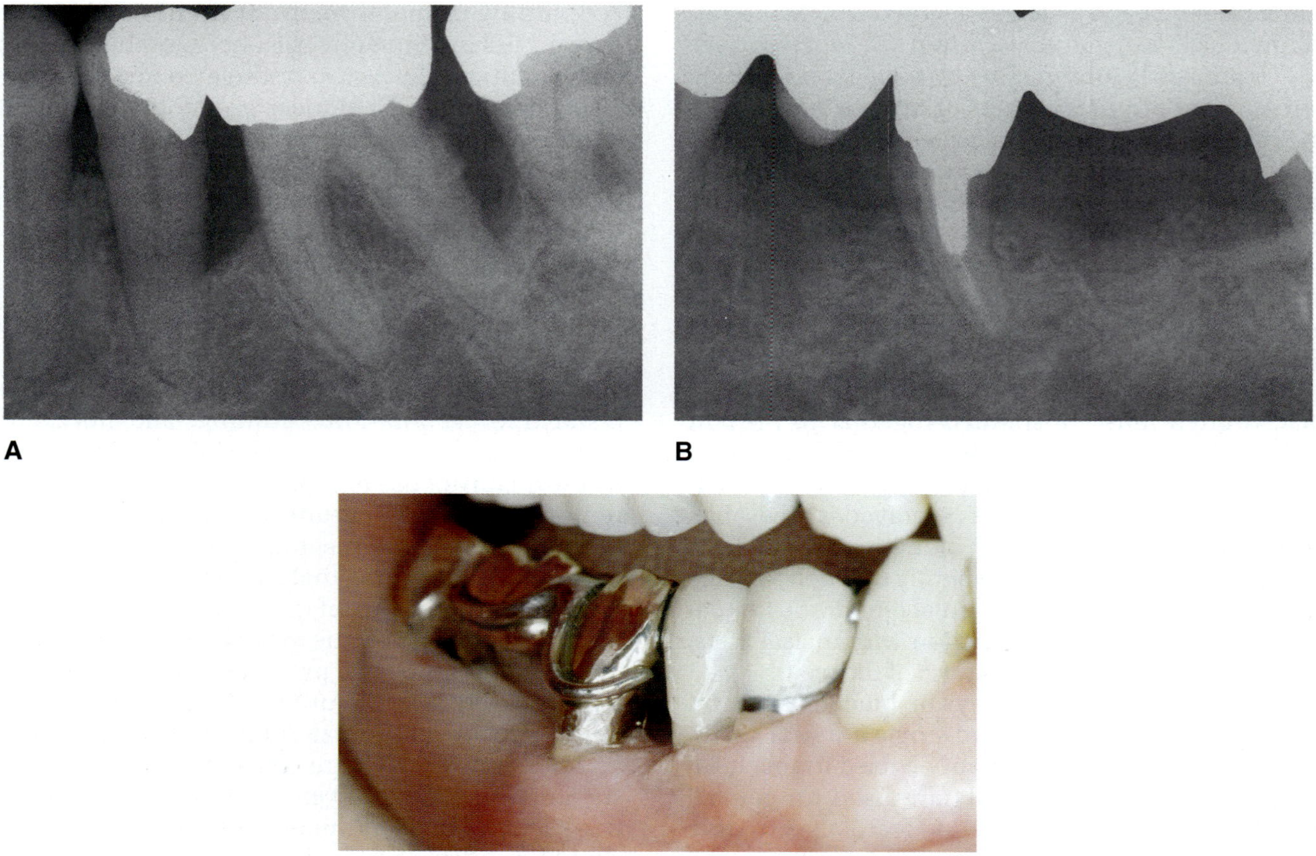

A B C

Figure 14-10 **A,** Periodontal disease required removal of #30 distal and #31 mesial roots. **B,** First premolar and hemi-sected roots were splinted using a 5-unit fixed partial denture. **C,** Fixed prosthesis provided cross-arch support, stability, and retention to a Kennedy Class II removable partial denture.

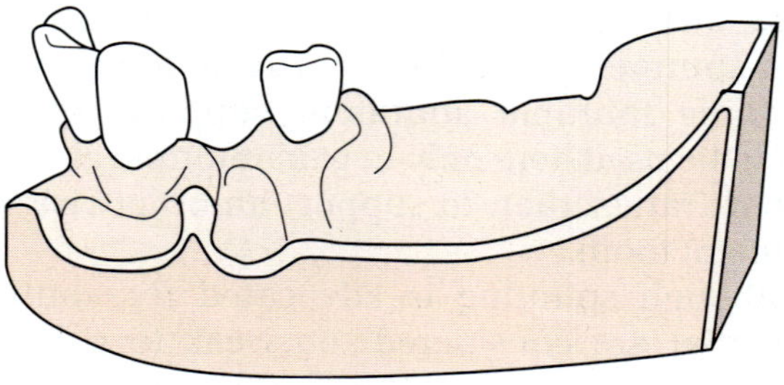

Figure 14-11 Lone standing premolar should be splinted to canine with fixed partial denture. Not only will design of removable partial denture be simplified, but longevity of abutment service by premolar will be greatly extended.

to the patient that an isolated tooth to be used as a terminal abutment be given the advantage of splinting by means of a fixed partial denture. If compromises are necessary, the patient must assume the responsibility for the use of the isolated tooth as an abutment.

The economic aspect of using fixed restorations as part of the mouth preparations for a removable partial denture is essentially the same as for any other splinting procedure. The best design of the fixed partial denture, which will ensure the longevity of its service, makes the additional procedure and expense necessary. Although it must be recognized that economic considerations, combined with a particularly favorable prognosis of an isolated tooth, may influence the decision to forego the advantages of using a fixed partial denture, the original treatment plan should include this provision even though the alternative method may be accepted for economic reasons.

MISSING ANTERIOR TEETH

When a removable partial denture is to replace missing posterior teeth, especially in the absence of distal abutments, any additional missing anterior teeth are best replaced by means of fixed restorations rather

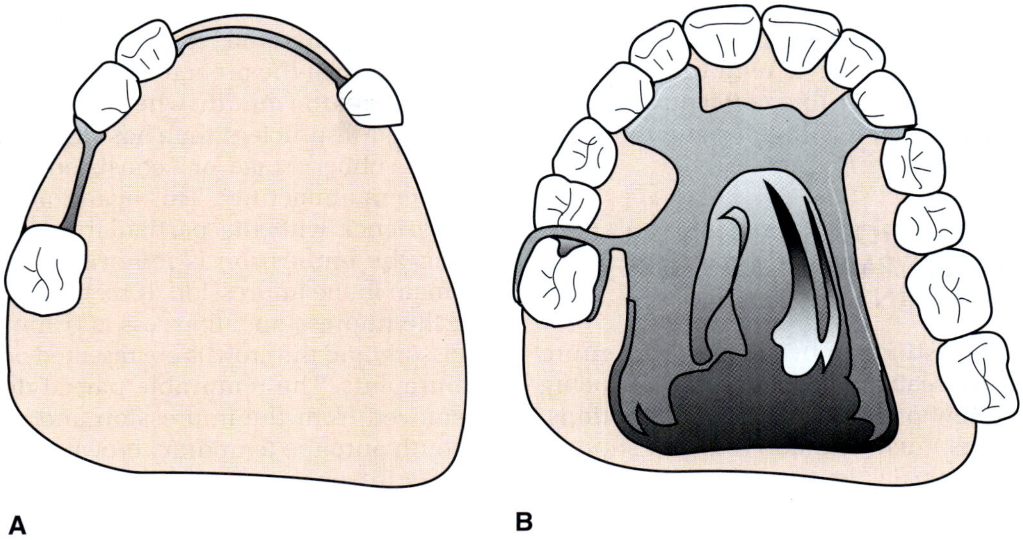

Figure 14-12 **A,** Isolated abutments have been splinted using splint bars. **B,** Removable partial denture is more adequately supported by splinting mechanism shown in **A** than could be realized with isolated abutments.

than included in the removable partial denture. In any distal extension situation, some anteroposterior rotational action will result from the addition of an anterior segment to the denture. The ideal treatment plan, which would consider the anterior edentulous space separately, may result in conflict with economic and esthetic realities. Each situation must be treated according to its own merits. Often the best esthetic result can be obtained by replacing missing anterior teeth and tissue with the removable partial denture rather than with a fixed restoration. From a biomechanical standpoint, however, it is generally advisable that a removable partial denture should replace only the missing posterior teeth after the remainder of the anterior arch has been made intact by fixed restorations.

Although the need for compromise is recognized, the decision to include an anterior segment on the denture depends largely on the support available for that part of the removable partial denture. The greater the number of natural anterior teeth remaining, the better the available support for the edentulous segment. If definite rest seats can be prepared on multiple abutments, the anterior segment may be treated as any other tooth-bounded modification space. Sound principles of rest support apply just as much as elsewhere in the arch. Inclined tooth surfaces should not be used for occlusal support, nor should rests be placed on unprepared lingual surfaces. The best possible support for an anterior segment is multiple support extending, if possible, posteriorly across prepared lingual rest seats on the canine teeth to mesioocclusal rest seats on the first premolars. Such support would permit the missing anterior teeth to be included in the removable partial denture, often with some cosmetic advantages over fixed restorations.

In some instances the replacement of anterior teeth by means of a removable partial denture cannot be prevented. However, without adequate tooth support, any such prosthesis will lack the stability that would exist from replacing only the posterior teeth with the removable partial denture and the anterior teeth with fixed restorations. When anterior teeth have been lost through accident or have been missing for some time, resorption of the anterior residual ridge may have progressed to the point that neither fixed nor removable pontics may be butted to the residual ridge. In such instances, for reasons of esthetics and orofacial tissue support, the missing teeth must be replaced with a denture base supporting teeth that are more nearly in their original position, considerably forward from the residual ridge. Although such teeth may be positioned to better cosmetic advantage, the contouring and coloring of a denture base to be esthetically pleasing require the maximum artistic effort of both the dentist and the technician. Such a removable partial denture, both from an esthetic and biomechanical standpoint, is one of the most difficult of all prosthetic restorations. However, a splint bar, connected by abutments on both sides of the edentulous space, will provide much-needed support and retention to the anterior segment of the removable partial denture. Because the splint bar will provide vertical support, rest seats on abutments adjacent to the edentulous area need not be prepared, thus simplifying an anterior restoration to some extent.

Recognition is given to the concept of dual path of placement to enhance the esthetic replacement of missing anterior teeth with a removable partial. Sources of information on this concept are made available in the Selected Reading Resources of this text under *Partial Denture Design.*

TEMPORARY CROWNS WHEN A REMOVABLE PARTIAL DENTURE IS BEING WORN

Occasionally an existing removable partial denture must remain serviceable while the mouth is being prepared for a new prosthesis. In such situations, temporary crowns must be made that will support the old removable partial denture and will not interfere with its placement and removal. Acrylic resin temporary crowns that duplicate the original form of the abutment teeth must be made.

The technique for making temporary crowns to fit direct retainers is similar to that for other types of acrylic resin temporary crowns. The principal difference is that an impression, using an elastic impression material, must be made of the entire arch with the existing removable partial denture in place. It is necessary that the removable partial denture remain in the impression, when it is removed from the mouth. If it remains in the mouth, it must be removed and inserted in the impression in its designated position. The impression, with the removable partial denture in place, is disinfected, wrapped in a wet paper towel (if irreversible hydrocolloid was used as the impression material), or placed in a plastic bag, and set aside while the tooth or teeth are being prepared for new crowns.

After the preparations are completed and the impressions and jaw relation records have been made, the prepared teeth are dried and lubricated. The original impression is trimmed to eliminate any excess, undercuts, and interproximal projections that would interfere with the replacement of the impression in the mouth.

The methyl methacrylate acrylic resins, composites, copolymers, and fiber-reinforced resins may serve as excellent materials for temporary crowns in conjunction with removable partial dentures. Making temporary crowns requires a small mixing cup or dappen dish; a cement spatula; and a small, disposable, plastic syringe. Autopolymerizing acrylic resin of the appropriate tooth color is placed in the cup or dappen dish, and monomer is added to make a slightly viscous mix. The volume should be slightly in excess of the amount estimated to fabricate the temporary restorations. The mix should be spatulated to a smooth consistency and the mix immediately poured into the barrel of the disposable syringe. A small amount of the mix should be injected over and around the margins of the prepared teeth. The remaining material should be injected into the impression of the prepared teeth. The impression is seated into the mouth, where the dentist holds it in place until sufficient time has elapsed for it to reach a stiff, rubbery stage, or a consistency recommended by the manufacturer. This again must be based on experience with the particular resin used. At this time the impression is removed. The crowns may remain in the impression. If so, they are stripped out of the impression, all excess is trimmed away with scissors, and the crowns are reseated on the prepared abutments. The removable partial denture is then removed from the impression and reseated in the mouth onto the temporary crowns, which should be in a stiff-rubbery state. The patient may bring the teeth into occlusion to reestablish the former position and occlusal relationship of the existing removable partial denture.

After the resin crown or crowns have polymerized, the removable partial denture is removed, and the crowns remain on the teeth. These are then carefully removed, contoured to accommodate oral hygiene access, trimmed, polished, and temporarily cemented. The result is a temporary crown that restores the original abutment contours and allows the removable partial denture to be placed and removed without interference, but providing the same support temporarily to the denture that existed before the teeth were prepared.

Cementation of Temporary Crowns

Cementation of temporary crowns may require slight relief of the internal surface of the crowns to accommodate the temporary cement and to facilitate removal. The temporary cement should be thin and applied only to the inside gingival margin of the crowns to ensure complete seating. As soon as the temporary cement has hardened, the occlusion should be checked and adjusted accordingly. Regardless of the type of temporary cement used, any excess that might irritate the gingivae should be removed.

FABRICATING RESTORATIONS TO FIT EXISTING DENTURE RETAINERS

It is often necessary that an abutment tooth be restored with a complete crown (or other restoration) that will fit the inside of the clasp of an otherwise serviceable removable partial denture. One technique for doing so is simple enough, but it requires that an indirect-direct pattern be made and therefore justifies a fee for service above that for the usual restoration.

The technique for making a crown to fit the inside of a clasp is as follows: An irreversible hydrocolloid impression of the mouth is made with the removable partial denture in place. This impression, which is used to make the temporary crown, is wrapped in a wet paper towel or placed in a plastic bag and set aside while the tooth is being prepared. Even though several abutment teeth are to be restored, it is usually necessary that each temporary restoration be completed before the next one is begun. This is necessary so that the original support and occlusal relationship of the removable partial denture can be maintained as each new temporary crown is being made. During the preparation of the abutment tooth, the removable partial denture is replaced frequently to ascertain that sufficient tooth structure is removed to allow for the thickness of the casting. When the preparation is completed, an individual impression of the tooth is obtained from which a stone die is made. A temporary crown is then made in the original irreversible hydrocolloid impression as outlined in the preceding paragraphs. It is trimmed, polished, and temporarily cemented, and the removable partial denture is returned to the mouth. The patient is dismissed after the excess cement has been removed.

On the stone die made from the individual impression, a thin, autopolymerizing resin coping will be formed with a brush technique. The stone die should first be trimmed to the finishing line of the preparation, which is then delineated with a pencil, and the die painted with a tinfoil substitute. A separating material, such as a tinfoil substitute, should be used and will form a thin film on a cold, dry surface. Not all tinfoil substitutes are suitable for this purpose. With autopolymerizing resin powder and liquid in separate dappen dishes and a fine brush, a coping of resin of uniform thickness is painted onto the die. This should extend not quite to the pencil line representing the limit of the crown preparation. After hardening, the resin coping may be removed, inspected, and trimmed if necessary. The thin film of foil substitute should be removed before the coping is reseated onto the die.

The wax pattern buildup on the resin coping is usually not begun until the patient returns. A sequence using a functional chew-in technique for occlusion would be followed, establishing proximal contact and contours appropriate for the clasp assembly as outlined below.

First, the occlusal portion of the wax pattern is established by having the patient close into maximum intercuspation, followed by excursive movements (Figure 14-13, *A*). The wax pattern is returned to the cast, and additions are made as required to dull areas. The process is repeated until a smooth occlusal registration has been obtained. Except for narrowing of the occlusal surface and the carving of grooves and spillways, this will be the occlusal anatomy of the finished restoration.

The second step is the addition of sufficient wax to establish contact relations with the adjacent tooth. At this time, the occlusal relation of the marginal ridges also must be established. Next, wax is added to buccal and lingual surfaces where the clasp arms will contact the crown, and the wax pattern is again reseated in the mouth. The clasp arms, minor connectors, and occlusal rests involved on the removable partial denture are carefully warmed with a needlepoint flame, carefully avoiding any adjacent resin, and the removable partial denture is positioned in the mouth and onto the wax pattern (Figure 14-13, *B*). Several attempts may be necessary until the removable partial denture is fully seated and the components of the clasp are clearly recorded in the wax pattern. Each time the removable partial denture is removed, the pattern will draw with it and must be teased out of the clasp.

When contact with the clasp arms and the occlusal relation of the removable partial denture have been established satisfactorily, the temporary crown may be replaced and the patient dismissed. The crown pattern is completed on the die by narrowing the occlusal surface buccolingually, adding grooves and spillways, and refining the margins.* Any wax ledge remaining below the reciprocal clasp arm may be left to provide some of the advantages of a crown ledge, which were described earlier in this chapter. Excess wax remaining below the retentive clasp arm, however, must be removed to permit the addition of a retentive undercut later (Figure 14-13, *C*).

If a veneer material is to be added, the veneer space must now be carved in the wax pattern. In such situations, the contour of the veneer may be recorded by making a stone matrix of the buccal surface, which can be repositioned on the completed casting to ensure the proper contour of the composite veneer.

The wax pattern must be sprued with care so that essential areas on the pattern are not destroyed. After casting, the crown should be subjected to a minimum of polishing, because the exact form of the axial and occlusal surfaces must be maintained.

*Margins on all crown and inlay wax patterns can be refined with S.S. White red casting wax, which contrasts with the blue or green wax used for the pattern and permits the carving of delicate margins with accuracy. The preferred wax for the body of crown and inlay patterns is Maves inlay wax. This wax is available in both cone and stick form and has excellent carving properties and color.

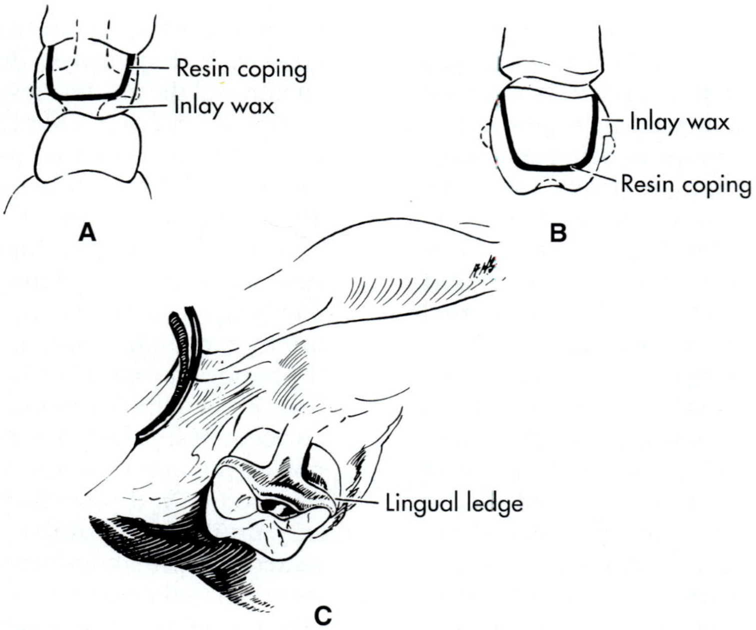

Figure 14-13 Making of cast crown to fit existing removable partial denture clasp. **A,** Thin acrylic resin coping is first made on individual die of prepared tooth. Inlay wax is then added and coping placed onto prepared tooth where occlusal surfaces and contact relations are established directly in mouth. Clasp assembly is warmed with needlepoint flame only enough to soften inlay wax, and removable partial denture is placed in mouth where it is guided gently into place by opposing occlusion. This step must be repeated several times and excess wax removed or wax added until full supporting contact with underside of clasp assembly has been established, with denture fully seated. Usually wax pattern withdraws with denture and must be gently teased out of clasp each time. **B,** Wax pattern is then placed back onto individual die to complete occlusal anatomy and refine margins. Excess wax remaining below impression of retentive clasp arm must be removed, but wax ledge may be left below reciprocal clasp arm. **C,** Finished casting in mouth. Terminus of retentive clasp is then readapted to engage undercut. It is frequently necessary to remove some interference from casting, as indicated by articulating paper placed between clasp and crown, until clasp is fully seated.

Because it is impossible to withdraw a clasp arm from a retentive undercut on the wax pattern, the casting must be made without any provision for clasp retention. After the crown has been tried in the mouth with the denture in place, the location of the retentive clasp terminal is identified by scoring the crown with a sharp instrument. Then the crown may be ground and polished slightly in this area to create a retentive undercut. The clasp terminal then may be carefully adapted into this undercut, thereby creating clasp retention on the new crown.

An alternate method for making crowns to fit existing retainers uses mounted casts with the removable prosthesis adapted to the working cast to develop the occlusal surfaces for the involved crowns.

Ideally, all abutment teeth would best be protected with complete crowns before the removable partial denture is fabricated. Except for the possibility of recurrent caries because of defective crown margins or gingival recession, abutment teeth so protected may be expected to give many years of satisfactory service in the support, stabilization, and retention of the removable partial denture. Economically a policy of insisting on complete coverage for all abutment teeth may well be justified from a long-term viewpoint. It must be recognized, however, that in practice complete coverage of all abutment teeth is not always possible at the time of treatment planning. Many factors influence the future health status of an abutment tooth, some of which cannot be foreseen. It is necessary that the dentist be able to treat abutment teeth that later become defective so that their service as abutments may be restored and serviceability of the removable partial denture maintained. Although not part of the original mouth preparations, this service accomplishes much the same objective by providing support, stability, and retention, and the dentist must be technically capable of providing this removable partial denture service when it becomes necessary.

SELF-ASSESSMENT AIDS

1. What does the use of a terminal molar abutment contribute to a removable partial denture?
2. Endodontic treatment of any tooth in the arch (when indicated) should be performed before making a final impression for a removable restoration. Why?
3. If one is faced with a single posterior abutment (second molar), and there is some doubt that it can be retained and used as one end of a tooth-supported base, what options are available for design of the denture?
4. Abutment preparations on sound enamel should be accomplished in a definite order with the altered and designed diagnostic cast used as a blueprint. Give the order of preparation, including a method to check this preparation.
5. What is the danger of preparing an occlusal rest seat before contouring the guiding plane?
6. Inlay preparations on teeth to be used as removable partial denture abutments differ from conventional inlay preparations in three requirements. What are they?
7. Where is the most vulnerable area on an abutment tooth, with regard to cleanliness?
8. Give the sequence of contouring wax patterns for abutment restorations to obtain ideal contours for optimum location of components by use of a dental cast surveyor.
9. A rest seat is carved on the occlusal surface of a complete coverage crown wax pattern for a posterior abutment. The occlusal morphology has been carved to satisfy occlusal requirements, and axial contours have also been accomplished. The rest seat preparation, however, is inadequate because of its shallowness, created by insufficient room between the preparation and opposing occlusion in the area of the rest seat. What options exist to prevent a compromised result?
10. Crown ledges, parallel to the path of placement, are often carved on the lingual surfaces of abutment crowns. How does this enhance the direct retainer assembly?
11. Contrast the quality of reciprocation afforded by a crown ledge on a molar abutment and that offered by the lingual surface of an unrestored molar abutment.
12. Explain the method of preparing a lingual ledge on the wax pattern for an abutment crown. Include its depth, width, extent, and definitive location.
13. How may the crown ledge be refined after the crown has been cast?
14. Describe the contour of the component of the direct retainer assembly that occupies the crown ledge preparation.
15. It is rare that the ceramic surface of a ceramometal crown can be fabricated and finished freehand to exhibit the exact planned height of contour for a retentive clasp arm. How may a surveyor be used to ensure that the planned location of the height of contour is established? At what stage in the fabrication of the crown should the procedure be undertaken?
16. Splinting of adjacent teeth is sometimes indicated as a means of gaining multiple abutment support. What examination data would indicate that splinting should be performed?
17. Where is the most common application of multiple abutments by splinting found in an arch?
18. Often the design of a restoration requires lingual rests on lower anterior teeth. How can orthodontic movement of these teeth be minimized?
19. Isolated abutments adjacent and anterior to edentulous residual ridges usually have a poor prognosis. What is the reason for this?
20. An isolated anterior abutment adjacent to a distal extension base, when splinted to the nearest tooth, provides two beneficial effects. What are these desirable effects?
21. An isolated abutment adjacent to an extension base may be splinted to the nearest tooth by either a fixed partial denture or a ______.
22. Missing anterior teeth should be replaced with fixed partial dentures rather than included in a removable restoration. What are the contraindications for the preceding treatment?
23. On rare occasions an abutment tooth supporting a removable partial denture will have to be restored with an inlay or crown. Describe a procedure whereby an abutment crown can be fabricated to fit an existing direct retainer.

15

IMPRESSION MATERIALS AND PROCEDURES FOR REMOVABLE PARTIAL DENTURES

Impression materials used in the various phases of partial denture fabrication may be classified as being rigid, thermoplastic, or elastic substances. Rigid impression materials are those that set to a rigid consistency. Thermoplastic impression materials are those that become plastic at higher temperatures and resume their original form when cooled. Elastic impression materials are those that remain in an elastic or flexible state after they have set and have been removed from the mouth.

Although rigid impression materials may be capable of recording tooth and tissue details accurately, they cannot be removed from the mouth without fracture and reassembly. Thermoplastic materials cannot record minute details accurately because they undergo permanent distortion during withdrawal from tooth and tissue undercuts. Elastic materials are the only ones that can be withdrawn from tooth and tissue undercuts without permanent deformation and are therefore most generally used for making impressions for removable partial dentures, immediate dentures, crowns, and fixed partial dentures when tooth and tissue undercuts and surface detail must be recorded with accuracy.

RIGID MATERIALS*

Plaster of Paris

One type of rigid impression material is plaster of Paris, which has been used in dentistry for over 200 years. Although all plaster of Paris impression materials are handled in approximately the same manner, the setting and flow characteristics of each manufacturer's product will vary. Some are pure and finely ground, with only an accelerator

*Some of the historical parts of this discussion have been quoted or paraphrased from McCracken WL: Impression materials in prosthetic dentistry, Dent Clin North Am, 2:671-684, 1958.

added to expedite setting within reasonable working limits. Others are modified impression plasters in which binders and plasticizers have been added to permit limited border manipulation while the material is setting. These do not set as hard or fracture as cleanly as pure plaster of Paris and therefore cannot be reassembled with as much accuracy if fracture occurs.

Plaster of Paris was once the only material available for removable partial denture impressions, but now elastic materials have completely replaced the impression plasters in this phase of prosthetic dentistry. It is still widely used for making accurate transfers of abutment castings or copings in the fabrication of fixed restorations and internal attachment dentures and for making rigid indexes and matrices for various purposes in prosthetic dentistry. Modified impression plasters are used by many dentists to record maxillomandibular relationships (see Figure 20-2, *M-O*).

Metallic Oxide Paste

A second type of rigid impression material is metallic oxide paste, which is usually some form of a zinc oxide–eugenol combination. A number of these pastes are available. However, they are not used as primary impression materials and should never be used for impressions that include remaining natural teeth. They are also not to be used in stock impression trays.

Metallic oxide pastes are manufactured with a wide variation of consistencies and setting characteristics. For convenience, most of them are dispensed from two tubes, which enables the dentist to dispense and mix the correct proportion from each tube on a mixing slab. The previously prepared tray for the edentulous ridge segments is loaded and positioned in the mouth with or without any attempt at border molding. Border molding with metallic oxide impression pastes is not advisable because wrinkles will occur if movement is permitted at the time the material reaches its setting state.

As with all impression techniques, the accuracy of the primary impression and of the impression tray has a great influence on the final impression. Some metallic oxide pastes remain fluid for a longer period than do others, and some manufacturers claim that border molding is possible. In general, however, all metallic oxide pastes have one thing in common with plaster of Paris impression materials: they all have a setting time during which they should not be disturbed and after which no further border molding is effective.

Metallic oxide pastes, being rigid substances, can be used as secondary impression materials for complete dentures and for extension base edentulous ridge areas of a removable partial denture if a custom impression tray has been properly designed and attached to the removable partial denture framework (see Chapter 16).

Metallic oxide pastes can also be used as an impression material for relining distal extension denture bases and may be used successfully for this purpose if the original denture base has been relieved sufficiently to allow the material to flow without displacement of either the denture or the underlying tissue.

THERMOPLASTIC MATERIALS*

Modeling Plastic

Like plaster of Paris, modeling plastic is among the oldest impression materials used in prosthetic dentistry. This material is most often used for border correction (border molding) of custom impression trays for Kennedy Class I and II removable partial denture bases. Modeling plastic is manufactured in several different colors, each color being an indication of the temperature range at which the material is plastic and workable. A common error in the use of modeling plastic is that it is often subjected to higher temperatures than intended by the manufacturer. It then becomes too soft and loses some of its favorable working characteristics. If a temperature-controlled water bath is not used, a thermometer should be used to maintain the water temperature. If modeling plastic is softened at a temperature above that intended by the manufacturer, the material becomes brittle and unpredictable. Also, there is the ever-present danger of burning the patient when the temperature used in softening the modeling plastic is too high.

The most commonly used modeling plastic for corrected impressions of extension base areas is the red (red-brown) material in cake form that softens at about 132° F. It should never be softened at temperatures much above this. Neither it nor any other modeling plastic should be immersed in the water bath for an indefinite period. It should be dipped and kneaded until soft and subjected to no more heat than necessary before loading the tray and positioning it in the mouth. Then it may be flamed with an alcohol torch for the purpose of border molding, but it should always be tempered by being dipped back into the water bath before its return to the mouth to prevent burning the patient. The modeling plastic then may be chilled using a water spray before removal from the mouth, although this

*Some of the historical parts of this discussion have been quoted or paraphrased from McCracken WL: Impression materials in prosthetic dentistry, Dent Clin North Am, 2:671-684, 1958.

is not necessary if care is used in removing the impression. During sectional flaming and border molding, the modeling plastic should be chilled in ice water after each removal from the mouth; then it may be trimmed with a sharp knife without danger of fracture or distortion.

The red, gray, and green modeling plastics are obtainable in stick form for use in border molding an impression or an impression tray. The green material is the lowest fusing of the modeling plastics. The red and gray sticks have a higher and broader working range than do the cakes of like color so that they may be flamed without harming the material. The gray material in stick form is preferred by some dentists for border molding because of its contrasting lighter color. The choice between the use of green and gray sticks is purely optional and entirely up to the dentist.

Some dentists still prefer to use modeling plastic as a secondary impression material to record edentulous ridges in removable partial denture fabrication. When this is done, it is generally used only as a means of building up the underside of the denture before recording the tissue with some secondary impression material (see Chapter 16).

Impression Waxes and Natural Resins

A second group of thermoplastic impression materials are those impression waxes and resins commonly spoken of as mouth-temperature waxes. The most familiar of these have been the Iowa wax* and the Korecta waxes,† all of which were developed for specific techniques. Knowledge of the characteristics of mouth-temperature waxes is important in using them correctly.

The Iowa wax was developed for use in recording the functional or supporting form of an edentulous ridge. It may be used either as a secondary impression material or as an impression material for relining the finished removable partial denture to obtain support from the underlying tissue. The mouth-temperature waxes lend themselves well to all relining techniques, as they will flow sufficiently in the mouth to prevent displacement of tissue. As with any relining technique, it is necessary that sufficient relief and venting be provided to give the material the opportunity to flow.

The difference between impression wax and modeling plastic is that impression waxes have the ability to flow as long as they are in the mouth and thereby permit equalization of pressure and prevent displacement. The modeling plastics flow only in proportion to the amount of flaming and tempering that can be done out of the mouth, and this does not continue after the plastic has approached mouth temperature. The principal advantage of mouth-temperature waxes is that given sufficient time they permit a rebound of tissue that may have been forcibly displaced.

The impression waxes also may be used to correct the borders of impressions made of more rigid materials, thereby establishing optimum contact at the border of the denture. All mouth-temperature wax impressions have the ability to record border detail accurately and include the correct width of the denture border. They also have the advantage of being correctable.

Mouth-temperature waxes vary in their working characteristics. They are designed primarily for impression techniques that attempt to record the tissue under an occlusal load. In such techniques the occlusion rim or the arrangement of artificial teeth is completed first. Mouth-temperature wax is then applied to the tissue side of the denture base, and the final impression is made under functional loading by using various movements to simulate functional activity. These mouth-temperature materials also may be used successfully in open-mouth impression techniques. Iowa wax will not distort after removal from the mouth at ordinary room temperatures, but the more resinous waxes must be stored at much lower temperatures to prevent flow when they are out of the mouth. Resinous waxes are not ordinarily used in removable partial denture impression techniques except for secondary impressions.

*Kerr Co., Romulus, MI.
†D-R Miner Dental, Concord, CA.

ELASTIC MATERIALS*

Reversible Hydrocolloids

Reversible (agar-agar) hydrocolloids, which are fluid at higher temperatures and gel upon reduction in temperature, are used primarily as impression materials for fixed restorations. They demonstrate acceptable accuracy when properly used. However, the reversible hydrocolloid impression materials offer few advantages over the irreversible (alginate) hydrocolloids when used as a removable partial denture impression material. Present-day irreversible hydrocolloids are sufficiently accurate for making master casts for removable partial dentures. However, border control of impressions made with these materials is difficult.

Irreversible Hydrocolloids

Irreversible hydrocolloids are used for making diagnostic casts, orthodontic treatment casts, and master

*Some of the historical parts of this discussion have been quoted or paraphrased from McCracken WL: Impression materials in prosthetic dentistry, Dent Clin North Am, 2:671-684, 1958.

casts for removable partial denture procedures. Because they are made of colloid materials, neither reversible nor irreversible hydrocolloid impressions can be stored for any length of time, but must be poured immediately.

These materials have low tear strength, provide less surface detail than other materials (e.g., mercaptan rubber base), and are not as dimensionally stable as other materials. They can, however, be used in the presence of moisture (saliva); are hydrophilic; pour well with stone; have a pleasant taste and odor; and are nontoxic, nonstaining, and inexpensive. The combination reversible-irreversible hydrocolloids have demonstrated a tendency to separate and should be used with that understanding. The hydrocolloids can be acceptably disinfected with a spray solution of 2% acid glutaraldehyde, stored in 100% humidity, and poured within 1 hour.

Mercaptan Rubber-Base Impression Materials

The mercaptan rubber-base (Thiokol) impression materials can also be used for removable partial denture impressions and especially for secondary corrected or altered cast impressions. To be accurate, the impression must have a uniform thickness that does not exceed 3 mm (1/8 inch). This necessitates the use of a carefully made individual impression tray of acrylic resin or some other material possessing adequate rigidity and stability. Those materials that are highly cross-linked (medium and heavy body) do not recover well from deformation and should not be used when large or multiple undercuts are present. For example, when large numbers of teeth with natural tooth contours that display multiple undercuts remain, these materials will be subjected to clinically significant distortion upon withdrawal. The long-term dimensional stability of these materials is poor because of the water loss after setting. The material must be held still during the impression-making procedure because it does not have a snap set. It should be allowed to rebound for 7 to 15 minutes after it is removed from the mouth and then should be poured immediately. Many of these materials have an unpleasant odor and can stain clothes. These materials are moderately inexpensive, have high tear strength, a long working and setting time (8 to 10 minutes), and can be disinfected in liquid, cold-sterilizing solutions. The accuracy of mercaptan rubber base is acceptable for making impressions for removable partial dentures. However, as with the hydrocolloid impression materials, certain precautions must be taken to prevent distortion of the impression. The mercaptan rubber-base impression materials do have an advantage over the hydrocolloid materials in that the surface of an artificial stone poured against them is of a smoother texture and therefore appears to be smoother and harder than one poured against a hydrocolloid material. This is probably because the rubber material does not have the ability to retard or etch the surface of the setting stone. Despite their accuracy, this has always been a disadvantage of all hydrocolloid impression materials. The fact that a smoother surface results does not, however, preclude the possibility of a grossly inaccurate impression and stone cast stemming from other causes. Rubber-base impression materials possess a longer setting time than the irreversible hydrocolloid materials and lend themselves better to border molding in adequate supporting trays.

Polyether Impression Materials

Polyether impression material is an elastic-type material, as are the polysulfide and silicone materials. These materials have demonstrated good accuracy in clinical evaluations and are thixotropic, which provides good surface detail and makes them useful as a border molding material. It should be noted, however, that these materials are not compatible with the addition reaction silicone impression materials and should not be used to border mold custom trays when the silicone impression materials are to be used as the final impression material. The polyethers are also hydrophilic, which produces good wettability for easy cast forming.

The polyethers have low-to-moderate tear strength and a much shorter working and setting time, which can limit the usefulness of the material. The flow characteristics and flexibility of the polyether materials are the lowest of any of the elastic materials. These characteristics can limit the use of polyethers in removable partial denture impression procedures. The stiffness of the material can result in cast breakage when removal of the cast from a custom tray is attempted. These materials have a higher permanent deformation than the addition reaction silicones. Some have an unpleasant taste, and because the material will absorb moisture, it cannot be immersed in disinfecting solutions or stored in high humidity for any extended period of time. The materials should be poured within 2 hours; however, manufacturers claim that if the impression is kept dry, clinically acceptable casts can be poured for up to 7 days.

Silicone Impression Materials

The silicone impression materials are more accurate and easier to use than the other elastic impression materials. The condensation silicones have a moderate (5 to 7 minutes) working time that can be altered by adjusting the amount of the accelerator. They have a pleasant odor, moderately high tear strength, and excellent recovery from deformation. These materials can be used with a compatible putty material to form fit a custom tray. Silicone impression materials are hydrophobic, which can make cast formation a problem. These materials can be disinfected in any of the disinfecting solutions with no alteration in accuracy. Ideally, these materials should be poured within 1 hour.

The addition reaction silicones are the most accurate of the elastic impression materials. They have less polymerization shrinkage, low distortion, fast recovery from deformation, and moderately high tear strength. These materials have a working time of 3 to 5 minutes, which can be easily modified with the use of retardants and temperature controls. They are available in both hydrophilic and hydrophobic forms, have no smell or taste, and also come in putty form to assist in form fitting the impression tray at chairside. Most of the addition reaction silicones are available in automixing devices, can be poured up to 1 week after impression making with acceptable clinical results, and are stable in most sterilizing solutions. Sulfur in latex gloves and in ferric and aluminum sulfate retraction solution may inhibit polymerization. Many of the hydrophobic types are difficult to pour with stone, and adhesion to acrylic resin trays is not good. The putties for these materials have a relatively short shelf life and they are more expensive than the other elastic impression materials.

IMPRESSIONS OF THE PARTIALLY EDENTULOUS ARCH

An impression of the partially edentulous arch must record accurately the anatomic form of the teeth and surrounding tissue. This is necessary so that the prosthesis may be designed to follow a definite path of placement and removal and so that support, stability, and retention derived from the abutment teeth may be precise and accurate.

Materials that could be permanently deformed by removal from tooth or tissue undercuts should not be used. The thermoplastic impression materials and metallic oxide pastes are therefore excluded for recording the anatomic form of the dental arch. Rubber-base materials that are highly cross-linked should not be used when large or multiple undercuts are present because these materials will be subjected to considerable distortion upon withdrawal. Plaster of Paris and modeling plastic are capable of recording tissue detail accurately, but they must be sectioned for removal and subsequently reassembled, which often leads to permanent deformation.

The introduction of hydrocolloids as impression materials was a giant step forward in dentistry. For the first time, impressions could be made of undercut areas with a material that was elastic enough to be withdrawn from those undercuts without permanent distortion. It permitted the making of a one-piece impression, which did not require the use of a separating medium, and was and still is an acceptably accurate material when handled properly.

The principal differences between reversible and irreversible hydrocolloids are as follows:

1. Reversible hydrocolloid converts from the gel form to a sol by the application of heat. It may be reverted to gel form by a reduction in temperature. This physical change is reversible.
2. Irreversible hydrocolloid becomes a gel via a chemical reaction as a result of mixing alginate powder with water. This physical change is irreversible.

Reversible hydrocolloid does have some disadvantages. It must be introduced into the mouth while warm enough to be a sol, and then it converts to an elastic gel on cooling. Therefore there is an ever-present danger of burning the tissue of the mouth—a burn that is painful and slow to heal. It requires warming and tempering equipment that is thermostatically controlled and necessitates the use of water-jacketed impression trays for cooling.

All hydrocolloids are dimensionally stable only during a brief period after removal from the mouth. If exposed to the air, they rapidly lose water content, with a resulting shrinkage and other dimensional changes. If immersed in water, they imbibe water, with accompanying swelling and dimensional changes. All hydrocolloid impressions should be poured immediately, but if they must be stored for a brief period, they should be in a saturated atmosphere rather than immersed in water. This can be accomplished simply by wrapping the impression in a damp paper towel or sealing it in a plastic bag.

Hydrocolloids also exhibit a phenomenon known as syneresis, which is associated with the giving off of a mucinous exudate. This mucinous exudate has a retarding effect on any gypsum material, which results in a soft or chalky cast surface. Sometimes this is only detected by a close examination of the impression after removal from the cast. Nevertheless, such a cast surface is inaccurate and ultimately will result in an inaccurate removable partial denture framework. Pouring the cast immediately and using some chemical accelerator, such as potassium sulfate, to counteract the retarding effect of the hydrocolloid can prevent this inaccuracy. All modern irreversible hydrocolloid impression materials have an accelerator incorporated into the powder and no longer need to be treated with a fixing solution.

Because no heat is used in the preparation of irreversible hydrocolloid, there is no danger of burning the patient. For this reason the patient should be more relaxed and cooperative during the positioning of the tray. However, some disadvantages are associated with the use of irreversible hydrocolloid. This material gels by means of a chemical reaction that is accelerated by the warmth of the tissue, whereas reversible hydrocolloid gels from the tray in toward the tissue, because of the cooling action of the water that circulates through the tray. In the irreversible hydrocolloid, gelation first takes place next to the tissue, and any movement of the tray during gelation will result in internal stresses that are released on removal of the impression from the mouth. A distorted and therefore inaccurate impression results from an irreversible hydrocolloid impression that is not held immobile during gelation.

Another disadvantage of irreversible hydrocolloid is that it must be introduced into the mouth at approximately 70° F, which results in an immediate increase in the viscosity and surface tension of the material. Air bubbles are therefore harder to dispel, and it is inevitable that more air will be trapped in an irreversible impression than in a reversible impression. Every precaution must be taken to prevent the entrapment of air in critical areas.

Important Precautions to Be Observed in the Handling of Hydrocolloid Impressions

Some important precautions to be observed in the handling of hydrocolloid are as follows:

1. Impression should not be exposed to air because some dehydration will inevitably occur and result in shrinkage.
2. Impression should not be immersed in water or disinfectants, because some imbibition will inevitably result, with an accompanying expansion.
3. Impression should be protected from dehydration by placing it in a humid atmosphere or wrapping it in a damp paper towel until a cast can be poured. To prevent volume change, this should be done within 15 minutes after removal of the impression from the mouth.
4. Exudate from hydrocolloid has a retarding effect on the chemical reaction of gypsum products and results in a chalky cast surface. This can be prevented by pouring the cast immediately or by first immersing the impression in a solution of accelerator, if an accelerator is not included in the formula.

Step-by-step Procedure for Making a Hydrocolloid Impression

The step-by-step procedure and important points to observe in the making of a hydrocolloid impression are as follows:

1. Select a suitable, sterilized, perforated or rim lock impression tray that is large enough to provide a 4- to 5-mm thickness of the impression material between the teeth and tissue, and the tray.
2. Build up the palatal portion of the maxillary impression tray with wax or modeling plastic to ensure even distribution of the impression material and to prevent the material from slumping away from the palatal surface (Figure 15-1, *A*). At this time, it is also helpful to pack the palate with gauze that has been sprayed with a topical anesthetic. This will serve to anesthetize the minor salivary glands and mucous glands of the palate and thus prevent secretions as a response to smell or taste or to the physical presence of the impression material. If gelation occurs next to the tissue while the deeper portion is still fluid, a distorted impression of the palate may result, which cannot be detected in the finished impression. This may result in the major connector of the finished casting not being in contact with the underlying tissue. The maxillary tray frequently has to be extended posteriorly to include the tuberosities and vibrating line region of the palate. Such an extension also aids in correctly orienting the tray in the patient's mouth when the impression is made.

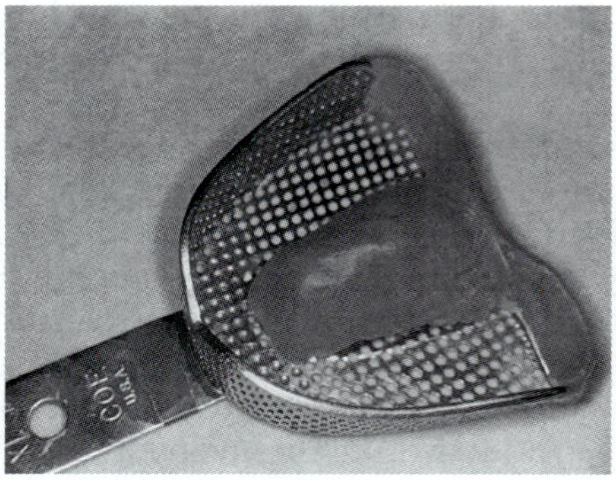
A

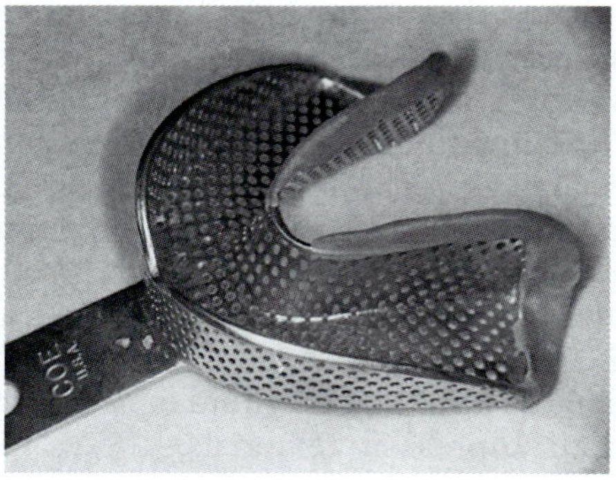
B

Figure 15-1 **A,** Maxillary impression tray with palatal portion built up with base-plate wax to prevent impression material from sagging away from palatal surface. Periphery wax is also added across posterior border of tray to cover maxillary tuberosities and to prevent impression material from being expelled posteriorly when impression is made. **B,** Mandibular impression tray with periphery wax added to lingual flanges to prevent tissues of floor of mouth from rising inside tray. Posterior end of tray is extended with periphery wax to cover retromolar pad regions.

3. The lingual flange of the mandibular tray may need to be lengthened with wax in the retromylohyoid area or to be extended posteriorly, but it rarely ever needs to be lengthened elsewhere. Wax may need to be added inside the distolingual flange to prevent the tissue of the floor of the mouth from rising inside the tray (Figure 15-1, *B*).
4. Place the patient in an upright position, with the arch to be impressed nearly parallel to the floor.
5. When irreversible hydrocolloid is used, place the measured amount of water (at 70° F) in a clean, dry, rubber mixing bowl (600-ml capacity). Add the correct measure of powder. Stir rapidly against the side of the bowl with a short, stiff spatula. This should be accomplished in less than 1 minute. The patient should rinse his or her mouth with cool water to eliminate excess saliva while the impression material is being mixed and the tray is being loaded.
6. In placing the material in the tray, avoid entrapping air. Have the first layer of material lock through the perforations of the tray or rim lock to prevent any possible dislodgment after gelation.
7. After loading the tray, remove the gauze with the topical anesthetic and quickly place (rub) some of the impression material on any critical areas using your finger (areas such as rest preparations and abutment teeth). If a maxillary impression is being made, place material in the highest aspect of the palate and over the rugae.
8. Use a mouth mirror or index finger to retract the cheek on the side away from you as the tray is rotated into the mouth from the near side.
9. Seat the tray first on the side away from you, next on the anterior area while reflecting the lip, and then on the near side, with the mouth mirror or finger for cheek retraction. Finally, make sure that the lip is draping naturally over the tray.
10. Be careful not to seat the tray too deeply, leaving room for a thickness of material over the occlusal and incisal surfaces.
11. Hold the tray immobile for 3 minutes with light finger pressure over the left and right premolar areas. To prevent internal stresses in the finished impression, do not allow the tray to move during gelation. Any movement of the tray during gelation will produce an inaccurate impression. If, for example, you allow the patient or the assistant to hold the tray in position at any time during the impression procedure, some movement of the tray will be inevitable during the transfer and the impression will probably be inaccurate. Do not remove the impression from the mouth until the impression material has completely set.
12. After releasing the surface tension, remove the impression quickly in line with the long axis of the teeth to prevent tearing or other distortion.
13. Rinse the impression free of saliva with slurry water, or dust it with plaster, and rinse gently. Then examine it critically. Spray the impression thoroughly with a suitable disinfectant, and cover it immediately with a damp paper towel.

A cast should be poured immediately into a disinfected hydrocolloid impression to prevent dimensional changes and syneresis. Circumstances often necessitate some delay, but this time lapse should be kept to a minimum. A delay of 15 minutes will satisfy the disinfection requirements and should not be deleterious if the impression is kept in a humid atmosphere.

Step-by-step Procedure for Making a Stone Cast From a Hydrocolloid Impression

The step-by-step procedure for making the stone cast from the impression is as follows:

1. A more abrasive resistant Type IV stone should be used to form removable partial denture casts. Have the measured dental stone at hand, along with the designated quantity of room temperature water, as recommended by the manufacturer. A clean, 600-ml rubber mixing bowl, a stiff spatula, and a vibrator complete the preparations. A No. 7 spatula also should be within reach.
2. First pour the measure of water into the mixing bowl and then add the measure of stone. Spatulate thoroughly for 1 minute, remembering that a weak and porous stone cast may result from insufficient spatulation. Mechanical spatulation under vacuum is preferred. After any spatulation, other than in a vacuum, place the mixing bowl on the vibrator and knead the material to permit the escape of any trapped air.
3. After removing the impression from the damp towel, gently shake out surplus moisture and hold the impression over the vibrator, impression side up, with only the handle of the tray contacting the vibrator. The impression material must not be placed in contact with the vibrator because of possible distortion of the impression.
4. With a small spatula, add the first cast material to the distal area away from you. Allow this first material to be vibrated around the arch from tooth to tooth toward the anterior part of the impression (Figure 15-2). Continue to add small increments of material at this same distal area, with each portion of added stone pushing the mass ahead of it. This prevents the entrapment of air. The weight of the material causes any excess water to be pushed around the arch and to be expelled ultimately at the opposite end of the impression. Discard this fluid material. When the impressions of all teeth have been filled, continue to add artificial stone in larger portions until the impression is completely filled.

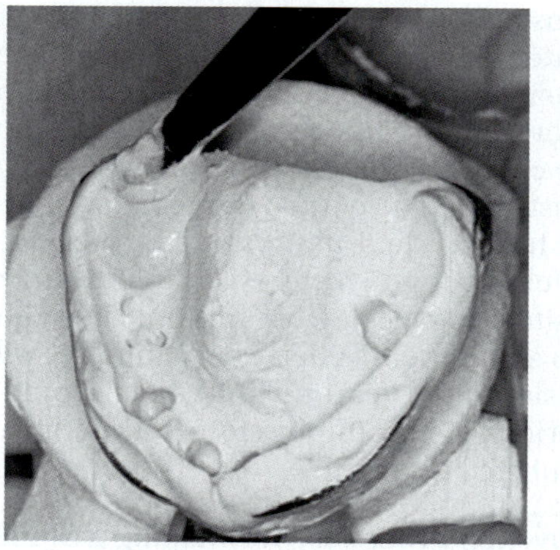

Figure 15-2 Small portions of mechanically spatulated stone are applied at posterior section of impression and vibrated around arch, pushing moisture and diluted stone ahead of mass. Stone is applied at this point only until impressions of teeth are filled and diluted stone is discarded at opposite end. Only then is remainder of impression filled with larger portions, using larger spatula. Only handle of impression tray should be allowed to touch vibrator so that distortion of impression material will be avoided. (Note that vibrator is protected as impression is filled.)

5. The filled impression should be placed so that its weight does not distort the hydrocolloid impression material. The base of the cast can be completed with the same mix of stone (Figure 15-3). The base of the cast should be 16 to 18 mm (⅔ to ¾ inch) at its thinnest portion and should be extended beyond the borders of the impression so that buccal, labial, and lingual borders will be recorded correctly in the finished cast. A distorted cast may result from an inverted impression.
6. As soon as the cast material has developed sufficient body, trim the excess from the sides of the cast. Wrap the impression and cast in a wet paper towel, or place it in a humidor, until the initial set of the stone has taken place. The impression is thus prevented from losing water by evaporation, which might deprive the cast material of sufficient water for crystallization. Chalky cast surfaces around the teeth are often the result of the hydrocolloids acting as a sponge and robbing the cast material of its necessary water for crystallization.
7. After the cast and impression have been in the humid atmosphere for 30 minutes, separate the impression from the cast. Thirty minutes is sufficient for initial setting. Any stone that interferes with separation from the tray must be trimmed away with a knife.
8. Clean the impression tray immediately while the used impression material is still elastic.
9. The trimming of the cast should be deferred until final setting has occurred. The sides of the cast then may be trimmed to be parallel, and any blebs or defects resulting from air bubbles in the impression may be removed. If this is a cast for a permanent record, it may be trimmed to orthodontic specification to present a neat appearance for demonstration purposes. Master casts and other working casts are ordinarily trimmed only to remove excess stone.

Possible Causes of an Inaccurate and/or a Weak Cast of a Dental Arch

The possible causes of an inaccurate cast are as follows:

1. Distortion of the hydrocolloid impression (a) by use of an impression tray that is not rigid; (b) by partial dislodgment from the tray; (c) by shrinkage caused by dehydration; (d) by expansion caused by imbibition (this will be toward the teeth and will result in an undersized rather than oversized cast); and (e) by attempting to pour the cast with stone that has already begun to set.
2. A ratio of water to powder that is too high. Although this may not cause volumetric changes in the size of the cast, it will result in a weak cast.
3. Improper mixing. This also results in a weak cast or one with a chalky surface.
4. Trapping of air, either in the mix or in pouring, because of insufficient vibration.
5. Soft or chalky cast surface that results from the retarding action of the hydrocolloid or the absorption of necessary water for crystallization by the dehydrating hydrocolloid.
6. Premature separation of the cast from the impression.
7. Failure to separate the cast from the impression for an extended period.

INDIVIDUAL IMPRESSION TRAYS

This chapter has previously dealt with making an impression in a rigid stock tray of the anatomic form of a dental arch for making a diagnostic cast, a working cast for restorations, or a master cast. There are times, however, when a stock tray is not suitable for making the final anatomic impression of the dental arch. Most tooth-supported removable partial dentures may be made on a master cast from such an impression. Some maxillary distal extension removable partial dentures with broad palatal coverage, particularly those for a Kennedy Class I arch, may also be made on an anatomic cast—but usually these necessitate the use of an individually made tray.

A stock tray must be sufficiently rigid to prevent distortion during the impression and cast forming procedures. It should fit the mouth with about

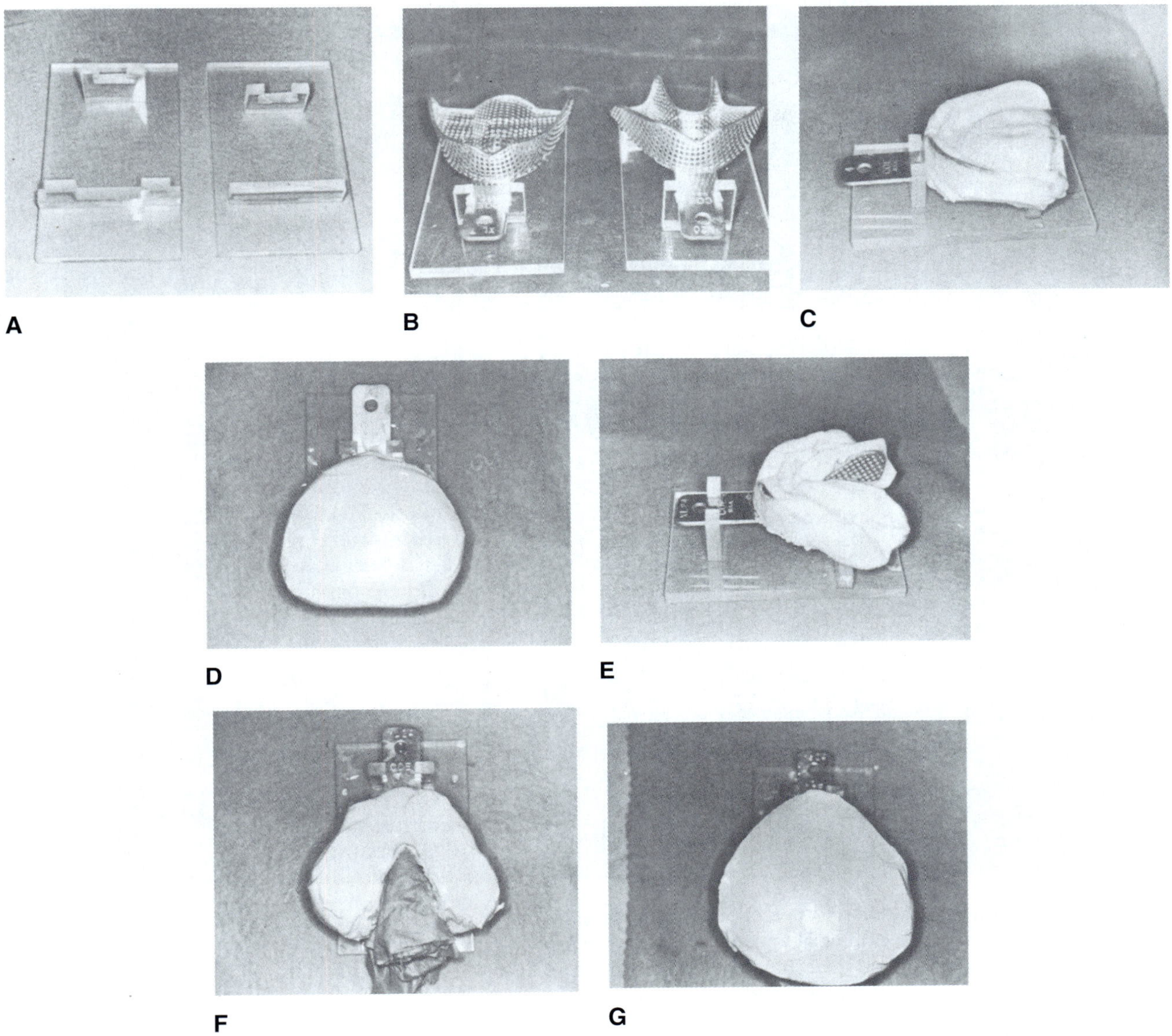

Figure 15-3 **A,** Homemade plastic jigs are used to support impressions. Handle of tray is placed in slotted portion, and posterior end of tray is supported by elevated cross-members. Jig used to support mandibular impression is on left. **B,** Note that impression trays are elevated and contact jigs at only three points. **C,** An impression could be easily distorted when cast is being poured if tray was placed on laboratory bench. Because impression is elevated by jig, distortion of impression is minimized. **D,** After impression is filled with stone, as previously demonstrated, it is placed in jig, and additional stone is added to form base of cast. **E,** Mandibular impression placed in jig to demonstrate support by jig. Note that impression is supported by contact of tray only at handle and on either side posteriorly. **F,** Impression is returned to supporting jig after being filled with stone. Wet paper is placed in tongue space to support stone base in this region and to avoid locking impression tray to cast. **G,** Additional stone is added to impression to form base for cast.

4 to 5 mm of clearance for the impression material without interfering with teeth or bordering tissue. Otherwise an individual tray made of some acrylic resin tray material should be used for the final anatomic impression.

Most stock or disposable removable partial denture trays are of either the rim lock or perforated varieties. Both are made in a limited selection of sizes and shapes. There are a wide selection of trays that can be used for partially edentulous patients, including trays for both bilateral and unilateral edentulous areas (Figure 15-4).

All of these trays have reinforced borders. Although a complete denture impression tray is, or should be,

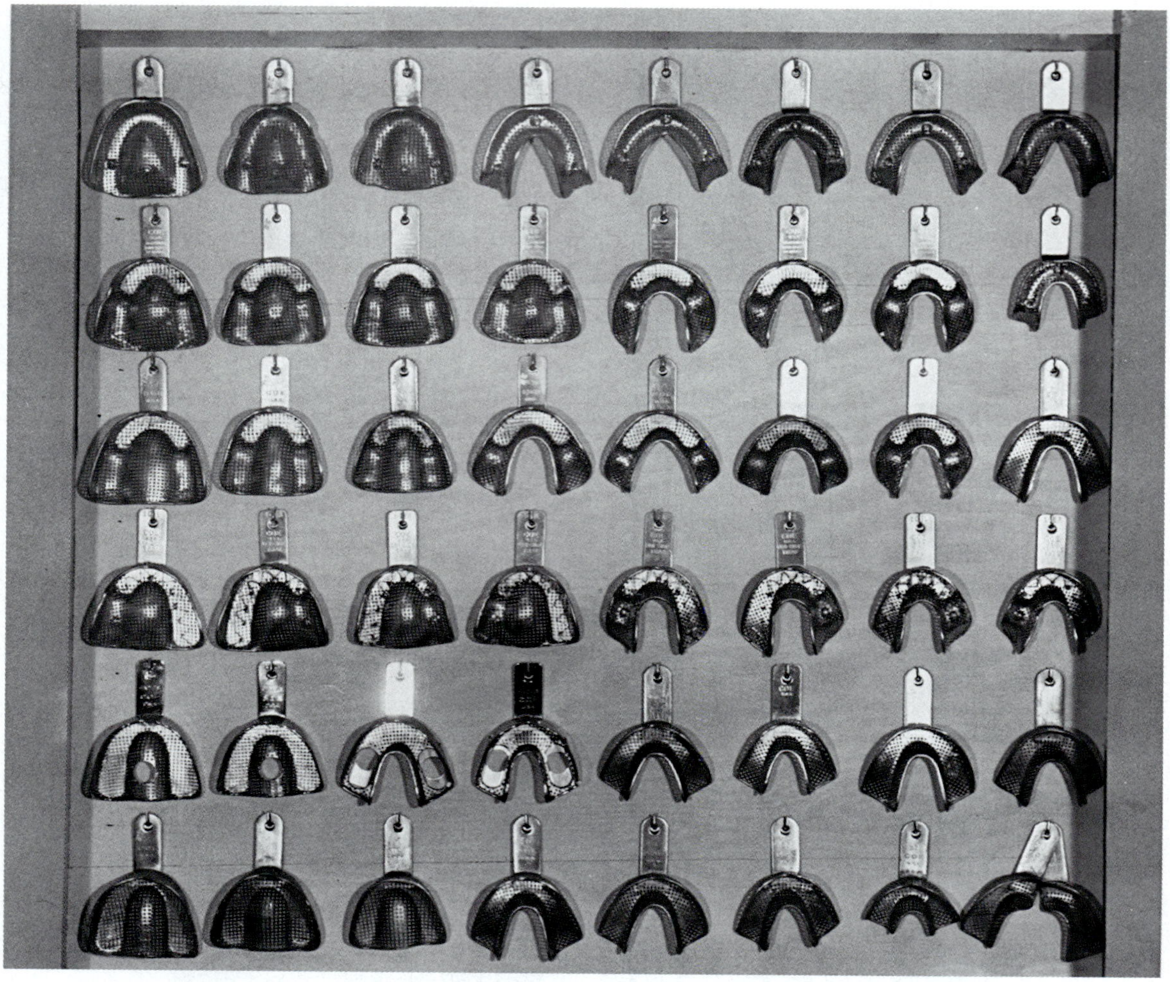

Figure 15-4 Wide selection of perforated impression trays for an irreversible hydrocolloid impression. Beginning at top are impression trays for completely edentulous mouths, depressed anterior trays, trays with unilateral occlusal stops, Hindels trays for use with double impression technique, and more commonly and regularly used perforated trays. All trays must be sterilized before use.

made of material that permits trimming and shaping to fit the mouth, the existence of a beaded border and the rigidity of a stock removable partial denture tray allow no trimming and little shaping. The resulting impression is often a record of border tissue distorted by an ill-fitting tray rather than an impression of tissue draping naturally over a slightly underextended impression tray.

An individual acrylic resin tray, on the other hand, can be made with sufficient clearance for the impression material and can be trimmed just short of the vestibular reflections to allow the tissue to drape naturally without distortion. The removable partial denture borders may then be made as accurately as complete denture borders with equal advantages.

Although techniques have been proposed for making individual impression trays that incorporate plastic tubing for water-cooling reversible hydrocolloid impressions, the final anatomic impression usually will be made with irreversible hydrocolloid, mercaptan rubber, or silicone impression materials.

Technique for Making Individual Acrylic Resin Impression Trays

The diagnostic cast is often adequate for the preparation of the individual tray. However, if extensive surgery or extractions were performed after making the diagnostic cast, a new impression in a rigid stock tray and a new cast must be made. The procedures for making the new cast are identical to those described previously.

A duplicate of the diagnostic cast, on which the individual tray can be fabricated, should be made because the cast on which an individual tray is made is often damaged or must be mutilated to separate the tray from the cast. Obviously the original diagnostic cast must be retained as a permanent record in the patient's file. There are several techniques for making individual impression trays. One technique for making an individual maxillary tray is described in Figures 15-5 and 15-6. This format could be used for both auto-polymerizing acrylic resin and visible light-cured (VLC) acrylic resin. The VLC custom tray materials are premixed sheet materials which, when polymerized, provide a highly stable, distortion-free custom impression tray that is ready to use in minutes. These materials are provided by the manufacturers in sheet forms of various sizes, thicknesses, and colors.

A technique for making an individual maxillary tray with light-polymerized resin is as follows:

1. Outline the extent of the tray on the cast with a pencil. The tray must include all teeth and tissue that will be involved in the removable partial denture.
2. Adapt one layer of baseplate wax over the tissue surfaces and teeth of the cast to serve as a spacer for impression material. The wax spacer should be trimmed 2 to 3 mm short of the outline drawn

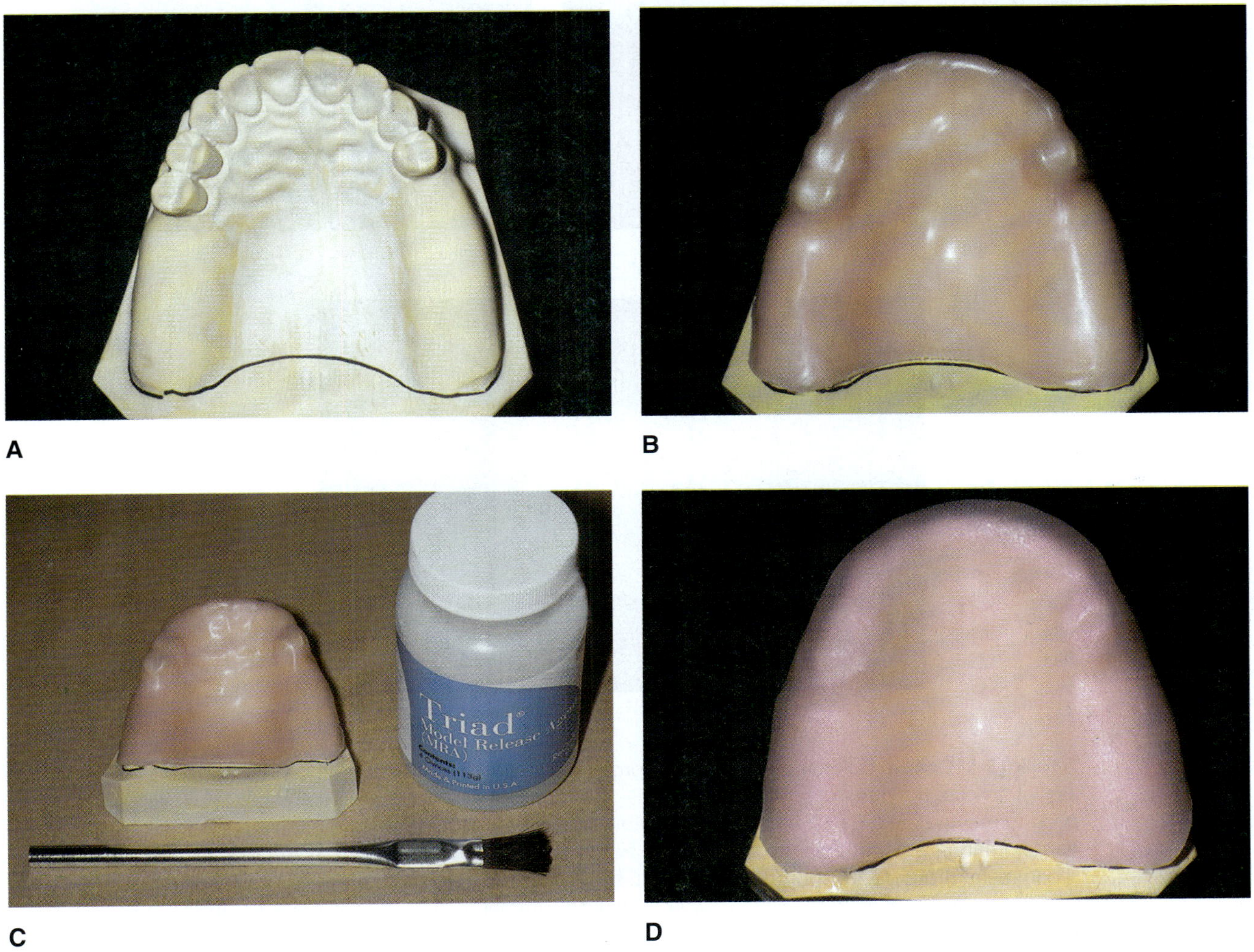

Figure 15-5 **A,** Desired outline of tray is drawn on diagnostic cast. The tray must include all teeth and tissues that will be involved in the removable partial denture. **B,** One thickness of baseplate wax is adapted to cast and is trimmed to penciled outline, which is 2–3 mm short of the desired border. The posterior palatal seal region is not covered by wax but will be included in finished tray. Two thicknesses of baseplate wax cover teeth. A window is created in wax spacer over incisal edges. **C,** Model Release Agent is painted on the stone surfaces of cast that will be contacted by the resin. **D,** The VLC resin tray material is removed from the light-proof wrap and shaped to the desired outline in a uniform manner.

Continued

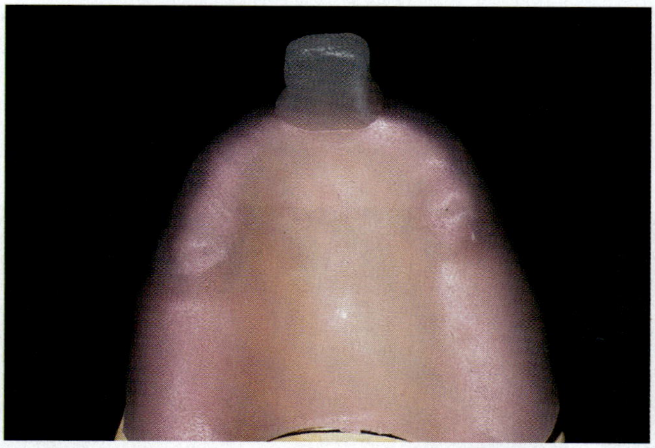

E

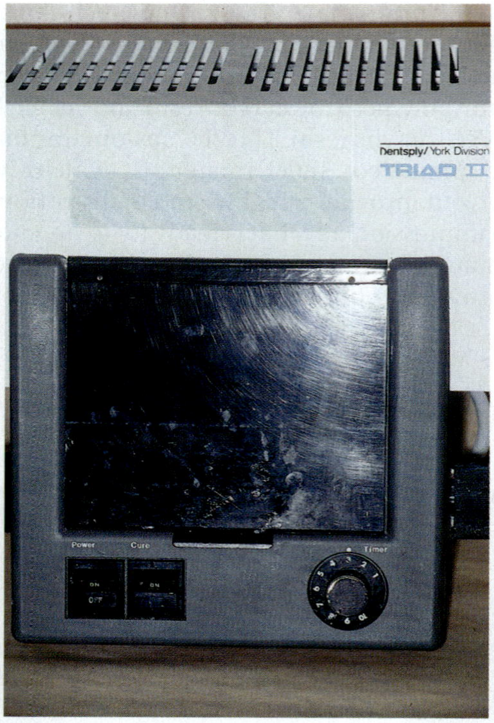

F

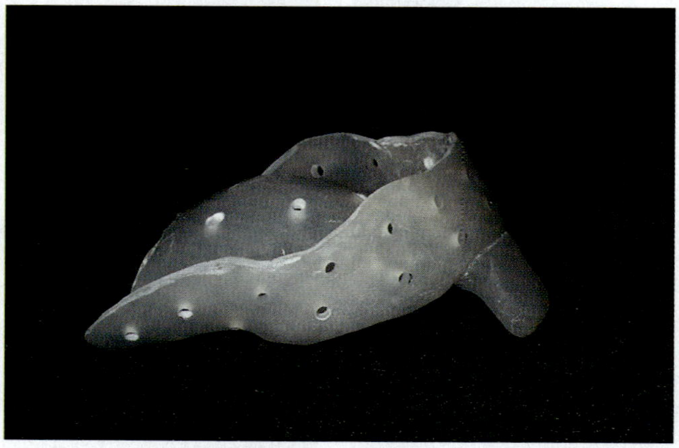

G

Figure 15-5 Cont'd **E,** A handle is added to provide a means to place and remove the tray, as well as pass the tray from assistant to dentist. Its form should consider the lip length and need to manipulate the peri-oral region. **F,** Prior to placing the tray in the curing oven, an air barrier coating is painted on the surface. The tray is then polymerized as per manufacturers' recommendations. **G,** As soon as tray material has hardened, tray is removed from cast, and wax spacer is removed from rough tray. Acrylic resin trimmer in lathe is used to rough finish the tray. Holes are drilled through tray, spaced approximately 4.5 mm apart. These holes will serve to lock impression material in tray. In addition, excess impression material is forced out of holes when impression is made, thereby minimally displacing soft oral tissues.

on the diagnostic cast. Wax covering the posterior palatal seal area should be removed so that intimate contact of the tray and tissue in this region may serve as an aid in correctly orienting the tray when making the impression. Expose portions of the incisal edges of the central incisors to serve as anterior stops when placing the tray in the mouth. Bevel the wax so that the completed tray will have a guiding incline that will help position the tray on the anterior stop. Other cast undercuts should be blocked out with wax or modeling compound. NOTE: Adapt an additional

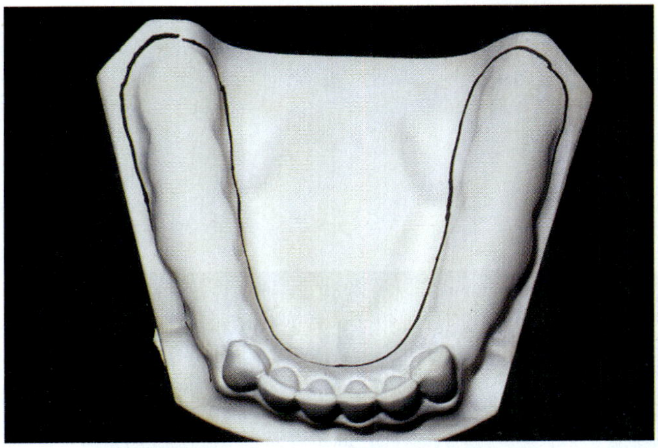

A

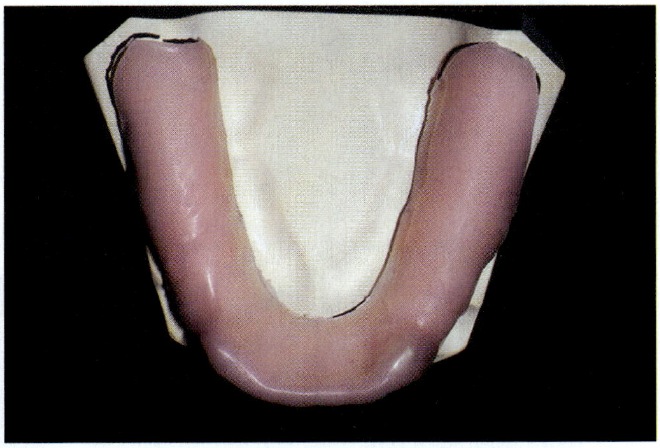

B

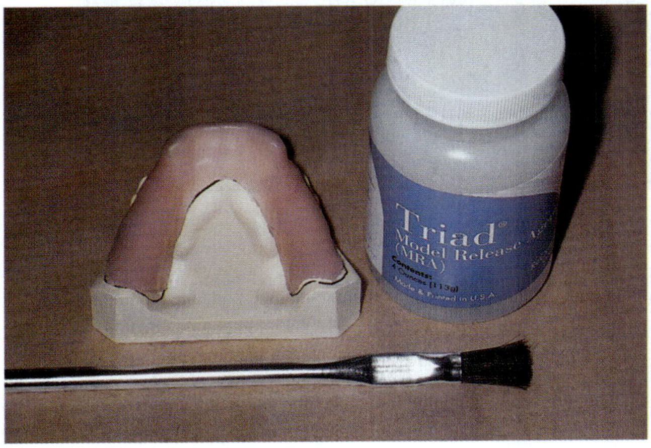

C

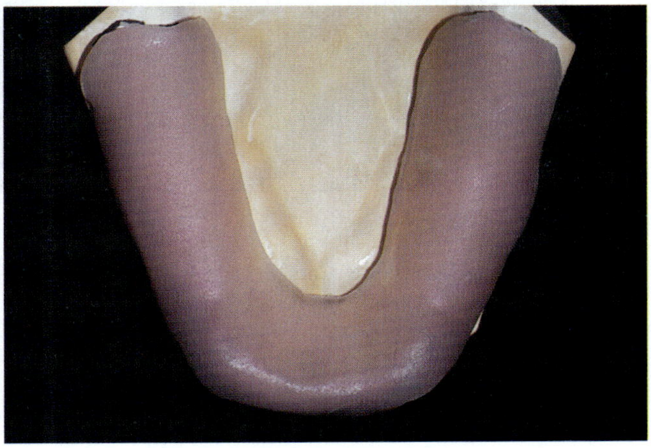

D

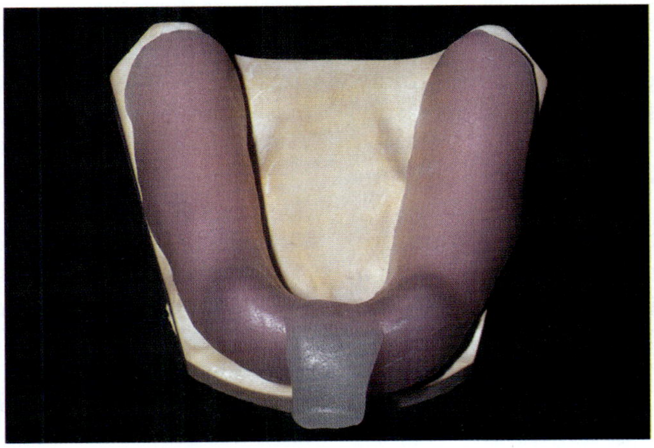

E

Figure 15-6 Similar technique used for fabrication of the maxillary tray in Figure 15-5 is used for the mandibular tray. **A,** Outline of tray is penciled on duplicate mandibular diagnostic cast. **B,** Single sheet of baseplate wax is adapted to outline of tray, and another sheet of baseplate wax is adapted over teeth. A window is cut in spacer to expose incisal edges of lower central incisors to serve as a stop in seating the tray. **C,** Model Release Agent is painted on regions of the cast to be in contact with the resin. **D,** VLC tray material wafer is adapted over cast and spacer. **E,** A handle is formed with excess tray material as previously described.

Continued

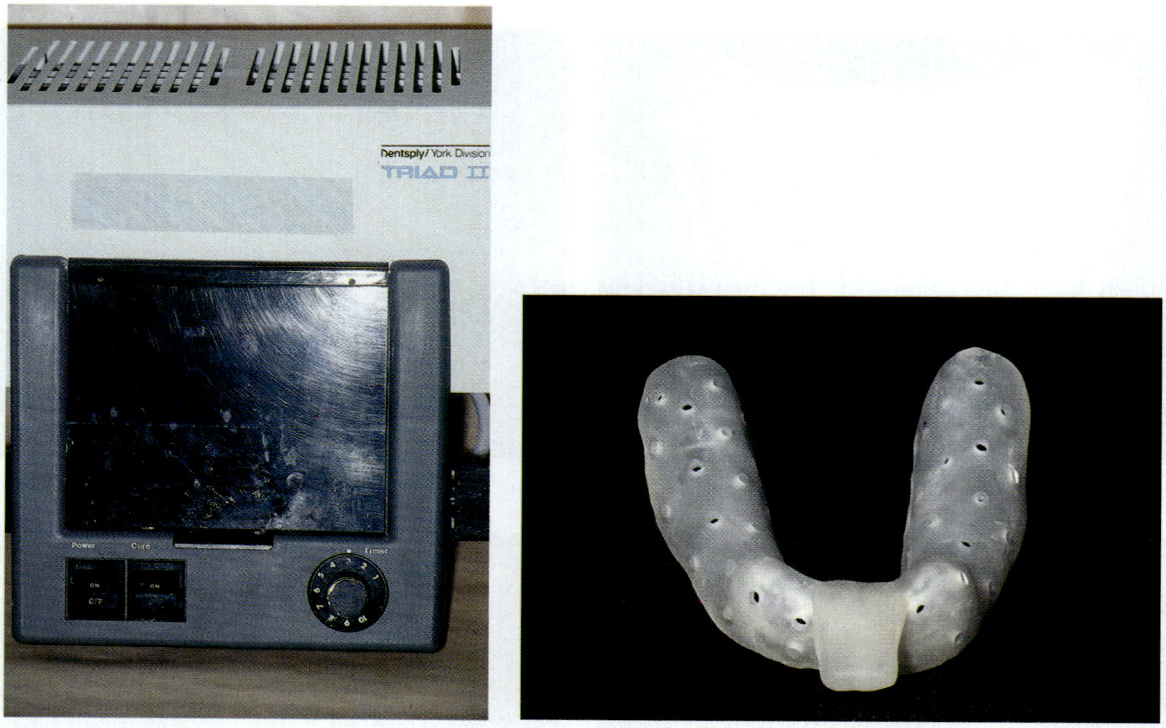

Figure 15-6 Cont'd **F,** An air barrier coating is painted on the tray material and it is processed as described in Figure 15-5. **G,** Following processing, multiple holes are placed throughout tray.

layer of baseplate wax over the teeth if the impression is to be made in irreversible hydrocolloid. This step is not necessary if the choice of impression material is a rubber-base or silicone type of material.

3. Paint the exposed surfaces of the cast that may be contacted by the light-polymerized resin tray material with a model release agent (MRA) to facilitate separation of the polymerized tray from the cast.
4. Remove the VLC tray material from the lightproof pouch and carefully cut the desired length with a knife or scalpel. Adapt the VLC material to the cast and trim it with a knife. Be sure not to thin the material over the teeth or the posterior border area.
5. Attach a handle by molding excess VLC material into the desired shape and blend it into the tray material in the cast. With some materials, a paper clip or similar wire may be shaped and used to reinforce the handle. Alternatively, some manufacturers make prefabricated metal custom tray handles that may be easily adapted.
6. Place the cast with the adapted tray in the light polymerizing unit and process according to the manufacturer's directions, usually a maximum of 1 minute.
7. Remove the cast from the unit and gently remove the tray from the cast. Peel the softened wax out of the tray while the wax is still warm.
8. Paint the entire impression tray with the manufacturer's air barrier coating material and return the tray to the unit turnstile for additional polymerizing tissue side up.
9. When the polymerizing cycle is completed, remove the tray from the unit and clean it with a brush and water.
10. Perfect the borders of the tray with rotary instruments (vulcanite burs, acrylic resin trimmers, etc.) and slightly polish the external surface of the tray.
11. Place perforations (No. 8 bur size) in the VLC resin tray at 5-mm intervals, with the exception of the alveolar groove areas, if using an irreversible hydrocolloid impression material.
12. The finished tray must be sanitized and tried in the mouth so that any necessary corrections to the tray can be accomplished before the impression is made.

The technique for making an individual mandibular VLC resin tray follows the same procedures. The wax spacer does not cover the buccal shelf regions on the mandibular cast, because these areas provide the primary support for the mandibular removable partial denture and serve as posterior stops in orienting the tray in the patient's mouth. During impression making, these areas will permit selective placement of tissue in the mandibular stress-bearing areas.

If mercaptan rubber is to be used, perforations are not usually necessary to lock the material in the tray, as the adhesive provided by the manufacturer provides reliable retention, and some confinement of these materials is desirable. However, a series of perforations are necessary in the median palatal raphe and incisive papilla areas of the maxillary tray so that excess impression material will escape through them, thus providing relief of the tissue in this area. For the same reasons, perforations are placed in the alveolar groove of the mandibular tray. With the use of adhesives, the impression material is not easily removed from the tray should a faulty impression have to be remade, but this is an inconvenience common to all newer elastic materials and does not prevent reuse of the impression tray. The opaque elastic impression materials and adhesives can prevent the detection of undesirable pressure areas when evaluating an impression.

Master casts made from impressions in individual acrylic resin trays are generally more accurate than are those made in rigid stock trays. The use of individual trays should be considered a necessary step in making the majority of removable partial dentures when a secondary impression technique is not to be used. Reasons and methods for making a secondary impression will be considered in Chapter 16.

Final impressions for maxillary tooth-supported removable partial dentures often may be made in carefully selected and recontoured rigid stock impression trays. However, an individual acrylic resin tray is preferred in those situations in the mandibular arch when the floor of the mouth closely approximates the lingual gingiva of remaining anterior teeth. Recording the floor of the mouth at the elevation it assumes when the lips are licked is important in selecting the type of major connector to be used (see Chapter 5). Modification of the borders of an individual tray to fulfill the requirements of an adequate tray is much easier than is the modification of a metal stock tray.

SELF-ASSESSMENT AIDS

1. Impression materials used in various phases of removable partial denture construction may be classified as rigid, thermoplastic, or elastic. Give two examples for each of the three categories.
2. Which type of impression material has been used the longest in prosthodontics?
3. Why should the metallic oxide paste types of impression material not be used for primary impressions of partially edentulous arches?
4. Modeling plastic (compound) may be used effectively in modifying impression trays to make secondary impressions of Class I and II partially edentulous arches. Describe how it is used. Why is it not used for primary impression for the removable partial denture patient?
5. What is an impression wax? Do its characteristics make it appropriate for use as a primary impression or for a secondary impression? Describe how it is used.
6. There are two types of hydrocolloid impression materials used in dentistry. Name them.
7. Are the hydrocolloid impression materials elastic or thermoplastic?
8. What is the advantage in using an elastic material versus a rigid material in making impressions of partially edentulous arches?
9. Briefly compare reversible and irreversible hydrocolloid impression materials from the standpoints of composition, gelation mechanism, trays, and relative accuracy.
10. Mercaptan rubber-base impression material may be used for primary or secondary impressions. Its characteristics make it best suited, however, for the ______ impression.
11. Does the use of mercaptan rubber-base material and silicone impression material require the use of a rigid stock tray or an individualized tray? Why?
12. Many different artificial stones are used in dentistry and equally as many impression materials. Are these varied materials necessarily compatible with each other when used to make casts? What precautions should be taken to ensure compatibility?
13. What is syneresis? What effect will this phenomenon have on a cast poured in a hydrocolloid impression?
14. What is meant by the word imbibition in relation to hydrocolloid impressions? What effect does it have on a hydrocolloid impression?
15. How long should you wait to pour a cast into a hydrocolloid impression after it is removed from the mouth? Why?
16. There are two types of silicone impression materials. Name them and describe how they differ.
17. The thickness of impression material when rubber-base material is used should be about 3 mm ($\frac{1}{8}$ inch) for accuracy and stability. Does this equally apply to a hydrocolloid impression material? If not, give a rule of thumb for the desired thickness of the hydrocolloid material in the impression.
18. What are the advantages of perforated stock trays versus nonperforated stock trays when making impressions of partially edentulous arches with an irreversible hydrocolloid?

19. Inaccuracies of a cast made from a hydrocolloid impression may result from many causes. Describe six causes of such inaccuracy.
20. Why should impressions into which stone casts have been poured not be inverted until the initial set of the stone has taken place?
21. An individual acrylic resin impression tray has two distinct advantages over any type of stock tray. What are these two advantages?
22. Describe the procedures for making individual maxillary and mandibular impression trays, paying special attention to relief of the casts with wax spacers.
23. Holes about 3 mm (⅛ inch) in diameter should be placed at strategic locations in both maxillary and mandibular individualized trays. Give the location of the holes and describe what is accomplished by their presence.
24. What is the advantage of drilling holes in acrylic resin trays with a bi-bevel drill rather than with fissure or round burs?
25. Under what circumstances would you use a stock tray in preference to an individual acrylic resin tray?
26. Does a stock or disposable impression tray have to be rigid? Why?
27. Rubber-base impression materials have some serious disadvantages for making final impressions for removable partial dentures. What are they?
28. What are specific advantages of (a) polyether; (b) condensation silicone; and (c) addition silicone impression materials when used to make removable partial denture impressions?
29. What are specific disadvantages of (a) polyether; (b) condensation silicone; and (c) addition silicone impression materials when used to make removable partial denture impressions?
30. Of the impression materials mentioned in this chapter, which ones can be immersed in a sterilizing solution without being damaged, and which ones must be sprayed only?

16

SUPPORT FOR THE DISTAL EXTENSION DENTURE BASE

In a tooth-supported removable partial denture, a metal base or the framework that supports an acrylic resin base is connected to and is part of a rigid framework that permits the direct transfer of occlusal forces to the abutment teeth through the occlusal rests. Even though the denture base of the modification space(s) in a Kennedy Class III removable partial denture provides support for the supplied teeth, the residual ridge beneath the base is not called on to aid in the support of the removable partial denture. Therefore the resiliency of the ridge tissue, the ridge configuration, and the type of bone that supports this tissue are not factors in denture support. Regardless of the length of the edentulous spans, if the framework is rigid, the abutment teeth are sound enough to carry the additional load, and the occlusal rests are properly formed, support comes entirely from the abutment teeth at either end of the span. Support may be augmented by splinting and by the use of additional abutments, but in any event the abutments are the sole support of the removable restoration.

An impression (and resultant stone cast) records the anatomic form of the teeth and their surrounding structures and is needed to make a tooth-supported removable partial denture. The impression should also record the moving tissue that will border the denture in an unstrained position so the relationship of the denture base to this tissue may be as accurate as possible. Although underextension of the denture base in a tooth-supported prosthesis is the lesser of two evils, an underextended base may lead to food entrapment and inadequate facial contours, particularly on the buccal and labial sides. To accurately record the moving tissue of the floor of the mouth, an individual impression tray should be used, rather than an ill-fitting or overextended stock tray. This has been discussed at length in Chapters 5 and 15.

DISTAL EXTENSION REMOVABLE PARTIAL DENTURE

The distal extension removable partial denture does not have the advantage of total tooth support because one or more bases are extensions covering the residual ridge distal to the last abutment. It therefore is dependent on the residual ridge for a portion of its support.

The distal extension removable partial denture must depend on the residual ridge for some support, stability, and retention. Indirect retention, to prevent the denture from lifting away from the residual ridge, should also be incorporated in the design. The tooth-supported base is secured at either end by the action of a direct retainer and supported at either end by a rest, whereas this degree of support and direct retention is lacking in the distal extension prosthesis. For this reason, a distal abutment should be preserved whenever possible. In the event of the loss or absence of a distal abutment tooth, the patient must be made aware of the movements to be expected with a distal extension removable partial denture and the limitations imposed on the dentist when the residual ridge must be used for support, stability, and retention for that part of the prosthesis.

FACTORS INFLUENCING THE SUPPORT OF A DISTAL EXTENSION BASE

Because one of the stated objectives of prosthodontic treatment is the restoration of function and comfort in an esthetically pleasing manner, maintenance of occlusal contact in distal extension removable partial dentures demands an understanding of the factors that influence residual ridge support. Support from the residual ridge becomes more important as the distance from the last abutment increases and will depend on the following several factors:

1. Contour and quality of the residual ridge
2. Extent of residual ridge coverage by the denture base
3. Type and accuracy of the impression registration
4. Accuracy of the fit of the denture base
5. Design of the removable partial denture framework
6. Total occlusal load applied

Contour and Quality of the Residual Ridge

The ideal residual ridge to support a denture base would consist of cortical bone that covers relatively dense cancellous bone with a broad rounded crest and high vertical slopes, and covered by firm, dense, fibrous connective tissue. Such a residual ridge would optimally support vertical and horizontal stresses placed on it by denture bases. Unfortunately, this ideal is seldom encountered.

Easily displaceable tissue will not adequately support a denture base, and tissue that is interposed between a sharp, bony residual ridge and a denture base will not remain in a healthy state. Not only must the nature of the bone of the residual ridge be considered in developing optimum support for the denture base, but the positional relationship of the bone to the direction of forces that will be placed on it must also be considered.

The crest of the bony mandibular residual ridge is most often cancellous. Because lining mucosa restricts both the buccal and lingual mucosa adjacent to teeth in the mandible, loss of firm mucosa overlying the residual ridge is common following tooth extraction in the posterior mandible. Pressures placed on tissue overlying the crest of the mandibular residual ridge usually result in irritation of this tissue, accompanied by the sequelae of chronic inflammation. Therefore the crest of the mandibular residual ridge cannot be a primary stress-bearing region. The buccal shelf region (bounded by the external oblique line and crest of alveolar ridge) seems to be better suited for a primary stress-bearing role, because it is covered by relatively firm, dense, fibrous connective tissue supported by cortical bone. In most instances this region bears more of a horizontal relationship to vertical forces than do other regions of the residual ridge (Figure 16-1). The slopes of the residual ridge then would become the primary stress-bearing regions to resist horizontal and off-vertical forces.

The immediate crest of the bone of the maxillary residual ridge may consist primarily of cancellous bone. Unlike in the mandible, oral tissue that overlies the maxillary residual alveolar bone is usually of a firm, dense nature (similar to the mucosa of the hard palate) or can be surgically prepared to support a denture base. The topography of a partially edentulous maxillary arch imposes a restriction on selection of a primary stress-bearing area. In spite of impression procedures, the crestal area of the residual ridge will become the primary stress-bearing area to vertically directed forces. Some resistance to these forces may come from the immediate buccal and

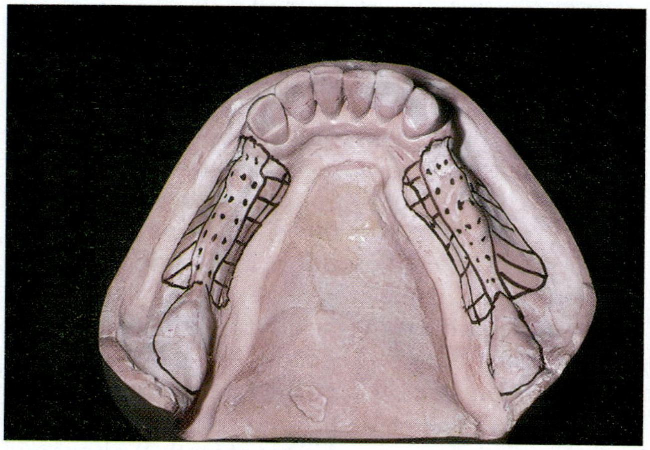

Figure 16-1 *Dotted portion* outlines crest of residual ridge, which should be recorded in its anatomic form in impression procedures. Similarly, retromolar pads should not be displaced by impression. Buccal shelf regions *(diagonal lines)* serve as primary support and therefore additional pressures may be placed on these regions for vertical support of denture base. Lingual slopes of residual ridge *(cross-hatched)* may furnish some vertical support to restoration; however, these regions principally resist horizontal rotational tendencies of denture base and should be recorded by impression in undisplaced form.

lingual slopes of the ridge. Palatal tissue between the medial palatal raphe and the lingual slope of the posterior edentulous ridge are readily displaceable and cannot be considered as primary stress-bearing sites (Figure 16-2). The tissue covering the crest of the maxillary residual ridge must be less displaceable than the tissue that covers palatal areas, or relief of palatal tissue must be provided either in the denture bases or for palatal major connectors.

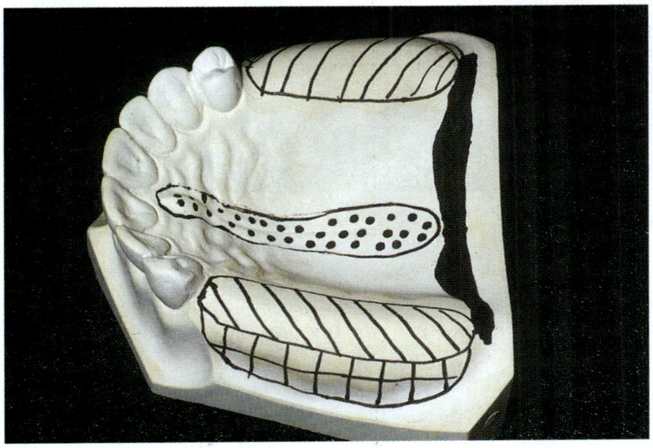

Figure 16-2 Crest of maxillary residual ridge *(diagonal lines)* is primary supporting region for maxillary distal extension denture base. Buccal and palatal slopes may furnish limited vertical support to denture base. It seems logical that their primary role is to counteract horizontal rotational tendencies of denture base. *Dotted portion* outlines incisive papilla and median palatal raphe. Relief must be provided for these regions, especially if tissues covering palatal raphe are less displaceable than those covering crest of residual ridge.

Extent of Residual Ridge Coverage by the Denture Base

The broader the residual ridge coverage the greater the distribution of the load, which results in less load per unit area (Figure 16-3). A denture base should cover as much of the residual ridge as possible and be extended the maximum amount within the physiological tolerance of the limiting border structures or tissue. Knowledge of this border tissue and the structures that influence its movement is paramount to the development of broad coverage denture bases. In a series of experiments, Kaires has shown that "maximum coverage of denture-bearing areas with large, wide denture bases is of the utmost importance in withstanding both vertical and horizontal stresses."

It is not within the scope of this text to review the anatomic considerations related to denture bases. The student is referred to several articles listed in the Selected Reading Resources concerning this subject.

Type and Accuracy of the Impression Registration

The residual ridge may be said to have two forms: the anatomic form and the functional form (Figure 16-4). The anatomic form is the surface contour of the ridge when it is not supporting an occlusal load. The functional form of the residual ridge is the surface contour of the ridge when it is supporting a functional load.

A soft impression material, such as a metallic oxide impression paste, records the anatomic form if the entire impression tray is uniformly relieved. Depending on the viscosity of the particular impression material used and the rigidity of the impression tray, it is also the form that can be recorded by mercaptan rubber, silicone, and hydrocolloid impression

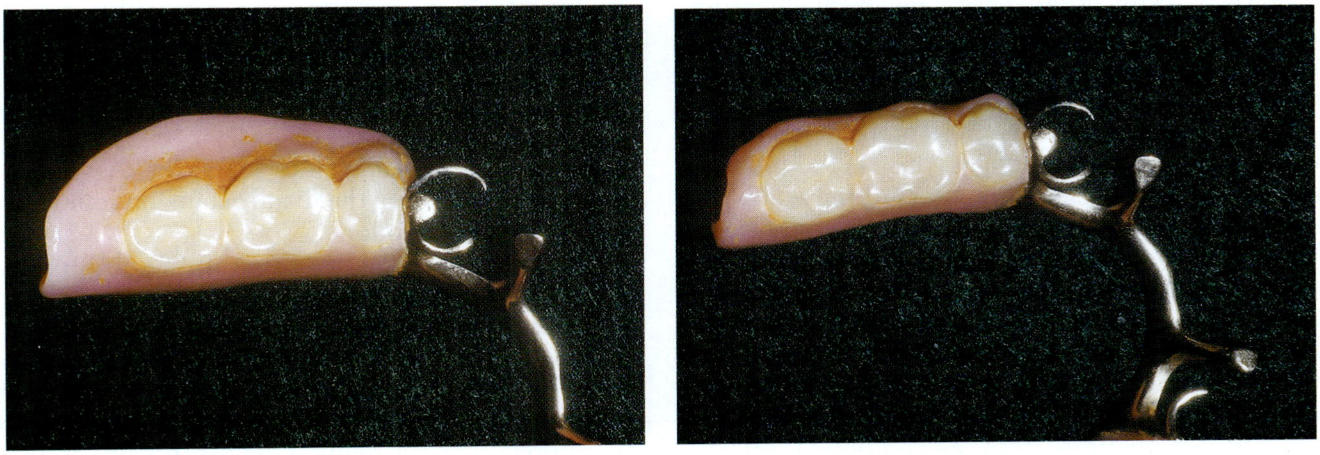

A **B**

Figure 16-3 Comparison of two removable partial dentures for same patient. **A,** A distal extension base that is adequately extended, as it covers both the buccal shelf and retromolar pad. **B,** Underextension of this base results in less support to the prosthesis from the residual ridge, which can cause increased instability of the prosthesis.

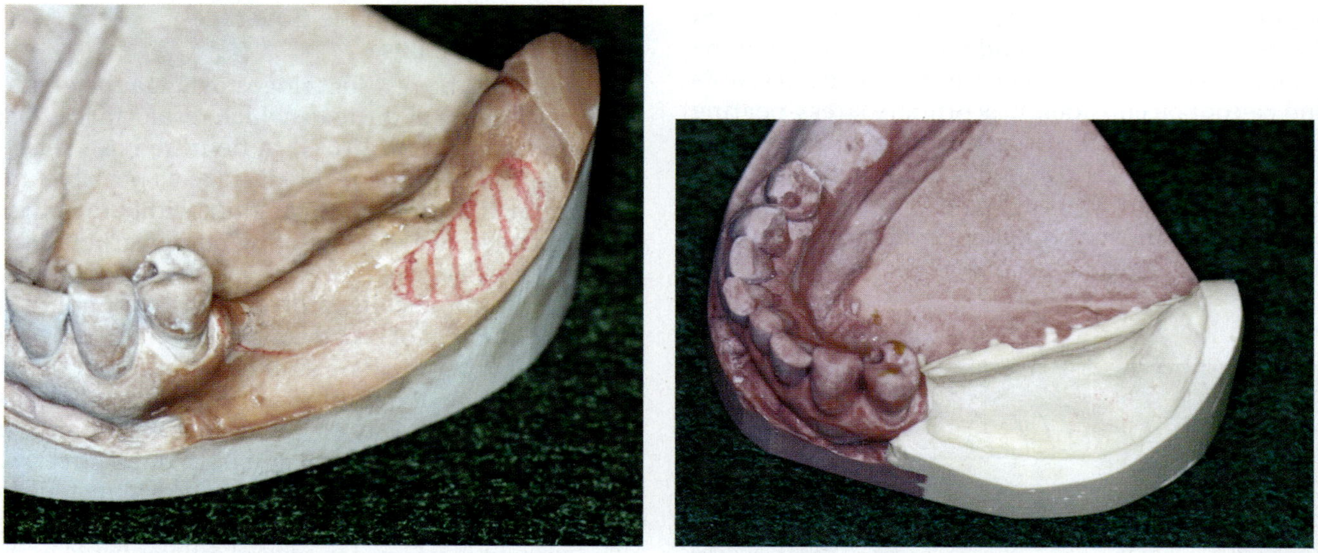

A B

Figure 16-4 Comparison of anatomic and functional ridge forms. **A,** Original mandibular cast showing left residual ridge area recorded in its anatomic form. Buccal shelf region is outlined. **B,** Same cast after left residual ridge area has been repoured to its functional form as recorded by secondary impression.

materials. Distortion and tissue displacement by pressure may result from confinement of the impression material within the tray and from insufficient thickness of impression material between the tray and the tissue, and from the viscosity of the impression material. However, none of these factors is selective or physiological in its action. These accidental distortions of the tissue occur because of faulty technique. The use of the anatomic form of the residual ridge in fabricating complete dentures is quite common because of a belief that this is the most physiological form for support of the dentures.

However, many other dentists believe that certain regions of the residual ridge(s) in a partially edentulous patient are more capable of supporting dentures than other regions. Their impression methods are directed to place more stress on primary stress-bearing regions with specially constructed individual trays and at the same time record the anatomic form of other basal seat tissue, which cannot assume a stress-bearing role. The form of the residual ridge recorded under some loading, whether by occlusal loading, finger loading, specially designed individual trays, or the consistency of the recording medium, is called the functional form. This is the surface contour of the ridge when it is supporting a functional load. How much it will differ from the anatomic form will depend on the thickness and structural characteristics of the soft tissue overlying the residual bone. It will also differ from the anatomic form in proportion to the total load applied to the denture base. Of the two philosophies, the latter seems to be more logical.

McLean and others recognized the need to record the tissue that supports a distal extension removable partial denture base in its functional form, or supporting state, and then relate them to the remainder of the arch by means of a secondary impression. This was called a *functional impression* because it recorded the ridge relation under simulated function.

Any method, whether it records the functional relationship of the ridge to the remainder of the arch or the functional form of the ridge itself, may provide acceptable support for the removable partial denture. On the other hand, those who use the anatomic ridge form for the removable partial denture should seriously consider the need for some mechanical stress-breaker to prevent the possible cantilever action of the distal extension base against the abutment teeth.

Steffel has classified advocates of the various methods for treating the distal extension removable partial denture as follows:

1. Those who believe that ridge and tooth supports can best be equalized by the use of stress-breakers or resilient equalizers
2. Those who insist on bringing about the equalization of ridge and tooth support by physiological basing, which is accomplished by a pressure impression or by relining the denture under functional stresses
3. Those who uphold the idea of extensive stress distribution for stress reduction at any one point

It would seem that there is little difference in the philosophy behind methods 2 and 3 as given by

Steffel because both the equalization of tooth and tissue support and stress distribution over the greatest area are objectives of the functional type of impression. Many of the requirements and advantages that are associated with the distributed stress denture apply equally well to the functionally or physiologically based denture. Some of these requirements are (1) positive occlusal rests; (2) an all-rigid, nonflexible framework; (3) indirect retainers to add stability; and (4) well-adapted, broad coverage bases.

Those who do not accept the theory of physiological basing, for one reason or another, should use some form of stress-breaker between the abutment and the distal extension base. The advantages and disadvantages of doing so have been given in Chapter 9.

Accuracy of the Fit of the Denture Base

Support of the distal extension base is enhanced by intimacy of contact of the tissue surface of the base and the tissue that covers the residual ridge. The tissue surface of the denture base must optimally represent a true negative of the basal seat regions of the master cast. Denture bases have been discussed in Chapter 9.

In addition, the denture base must be related to the removable partial denture framework in the same manner as the basal seat tissue was related to the abutment teeth when the impression was made. Every precaution must be taken to ensure this relationship when the altered cast technique of making a master cast is used.

Design of the Removable Partial Denture Framework

Some rotation movement of a distal extension base at the distal abutment is inevitable under functional loading. It must be remembered that the extent to which abutments are subjected to rotational and torquing forces that result from masticatory function is directly related to the position and resistance of the food bolus. The greatest movement takes place at the most posterior extent of the denture base. The retromolar pad region of the mandibular residual ridge and the tuberosity region of the maxillary residual ridge therefore are subjected to the greatest movement of the denture base (Figure 16-5). Steffel and Kratochvil have suggested that as the rotational axis is moved from a distal-occlusal rest to a more anterior location, more of the residual ridge receives vertically directed occlusal forces to support the denture base (Figure 16-6). They have suggested that occlusal rests may be moved anteriorly to better use the residual ridge for support without jeopardizing either vertical or horizontal support of the denture by occlusal rests and guiding planes (Figure 16-7).

It is possible, however, that the proximal plate minor connector adjacent to the edentulous area will

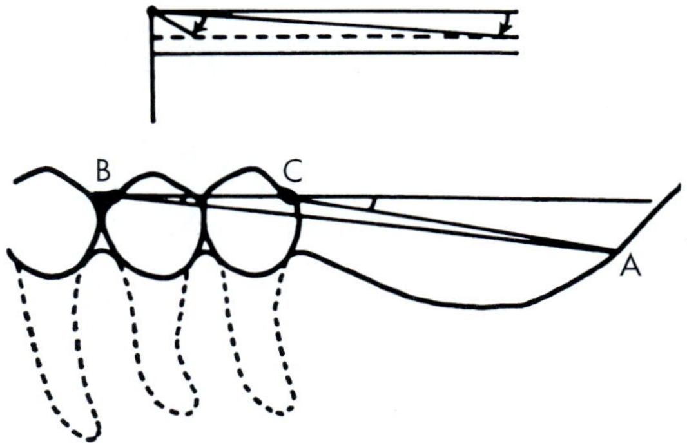

Figure 16-5 Acute dip of short denture base is compared with that of long one in upper figure. In lower figure, when point of rotation is changed from *C* to *B* by losing more teeth, it can be seen that proportionally greater area of residual ridge is used to support denture base than occurs when fulcrum line passes through *C*. Amount of movement is directly related to quality of tissue support. Line *AC* represents length of denture base. (See also Figure 10-3.)

not disengage from or break contact with the guiding plane. When one considers impression and cast formation variables—such as waxing, investing, and casting discrepancies, and finishing and polishing procedures—it may be somewhat philosophical to assume that the minor connector proximal plate will have contact. And if it does, it will disengage its contact with the guiding plane, especially if the tissue that supports the extension denture base is healthy and demonstrates favorable contour. It is more likely that the abutment tooth will move physiologically to contact the minor connector and that the disengagement will depend on the amount of tissue displacement. Figure 10-4 demonstrates geometrically that the actual amount of tissue displacement in the extension base area under occlusal load may not be enough to cause the minor connector to break contact with the guiding plane.

Total Occlusal Load Applied

Patients with distal extension removable partial dentures generally orient the food bolus over natural teeth rather than prosthetic teeth. This is likely because of the more stable nature of the natural dentition, the proprioceptive feedback they provide for chewing, and the possible nociceptive feedback from the supporting mucosa. This has an effect on the direction and magnitude of the occlusal load to the removable partial denture, and thus on the load transferred to the abutments. Given this, the support from the residual ridge should be optimized and shared appropriately with the remaining natural dentition.

The number of artificial teeth, the width of their occlusal surfaces, and their occlusal efficiency influence the total occlusal load applied to the removable

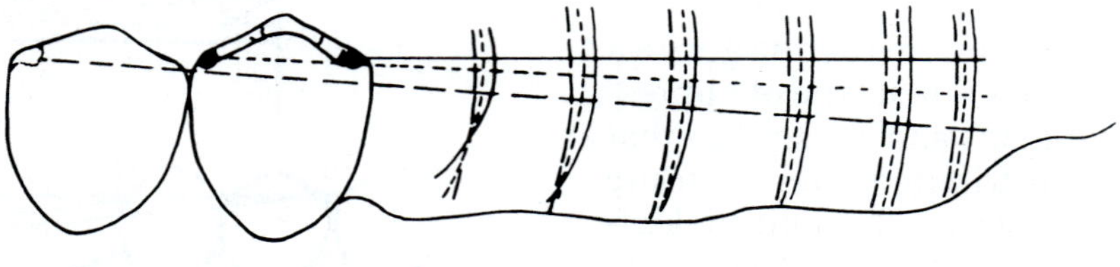

Figure 16-6 If rotation of distal extension base occurs around nearest rest; as rest is moved anteriorly, more of residual ridge will be used to resist rotation. Compare vertical arcs of long-dash broken line with arcs of solid line. (See also Figure 10-4.)

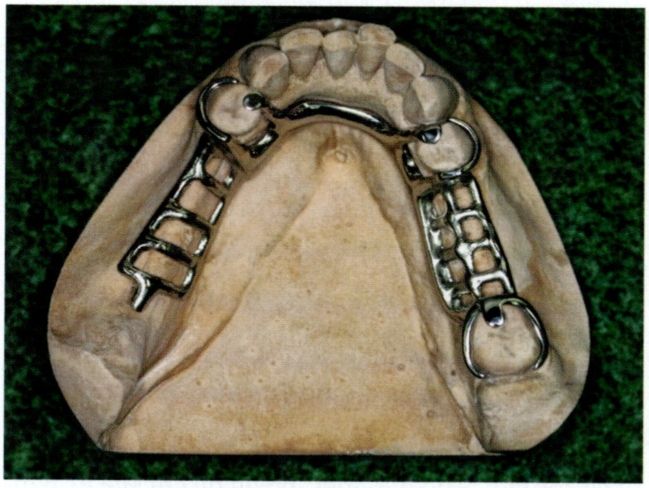

Figure 16-7 Occlusal rest is placed on mesioocclusal surface of left mandibular first premolar, which will move point of rotation anterior to conventionally placed disto-occlusal rest if contact of proximal minor connector on distal guiding plane is designed to release under function. Occlusal rest is connected to lingual bar by minor connector, which contacts small mesiolingual prepared guiding plane.

partial denture. Kaires conducted an investigation under laboratory conditions and concluded "the reduction of the size of the occlusal table reduces the vertical and horizontal forces that act on the removable partial dentures and lessens the stress on the abutment teeth and supporting tissue."*

ANATOMIC FORM IMPRESSION

The anatomic form impression is a one-stage impression method using an elastic impression material that will produce a cast that does not represent a functional relationship between the various supporting structures of the partially edentulous mouth. It will only represent the hard and soft tissue at rest. With the removable partial denture in position in the dental arch, the occlusal rest(s) will fit the rest seat(s) of the abutment teeth, whereas the denture base(s) will fit the surface of the mucosa at rest. When a masticatory load is applied to the extension base(s) with a food bolus, the rest(s) will act as a definite stop, which will limit the part of the base near the abutment tooth from transmitting the load to the underlying anatomic structures. The distal end of the base(s) that is able to move more freely, however, will transmit more of the masticatory load to the underlying extension base tissue and will transmit more torque to the abutment teeth through the rigid removable partial denture framework.

It is obvious that the soft tissue that covers the ridge cannot by itself carry any load applied to it. The soft tissue acts as a protective padding for the bone, which in the final analysis is the structure that receives and resists the masticatory load. Distribution of this load over a maximum area of bone is a prime requisite in preventing trauma both to the tissues of the extension base areas and to the abutment teeth.

A removable partial denture fabricated from a one-stage impression, which only records the anatomic form of basal seat tissue, places more of the masticatory load on the abutment teeth and that part of the bone that underlies the distal end of the extension base. The balance of the bony ridge will not function in carrying its share of the load. The result will be a traumatic load to the bone underlying the distal end of the base and to the abutment tooth, which in turn can result in bone loss and loosening of the abutment tooth. The use of a properly prepared, individualized impression tray can be a means to record the primary stress-bearing areas in a functional form and the nonstress-bearing areas in an anatomic form, just as is often accomplished in making impressions for complete dentures.

Some dentists believe that every removable partial denture should be relined before its final placement in the mouth. Some believe that tissue can be evenly displaced and use impression materials of heavy consistency. This latter practice can introduce traumatic stresses to the underlying tissue. Some dentists use free-flowing pastes that produce an impression of the soft tissue at rest. A removable partial denture

*From Kaires AK: Effect of partial denture design on bilateral force distribution, J Prosthet Dent 6:373-389, 1956.

made according to this technique will be similar to a removable partial denture fabricated from a one-piece impression. The occlusal rest will act as a stop and prevent an even distribution of the masticatory load by the base to the edentulous ridge.

METHODS FOR OBTAINING FUNCTIONAL SUPPORT FOR THE DISTAL EXTENSION BASE

The objective of any functional impression technique is to provide maximum support for the removable partial denture bases. This allows for the maintenance of occlusal contact between both natural and artificial dentition and, at the same time, minimum movement of the base, which would create leverage on the abutment teeth. Although some tissueward movement of the distal extension base is unpreventable and dependent on the six factors listed previously, it can be minimized by providing the best possible support for the denture base.

A thorough understanding of the characteristics of each of the impression materials and impression methods leads to the conclusion that no single material can record both the anatomic form of the teeth and tissue in the dental arch and, at the same time, the functional form of the residual ridge. Therefore some secondary or corrected impression method must be used.

The method selected is greatly influenced by a determination of the support potential of the residual ridge mucosa. Mucosa that is firm and minimally displaceable provides a different support potential than mucosa that is more easily displaced. Methods for obtaining functional support for either should satisfy the two requirements for providing adequate support to the distal extension removable partial denture base. These are (1) that it records and relates the supporting soft tissue under some loading and (2) that it distributes the load over as large an area as possible.

Selective Tissue Placement Impression Method

Soft tissue that covers basal seat areas may be placed, displaced, or recorded in their resting or anatomical form. Placed and displaced tissue differs in the degree of alteration from their resting form and in their physiological reaction to the amount of displacement. For example, the palatal tissue in the vicinity of the vibrating line can be slightly displaced to develop a posterior palatal seal for the maxillary complete denture and will remain in a healthy state for extended periods. On the other hand, this tissue develops an immediate inflammatory response when it has been overly displaced in developing the posterior palatal seal.

Oral tissues that have been overly displaced or distorted attempt to regain their anatomic form. When they are not permitted to do this by the denture bases, the tissues become inflamed and their physiological functions become impaired, accompanied by bone resorption. Tissues that are minimally displaced (placed) by impression procedures for definitive border control respond favorably to the additional pressures placed on them by the resultant denture bases if these pressures are intermittent rather than continuous.

The selective tissue placement impression method is based on these clinical observations, the histological nature of tissue that covers the residual alveolar bone, the nature of the residual ridge bone, and its positional relationship to the direction of stresses that will be placed on it. It is further believed that by use of specially designed individual trays for impressions, denture bases can be developed that will use those portions of the residual ridge that can withstand additional stress and at the same time relieve the tissue of the residual ridge that cannot withstand functional loading and remain healthy.

There should be no philosophical difference in the requirement of support and coverage by bases of distal extension removable partial dentures and complete dentures, either maxillary or mandibular, because the objective of maximum support is the same (Figure 16-8). The tray is unquestionably the most important part of an impression. However, a tray must be so formed and modified that the impression philosophy of the dentist can be carried out. Making individualized acrylic resin impression trays is described in Chapter 15, and the method of attaching custom trays to a removable partial denture framework is illustrated in Figure 16-9.

Since the goal is to maximize soft tissue support and also use teeth to their supportive advantage, the framework fitted to the teeth while registering soft tissue support is a means to coordinate both. This means that before the trays are attached, the framework must be fitted in the mouth as illustrated in Figure 16-10. Fitting the framework involves the following steps:

1. Use of a disclosing media to identify interferences to completely seating the removable partial denture framework
2. Use of disclosing media to identify the appropriate contact(s) of the component parts of the framework during the seating of the framework and when the framework is completely seated in its designated terminal position
3. Adjusting the seated framework to the opposing occlusion

If there are opposing frameworks, the maxillary framework is removed from the mouth and the mandibular framework is adjusted to the natural maxillary dentition. Then the maxillary framework is replaced and it is adjusted to the mandibular

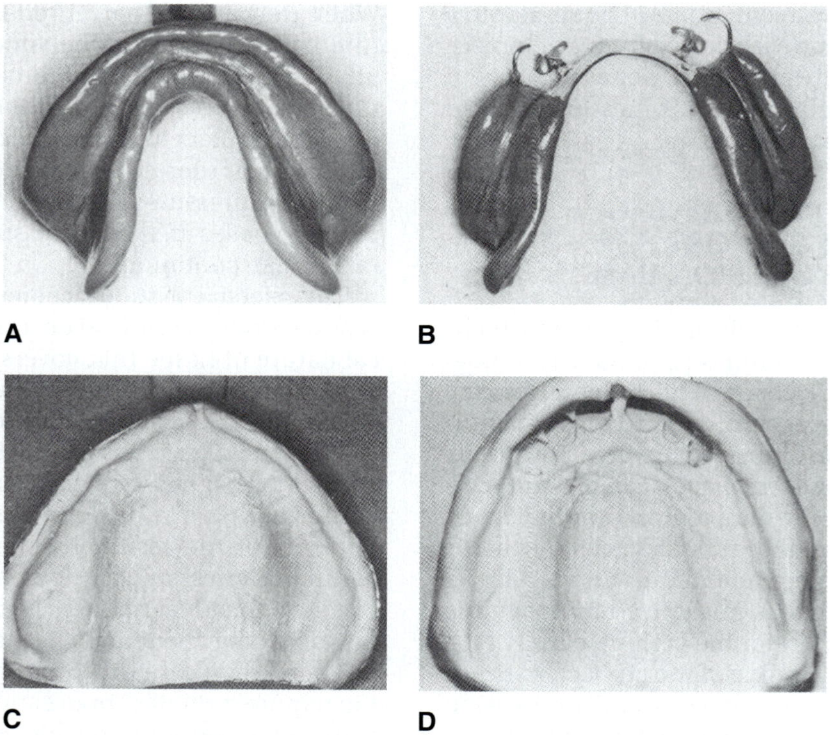

Figure 16-8 **A,** Impression of mandibular edentulous arch using individualized tray and rubber-base impression material. Tray was constructed and impression made so buccal shelves of mandible could assume primary stress-bearing role. **B,** Rubber-base secondary impression of Class I partially edentulous arch made in individualized trays attached to framework. Just as in **A,** buccal shelves will assume primary stress-bearing role. Note similarity of two impressions. In each instance, individualized acrylic resin impression trays permitted dentist to carry out his philosophy of impression making for support of denture bases. **C,** Impression of edentulous maxillary arch made with impression plaster in individualized tray. **D,** Impression of Class I partially edentulous arch made with irreversible hydrocolloid material in individualized tray. Again, without properly constructed individualized tray, a philosophy of impression making is most difficult to carry out.

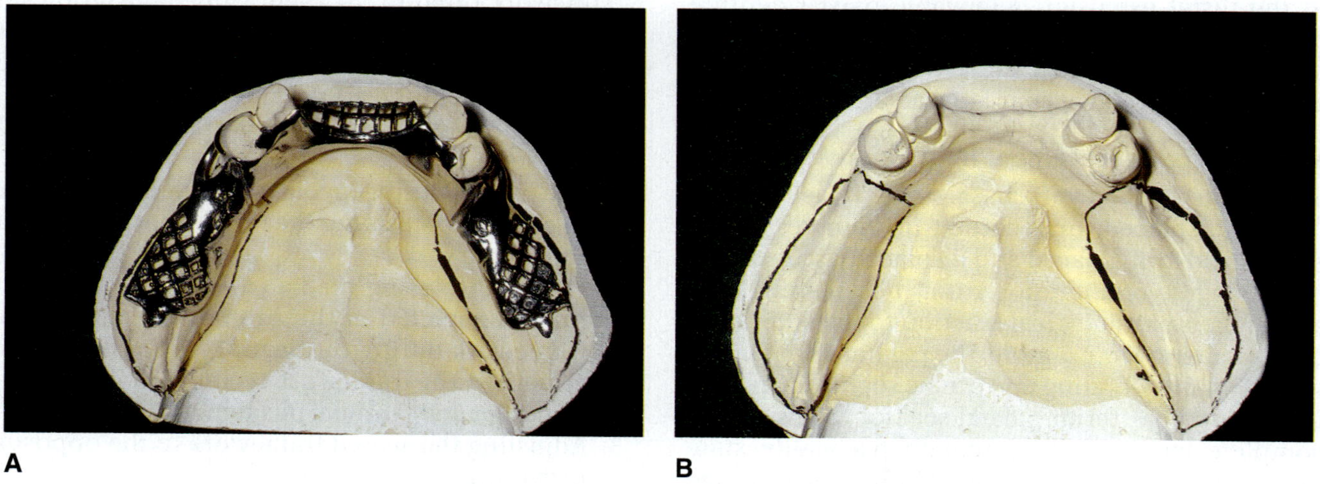

Figure 16-9 Secondary impression for distal extension mandibular removable partial denture is made using individual trays attached to distal extension minor connectors of removable partial denture framework. **A,** Framework has been tried in and fitted to the mouth. **B,** The cast has had the tray outline marked to outline the tray extension.

Continued

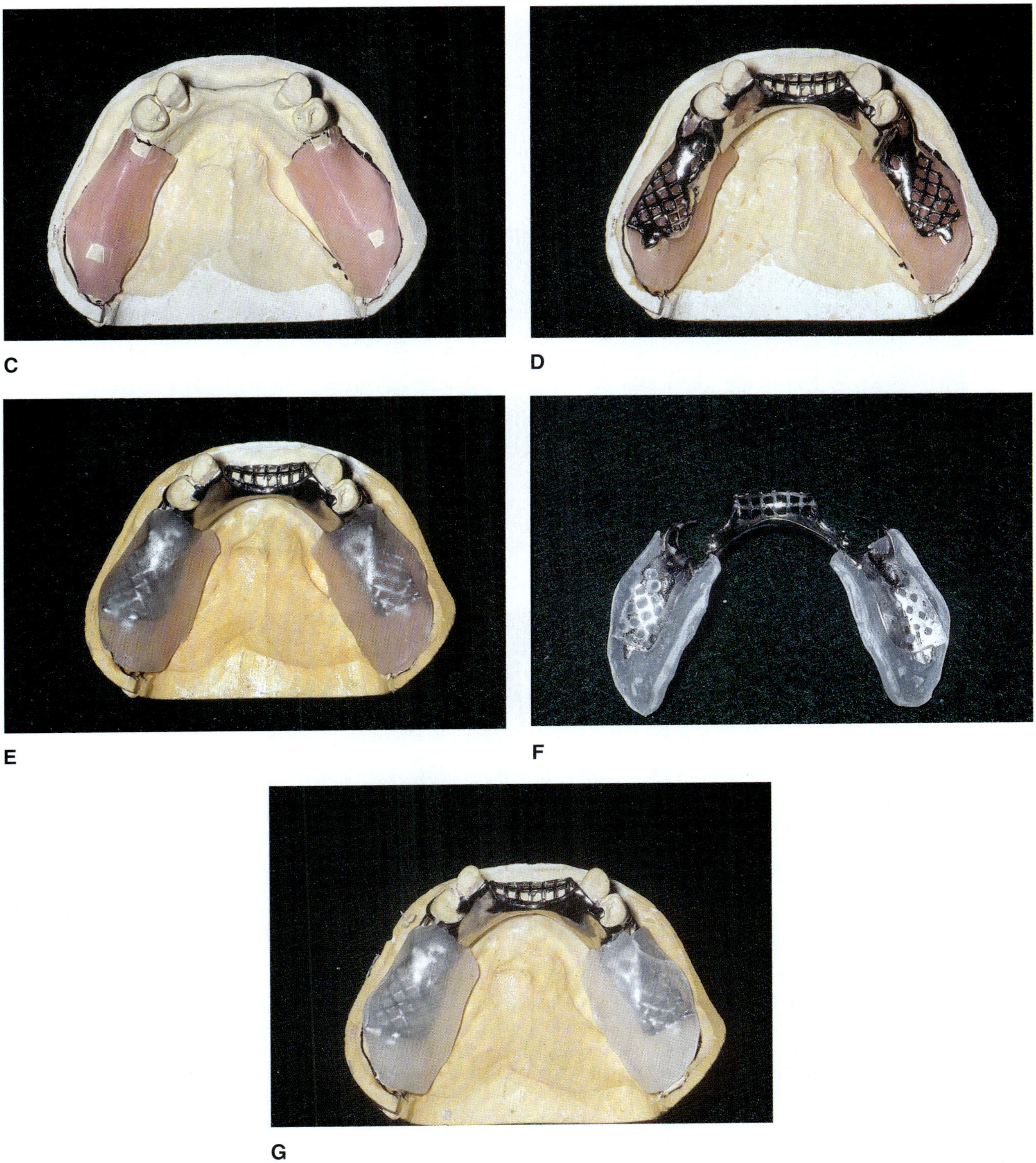

Figure 16-9 Cont'd **C,** A single sheet of baseplate wax relief provided with a window for the posterior tissue stop and anterior tissue index. **D,** The framework is warmed and pressed to position on cast. All regions of cast that will be contacted by autopolymerizing acrylic resin or VLC resin are painted with tinfoil substitute (Alcote) or model release agent (MRA). **E,** A sheet of VLC resin material is adapted to cast and over the framework with finger pressure. Excess material over borders of cast is removed with sharp knife while material is still soft. **F,** The cured acrylic resin trays with framework are removed from cast, and trays are trimmed to outline of wax spacer. **G,** Borders of trays will be adjusted to extend 2 mm short of tissue reflections. Holes will be placed in trays corresponding to crest of residual ridge and retromolar pads to allow escape of excess impression material when impression is made.

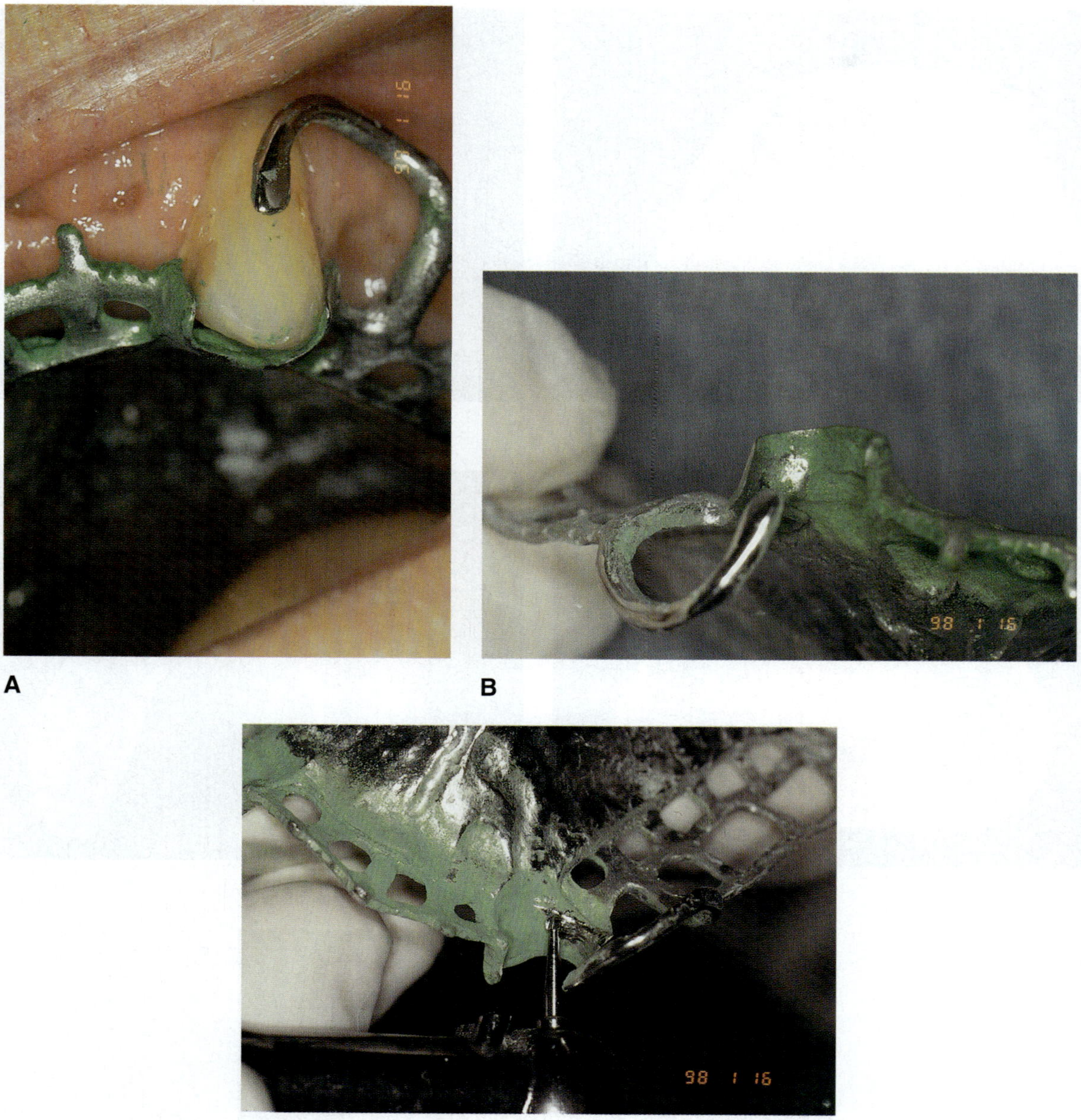

Figure 16-10 The framework must be evaluated to assure complete seating, full contact with the remaining dentition for stabilization, support, and retention as planned, and to allow full natural tooth contact. **A,** Several types of disclosing media may be used, such as stencil correction fluid, rouge and chloroform, and disclosing fluids, pastes, and waxes. Here, a spray disclosing medium has been applied and the framework is placed with mild pressure. Incomplete seating is seen when the framework binds. It is imperative that the framework not be forced to place at this initial seating. **B,** Upon removal it is seen that a portion of the proximal plate is preventing complete seating. **C,** The framework is carefully adjusted since over-adjustment can result in a poorly adapted framework.

Continued

dentition with its framework in place. It is important to remember that the metal frameworks must allow all of the natural dentition to maintain the same designed contact relationship with the opposing arch as when the frameworks are out of the mouth. After the framework has been fitted and the custom trays have been attached, the selective tissue placement impression and cast formation can be accomplished as described in Figure 16-11.

The altered cast method of impression making is most commonly used for the mandibular distal extension partially edentulous arch (Kennedy Class I

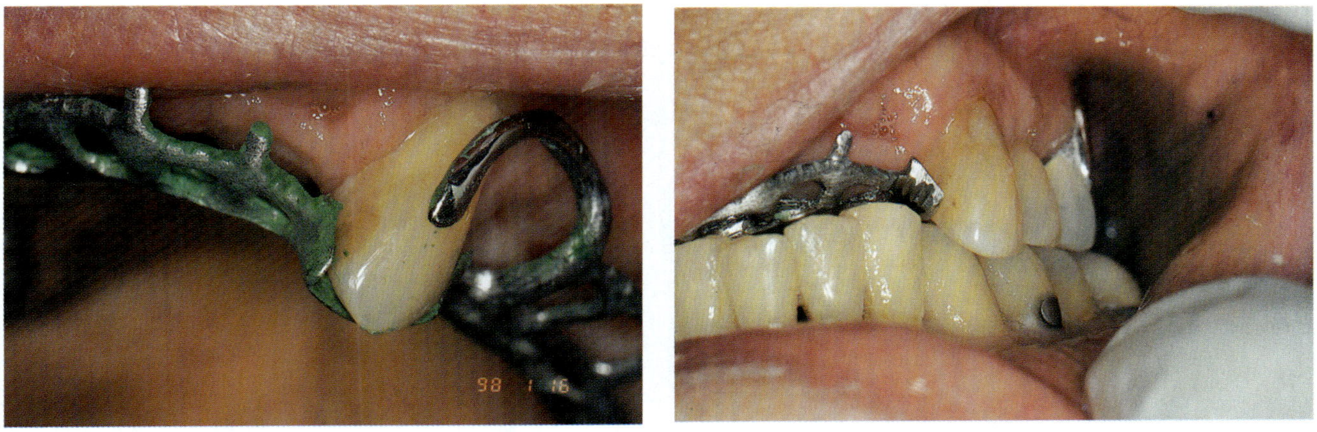

D E

Figure 16-10 Cont'd **D,** The framework is seen to completely seat following adequate adjustment. This may require disclosing and careful adjustment repeated times; however, if improvement is not seen with each framework modification there should be a concern regarding frame accuracy. **E,** Following complete seating and verification of appropriate tooth contacts by component parts (i.e., rests, proximal plates, stabilizing components) the occlusion must be checked and the framework adjusted until natural tooth contacts that exist without the framework seated are achieved with the framework in place. All adjusted regions can be carefully polished with rotary rubber points.

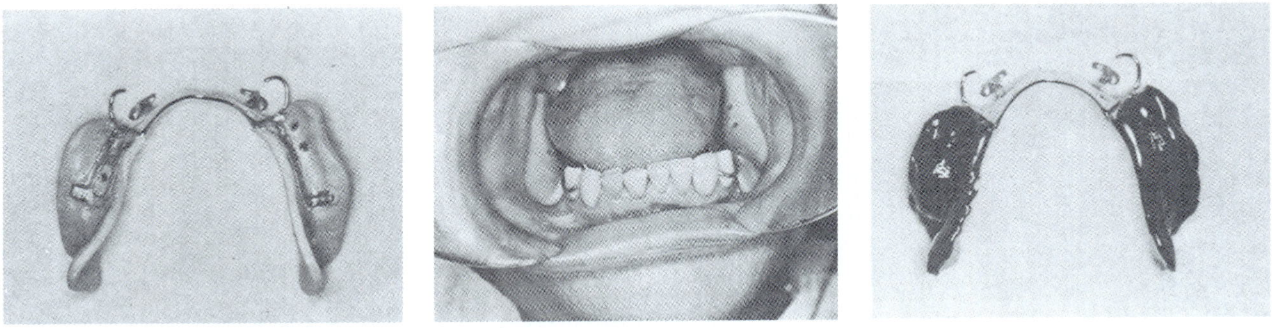

A B C

Figure 16-11 Selective tissue placement impression method (corrected impression). **A,** Individual acrylic resin impression trays are attached to framework. Holes are placed in trays along alveolar grooves to allow escape of excess impression material. **B,** Framework and attached trays are tried in patient's mouth. Borders of trays are adjusted so that they are 2 to 3 mm short of all reflections but cover retromolar pads. **C,** Thin layer of red stick modeling plastic is painted on tissue sides of impression trays by first softening modeling plastic with flame.

Continued

and II arch forms). A common clinical finding in these situations is a greater variation in tissue mobility and tissue distortion or displaceability, which necessitates some selective tissue placement to obtain the desired support from this tissue. This variability in tissue mobility is probably related to the pattern of mandibular residual ridge resorption. Altered cast impression methods are seldom used in the maxillary arch because of the nature of the masticatory mucosa and the amount of firm palatal tissue present to provide soft tissue support. This tissue seldom requires placement to provide the required support. If excessive tissue mobility is present, it is often best managed by surgical resection as this is a primary supporting area.

Obtaining support from the primary support areas is achieved by the manner in which the flow of the impression material is controlled during the impression-making procedure. Restricting the flow of the material in the primary stress-bearing areas (by minimizing the amount of relief over the area when the custom tray was made) causes greater pressure to be exerted on the tissue in this area

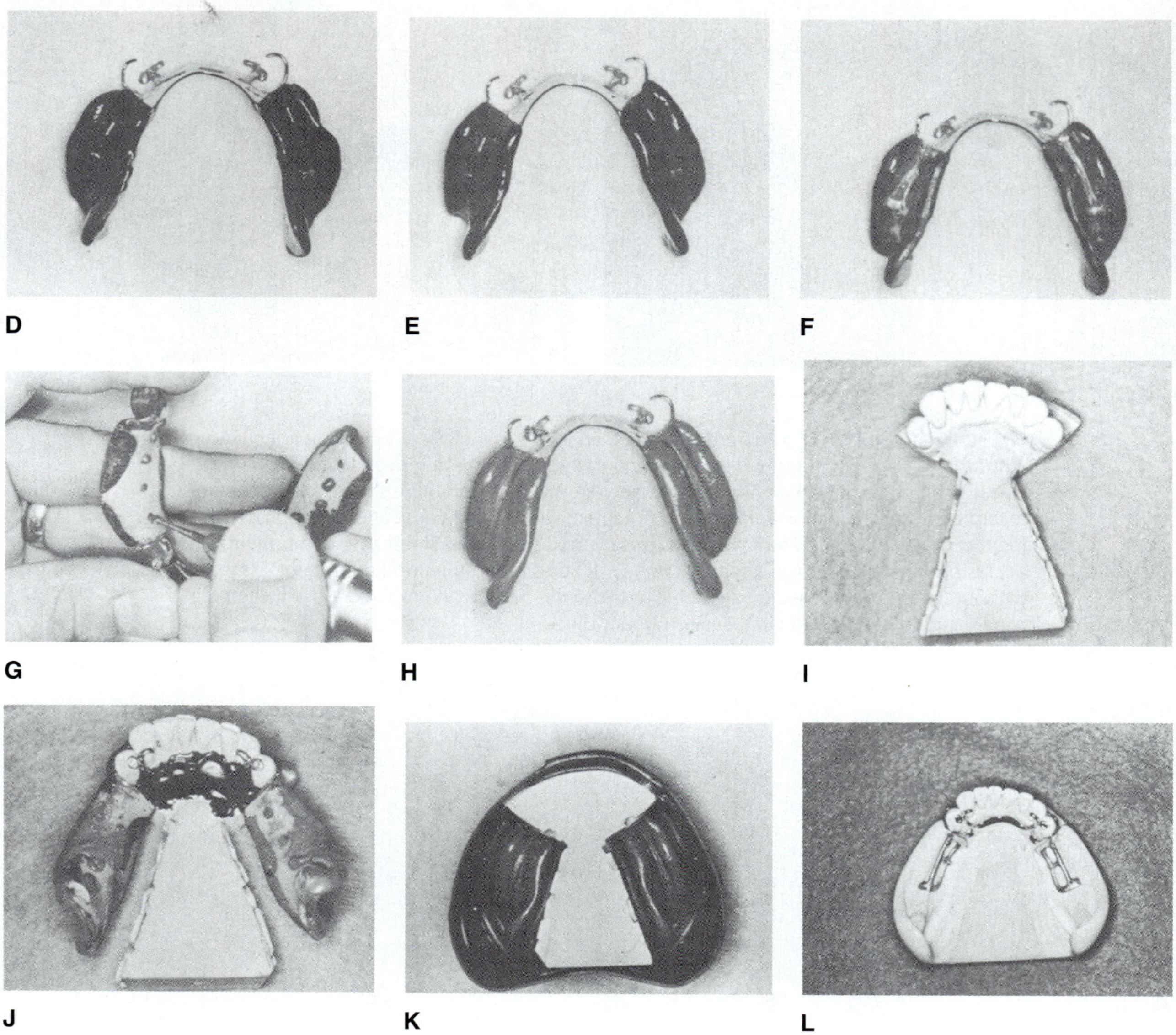

Figure 16-11 Cont'd **D,** Modeling plastic has been softened by flame, tempered in 135° F water, and placed in patient's mouth. This procedure is repeated several times until basal seat tissues are selectively displaced and framework is correctly positioned. Impression trays will be stable at this time and border-molding procedures can begin. **E,** Borders are perfected by heating individual areas, placing tempered tray in mouth, manipulating cheeks, and having patient form lingual borders by tongue movements. Note that lingual flanges have assumed an S shape. This S shape has been formed by action of mylohyoid muscle. Note also that lingual flanges have been extended into retromylohyoid fossas. There would be no difference in form of impression of edentulous regions at this stage from complete denture impression of same regions if patient were edentulous. **F,** Borders of compound impression are shortened 1 to 1.5 mm, and whole inside of impression, with exception of buccal shelf region, is relieved approximately 1 mm. **G,** Modeling plastic is removed from holes in trays. **H,** Final impression is completed with elastic impression material wash. Framework must be perfectly seated and maintained in position while impression material is setting. **I,** Edentulous regions of cast are eliminated. Cut surfaces are grooved for additional retention of stone poured to make altered cast. **J,** Framework and impression are returned to cast and are luted with sticky wax to avoid displacement during boxing and pouring procedures. **K,** Utility wax is used to box impression. **L,** Altered master cast with framework in position. Buccal shelf regions have been recorded in functional form. Other regions of basal seats have been recorded in anatomic form.

(compared with other areas of unrestricted flow where a greater amount of relief or venting of the impression tray was provided). This is often referred to as the "selected pressure" or "dynamic" impression method. By controlling the flow of the impression material with wax relief and venting, one can place or displace the soft tissues over the primary support areas so that they are the primary areas to provide support to the denture base when a removable partial denture is functionally loaded.

An impression for a mandibular distal extension partially edentulous arch may also be adequately made in an individualized, complete arch tray. To do so, not only must the tray be formed to provide proper space for the particular impression materials but also provision must be made so that the functional form of primary stress-bearing areas can be recorded. Such an impression procedure, properly executed, can be used when metal bases are to be incorporated in the design of the restoration. There is little difference if any between recording the basal seats in the partially edentulous arch and recording like areas for complete dentures on an edentulous arch. A secondary impression made in custom trays attached to the framework only makes definitive border control and tissue placement a bit easier compared with the individualized complete arch tray.

Functional Impression Technique

When the residual ridge mucosa demonstrates a uniformly firm consistency, an impression technique that involves capturing the tissue form while the patient is in occlusion can be considered. Such a technique records the mucosal position and shape under the influence of a static closure force, similar to functional masticatory forces. The more the mucosa displaces under function, the more rebound there is likely to be. Since the prosthesis will be under occlusal load for only a portion of a day, minimal rebound is desired so as to maintain the clasp assembly tooth relationship. When such a technique is applied to firm, minimally displaceable mucosa, there is minimal rebound effect on prosthesis position. The selective pressure technique described above can be applied to all varieties of residual ridges as it is customized to mucosal conditions, whereas the functional impression technique has limited application to a uniformly firm ridge consistency.

SELF-ASSESSMENT AIDS

1. Support for a tooth-supported removable partial denture is provided by what oral structures?
2. Support for a distal extension denture is provided by what oral structures?
3. Residual ridges may be recorded by an impression in their anatomic form or functional form. A Class III arch may be recorded in its ______ form; however, the residual ridges in Class I or II arches should be recorded in their ______ form.
4. There are at least six important factors that influence the support of a distal extension denture base by the residual ridges. State them.
5. Describe what is considered to be an ideal residual ridge to support a distal extension denture base.
6. What areas of the residual ridge are considered to be the primary stress-bearing areas for a mandibular distal extension base? A maxillary distal extension base?
7. Why can the crest of the mandibular residual ridge not assume a stress-bearing role?
8. Which type of tissue interposed between a denture base and the underlying bone would probably afford a more favorable reaction to stress: firm, dense, fibrous connective tissue or easily displaceable connective tissue? Defend your choice.
9. The space that is available for a distal extension denture base is controlled by the moving structures that surround the space. True or false?
10. A denture base should cover as much of the residual ridge as possible and be extended the maximum amount within the physiological tolerance of the limiting border structures. True or false?
11. The objective of any functional impression technique is to provide maximum support for the removable partial denture base. When this objective is attained, what advantages accrue to the denture environment?
12. How does accuracy or inaccuracy of the denture base influence the quality of support by the residual ridge?
13. Because some rotational movement of the extension denture is bound to occur, and because use of as much of the primary stress-bearing areas as possible is desirable, in what manner may the design of the framework (location of rests and minor connectors) influence the greatest use of the primary stress-bearing areas? Illustrate with a simple diagram.
14. Total occlusal load applied to a denture base certainly influences the quality of support from the base. What can be done to lessen the total occlusal applied load in relation to the prosthetically supplied teeth?
15. Many approaches can record the functional form of residual ridges in Class I and II arches and relate this form accurately to the rest of the dental arch. The various methods are only means to an end. A basic understanding of anatomy, histology, physiology, materials, and principles

will permit each dentist to develop an individual philosophy and a technique of impression making. Rationalize the functional relining method and the selective tissue placement method (whether with fluid waxes or other materials) and how they are related to the anatomic form under functional loading to the rest of the arch.

16. What are the risks involved in a closed-mouth method while performing a functional impression procedure?
17. It is noted in some of the various methods of making functional impressions of residual ridges that a series of holes are placed in the alveolar groove of the trays. What is accomplished by such a procedure?
18. What is the most important part of an impression? If you answered the tray, that is correct. Describe why this must be true in relation to what one tries to accomplish in an impression procedure.
19. Should there be any difference in the support characteristic, extension, and form of a removable partial denture extension base and a complete denture base occupying the same area? Explain.
20. One procedure discussed in the text is the selective tissue placement of impression making. What is meant by tissue placement?
21. Fully describe a selective tissue placement procedure for making impressions of mandibular extension residual ridges.
22. What is meant by a secondary impression?
23. What does an altered cast in relation to impression making mean?

17

OCCLUSAL RELATIONSHIPS FOR REMOVABLE PARTIAL DENTURES

The fourth phase* in the treatment of patients with removable partial dentures is the establishment of a functional and harmonious occlusion. Occlusal harmony between a removable partial denture and the remaining natural teeth is a major factor in the preservation of the health of their surrounding structures. In the treatment of patients with complete dentures, the inclination of the condyle path is the only factor not within the control of the dentist. All other factors may be altered to obtain occlusal balance and harmony in eccentric positions to conform to a particular concept and philosophy of occlusion.

Balanced occlusion is desirable with complete dentures because unbalanced occlusal stresses may cause instability of the dentures and trauma to the supporting structures. These stresses can reach a point that causes movement of the denture bases. In removable partial dentures, however, because of the attachment of the removable partial denture to the abutment teeth, occlusal stresses can be transmitted directly to the abutment teeth and other supporting structures, resulting in sustained stresses that may be more damaging than those transient stresses found in complete dentures. Failure to provide and maintain adequate occlusion on the removable partial denture is primarily a result of: (1) lack of support for the denture base, (2) the fallacy of establishing occlusion to a single static jaw relation record, and (3) an unacceptable occlusal plane.

In establishing occlusion on a removable partial denture the influence of the remaining natural teeth is usually such that the occlusal forms of the teeth on the removable partial denture must be made to conform to an already established occlusal pattern. Occlusal adjustment or restoration may have altered this pattern. However, the pattern present at the time the removable partial denture is made dictates the occlusion on the removable partial denture. The only exceptions are those in which an opposing complete denture can be made to function harmoniously with the removable partial denture or in which only anterior teeth remain in both arches and the incisal relationship can be made so that tooth contacts do not disturb denture stability or retention. In these situations jaw relation records and the arrangement of the teeth may proceed in the same manner as with complete dentures, and the same general principles apply.

*See Chapter 2, under discussion on the six phases of removable partial denture service.

With all other types of removable partial dentures the remaining teeth dictate the occlusion. The dentist should strive for planned contacts in centric occlusion and no interferences in lateral excursions. While a functional relationship of the removable partial denture to the natural dentition sometimes may be adjusted satisfactorily in the mouth, extraoral adjustment is often easier for both dentist and patient, more accurate, and can be accomplished in a more comprehensive manner.

The establishment of a satisfactory occlusion for the removable partial denture patient should include the following: (1) an analysis of the existing occlusion; (2) the correction of existing occlusal disharmony; (3) the recording of centric relation or an adjusted centric occlusion; (4) the recording of eccentric jaw relations or functional eccentric occlusion; and (5) the correction of occlusal discrepancies created by the fit of the framework and in processing the removable partial denture.

DESIRABLE OCCLUSAL CONTACT RELATIONSHIPS FOR REMOVABLE PARTIAL DENTURES

The following occlusal arrangements are recommended to develop a harmonious occlusal relationship of removable partial dentures and to enhance stability of the removable partial dentures:

1. Simultaneous bilateral contacts of opposing posterior teeth must occur in centric occlusion.
2. Occlusion for tooth-supported removable partial dentures may be arranged similar to the occlusion seen in a harmonious natural dentition, since stability of such removable partial dentures results from the effect of the direct retainers at both ends of the denture base (Figure 17-1).
3. Bilateral balanced occlusion in eccentric positions should be formulated when a maxillary complete denture (Figure 17-2) opposes the removable partial denture. This is accomplished primarily to promote the stability of the complete denture. However, simultaneous contacts in a protrusive relationship do not receive priority over appearance, phonetics, and/or a favorable occlusal plane.
4. Working side contacts should be obtained for the mandibular distal extension denture (Figure 17-3). These contacts should occur simultaneously with working side contacts of the natural teeth to distribute the stress over the greatest possible area. Masticatory function of the denture is improved by such an arrangement.
5. Simultaneous working and balancing contacts should be formulated for the maxillary bilateral distal extension removable partial denture whenever possible (Figure 17-4). Such an arrangement will compensate in part for the unfavorable position the maxillary artificial teeth must occupy in relation to the residual ridge, which is usually lateral to the crest of the ridge. However, this desirable relationship must often be compromised when the patient's anterior teeth have an excessively steep vertical overlap with little or no horizontal overlap. Even in this situation, working side contacts can be obtained without resorting to excessively steep cuspal inclinations.
6. Only working contacts need to be formulated for either the maxillary or mandibular unilateral distal extension removable partial denture (Figure 17-5). Balancing side contacts would not enhance the stability of the denture because it is entirely tooth supported by the framework on the balancing side.

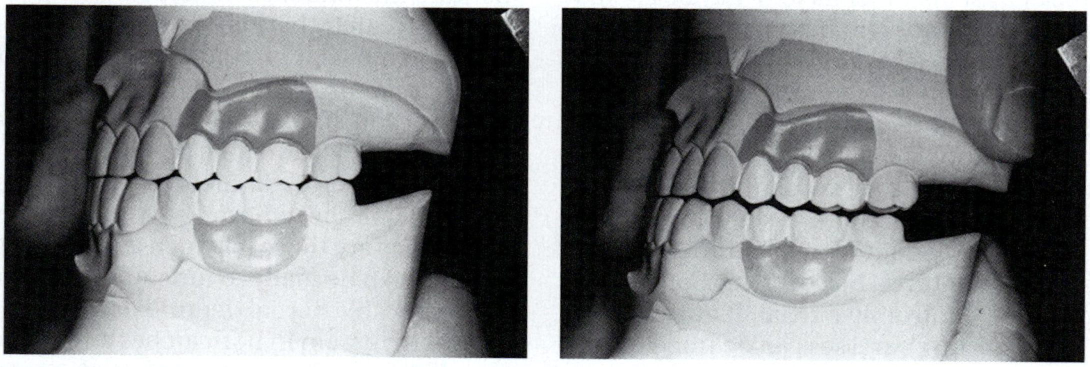

A B

Figure 17-1 Opposing partially edentulous arches having prospective abutments bounding all edentulous spaces. **A,** Linear working contacts may be developed if group function does not take molars out of contact in working position. **B,** Posterior balancing and protrusive contacts would not add to stability of either restoration and should be avoided.

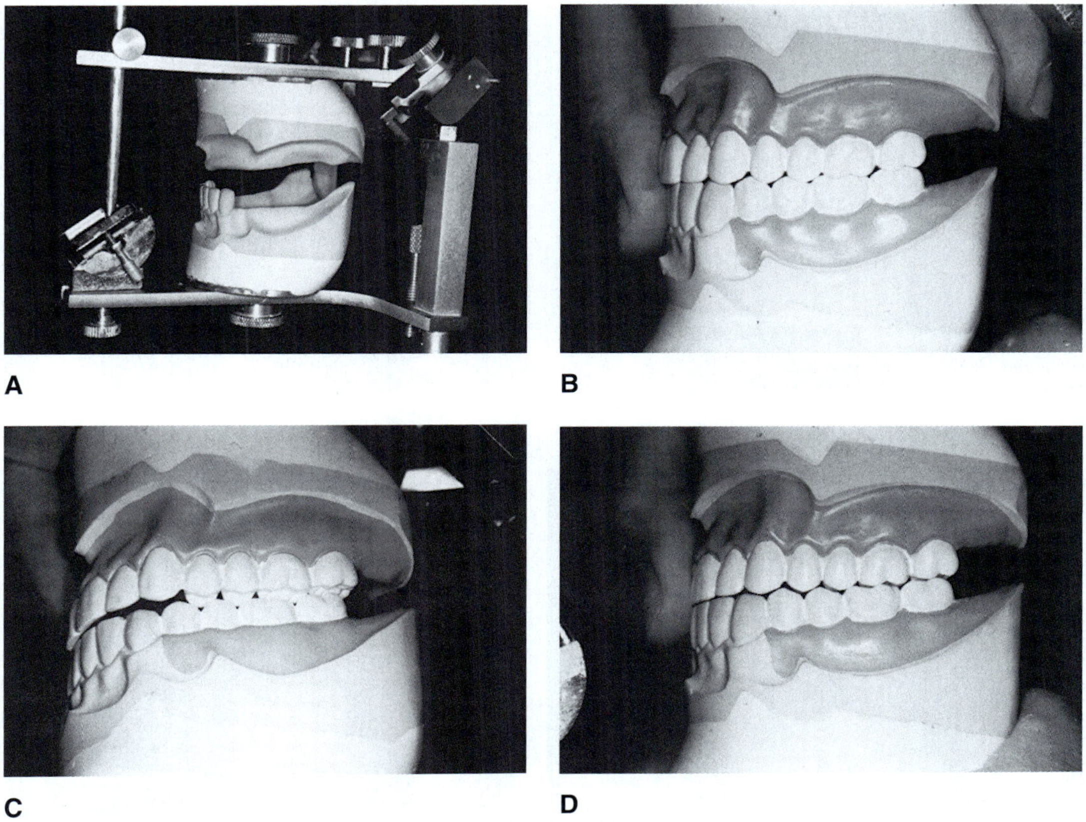

Figure 17-2 **A,** Class I partially edentulous arch opposed by edentulous maxillary arch. Stability of maxillary complete denture can be promoted by developing balanced occlusion. **B,** Linear working contacts. **C,** Balancing contacts are arranged, thus minimizing tipping stresses to complete denture. **D,** Protrusive contact of posterior teeth will better distribute forces to entire basal seat of complete denture in contrast to contacts only by opposing anterior teeth.

7. In the Kennedy Class IV removable partial denture configuration, contact of opposing anterior teeth in the planned intercuspal position is desired to prevent a continuous eruption of the opposing natural incisors (Figure 17-6), unless they are otherwise prevented from extrusion by means of a lingual plate, auxiliary bar, or by splinting. Contact of the opposing anterior teeth in eccentric positions can be developed to enhance incisive function but should be arranged to permit balanced occlusion without excursive interferences.
8. Balanced contact of opposing posterior teeth in a straightforward protrusive relationship and functional excursive positions is desired only when an opposing complete denture or bilateral distal extension maxillary removable partial denture is placed (see Figures 17-2 and 17-4).
9. Artificial posterior teeth should not be arranged farther distally than the beginning of a sharp upward incline of the mandibular residual ridge or over the retromolar pad (Figure 17-7). To do so would have the effect of shunting the denture anteriorly.

A harmonious relationship of opposing occlusal and incisal surfaces alone is not adequate to ensure stability of distal extension removable partial dentures. In addition, the relationship of the teeth to the residual ridges must be considered. Bilateral eccentric contact of the mandibular distal extension removable partial denture need not be formulated to stabilize the denture. The buccal cusps, however, must be favorably placed to direct stress toward the buccal shelf, which is the primary support area in the mandibular arch. In such positions the denture is not subjected to excessive tilting forces (Figure 17-8). On the other hand, the artificial teeth of the bilateral, distal extension, maxillary removable partial denture often must be placed laterally to the crest of the residual ridge (Figure 17-9). Such an unfavorable position can cause tipping of the denture, which is restrained only by direct retainer action on the balancing side. To enhance the stability of the denture, it seems logical to provide simultaneous working and balancing contacts in these situations if possible.

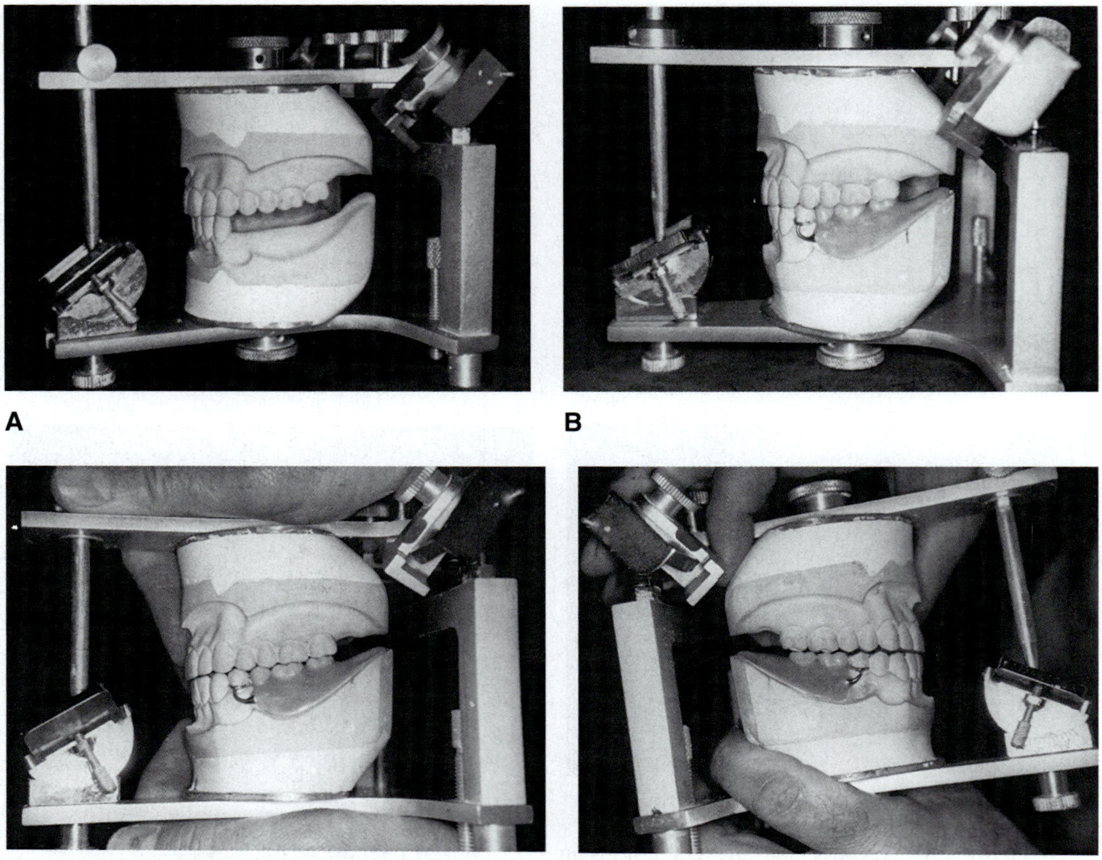

A B C D

Figure 17-3 **A,** Bilateral distal extension mandibular arch opposed by natural dentition in maxillary arch. Master casts have been oriented in articulator in centric relation. **B,** Acrylic resin record bases attached to framework are used to support artificial teeth that have been arranged in maximum intercuspation. **C,** Working contacts have been developed after articulator was programmed with eccentric records. **D,** Balancing contacts are purposefully avoided because they would not enhance stability of restoration. Protrusive balance is also avoided in order to achieve an acceptable appearance, phonetics, and a favorable occlusal plane.

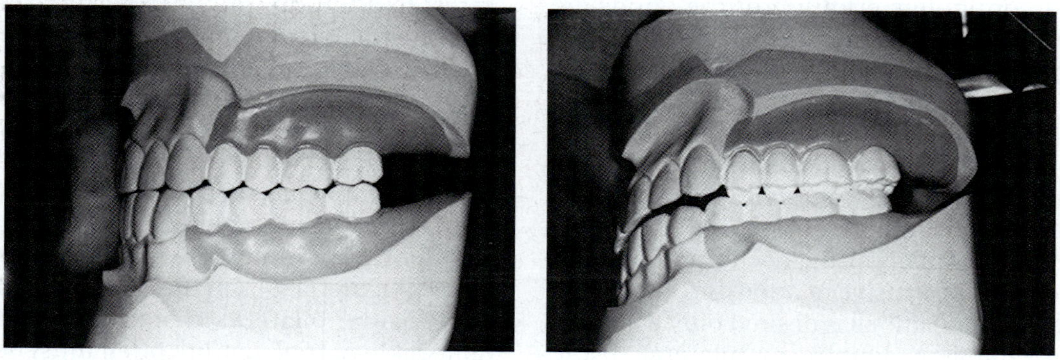

A B

Figure 17-4 Casts of opposing Class I partially edentulous arches correctly oriented on programmed articulator. **A,** Resultant restoration has linear working side contacts of opposing posterior teeth occurring simultaneously with contact of opposing canines on working side. **B,** Balancing contact should be arranged to minimize tipping of maxillary removable partial denture and to broadly distribute forces accruing to its supporting structures (abutments and residual ridges).

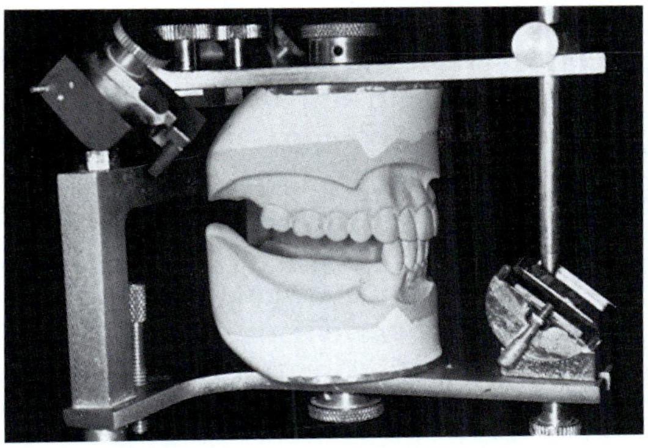

A

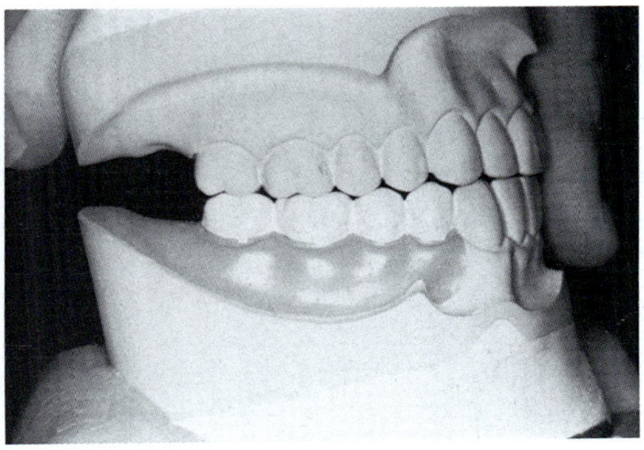

B

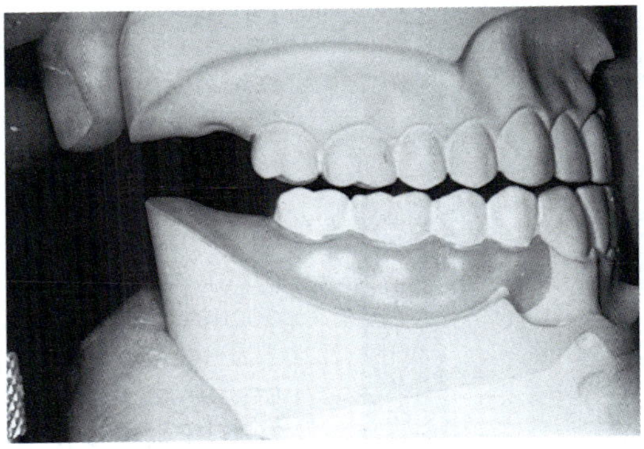

C

Figure 17-5 **A,** Class III (skeletal classification) mandibular arch opposed by natural dentition. **B,** Artificial teeth were arranged for maximum intercuspation in centric occlusion with linear working contacts. **C,** Posterior protrusive and balancing contacts have been avoided because such arrangement would not enhance stability of the unilateral restoration.

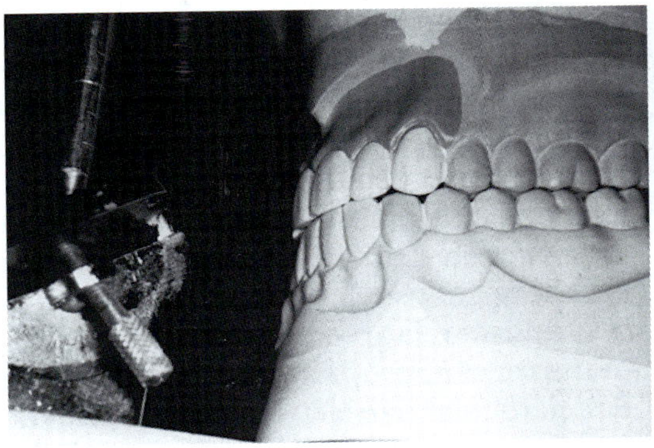

A

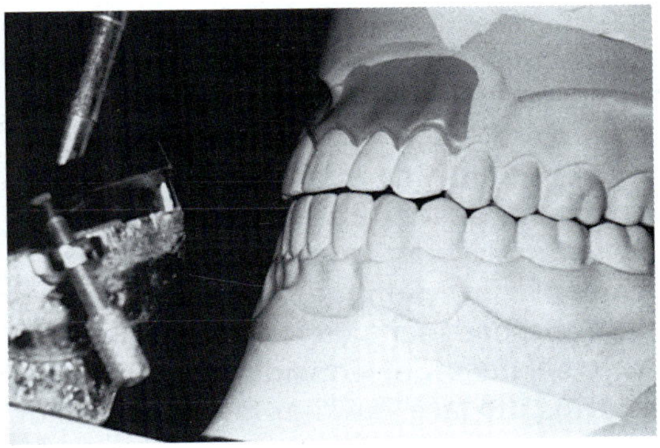

B

Figure 17-6 Class IV maxillary arch opposed by mandibular dentulous arch. **A,** Contact of prosthetically supplied teeth and opposing mandibular teeth has been developed in the planned intercuspal position to prevent continued eruption of mandibular teeth. **B,** Contact of anterior teeth in eccentric positions is avoided to eliminate unfavorable forces to maxillary anterior residual ridge.

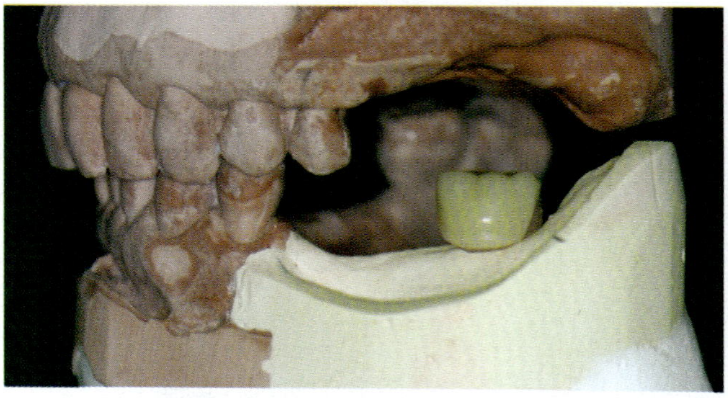

Figure 17-7 Mandibular posterior teeth should not be arranged distal to the upward incline *(ascending ramus)* of residual ridge. The molar tooth has been placed just anterior to a mark on the cast land area designating the beginning incline.

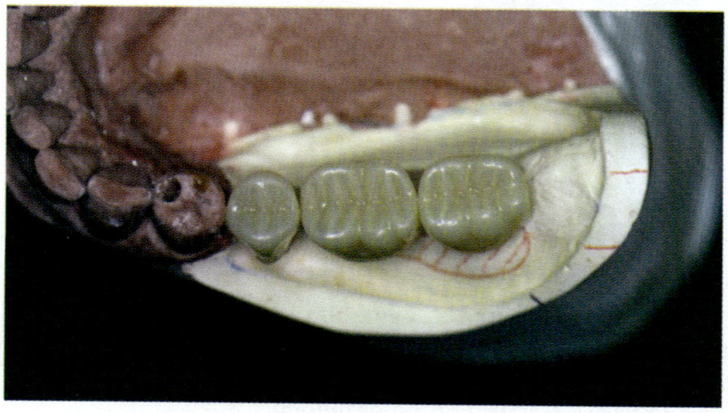

Figure 17-8 The posterior teeth in this distal extension have been selected with a narrower buccal-lingual width than the original teeth, and they are placed relative to the primary support *(buccal shelf)* to distribute the functional load to the most anatomically favorable location in a manner that reduces leverage effects.

METHODS FOR ESTABLISHING OCCLUSAL RELATIONSHIPS

Five methods of establishing interocclusal relations for removable partial dentures will be briefly described. Before describing any of these, it is necessary that the use of a face-bow mounting of the maxillary cast and the pertinent factors in removable partial denture occlusion be considered. The technique for applying the face-bow has been described briefly in Chapter 12.

Although a hinge axis mounting may be desirable for complete oral rehabilitation procedures, any of the common types of face-bow will facilitate mounting of the maxillary cast in relation to the condylar axis in the articulating instrument with reasonable accuracy and are acceptable for a removable partial denture. As suggested in Chapter 12, it is still better that the plane of occlusion be related to the axis-orbital plane. Because the dominant factor in removable partial denture occlusion is the remaining natural teeth and their proprioceptive influence on occlusion, a comparable radius at the oriented plane of occlusion in an acceptable instrument will allow reasonably valid mandibular movements to be reproduced.

Semiadjustable articulators can simulate but not duplicate jaw movement. A realization of the limitations of a specific instrument and knowledge of the procedures that can overcome these limitations are necessary if an adequate occlusion is to be created.

The recording of occlusal relationships for the partially edentulous arch may vary from the simple apposition of opposing casts (by occluding sufficient remaining natural teeth) to the recording of jaw relations in the same manner as for a completely edentulous patient. As long as there are natural teeth that remain in contact, however, the cuspal influence that those teeth will have on functional jaw movements dictates the placement of the artificial teeth and the occlusal scheme.

The horizontal jaw relation (planned intercuspal position or centric relation) in which the restoration is to be fabricated should have been determined during diagnosis and treatment planning. Mouth preparations also should have been accomplished based on this determination, including occlusal adjustment of the natural dentition, if such was indicated. Therefore one of the following conditions should exist: (1) centric relation and planned intercuspal position coincide with no evidence of occlusal pathological conditions, therefore the decision should be to fabricate the restoration in centric relation; (2) centric relation and the planned intercuspal position do not coincide, but the planned intercuspal position is clearly defined and the decision has been made to fabricate the restoration in the planned intercuspal position; (3) centric relation and the planned intercuspal position do not coincide and the intercuspal position is not clearly defined, therefore the decision should be made to fabricate the restoration in centric relation; and (4) posterior teeth are not present in one or both arches and the denture will be fabricated in centric relation.

Occlusal relationships may be established by use of the most appropriate of the following methods to fit a particular partially edentulous situation.

Direct Apposition of Casts

The first method is used when there are sufficient opposing teeth that remain in contact to make the existing jaw relationship obvious or when only a few teeth are to be replaced on short denture bases and there is no evidence of occlusal abnormalities. In this method, opposing casts may be occluded by hand. The occluded casts should be held in apposition with

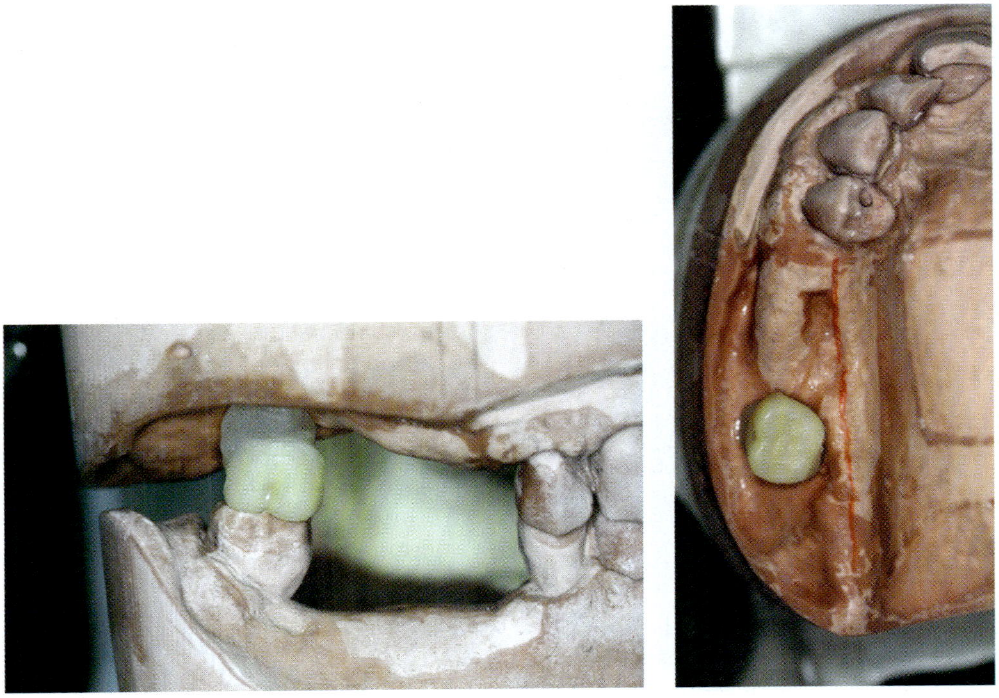

A B

Figure 17-9 **A,** Maxillary molar occluded in a normal horizontal relationship to the opposing molar. **B,** The resultant position is lateral to the supporting crest of the residual ridge. This position is functionally unfavorable due to the potentially unstable leverage effects; however, stability can be improved by arranging simultaneous working and balancing contacts in occlusal scheme.

rigid supports attached with sticky wax to the bases of the casts until they are securely mounted in the articulator.

At best, this method can only perpetuate the existing occlusal vertical dimension and any existing occlusal disharmony present between the natural dentition. Occlusal analysis and the correction of any existing occlusal disharmony should precede the acceptance of such a jaw relation record. The limitations of such a method should be obvious. Yet, such a jaw relation record is better than an inaccurate interocclusal record between the remaining natural teeth. Unless a record is made that does not influence the closing path of the mandible because of its bulk and/or the consistency of the recording medium, direct apposition of opposing casts at least eliminates the possibility of the patient giving a faulty jaw relationship.

Interocclusal Records With Posterior Teeth Remaining

A second method, which is a modification of the first, is used when sufficient natural teeth remain to support the removable partial denture (Kennedy Class III or IV), but the relation of opposing natural teeth does not permit the occluding of casts by hand. In such situations, jaw relations must be established the same as fixed restorations that use some type of interocclusal record.

The least accurate of these methods is the interocclusal wax record. The bulk, consistency, and accuracy of the wax will influence the successful recording of centric relation with an interocclusal wax record after chilling. Excess wax that contacts mucosal surfaces may distort soft tissue, thereby preventing accurate seating of the wax record onto the stone casts. Distortion of wax during or after removal from the mouth may also interfere with accurate seating. Therefore a definite procedure for making interocclusal wax records is given as follows.

A uniformly softened, metal-reinforced wafer of baseplate or set-up wax is placed between the teeth, and the patient is guided to close in centric relation (Figure 17-10). Correct closure should have been rehearsed before placement of the wax so that the patient will not hesitate or deviate in closing. The wax is then removed and immediately chilled thoroughly in room-temperature water. It should be replaced a second time to correct the distortion that results from chilling and then again chilled after removal.

All excess wax should now be removed with a sharp knife. It is most important at this time that all

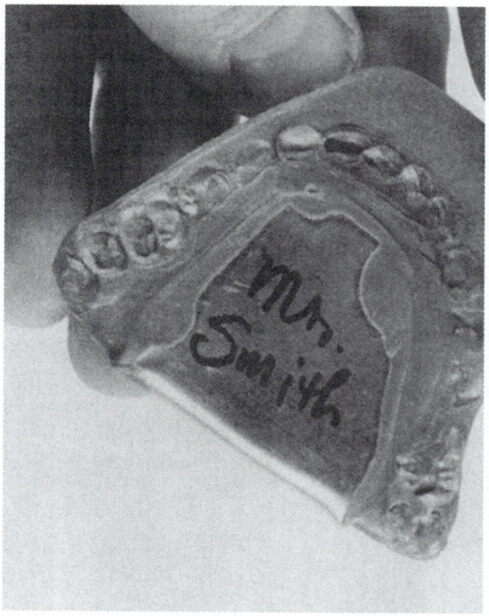

Figure 17-10 Aluwax wafer shaped to just clear lingual surfaces of teeth in lower arch. Water bath is used to uniformly soften Aluwax. Wax record is corrected with impression paste or bite registration paste.

wax that contacts mucosal surfaces be trimmed free of contact. The chilled wax record again should be replaced to make sure that no contact with soft tissue exists.

A wax record can be further corrected with a freely flowing occlusal registration material, such as a metallic oxide paste, which is used as the final recording medium. In making such a corrected wax record, the opposing teeth (and also the patient's lips and the dentist's gloves) should first be lightly coated with petroleum jelly or a silicone preparation. The occlusal registration material is then mixed and applied to both sides of the metal-reinforced wax record. It is quickly placed, and the patient is assisted with closing in the rehearsed path, which will be guided by the previous wax record. After the occlusal registration material has set, the corrected wax record is removed and inspected for accuracy. Any excess projecting beyond the wax matrix should be removed with a sharp knife until only the registration of the cusp tips remains. Such a record should seat on accurate casts without discrepancy or interference and will provide an accurate interocclusal record. When an intact opposing arch is present, use of an opposing cast may not be necessary. Instead a hard stone may be poured directly into the occlusal registration material record to serve as an opposing cast. However, although this may be an acceptable procedure in the fabrication of a unilateral fixed partial denture, the advantages of having casts properly oriented in a suitable articulator contraindicate the practice. The only exception to this is if the maxillary cast on which the removable partial denture is to be fabricated has been mounted previously with the aid of a face-bow. In such an instance, an intact mandibular arch may be reproduced in stone by pouring a cast directly into the interocclusal record.

An interocclusal record also may be made with an adjustable frame. Reference to this method was made in Chapter 12 (see Figure 12-13). The adjustable frame was devised for use with materials that offer no resistance to closure, such as zinc oxide and eugenol impression pastes.

Some of the advantages of using a metallic oxide paste over wax as a recording medium for occlusal records are: (1) uniformity of consistency; (2) ease of displacement on closure; (3) accuracy of occlusal surface reproduction; (4) dimensional stability; (5) the possibility of some modification in occlusal relationship after closure, if it is made before the material sets; and (6) less likelihood of distortion during mounting procedures.

Three important details to be observed when one uses such a material are:

1. Make sure that the occlusion is satisfactory before making the interocclusal record.
2. Be sure that the casts are accurate reproductions of the teeth being recorded.
3. Trim the record with a sharp knife wherever it engages undercuts, soft tissue, or deep grooves.

Occlusal Relations Using Occlusion Rims on Record Bases

A third method is used when one or more distal extension areas are present, when a tooth-supported edentulous space is large, or when opposing teeth do not meet. In these instances, occlusion rims on accurate jaw relation record bases must be used. Simple wax records of edentulous areas are never acceptable. Any wax, however soft, will displace soft tissue. It is impossible to accurately seat such a wax record on a stone cast of the arch.

In this method the recording proceeds much the same as in the second method, except that occlusion rims are substituted for missing teeth (Figure 17-11). It is essential that accurate bases be used to help support the occlusal relationship. Visible light-cured (VLC) bases may be adapted to the casts following the same technique described in Chapter 15 for making impression trays. Utilizing the master cast, block out undesirable undercuts. However, do not add any wax for spacing. Paint a thin layer of the model release agent on the cast and the relief wax to aid in removal of the base from the cast after the designated time of polymerization recommended by the manufacturer. Carefully, adapt the VLC base material to the cast. Do not thin the material, and do not adapt the VLC base material over the remaining teeth. Process the base in the polymerization to set

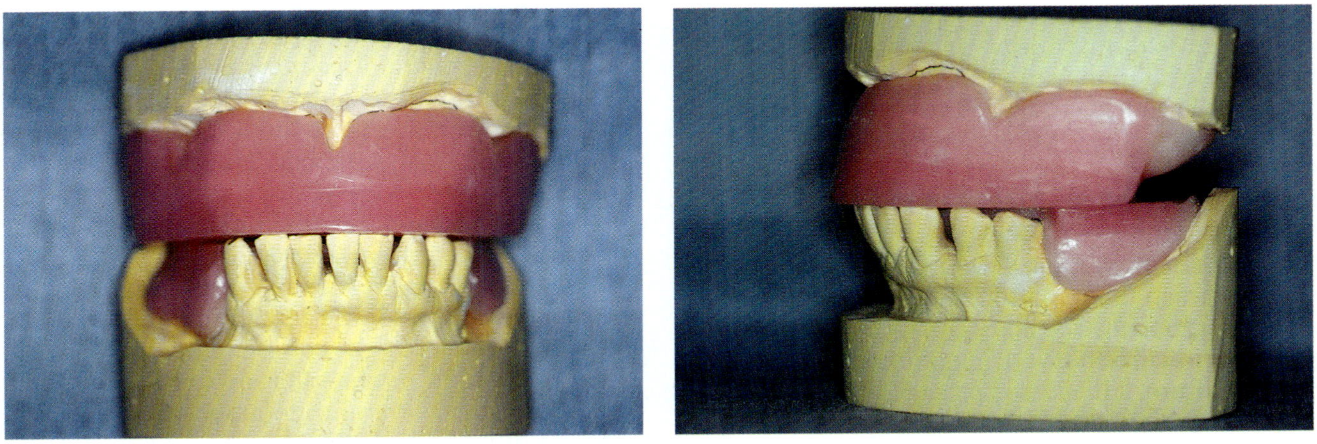

A

B

Figure 17-11 Relationship and distribution of remaining teeth for this patient require that record bases and occlusion rims be used for accurate mounting of casts. **A,** Acrylic resin record bases and hard baseplate wax occlusion rims for an edentulous maxilla and Kennedy Class I mandibular arch. These record bases are stable and were formed by sprinkling autopolymerizing acrylic resin. **B,** Occlusion rims substitute for missing posterior teeth and provide an opportunity for posterior support when making interocclusal records, which is most critical for the longer edentulous span on the mandibular right.

the material, then separate the record base from the cast and remove any remaining blockout wax. Clean the base and apply the air barrier coating over the entire record base and process (tissue side up) as directed.

Record bases may also be made entirely of autopolymerizing acrylic resin. Those materials used in dough form lack sufficient accuracy for this purpose unless they are corrected by relining. An acrylic resin base may be formed by sprinkling monomer and polymer into a shallow matrix of wax or clay after any undercuts are blocked out. If the matrix and blockout have been formed with care, interference to removal will not occur, and little trimming will be necessary. When the sprinkling method is used and sufficient time is allowed for progressive polymerization to occur, such bases are stable and accurate. Other record bases include the use of cast metal and compression molded or processed acrylic resin bases for jaw relation records.

Relative to the third method, some mention must be made of the ridge on which the record bases are formed. If the prosthesis is to be tooth supported or if a distal extension base is to be made on the anatomic ridge form, the bases will be made to fit that form of the residual ridge. But if a distal extension base is to be supported by the functional form of the residual ridge, it is necessary that the recording of jaw relations be deferred until the master cast has been corrected to that functional form.

Record bases must be as nearly identical as possible to the bases of the finished prosthesis. Jaw relation record bases are useless unless they are made on the same cast or a duplicate cast on which the denture will be processed, or are themselves the final denture bases. The latter may be either a cast alloy or a processed acrylic resin base.

Jaw relation records made by this method accomplish essentially the same purpose as the two previous methods. The fact that record bases are used to support edentulous areas does not alter the effect. In any method, the skill and care used by the dentist in making occlusal adjustments on the finished prosthesis will govern the accuracy of the resulting occlusion.

Methods for Recording Centric Relation on Record Bases

There are many ways by which centric relation may be recorded when record bases are used. The least accurate is the use of softened wax occlusion rims. Modeling plastic occlusion rims, on the other hand, may be uniformly softened by flaming and tempering, resulting in a generally acceptable occlusal record. This method is time proved, and when competently done, it is equal in accuracy to any other method.

When wax occlusion rims are used, they should be reduced in height until just out of occlusal contact at the desired vertical dimension of occlusion. A single stop is then added to maintain their terminal position as a jaw relation record is made in some uniformly soft material, which sets to a hard state. Quick-setting impression plaster, bite registration paste, or autopolymerizing resin may be used. With any of these materials, opposing teeth must be lubricated to facilitate easy separation. Whatever the recording medium, it must permit normal closure into centric relation without resistance and must be transferable with accuracy to the casts for mounting purposes.

Jaw Relation Records Made Entirely on Occlusion Rims

The fourth method is used when no occlusal contact exists between the remaining natural teeth, such as when an opposing maxillary complete denture is to be made concurrently with a mandibular removable partial denture. It may also be used in those rare situations in which the few remaining teeth do not occlude and will not influence eccentric jaw movements. Jaw relation records are made entirely on occlusion rims when either arch has only anterior teeth present (Figure 17-12).

In any of these situations, jaw relation records are made entirely on occlusion rims. The occlusion rims must be supported by accurate jaw relation record bases. Here the choice of method for recording jaw relations is much the same as that for complete dentures. Either some direct interocclusal method or a stylus tracing may be used. As with complete denture fabrication, the use of a face-bow, the choice of articulator, the choice of method for recording jaw relations, and the use of eccentric positional records are optional based on the training, ability, and desires of the individual dentist.

Establishing Occlusion by the Recording of Occlusal Pathways

The fifth method of establishing occlusion on the removable partial denture is the registration of occlusal pathways and the use of an occluding template rather than a cast of the opposing arch. When a static jaw relation record is used, with or without eccentric articulatory movements, the prosthetically supplied teeth are arranged to occlude according to a specific concept of occlusion. On the other hand, when a functional occlusal record is used, the teeth are modified to accept every recorded eccentric jaw movement.

These movements are made more complicated by the influence of the remaining natural teeth. Occlusal harmony on complete dentures and in complete mouth rehabilitation may be obtained by the use of several different instruments and techniques. Schuyler has emphasized the importance of establishing first the anterior tooth relation and incisal guidance before proceeding with any complete oral rehabilitation. Others have shown the advantages of establishing canine guidance as a key to functional occlusion before proceeding with any functional registration against an opposing prosthetically restored arch. This is done on the theory that the canine teeth serve to guide the mandible during eccentric movements when the opposing teeth come into functional contact. It also has been pointed out that the canine teeth transmit periodontal proprioceptor impulses to the muscles of mastication and thus have an influence on mandibular movement even without actual contact guidance. However, as long as the occlusal surfaces of unrestored natural teeth remain in contact, as in many a partially dentulous mouth, these teeth will always be the primary influence on mandibular movement. The degree of occlusal harmony that can be obtained on a fixed or removable restoration will depend on the occlusal harmony that exists between these teeth.

Regarding occlusion, Thompson has written: "Observing the occlusion with the teeth in static relations and then moving the mandible into various eccentric positions is not sufficient. A dynamic concept is necessary to produce an occlusion that is in functional harmony with the facial skeleton, the musculature, and the temporomandibular joints."* By adding "and with the remaining natural teeth," the requirements for removable partial denture occlusion are more completely defined.

Some of the methods described previously may be applied to the fabrication of removable partial dentures in both arches simultaneously, whereas the registration of occlusal pathways necessitates

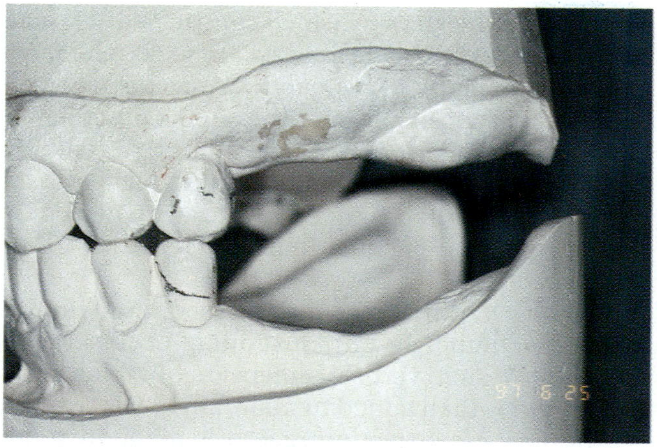

Figure 17-12 Opposing Kennedy Class I dental arches with remaining anterior teeth only. Recording of maxillomandibular relations was accomplished by using stable record bases and occlusion rims.

*From Thompson JR: Temporomandibular disorders: diagnosis and dental treatment in the temporomandibular joint. In Sarnat B, ed: The temporomandibular joint, ed, 2, Springfield, IL, 1964, Bernard G. Sarnat and Charles C. Thomas, pp. 146-184.

that an opposing arch be intact or restored to the extent of planned treatment. A diagnostic wax-up of both maxillary and mandibular arches will facilitate visualization of the proposed mouth preparation and restorative procedures required to accommodate the planned occlusal scheme, correct orientation of the occlusal plane, correct arch form, and complete tooth modifications to accommodate the removable partial denture design, all at the desired vertical dimension of occlusion. If removable partial dentures are planned for both arches, a decision is necessary as to which denture is to be made first and which is to bear a functional occlusal relation to the opposing arch. Generally the mandibular arch is restored first and the maxillary removable partial denture occluded to that restored arch. If the maxillary arch is to be restored with a complete denture or a fixed partial denture or crowns, a full diagnostic wax-up must be done before establishing the occlusion on the opposing removable partial denture. If opposing fixed partial dentures or opposing occluding crowns are to be fabricated, it may be advantageous to develop the occlusion and fabricate them simultaneously to ensure optimal positioning, cuspal relationship, and functional integrity.

Regardless of the method used for recording jaw relations, when one arch is completely restored first, that arch is treated as an intact arch even though it is wholly or partially restored by prosthetic means. The dentist must consider at the time of treatment planning the possible advantages of establishing the final occlusion to an intact arch.

Step-by-step Procedure for Registering Occlusal Pathways

After the framework has been adjusted to fit the mouth, the technique for the registration of occlusal pathways is as follows:

1. Support the wax occlusion rim by a denture base having the same degree of accuracy and stability as the finished denture base. Ideally, this would be the final denture base, which is one of the advantages of making the denture with a metal base. Otherwise, make a temporary base of VLC resin or sprinkled autopolymerizing acrylic resin (see Figures 18-34 through 18-38), either of which is essentially identical to the final acrylic resin base. In any distal extension removable partial denture, make this base on a cast that has been corrected to desired functional or supporting forms of the edentulous ridge. Place a film of hard sticky wax on the base before the wax occlusion rim is secured to it. The wax used for the occlusion rim should be hard enough to support biting stress and should be tough enough to resist fracture. Hard inlay wax has proved to be suitable for the majority of patients. However, some individuals with weak musculature or tender mouths may have difficulty in reducing this wax. In such situations use a slightly less hard wax. Make the occlusion rim wide enough to record all extremes of mandibular movement.
2. Inform the patient that the occlusion rim must be worn for 24 hours or longer. It should be worn constantly, including nighttime, except for removal during meals. By wearing and biting into a hard wax occlusion rim, a record is made of all extremes of jaw movement (Figure 17-13). The wax occlusion rim must maintain positive contact with the opposing dentition in all excursions and must be left high enough to ensure that a record of the functional path of each cusp will be carved in wax. This record should include not only voluntary excursive movements but also involuntary movements and changes in jaw movement caused by changes in posture. Extreme jaw positions and habitual movements during sleep should also be recorded.

   The occlusal paths, thus recorded, will represent each tooth in its three-dimensional aspect. Although the cast poured against this will resemble the opposing teeth, it will be wider than the teeth that carved it because it represents those teeth in all extremes of movement. The recording of occlusal paths in this manner

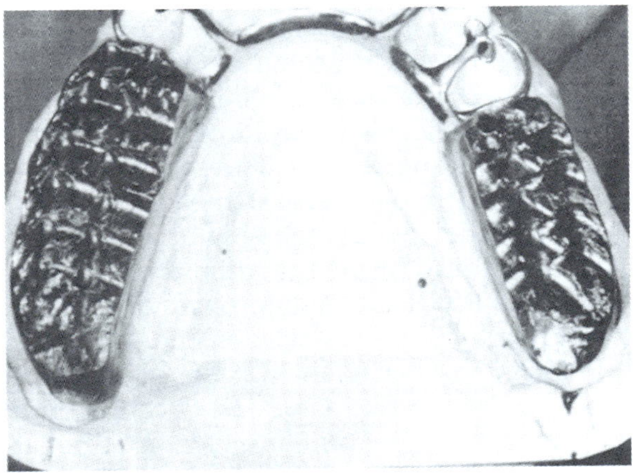

Figure 17-13 Example of completed occlusal registration in hard inlay wax supported by accurate record bases. Note that width of each cusp in all extremes of mandibular movement is recorded as continuous glossy surface. Yet, anatomy of each opposing tooth is well defined. Completed registration must be placed back onto master cast without intervening debris or discrepancy and secured there with sticky wax so that accuracy of occlusal registration will be maintained.

eliminates entirely the need to reproduce mandibular movement on an instrument.

Instruct the patient in the removal and placement of the removable partial denture that supports the occlusion rim and explain that by chewing in all directions, the wax will be carved by the opposing teeth. The opposing teeth must be cleaned occasionally of accumulated wax particles. It is necessary that the patient comprehend what is to be accomplished and understand that both voluntary and involuntary movements must be recorded.

Before dismissing the patient, add or remove wax where indicated to provide continuous contact throughout the chewing range. To accomplish this, repeatedly warm the wax with a hot spatula and have the patient close and chew into the warmed wax rim with the opposing dentition, each time adding to any areas that are deficient. Any area left unsupported by its flow under occlusal forces must be reinforced with additional wax. It is important that the wax rim be absolutely dry and free of saliva before additional wax is applied. Each addition of wax must be made homogeneous with the larger mass to prevent separation or fracture of the occlusion rim during the time it is being worn. Leave the wax occlusion rim from 1- to 3-mm high, depending on whether the occlusal vertical dimension is to be increased.

3. After 24 hours, the occlusal surface of the wax rim should show a continuous gloss, which indicates functional contact with the opposing teeth in all extremes of movement (see Figure 17-13). Any areas deficient in contact should be added to at this time. The reasons for maintaining positive occlusal contact throughout the time the occlusion rim is being worn are that (a) all opposing teeth may be placed in function; (b) an opposing denture, if present, will become fully seated; and (c) vertical dimension of occlusion in the molar region will be increased, thus the head of the mandibular condyle will be repositioned and temporomandibular tissue can return to a normal relationship.

   If during this period the wax occlusion rim has not been reduced to natural tooth contact, warm it by directing air from the air syringe through a flame onto the surface of the wax. By holding the wax rim with the fingers while warming it, a gradual softening process will result, rather than a melting of the surfaces already established. Repeatedly warm the occlusion rim and replace it in the mouth until the occlusal height has been reduced and lateral excursions have been recorded. At this time, use additional wax to support those areas left unsupported by the flow of the wax to the buccal or lingual surfaces. Trim the areas obviously not involved, thus narrowing the occlusion rim as much as possible. Remove those areas projecting above the occlusal surface, which by their presence might limit functional movement.

   Having accomplished seating of the denture and changes in mandibular position by the previous period of wear, it is possible to complete the occlusal registration in an operatory. However, if all involuntary movements and those caused by changes in posture are to be recorded, the patient should again wear the occlusion rim for a period of time.

4. After a second 24- to 48-hour period of wear, the registration should be complete and acceptable. The remaining teeth that serve as vertical stops should be in contact, and the occlusion rim should show an intact glossy surface representing each cusp in all extremes of movement.

Natural teeth formerly in contact will not necessarily be in contact on completion of the occlusal registration. Those teeth that have been depressed over a period of years and those that have been moved to accommodate overclosure or mandibular rotation may not be in contact upon reestablishment of mandibular equilibrium. Such teeth may possibly return to occlusal contact in the future or may have to be restored to occlusal contact after initial placement of the denture. Because the mandibular position may have been changed during the process of occlusal registration, the cuspal relation of some of the natural teeth may be different from before. This fact must be recognized in determining the correct restored vertical dimension of occlusion.

Occlusion thus established on the removable partial denture will have more complete harmony with the opposing natural or artificial teeth than can be obtained by adjustments in the mouth alone, because occlusal adjustment to accommodate voluntary movement does not necessarily prevent occlusal disharmony in all postural positions or during periods of stress. Furthermore, occlusal adjustment in the mouth without occlusal analysis is limited by the dentist's ability to correctly interpret occlusal markings made intraorally, whether by articulating ribbon or by other means.

The registration of occlusal pathways has additional advantages. It makes obtaining jaw relations possible under actual working conditions, with the denture framework in its terminal position, the opposing teeth in function, and an opposing denture, if present, fully seated. In some

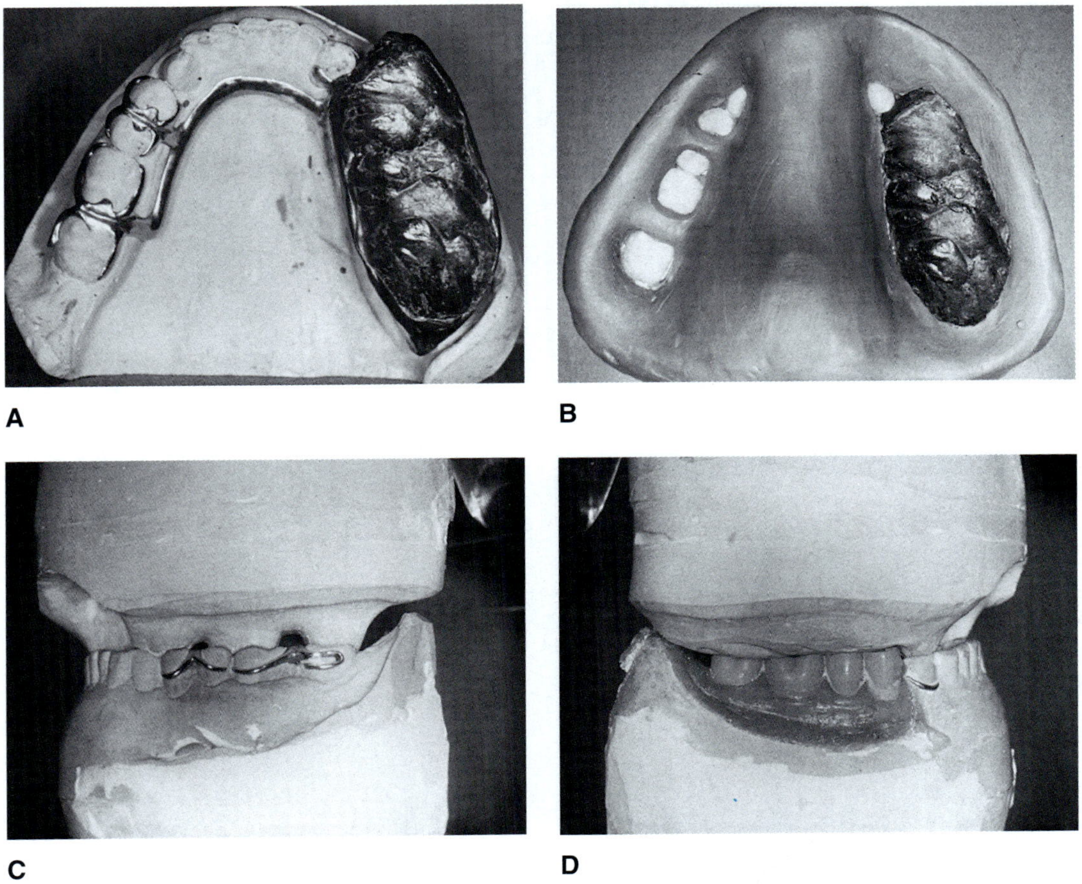

Figure 17-14 Four views of occlusal registration for lower Class II removable partial denture. **A,** Occlusal registration in wax returned to master cast. Note extreme horizontal movement recorded. **B,** Same cast boxed with clay, leaving multiple occlusal surfaces exposed as vertical stops. **C,** Effect of occlusal stops, eliminating any possible changes in vertical dimension of occlusion on articulator. **D,** Processed denture remounted for occlusal readjustment. Note modification in occlusal anatomy of stock artificial teeth and slight increase in height of occlusal plane. This is in harmony with natural tooth contact elsewhere in arch.

instances it also makes possible the recovery of lost vertical dimension of occlusion, either unilaterally or bilaterally, when overclosure or mandibular rotation has occurred.

The completed registration is now ready for conversion to an occluding template. This is usually done by boxing the occlusal registration with modeling clay after it has been reseated and secured onto the master or processing cast (Figures 17-14 through 17-16). Only the wax registration and areas for vertical stops are left exposed. It is then filled with a hard die stone to form an occluding template (see Chapter 18).

It is necessary that stone stops be used to maintain the vertical relation rather than relying on some adjustable part of the articulating instrument, which might be changed accidentally (Figure 17-17). Also, by using stone stops and by mounting both the denture cast and the template before separating them, a simple hinge instrument may be used.

MATERIALS FOR ARTIFICIAL POSTERIOR TEETH

The improved acrylic resin teeth are generally preferred to porcelain teeth, because they are more readily modified and thought to more nearly resemble enamel in their abrasion potential against opposing teeth. Improved acrylic resin teeth with gold occlusal surfaces are preferably used in opposition to natural teeth restored with gold occlusal surfaces, whereas porcelain teeth are generally used in opposition to other porcelain teeth.

Acrylic resin tooth surfaces, however, may in time become impregnated with abrasive particles, thereby becoming an abrasive substance themselves. This may explain why acrylic resin teeth are sometimes

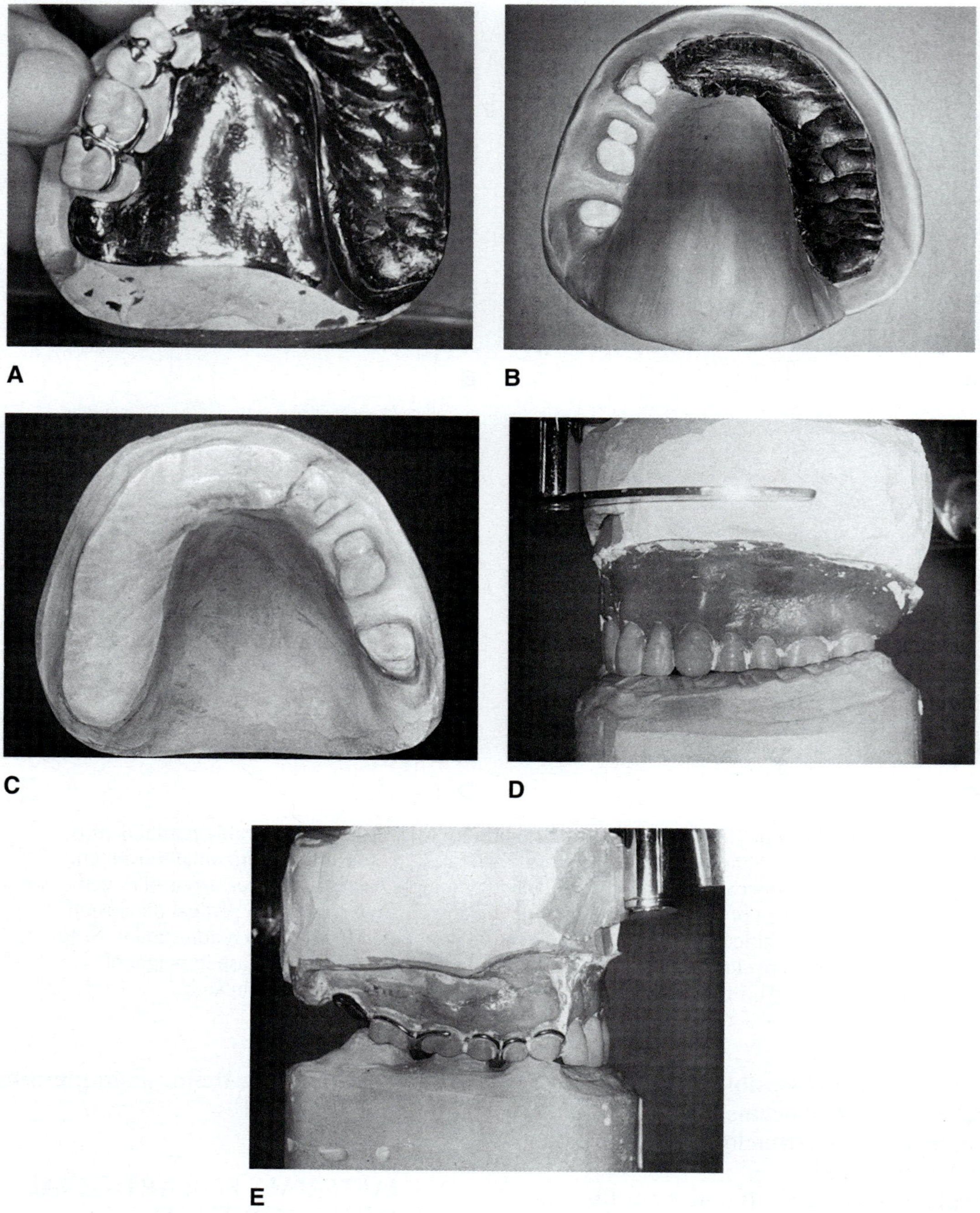

Figure 17-15 Five views of occlusal registration for maxillary Class II removable partial denture. Anterior teeth must be tried in mouth and positioned for esthetics before posterior teeth are arranged. **A,** Partial view of occlusal registration returned to master cast. Again, note extreme horizontal movement recorded. **B,** Same cast boxed with clay, leaving multiple occlusal surfaces exposed as vertical stops. **C,** Occlusal view of occluding template. **D,** Processed denture remounted for occlusal readjustment. **E,** Occlusal stops in full contact after processing and occlusal readjustment following remounting.

capable of wearing opposing gold surfaces. An evaluation of occlusal contact or lack of contact, however, should be meticulously accomplished at each 6-month recall appointment regardless of the choice of material for posterior tooth forms.

Although some controversy may still exist in regard to the use of porcelain or acrylic resin artificial teeth, there is broad agreement that narrow (reduced buccolingual) occlusal surfaces are desirable. Posterior teeth that will satisfy this requirement should be

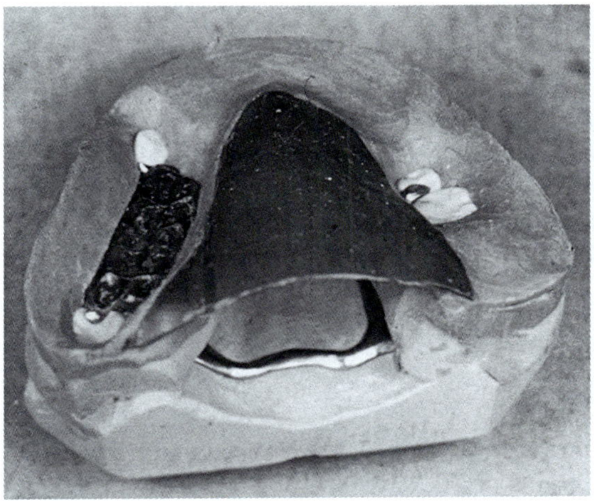

Figure 17-16 Rather than use clay to span the arch from one side to another, same may be done with wax with less time and material. Wax should form an acute angle with occlusal wax registration and exposed occlusal surfaces.

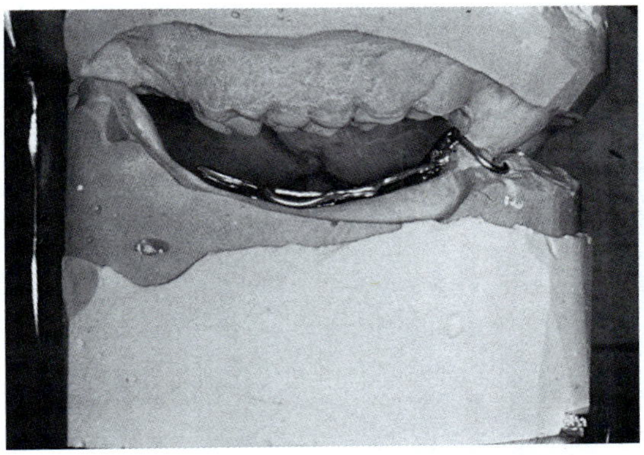

Figure 17-17 Profile view of occlusal template and one of its vertical stops. Despite fact that this is a record of all extremes of mandibular movement for this patient, anatomy of occluding teeth can easily be identified.

selected, and the use of tooth forms having excessive buccolingual dimension should be avoided.

Acrylic resin teeth are easily modified and readily lend themselves to construction of cast gold surfaces on their occlusal portions. A simple procedure for fabricating gold occlusal surfaces and attaching them to acrylic resin teeth is described in Chapter 18 under posterior tooth forms.

Arranging Teeth to an Occluding Template

The occlusal surface of the artificial teeth, porcelain or resin, must be modified to occlude with the template. In this method they are actually only raw materials from which an occlusal surface is developed that is in harmony with an existing occlusal pattern. Therefore the teeth must be occluded too high and then modified to fit the template at the established vertical dimension of occlusion.

Teeth arranged to an occluding template ordinarily should be placed in the center of the functional range. Whenever possible, the teeth should be arranged buccolingually in the center of the template. When natural teeth have registered the functional occlusion, this may be considered the normal physiological position of the artificial dentition regardless of its relation to the residual ridge. On the other hand, if some artificial occlusion in the opposing arch has been recorded, such as that of an opposing denture, the teeth should be arranged in a favorable relation to their foundation, even if this means arranging them slightly buccally or lingually from the center of the template.

The teeth are usually arranged for intercuspation with the opposing teeth in a normal cuspal relationship. Whenever possible, the mesiobuccal cusp of the maxillary first molar should be located in relation to the buccal groove of the mandibular first molar and all other teeth arranged accordingly. With a functionally generated occlusion, however, it is not absolutely necessary that normal opposing tooth relationships be reestablished (Figure 17-18). In the first place, the opposing teeth in a dental arch that is not contiguous may not be in normal alignment, and intercuspation may be difficult to accomplish. In the second place, the occlusal surfaces will need to be modified so that they will function favorably regardless of their anteroposterior position (Figure 17-19). Because cusps modified to fit an occlusal template will be in harmony with the opposing dentition, it is not necessary that the teeth themselves be arranged to conform to the usual concept of what constitutes a normal anteroposterior relationship.

ESTABLISHING JAW RELATIONS FOR A MANDIBULAR REMOVABLE PARTIAL DENTURE OPPOSING A MAXILLARY COMPLETE DENTURE

It is common for a mandibular removable partial denture to be made to occlude with an opposing maxillary complete denture. The maxillary denture may already be present, or it may be made concurrently with the opposing removable partial denture. In any event, the establishment of jaw relations in this situation may be accomplished by one of several previously outlined methods.

If an existing maxillary complete denture is satisfactory and the occlusal plane is oriented to an acceptable anatomic, functional, and esthetic position (which rarely occurs), then the complete denture

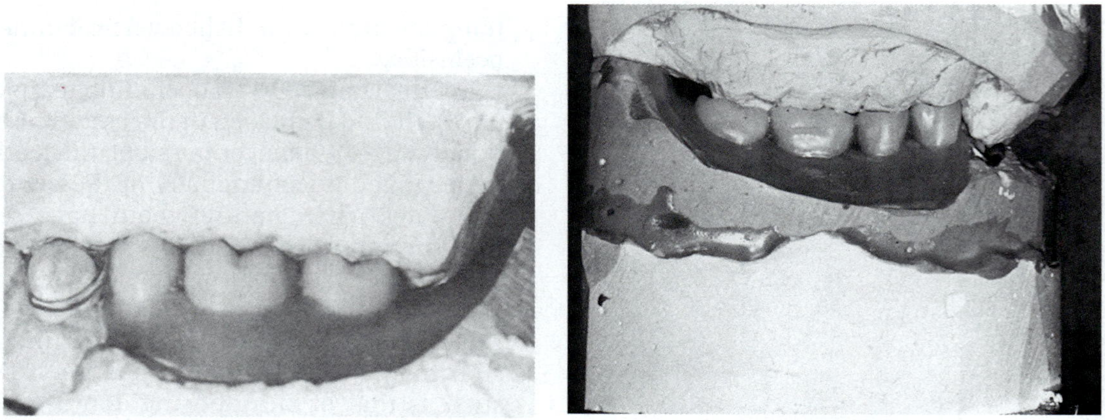

A B

Figure 17-18 **A,** View of intercuspation sometimes possible when teeth are arranged to occlusal template. This is possible only when gross migration of opposing teeth has not occurred. **B,** View of modification to occlusal surfaces necessary when customary intercuspation would create objectionable spaces. Note that original cusp-to-cusp relation of artificial teeth has been altered until marginal ridges have actually become cusps. Such occlusal relationship is entirely permissible and effective.

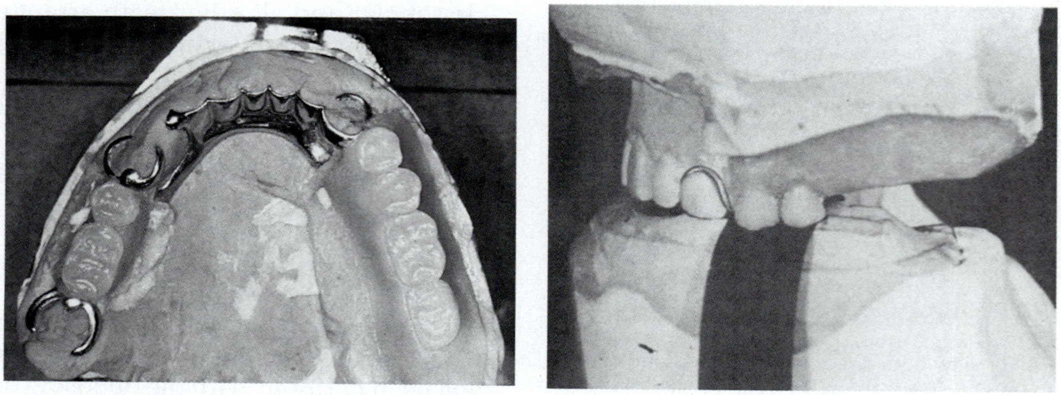

A B

Figure 17-19 **A,** Occlusal surfaces after remounting and final occlusal readjustment to template. Note functional occlusal anatomy resulting. This is entirely different occlusal surface from that which was present on stock artificial teeth as manufactured. **B,** When dentist is arranging teeth to occluding template, thin marking tape should be used in positioning and modifying each tooth to fit template. Note that at this early stage articulator has been opened approximately 0.5 mm, as evidenced by slight space at vertical stop.

need not be replaced and the opposing arch is treated as an intact arch as though natural teeth were present. A face-bow transfer is made of that arch, and the cast is mounted on the articulator. To accomplish this, a face-bow record is made with the complete denture in place. After the face-bow apparatus is removed from the patient, the complete denture is removed and an irreversible hydrocolloid impression of the denture is made. When the impression material has set, the denture is removed, cleaned, and returned to the patient. A cast is formed in the impression and then mounted on the articulator with the face-bow record. Maxillomandibular relations may be recorded on accurate record bases attached to the mandibular removable partial denture framework by use of a suitable recording medium. Centric relation is recorded and transferred to the articulator. Eccentric records can then be made to program the articulator.

In rare instances, when the mandibular removable partial denture replaces all posterior teeth and the anterior teeth are noninterfering, a central bearing point tracer may be mounted in the palate of the maxillary denture and centric relation recorded by means of an intraoral stylus tracing against a stable mandibular base. If a stylus jaw relation recording method is used, the stylus must be carefully removed from the denture and attached to the same palatal location of the stone cast that was transferred to the articulator via the face-bow. The mandibular cast can then be oriented by way of the horizontal jaw relation record and attached to the articulator.

When an existing complete denture is opposing the arch on which a removable partial denture is fabricated, a cast of the complete denture may be used during the fabrication procedures. However, when the occlusion is corrected after processing, and the removable partial denture is finalized during initial placement, the complete denture should be retrieved and mounted on the articulator with a centric relation record at the desired vertical dimension of occlusion. This will ensure a more accurate cuspal relationship and will prevent abrasion of the cusp contacts that would occur by using a stone cast of the denture. This procedure is completed when the patient is in the office so as not to deprive the patient of use of the existing complete denture.

If the relationship of the posterior teeth on the maxillary denture to the mandibular ridge is favorable and the complete denture is stable, jaw relations may be established by recording occlusal pathways in the mandibular arch just as for any opposing intact arch. The success of this method depends on the stability of the denture bases, the quality of tissue support, the relation of the opposing teeth to the mandibular ridge, and the interrelation of existing artificial and natural teeth.

More often than not, the existing maxillary complete denture will not be acceptable to use because of poor tooth position. The denture will have been made to occlude with malpositioned mandibular teeth, which have since been lost, or the teeth will have been arranged without consideration for the future occlusal relation with a mandibular removable partial denture. Too often one sees a maxillary denture with posterior teeth arranged close to the residual ridge without regard for the interarch relationship and with an occlusal plane that is too low. Usually, however, a new maxillary denture must be made concurrently with the mandibular removable partial denture, and jaw relations may be established in one of two ways.

If the mandibular removable partial denture will be tooth supported (a Kennedy Class III arch accommodating a bilateral removable prosthesis), the mandibular arch is restored first. The same applies to a mandibular arch being restored with fixed partial dentures. In either situation the mandibular arch is completely restored first, and jaw relations are established, as they would be to a full complement of opposing teeth. Thus the maxillary complete denture is made to occlude with an intact arch.

On the other hand, as is more often the situation, the mandibular removable partial denture may have one or more distal extension bases. The situation then necessitates that the occlusion be established on both dentures simultaneously.

All mouth preparations and restorative procedures required to correctly orient the occlusal plane, correct the arch form, accommodate the desired occlusal scheme, and accommodate the removable partial denture design must be accomplished on the remaining natural teeth. In addition, all supporting *tissue* must be in an acceptable state of health before making the final impression. After making final impressions, which include the altered cast impression or the corrected cast impression, the maxillary occlusion rim is contoured, occlusal vertical relation with the remaining lower teeth is established, and a face-bow transfer of the maxillary arch is made. The maxillomandibular relations may be recorded by any one of the several methods previously outlined and the articulator mounting completed. Occlusion may be established as for complete dentures, taking care to establish a favorable tooth-to-ridge relationship in both arches, an optimum occlusal plane, and cuspal harmony between all occluding teeth.

After try-in, several methods may be used to complete the restorations. Both dentures may be processed concurrently and remounted for occlusal correction, or the removable partial denture may be processed first. After the dentures are completed and remounted, the teeth—still in wax on the complete denture—are adjusted to any discrepancies occurring.

Correction of occlusal discrepancies created during processing must be accomplished before the patient is permitted to use the denture(s). Methods by which these discrepancies may be corrected are discussed in Chapter 18.

SELF-ASSESSMENT AIDS

1. Occlusal harmony exists when the masticating mechanism can carry out its physiological functions while the factors of occlusion remain in a healthy state—the factors of occlusion being the temporomandibular joints, the neuromuscular mechanism, and the teeth and their supporting structures. True or false?
2. Occlusal harmony between a removable partial denture and the remaining natural teeth is a major factor in preserving the health of the supporting structures of the natural teeth. True or false?
3. The establishment of a satisfactory occlusion for a removable partial denture patient should include five considerations or procedures by the dentist. List the five musts.
4. Define centric relation in your own words.
5. What is maximum planned intercuspation and how does it relate to centric occlusion?

6. What is meant by eccentric occlusion?
7. Describe a balanced occlusion.
8. Two methods are commonly used to develop an acceptable occlusion for a removable partial denture patient. Give a brief description of these two methods.
9. What records are necessary to correctly orient casts to an arcon-type articulator and to program the articulator?
10. A harmonious relationship of opposing occlusal and incisal surfaces, in itself, is not adequate to ensure stability of distal extension removable partial dentures. What other factor must be recognized and dealt with to minimize unwanted leverages?
11. There are differences among dentists in developing contacts of opposing teeth in centric and eccentric positions for partially edentulous patients. Answer the following queries correctly and try to rationalize the recommendations contained in this text:
    a. Simultaneous contacts of opposing posterior teeth must occur in the intercuspal position. True or false?
    b. Occlusion for tooth-supported removable partial dentures may be arranged to duplicate the occlusion seen in a harmonious natural dentition. True or false?
    c. Under what circumstances is a balanced occlusion desirable for the partially edentulous patient?
    d. Should working side contacts be developed when a mandibular distal extension denture is opposed by natural teeth (assuming all mandibular posterior teeth are missing)?
    e. A patient with a Kennedy Class I maxillary arch is being treated with a removable partial denture. Is it beneficial to develop balancing and working contacts? Explain. What about protrusive contacts?
    f. Are balancing-side contacts for a Kennedy Class II maxillary arch desirable? Why or why not?
    g. What are the desirable contact relationships of artificial and natural teeth when one arch is a Kennedy Class IV arch?
    h. What is the most distal extent that an artificial tooth should be arranged in a Kennedy Class I or II mandibular arch?
12. A patient requires a tooth-supported mandibular removable partial denture. The remaining teeth are maximum intercuspation; however, this position does not coincide with centric relation. There is no temporomandibular joint pathological process, no neuromuscular disorder, and no periodontal condition aggravated by occlusion. Would one insist that the patient be restored to have maximum intercuspation coincide with centric relation? Why or why not?
13. Under what circumstances would one develop an occlusion for a partially edentulous patient so that maximum intercuspation coincided with centric relation?
14. When must the dentist determine the horizontal jaw relation in which to develop the occlusion for the partially edentulous patient? Why?
15. After the horizontal relationship of the jaws to which the occlusion will be developed has been determined, occlusal relationships may be established by five methods. The choice of method will be determined by the existing partially edentulous situation of the patient, location of remaining teeth in each arch, and the prior correction of any existing occlusal discrepancies. These five methods are: (a) direct opposition of casts, (b) interocclusal records with posterior teeth remaining, (c) occlusal relations using occlusal rims, (d) jaw relation records made entirely on occlusion rims, and (e) recording functionally generated paths. Justify and briefly discuss the use of each of the five methods.
16. What are the disadvantages of using only wax for making interocclusal records?
17. What are the disadvantages in developing an occlusion to a stone template or stone teeth on a cast?
18. Materials of which the occlusal surfaces of artificial posterior teeth are made deserve serious consideration by the dentist. These considerations should be based on minimizing attrition of occlusal surfaces, maintaining the established vertical dimension of occlusion, and maintaining positive planned contact of posterior teeth. To best accomplish the preceding, please give the material of choice for occlusal surfaces that oppose (a) porcelain, (b) enamel, (c) restored natural teeth, and (d) fixed partial denture pontics with gold occlusal surfaces.
19. Acrylic resin posterior teeth lend themselves to easier modification than do porcelain teeth when the interresidual ridge distance is small or when an edentulous space to be restored with the denture is grossly restricted. However, acrylic resin teeth have one big drawback when occluded against any other occlusal surface, including acrylic resin. What is this drawback?
20. The occlusal surfaces of acrylic resin teeth attached to a denture may be duplicated in gold and attached to the same teeth. Describe this technique.
21. Occlusal discrepancies created during processing procedures must be corrected before the patient is given possession of the dentures. When should this be accomplished? Why is it necessary?

18

LABORATORY PROCEDURES

This chapter covers only those phases of dental laboratory procedures that are directly related to removable partial denture fabrication. Familiarity with laboratory procedures relative to making fixed restorations and complete dentures is presumed. Such information is available in numerous textbooks on those subjects and is not duplicated here. For example, the principles and techniques involved in the waxing, casting, and finishing of single inlays, crowns, and fixed partial dentures are adequately covered in lecture material and textbooks and in manuals available to the dental student, the dental laboratory technician, and the practicing dentist. Similarly, knowledge of the principles and techniques for mounting casts, articulating teeth, and waxing, processing, and polishing complete dentures is presumed as a necessary background for the laboratory phases of removable partial denture fabrication. Therefore this chapter is directed specifically toward the laboratory procedures involved in the fabrication of a removable partial denture.

DUPLICATING A STONE CAST

A stone cast may be duplicated for several purposes. One is the duplication in stone of the original or corrected master cast to preserve the original. One use of such a cast is for fitting a removable partial denture framework without danger of fracture or abrading the surface of the original master cast. Another use might be for processing a temporary prosthesis where wax relief and blockout on the original cast allow production of a duplicate, which following processing will make insertion of the prosthesis easier.

Another reason to duplicate a cast is to allow formation of an investment cast for framework fabrication. The careful preparation of the master cast for production of this investment cast involves consideration of the defined path of insertion, heights of contour, retentive, and stabilization areas designed into the mouth preparations. The framework produced should be carefully evaluated on the cast for fit, just as a fixed partial denture is evaluated on a working cast with dies (Figure 18-1).

Blockout should be accomplished on the master cast before making an investment cast. On this investment cast, the wax or plastic pattern is formed. The use of preformed plastic patterns eliminates some of the danger of damaging the surface of the investment cast in the process of forming the pattern. With freehand waxing, considerable care must be taken not to score or abrade the investment cast. The metal framework is ultimately cast against its surface, and the finished casting and the original cast are then returned to the dentist after all fitting has been completed on the duplicate cast.

Duplicating Materials and Flasks

Duplicating materials include both colloidal and silicone materials. The colloidal materials are made fluid by heating and return to a gel while cooling. The cast to be duplicated must be placed in the bottom of a suitable flask, called a duplicating flask. It is necessary that a duplicating flask contain the fluid material to facilitate its cooling, to support the mold while it is being filled with the cast material, and to facilitate removal of the cast from the mold without permanent deformation or damage to the mold. Numerous duplicating flasks are on the market.

The technique for duplicating is the same for any cast, whether or not blockout is present. However, if wax or clay blockout is present, the temperature of the duplicating material must not be any higher than recommended by the manufacturer to prevent melting and distorting the blockout material.

Ordinary baseplate wax may be used for parallel blockout and ledges, but care must be taken that the temperature of the duplicating material is not too high because it will then melt the wax. The use of prepared blockout material may be preferred, such as Ney blockout wax or Wills undercut material.

Duplicating Procedure

The equipment needed and the steps required for duplication using a silicone material are described in Figures 18-2 through 18-6.

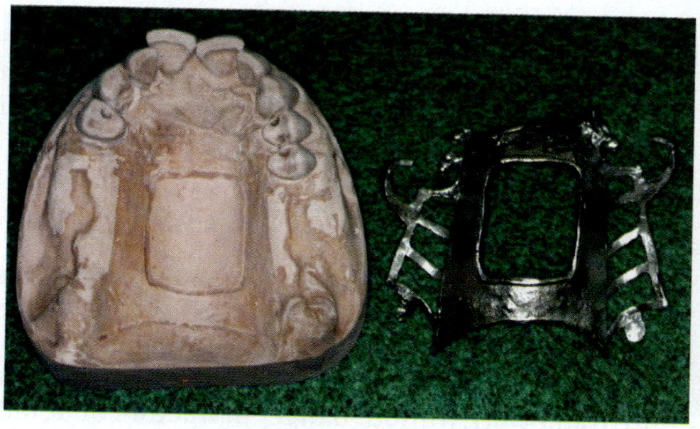

A

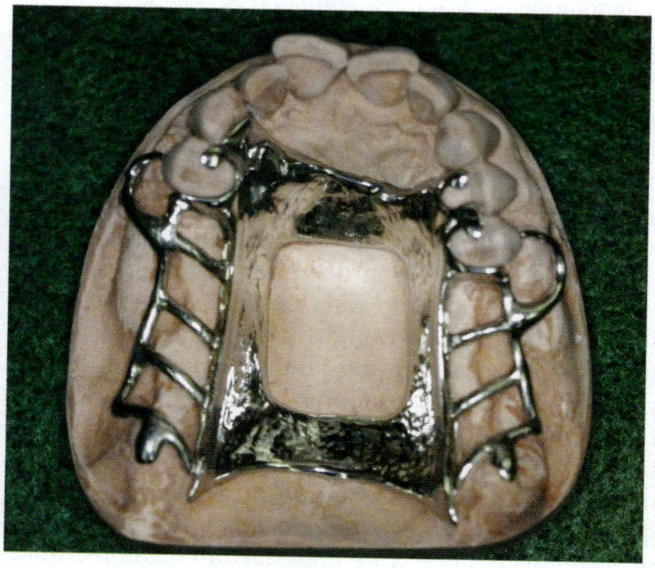

B

Figure 18-1 **A,** Framework returned from the laboratory with the master cast. **B,** Replacement on the cast reveals areas of contact that can erode the cast surface. Careful fitting to the cast will allow determination of potential framework adjustment regions prior to fitting in the mouth. If the framework is indiscriminately finished in the laboratory or prior to intraoral placement, critical tooth contact regions may be lost, resulting in a poorly retained and stabilized prosthesis. Most often, such an overly adjusted framework is poorly stabilized, not poorly retained.

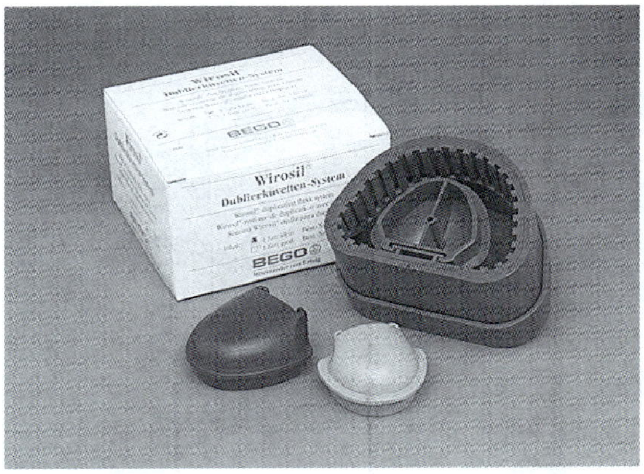

Figure 18-2 Wirosil duplicating flask with its stabilizing insert and three replaceable palate formers of different sizes ensure extremely low silicone consumption through flexible positioning. *(Courtesy Bego, Bremen, Germany.)*

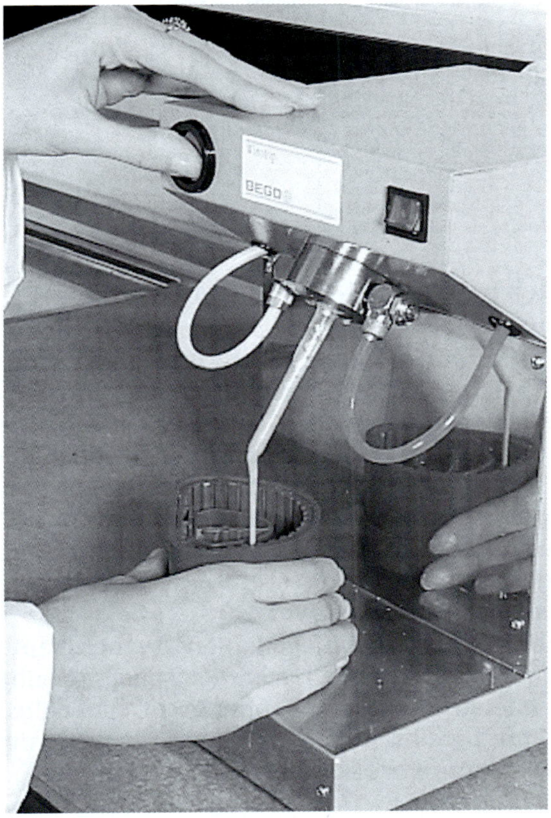

Figure 18-3 Wirotop automatic mixing and metering unit ensures the two components are mixed to prevent formation of bubbles. *(Courtesy Bego, Bremen, Germany.)*

WAXING THE REMOVABLE PARTIAL DENTURE FRAMEWORK

When preformed plastic patterns are used (Figure 18-7), parts of the denture framework must be waxed freehand to prevent excessive bulk and to create the desired contours for a

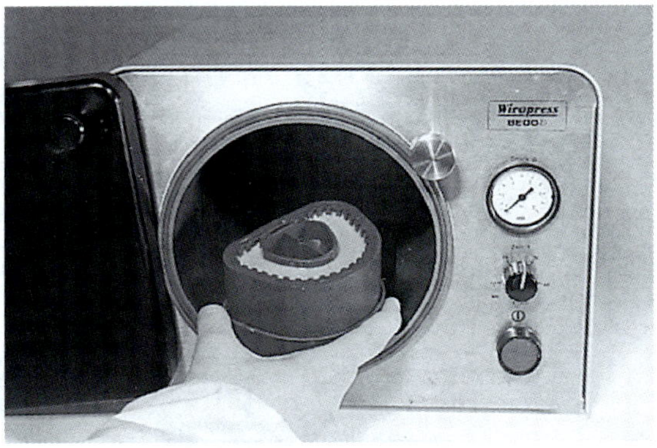

Figure 18-4 In Wiropress pressure compaction unit, duplicating silicone is forced into critical areas under pressure, thereby reducing number of bubbles. *(Courtesy Bego, Bremen, Germany.)*

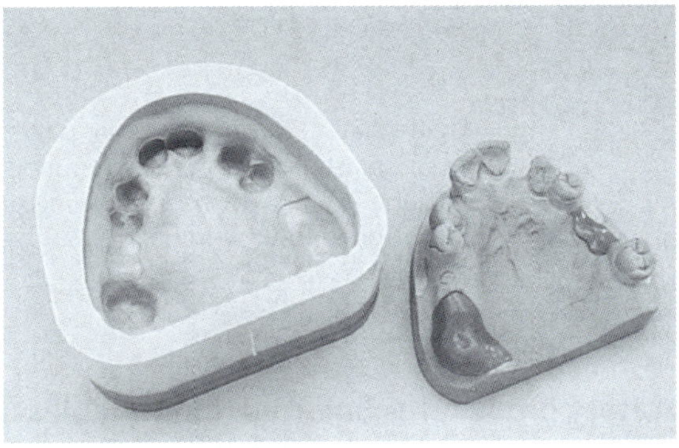

Figure 18-5 After hardening under pressure, cast is detached by blowing compressed air between cast and mold. *(Courtesy Bego, Bremen, Germany.)*

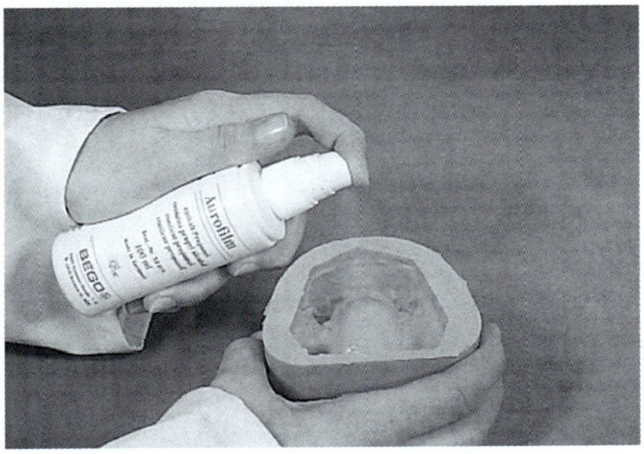

Figure 18-6 Spraying with surfactant eliminates any reaction with investment material and ensures more accurate casting surface. *(Courtesy Bego, Bremen, Germany.)*

satisfactory custom-made removable partial denture framework (Figure 18-8).

While most dentists do not fabricate their own removable partial denture castings, it is essential that they have an understanding of the dental

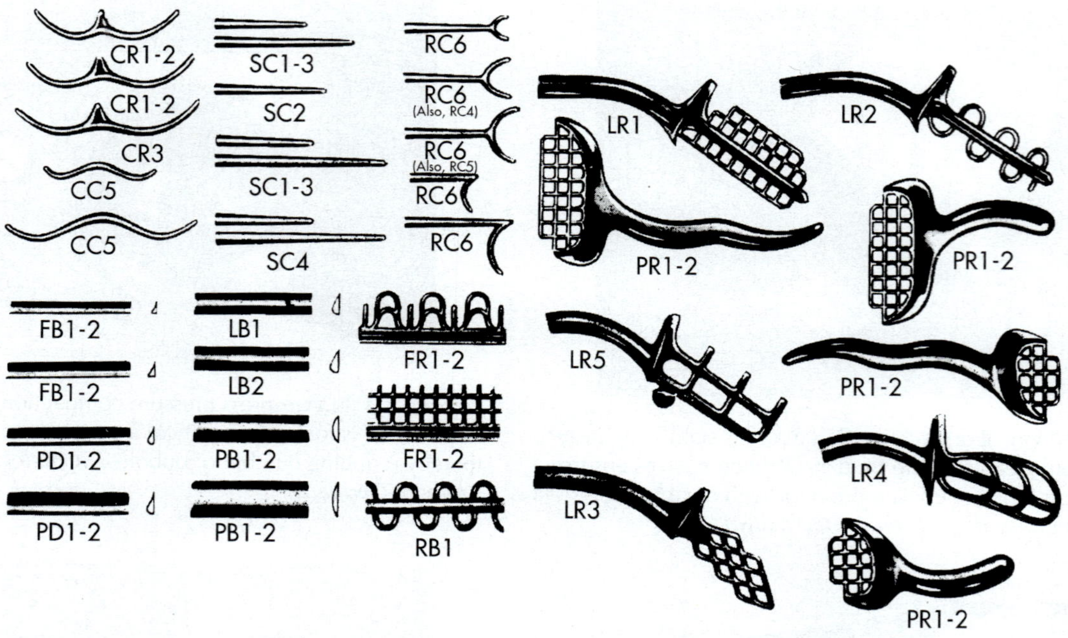

Figure 18-7 Preformed plastic patterns are available in many shapes and sizes. Being made of soft plastic material, they tend to stretch on removal from their backing. Therefore care must be exercised when removing patterns. Their use generally requires that tacky liquid be first applied to investment cast at their area of placement. *(Courtesy JF Jelenko & Company, Armonk, NY.)*

laboratory procedures involved. This enables them to design the removable partial denture framework, complete a laboratory work authorization that communicates the desired design and authorizes its fabrication, and evaluate the quality of the framework (Figure 18-9). An understanding and evaluation of the key features required in a completed removable partial denture framework ensure the patient of a chance to function comfortably with the finished product (Figure 18-10). The contrary is also true.

Forming the Wax Pattern for a Mandibular Class II Removable Partial Denture Framework

Examples that illustrate many of the essentials of waxing a removable partial denture framework are illustrated in Figures 18-11 through 18-20. This exercise includes the waxing of three types of direct retainers (circumferential, combination, and bar type), a mandibular lingual bar major connector, a maxillary anterior-posterior palatal strap major connector, both distal extension and tooth-bound modification spaces, and adaptation of round, 18-gauge, wrought-wire retentive arms for combination-type direct retainers.

Attaching Wrought-Wire Retainer Arms by Soldering

Wrought-wire retainers may be attached to a removable partial denture framework after it has been cast and finished (Figures 18-21 and 18-22). The soldering procedure may be accomplished by electric soldering or by a direct-heat method with an oxygen-gas flame. In either method, care must be taken to use compatible alloys, appropriate solder, and flux in conjunction with the careful application of controlled heat.

Students are encouraged to review the Chapter 12 discussion of the selection of metal alloys to enhance an understanding of the properties of solder, flux, the effect of heat on metal alloys, and the necessity for quality control in soldering procedures.

Waxing Metal Bases

A technique for forming the retentive framework for the attachment of acrylic resin bases has been given. Two basic types of metal bases may be used instead of the resin base. The advantages of cast metal bases in preference to acrylic resin bases have been discussed in Chapter 9. The type of base to be used must be determined before blockout and duplication so that the relief over each edentulous ridge may be provided or eliminated as required.

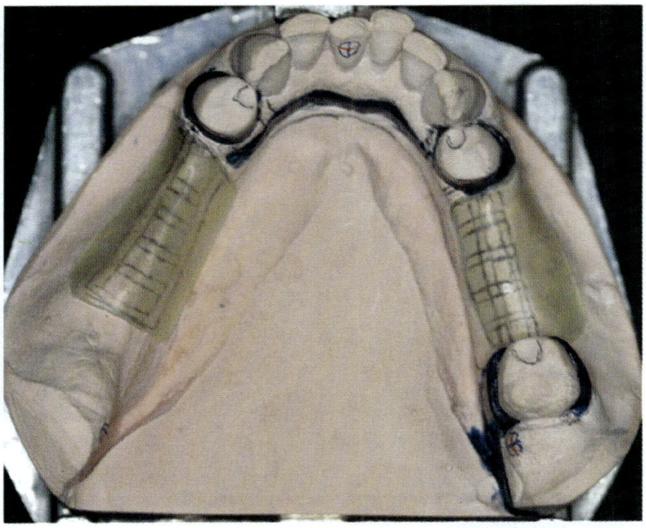

A

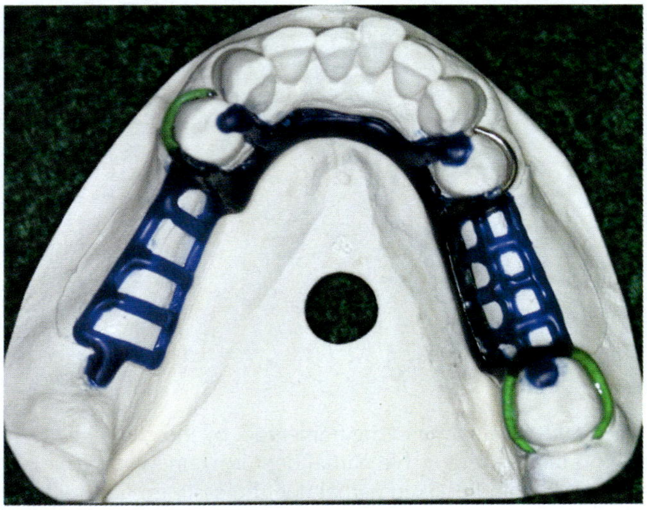

B

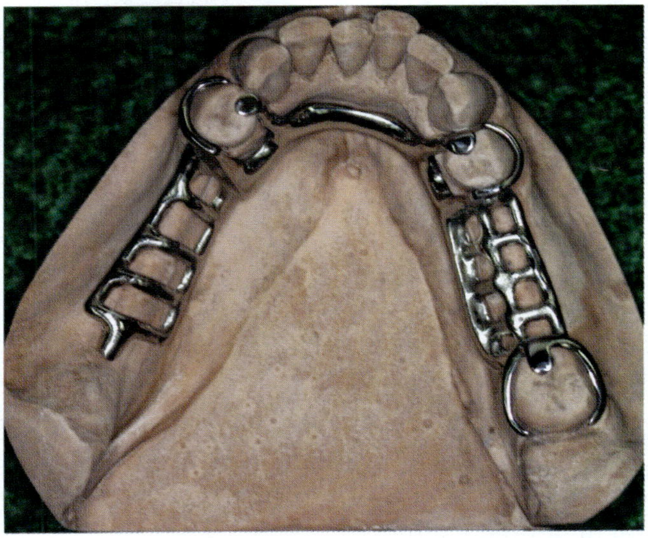

C

Figure 18-8 Three steps in making denture framework using relief, blockout ledges, and ready-made pattern forms. **A,** Master cast with relief, blockout of undercuts at posterior right and anterior lingual regions, and shaped blockout ledges for location of retentive and nonretentive clasp arms. **B,** Completed pattern using lingual bar major connector pattern, plastic clasp forms resting on investment ledges, wrought wire, and open retention mesh. **C,** Finished casting returned to master cast.

For an acrylic resin base, relief for the retentive frame must be provided. No relief over the residual ridge is used for a complete metal base. For a partial metal base, the junction between metal and acrylic resin must be clearly defined by trimming the relief along a definite, previously determined line.

One type of metal base is the complete base with a metal border to which tube teeth, cast copings, or an acrylic resin superstructure may be attached. If porcelain or plastic tube or grooved teeth are used, they must be positioned first and the pattern waxed around them to form a coping. The teeth are then attached to the metal base by cementation or, with the use of resin teeth, attached with additional acrylic resin under pressure, a so-called pressed-on method of attaching acrylic resin teeth to a metal base. Another method of attaching teeth is to wax the base to form a coping for each tooth, either by carving

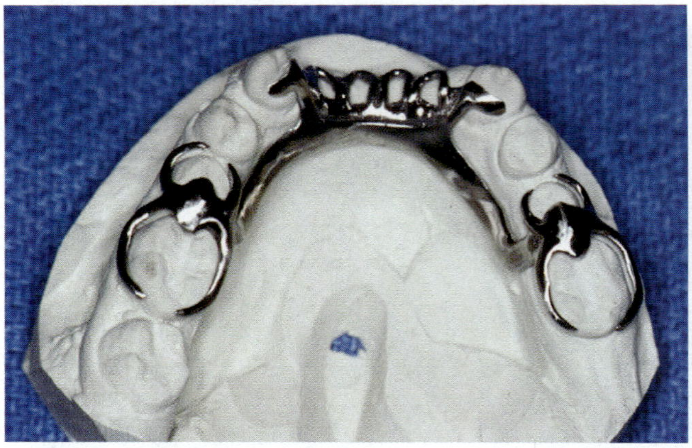

Figure 18-9 Evaluation of the framework by the clinician is as important for removable partial denture frameworks as it is for implant and/or fixed partial denture castings. Careful scrutiny of the attention to detail in following the design specifications is necessary, as well as evaluation of the fit of the framework to the cast. On this cast, initial seating of the framework reveals interference to complete seating bilaterally from the embrasure clasps. Only minor adjustment should be required to completely seat the framework. If major adjustment is needed, or if after completely seating the framework the clasp assemblies do not contact the teeth as prescribed, the framework should be re-made.

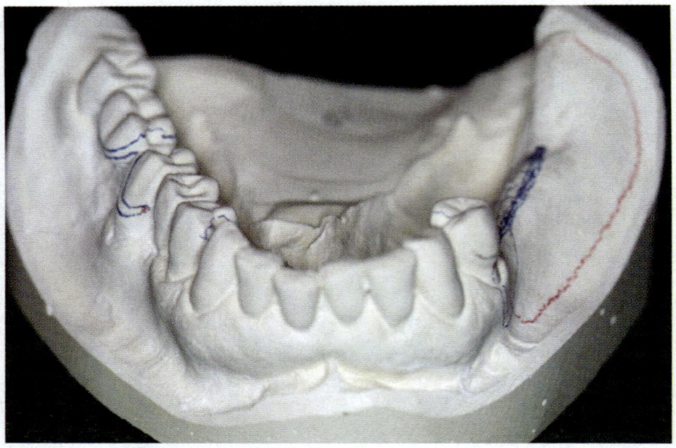

A

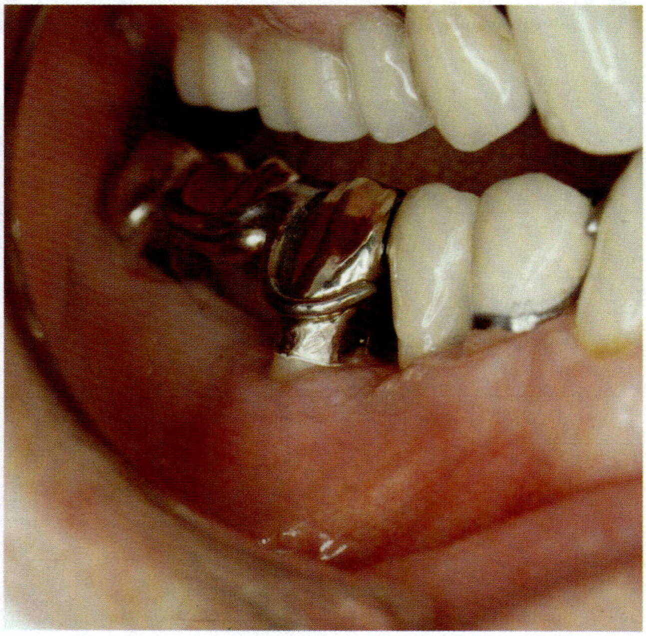

B

Figure 18-10 A, Design of mandibular removable partial denture framework is outlined on master cast for technician to follow in waxing and casting framework. B, Cast framework as returned from laboratory is evaluated intra-orally. It reveals sufficiently accurate adaptation and design identical to the embrasure clasp and mesio-occlusal rest #28 as shown on the design cast in A.

recesses in the wax or by waxing around artificial teeth. Rather than attaching a stock tooth, the full tooth may be waxed into occlusion, the base invested, and the wax patterns replaced with heat-polymerized acrylic resin. This method permits some variation in the dimension and form of the supplied teeth not possible with stock teeth. It is particularly applicable to abnormally long or short spaces or when a stock tooth of desired width is not available. With modern cross-linked acrylic resins, such processed teeth are fairly durable; however, the addition of gold occlusal surfaces is an option.

When artificial teeth are to be arranged to occlude with an opposing cast or an opposing template, the metal base must be formed for the attachment of the tissue-colored denture resin supporting the teeth. This is the most common method of attaching teeth to a metal base. The wax pattern for the base is formed from one thickness of 24-gauge casting wax, which is then reinforced at the border, and forming the retention of the acrylic resin superstructure. Because metal borders are more difficult to adjust than acrylic resin, they are usually made somewhat short of the area normally covered with an acrylic resin base. Also, because border thickness adds objectionable weight to the denture, it is made with only a slight border roll. This is one disadvantage of the complete metal base, because the border accuracy of the impression registration cannot be used to fullest advantage, and contouring facial and lingual surfaces cannot be as effective as with an acrylic resin base in which added bulk can sometimes be used to advantage.

The border is first penciled lightly on the investment cast, and then the 24-gauge sheet casting wax is smoothly adapted. Considerable care must be taken not to stretch and thin the

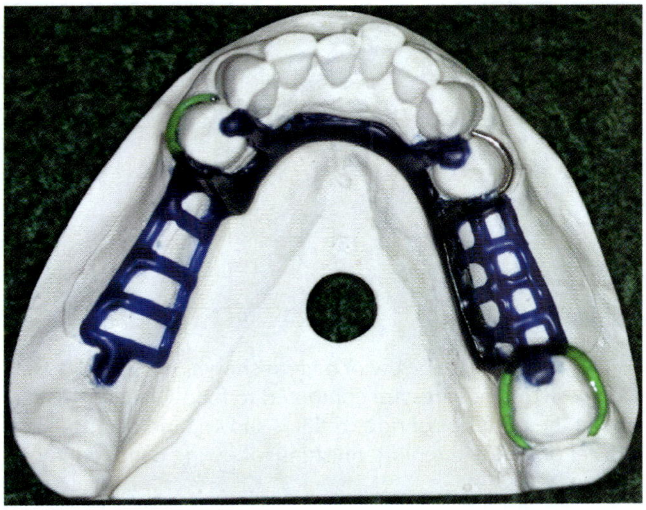

Figure 18-11 Occlusal view of mandibular Kennedy Class I, mod 1 wax pattern on a refractory cast. The lingual bar major connector joins 3 clasp assemblies (RPA, wrought wire, and cast circumferential).

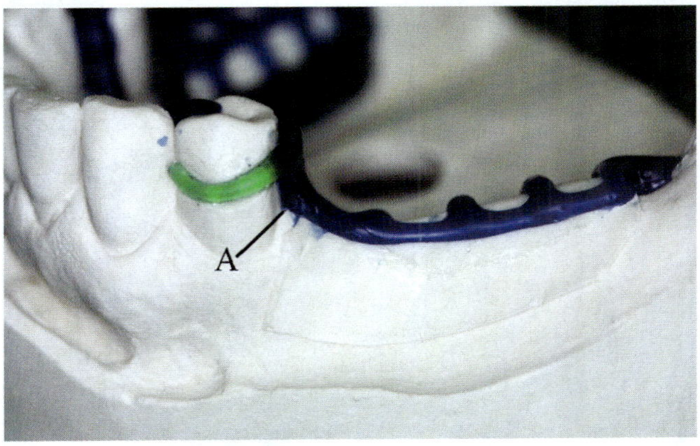

Figure 18-12 Buccal view of left side of pattern shown in Figure 18-11. Tapered retainer clasp pattern is placed on refractory cast ledge produced by duplication of shaped blockout ledges. Cast illustrates relief provided beneath minor connector, which retains denture base resin. Tissue index *(arrow)* at gingival region of proximal plate will provide an easily identifiable finish line for resin finishing and future trimming of altered cast impression.

sheet wax in adapting it to the cast. To prevent wrinkling, the wax should be adapted in at least two longitudinal pieces and joined and sealed together at the ridge crest. The wax is then trimmed along the penciled outline with a warm, dull instrument to prevent scoring the investment cast.

A single piece of 14-gauge round wax is now adapted around the border over the sheet wax. With a hot spatula, the round wax must be sealed

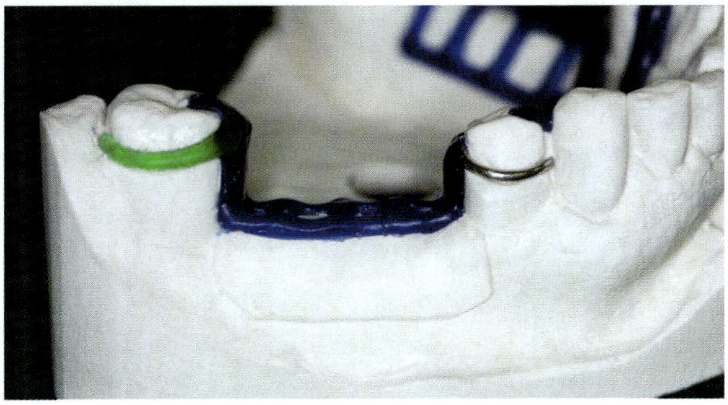

Figure 18-13 Buccal view of modification space of pattern shown in Figure 18-11. Wrought-wire clasp is contoured at anterior extent of modification space. Such a retainer will not overly stress the tooth if opposite denture base movement causes rotation across the fulcrum (see Figure 18-11, occlusal rests at #21 and #31). Tapered cast circumferential clasp follows shaped ledge to a distal buccal 0.01-inch undercut. Both proximal plates have been waxed with sufficient bulk to provide a complete casting. If thickness presents a problem with tooth placement, some finishing can be accomplished at a later time.

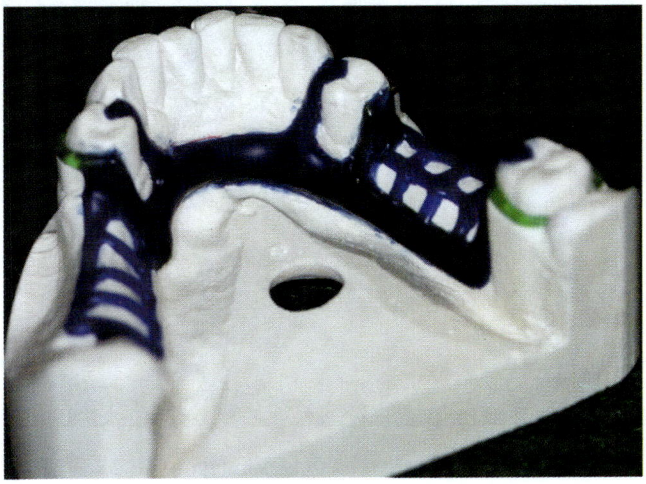

Figure 18-14 Lingual view of pattern shown in Figure 18-11. Lingual bar major connector rigidly connects components cross-arch. Minor connector for resin retention on left has buccal and lingual struts to allow unimpeded tooth placement. Tapered proximal plate on right (tooth #28) is thicker on the lingual and thinner on the buccal to allow close placement of buccal surface of denture tooth to #28. Finish line of modification space is positioned below adjacent tooth gingival margins to allow normal lingual contour of resin matrix.

to the cast along its outer border. Sufficient wax is flowed onto the round wax to blend it smoothly into the sheet wax, thus completing a border roll. The inner half of the round wax form remains untouched. Wax is added when needed to facilitate carving without trimming the original 24-gauge

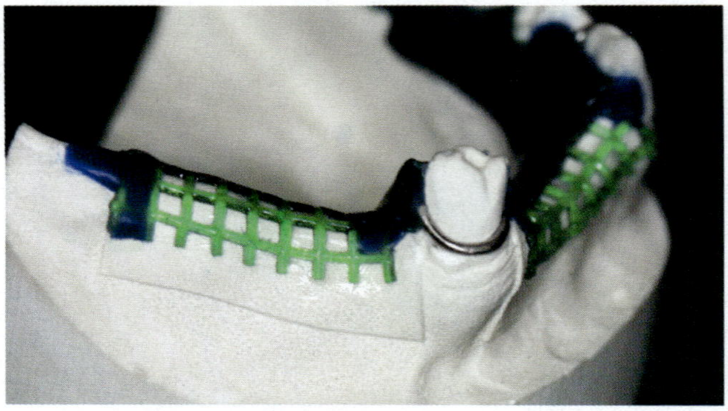

Figure 18-15 Another example of a wax pattern for a mandibular framework. A wrought wire has been adapted to tooth #27. The clasp demonstrates an appropriate circlet shape allowing maximum length. The circlet shape also allows the undercut to be approached from below, which improves retention—push retention is more efficient than pull retention. Ridge relief is evident beneath the resin minor connector, and the proximal plate housing the wire has been waxed with bulk to facilitate casting. The plate may require adjusting at a later time.

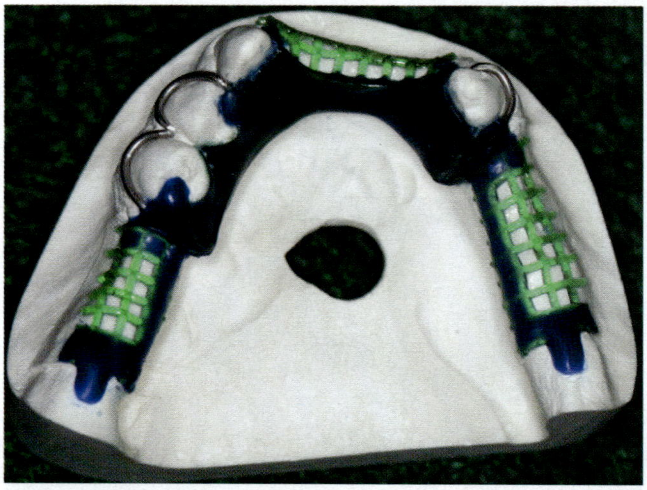

Figure 18-16 Same pattern as shown in Figure 18-15. Includes a lingual plate major connector design. The external finishing line at the anterior modification space is lingual to the anticipated tooth and resin position, allowing a natural contour to be developed in the completed prosthesis. The posterior denture base minor connector patterns have been reinforced with additional wax to add stiffness at the junction with the proximal plate and major connector. Because of the potential for repeated flexure in this region under function, such reinforcement is critical to long-term success with patterns such as this. Since the wrought wire retainers are not cast, it is important that they be contoured to contact the teeth as accurately as possible, as shown.

thickness. The result should be a rounded border blending smoothly into the sheet wax.

The boxing for the resin, which will in turn support the artificial teeth, is now added, again using 14-gauge round wax. The proposed outline for the boxing is identified by lightly scoring the sheet wax. On this scored line, the 14-gauge round wax is adapted, thus forming the outline of the boxing.

With additional wax, the ditch between the sheet wax and the outer border of the round wax is filled in and blended smoothly onto the sheet wax. This is done in the same manner as the border, adding sufficient wax to allow for smoothing

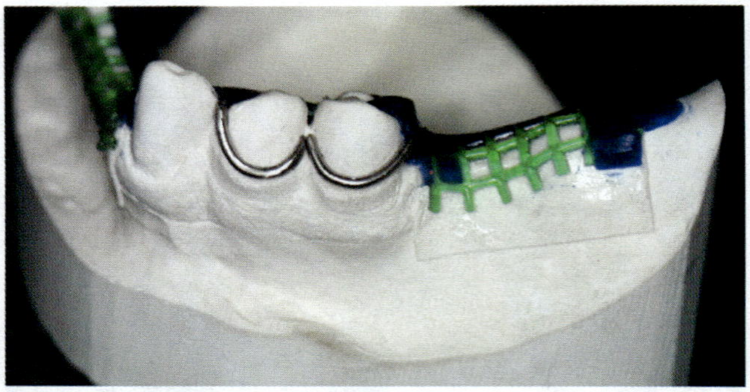

Figure 18-17 Buccal view of pattern shown in Figure 18-16. Double wrought wires are contoured to follow ledges, tissue stop at the posterior of ridge relief is shown, and occlusal rest a distal of #20 will require finishing following completion of casting.

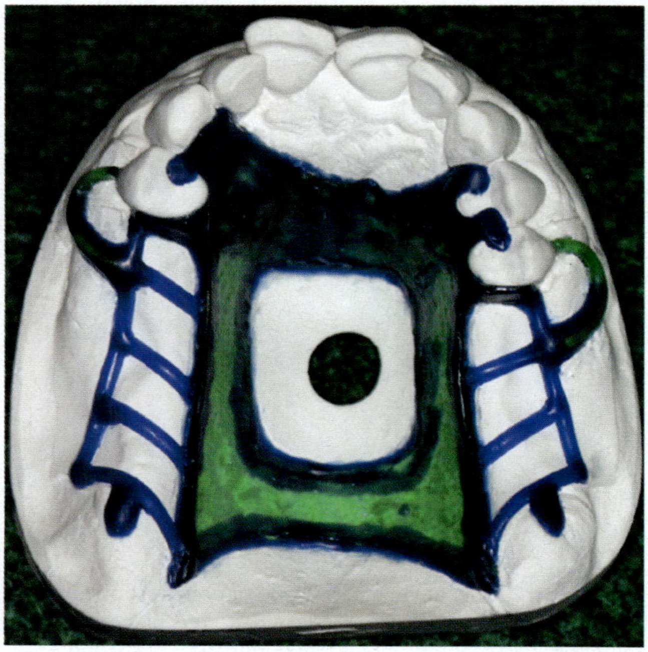

Figure 18-18 Occlusal view of maxillary refractory cast with wax pattern. Anatomic replica has been used to develop an anterior-posterior palatal strap major connector with beading evident at the anterior, posterior, and internal edges. Bilateral, tapered I-bar retainers have been waxed as extensions of the resin retaining minor connectors, and double rests were incorporated into the design on each side.

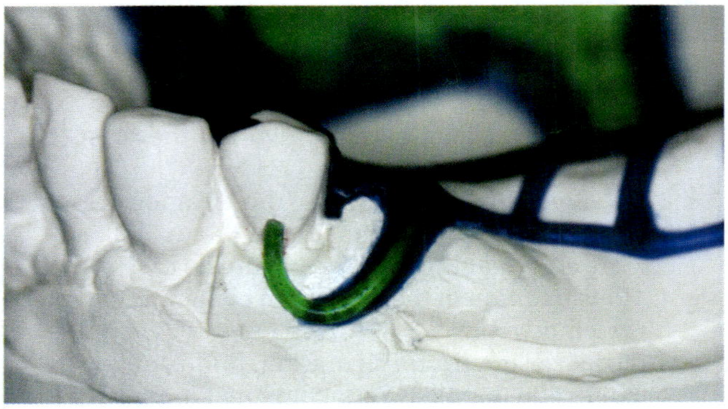

Figure 18-19 Buccal view of right I-bar shown in Figure 18-18. The tissue index is demonstrated gingival to the proximal plate, tissue relief is provided beneath the denture base minor connector, and the I-bar shows a taper as it approaches the mid-buccal 0.01-inch undercut.

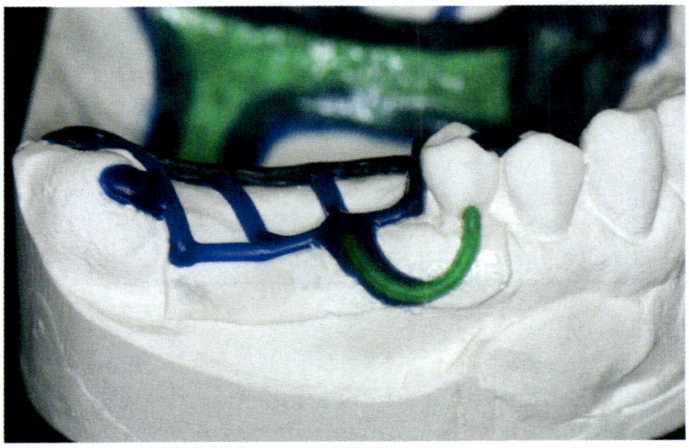

Figure 18-20 Buccal view of I-bar opposite to that shown in Figure 18-19. Many of the same features seen in Figure 18-19 are evident in this example. The tissue stop distal to the ridge relief is shown and the palatal external finishing line continues distal to the junction of the hard and soft palate (which is the terminus of the posterior palatal strap).

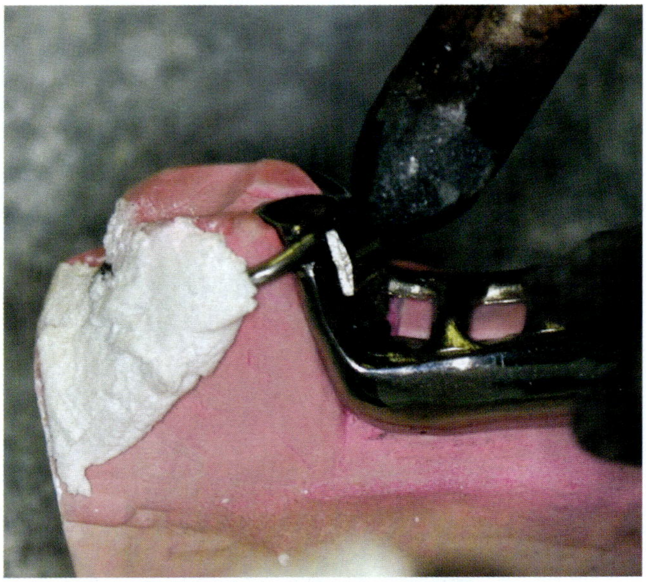

Figure 18-21 Wrought wire can be soldered to cast frameworks as an alternative method to incorporation in the wax pattern and casting procedure. Electric soldering is a common method for soldering and does not require heating the entire framework. Following preparation of the minor connector where the wire will be soldered, an 18-gauge, round wrought-wire clasp is carefully adapted and then secured to the framework and duplicate stone cast using refractory investment. In this situation a disto-lingual molar undercut will be used bilaterally for retention. The flux is placed at the proximal plate, followed by placement of sufficient solder, and the electric heat element tip is placed into contact with the solder while the frame is grounded at another location.

and carving. As mentioned previously, the pattern should not be flamed or polished with a cloth. Instead the pattern must be smoothed by carving.

The result thus far should be a pattern reinforced at the border and at the boxing and slightly concave in between, with some of the original sheet wax exposed. The inside of the boxing is not sealed to the sheet wax, thus leaving a slight undercut for the attachment of the acrylic resin. With a sharp blade, the margins of the boxing are then carved to a knife-edge finishing line. With the backside of the large end of the No. 7 wax spatula, this margin may be lifted slightly, further deepening the undercut beneath the finishing line.

In addition to the undercut finishing line, retention spurs, loops, or nail heads are added for retention of the acrylic resin to be added later. Spurs are usually made of 18-gauge or smaller round wax attached at one end only at random acute angles to the sheet wax. Loops are small-gauge round (wax, resin, or metal) circles attached either vertically or horizontally with space beneath for the acrylic resin attachment. Nail heads are made of short pieces of 18-gauge round wax attached vertically to the sheet wax, with the head flattened by a slightly warmed spatula. Any method of providing retention is acceptable if it permits positive attachment of the acrylic resin and will not interfere with the placement of artificial teeth.

A metal base waxed as described will provide optimum contours with a minimum of bulk and weight, and with adequate provision for the attachment of artificial teeth to the metal base. Properly designed, the more visible portions of the metal base will be covered with the acrylic resin supporting the supplied teeth.

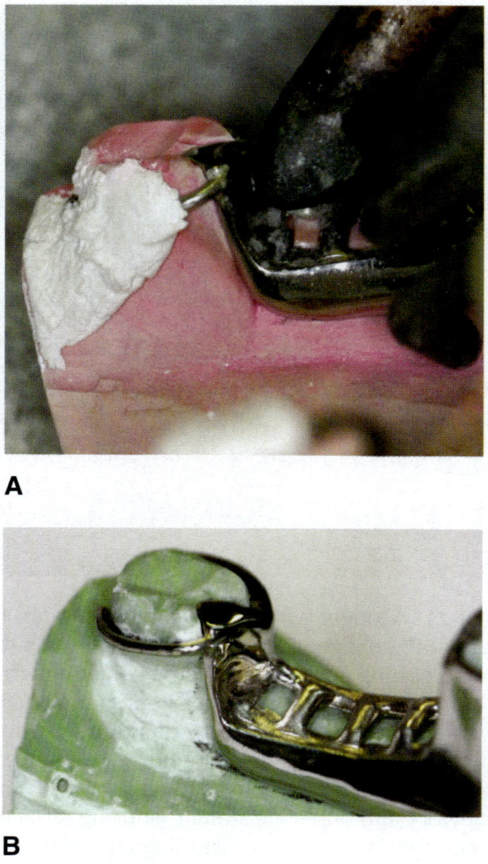

Figure 18-22 **A,** Electric soldering technique has been used to solder the wrought wire. The solder has flowed into the space between the framework and wire as well as around the wire to assure its secure attachment to the framework. **B,** Finished and polished wrought wire retainer.

BOX 18-1 Factors That Influence the Excellence of a Dental Casting

1. Care and accuracy with which the cast is reproduced
2. Intelligence with which the framework is designed and proportioned
3. Care and cleanliness in waxing up the cast
4. Consideration of the expansion of the wax caused by temperature
5. The size, length, configuration, points of attachment, and manner of attachment of the sprues
6. Choice of investment
7. The location of the pattern in the mold
8. The mixing water: amount, temperature, and impurities
9. The spatulation of the investment during mixing
10. The restraint offered to the expansion of the investment because of the investment ring
11. Setting time
12. Burn-out temperature and time
13. Method of casting
14. Gases: adhered, entrapped, and absorbed
15. Force used in throwing the metal into the mold
16. Shrinkage on cooling
17. Removal from the investment after casting
18. Scrubbing, pickling, and so on
19. Polishing and finishing
20. Heat handling

SPRUING, INVESTING, BURNOUT, CASTING, AND FINISHING OF THE REMOVABLE PARTIAL DENTURE FRAMEWORK

Brumfield has listed factors that influence the excellence of a dental casting (Box 18-1).

Spruing

Brumfield described the function of the sprues as follows:

The sprue channel is the opening leading from the crucible to the cavity in which the framework is to be cast. Sprues have the purpose of leading the molten metal from the crucible into the mold cavity. For this purpose, they should be large enough to accommodate the entering stream and of the proper shape to lead the metal into the mold cavity as quickly as possible, but with the least amount of turbulence. The sprues have the further purpose of providing a reservoir of molten metal from which the casting may draw during solidification, thus preventing porosity caused by shrinkage. The spruing of the cast may be roughly summarized in the following three general rules.

The sprues should be large enough that the molten metal in them will not solidify until after the metal in the casting proper has frozen (8- to 12-gauge round wax is usually used for multiple spruing of removable partial denture castings). The sprues should lead into the mold cavity as directly as possible and still permit a configuration that will induce a minimal amount of turbulence in the stream of molten metal. Sprues should leave the crucible from a common point and be attached to the wax pattern at its bulkier sections. That is, no thin sections of casting should intervene between two bulky, unsprued portions. The configuration of the sprues, from their point of attachment at the crucible until they reach the mold cavity, may be influential in reducing turbulence. One of the more important sources of difficulty in casting is the entrapment of gases in the mold cavity before they have a chance to escape. If the sprue channels contain sharp right-angle turns, great turbulence is induced, which is calculated to entrap such gases and so lead to faulty castings. Sprue channels should make long radii and easy turns, and also enter the mold cavity from a direction designed to prevent splashing at this point.

As previously stated, the sprues should be attached to the bulky points of the mold pattern. If two bulky points exist with a thin section between them, each of the bulky spots should be sprued. The points of attachment should be flared out and local constrictions avoided. If this practice is followed, the sprue—being bulky enough to freeze after the case framework has frozen—will continue to feed molten metal to the framework until it has entirely solidified. This provides sound metal in the casting proper with all shrinkage porosity forced into the sprue rod, which is later discarded.*

The laboratory procedure for multiple spruing is essentially the same for all mandibular and maxillary castings, except those with a palatal plate. Typical examples are illustrated in Figures 18-23 and 18-24.

There are two basic types of sprues: multiple and single. The majority of removable partial denture castings require multiple spruing, using 8- to 12-gauge round wax shapes for the main sprues and 12- to 18-gauge round wax shapes for auxiliary sprues. Occasionally, however, a single sprue is preferred for cast palates and cast metal bases for the mandibular arch when these are used as complete denture bases. With removable partial dentures, the use of a single sprue is limited to those maxillary frameworks in which—because of the presence of a palatal plate—it is impossible to locate multiple sprues centrally. In such situations the single sprue may be used advantageously. A single sprue must be attached to the wax pattern so that the direction of flow of the molten metal will be parallel to the long axis of the single sprue. In some instances the investment cast may have to be cut away anteriorly to make room for the attachment of the sprue; in others the sprue may be attached posteriorly. One disadvantage of using a single sprue for large castings is that an extra long investment ring must be used.

Some important points to remember in multiple spruing are as follows:

1. Use a few sprues of large diameter rather than several smaller sprues.
2. Keep all sprues as short and direct as possible.
3. Avoid abrupt changes in direction; avoid T-shaped junctions as much as possible.

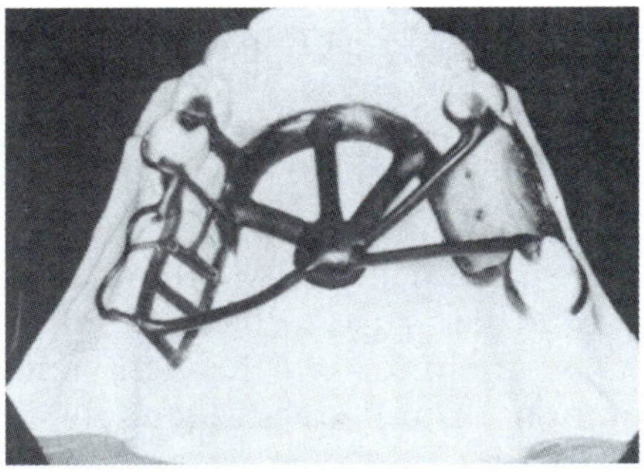

Figure 18-23 Illustration of mandibular sprued wax pattern. Three 8-gauge sprues attached to lingual bar and three 12-gauge sprues attached to denture base minor connector and direct retainer assemblies are joined at central sprue hole in investment cast.

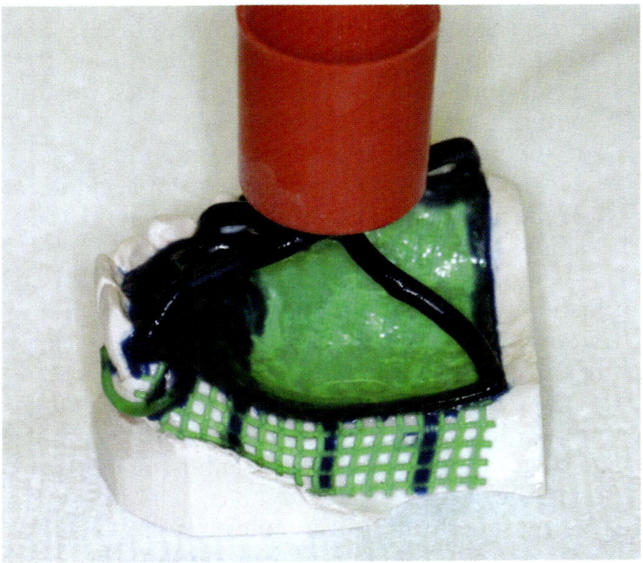

Figure 18-24 For a maxillary framework, either multiple 8-gauge sprues or a single main sprue located posteriorly can be used. When a single main sprue is used, additional sprues can feed critical regions for casting completeness.

4. Reinforce all junctions with additional wax to prevent constrictions in the sprue channel and to prevent V-shaped sections of investment that might break away and be carried into the casting.

Investing the Sprued Pattern

The investment for a removable partial denture casting consists of two parts: the investment cast on which the pattern is formed and the outer investment surrounding the cast and pattern (see Figures 18-41 through 18-44). The latter is confined within a metal ring, which may or may not be removed after the outer investment has set. If the metal ring is not to be removed, it must be

*From Brumfield RC: Dental gold structures, analysis and practicalities, New York, 1949, JF Jelenko.

lined with a layer of cellulose, asbestos substitute, or ceramic fiber paper to allow for both setting and thermal expansion of the mold in all directions.

The investment must conform accurately to the shape of the pattern and must preserve the configuration of the pattern as a cavity after the pattern itself has been eliminated through vaporization and oxidation. Brumfield has listed the purposes of the investment as follows:

1. It provides the strength necessary to hold the forces exerted by the entering stream of molten metal until this metal has solidified into the form of the pattern.
2. It provides a smooth surface for the mold cavity so that the final casting will require as little finishing as possible; in some situations a deoxidizing agent is used to keep surfaces bright.
3. It provides an avenue of escape for most of the gases entrapped in the mold cavity by the entering stream of molten metal.
4. It, together with other factors, provides necessary compensation for the dimensional changes of the alloy* from the molten to the solid, cold state.†

The investment for casting gold alloys is a plaster-bound silica material, so compounded that the total mold expansion will offset the casting shrinkage of the alloy, which varies from 1% to 1.74% (the highest figure being the shrinkage of pure gold). Generally the higher the percentage of gold in the alloy, the greater the contraction of the casting on solidifying.

Only one chromium-cobalt alloy has a sufficiently low melting temperature to be cast into a plaster-silica investment mold. According to Peyton, for the other alloys that have a higher melting temperature, an investment that contains quartz powder that is held together by an ethyl silicate or sodium silicate binder is generally used. Expansion to offset casting shrinkage for the chromium-cobalt alloys is accomplished primarily through thermal expansion of the mold and must be sufficient to offset their greater casting shrinkage, which is in the order of 2.3%. For this reason the casting ring is usually removed after the mold has hardened to allow for the greater mold expansion necessary with these alloys. Because the investments for chromium-cobalt alloys are generally less porous, there is greater danger of entrapping gases in the mold cavity by the molten metal. Spruing must be done with greater care, and in some instances, provision for venting the mold is necessary to prevent defective castings.

Step-by-step Procedure

The technique for applying the outer investment is usually referred to as investing the pattern. Actually the cast on which the pattern is formed is part of the investment also. This investment technique is presented in Figures 18-25 through 18-27.

Burnout

The burnout operation serves three purposes: it drives off moisture in the mold; it vaporizes and thus eliminates the pattern, leaving a cavity in the mold; and it expands the mold to compensate for contraction of the metal on cooling.

For the investment to heat uniformly, it should be moist at the start of the burnout cycle. Steam will then carry the heat into the investment during the early stages of the burnout. Therefore if the investment is not burned out on the same day that it is poured, it should be soaked in water for a few minutes before it is placed in the burnout furnace.

Just before it is placed in the furnace, the mold should be placed in the casting machine to balance the weight against the weight of the mold. At this time the mold should be properly oriented to the machine and its crucible, and a scratch line

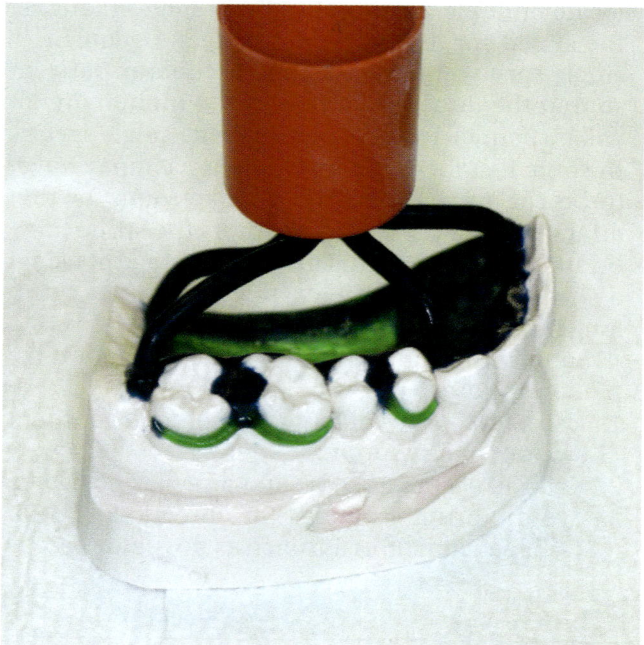

Figure 18-25 Wax pattern sprued and ready to invest.

*Note the substitution of the word alloy, as the same principles apply whether the metal is a precious metal alloy or a chromium-cobalt alloy. In some of the latter alloys, the cobalt is partially replaced by nickel; such alloys are sometimes decribed as Stellite alloys.

†From Brumfield RC: Dental gold structures, analysis and practicalities, New York, 1949, JF Jelenko.

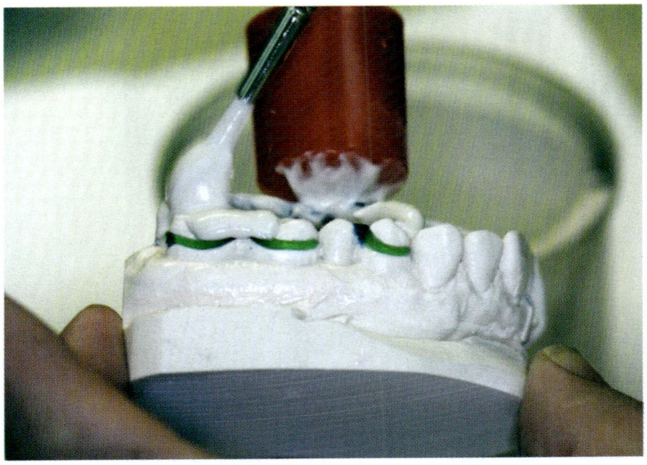

Figure 18-26 Applying the investment with a soft moistened brush to assure complete adaptation of the investment. This will help reduce the number of bubbles and make for a smoother cast surface.

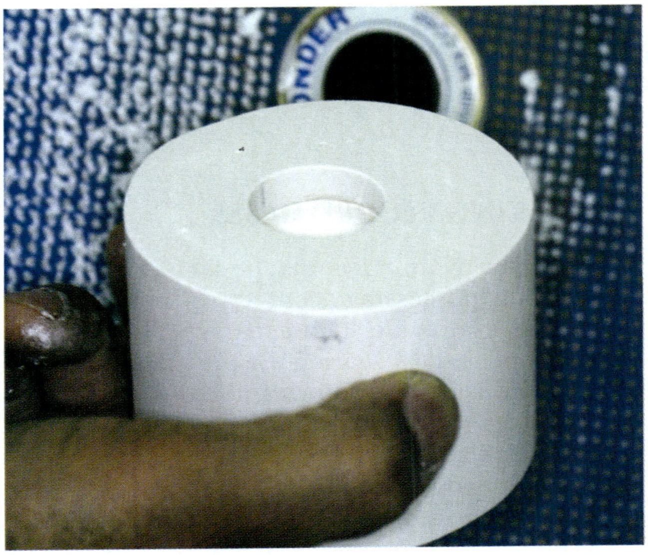

Figure 18-27 Investment mold has been trimmed to prepare the sprue end for burnout and subsequent complete adaptation to the casting machine.

should be made at the top for later repositioning of the hot mold.

The mold should be placed in the oven with the sprue hole down and the orientation mark forward. Burnout should be started with a cold oven, or nearly so. Then the temperature of the oven should be increased slowly to a temperature recommended by the manufacturer. This temperature then should be maintained for the period recommended by the manufacturer to ensure uniform heat penetration. More time must be allowed for plastic patterns, particularly palatal anatomic replica patterns. It is important that the peak temperature recommended by the manufacturer not be exceeded during the burnout period. (When a high-heat investment is used, follow the manufacturer's instructions as to burnout temperature.)

Casting

The method of casting will vary widely with the alloy and equipment being used. All methods use force to quickly inject the molten metal into the mold cavity. This force may be either centrifugal or air pressure; the former is more commonly used. In any case, either too much or too little force is undesirable. If too little force is used, the mold is not completely filled before the metal begins to freeze. If too much force is used, excessive turbulence may result in the entrapment of gases in the casting. With centrifugal casting machines, this is regulated by the number of turns put on the actuating spring.

The metal may be melted with a gas-oxygen blowtorch or by an electric muffle surrounding the metal. In some commercial casting procedures and in some dental laboratories, the induction method may be used (Figure 18-28), which provides a rapid and accurate method of melting the metal. Currently available casting machines include those that are electrically controlled to heat alloys to a specified temperature and to release the molten metal at precisely the correct casting temperature. These machines are relatively expensive and are primarily located in commercial laboratories or institutions where casting volume is high.

Removing the Casting From the Investment

Chromium-cobalt alloys are usually allowed to cool in the mold, are divested (Figure 18-29), and are not cleaned by pickling. Finishing (Figure 18-30) and polishing (Figure 18-31), which are done with special high-speed equipment, require a technical skill in the use of bench lathes. Just before being polished (high-shine), chromium-cobalt castings are electropolished, which is a controlled deplating process (Figure 18-32).

Finishing and Polishing

Some authorities hold that the sprues should not be removed from the casting until most of the polishing is completed. Although it is true that this policy may prevent accidental distortion, it is difficult to adhere to and is therefore somewhat impractical. Instead, reasonable care should be exercised to prevent any distortion resulting from careless handling. A specific precaution is that a cast clasp arm should not be indiscriminately polished and then pliered to place. The waxing

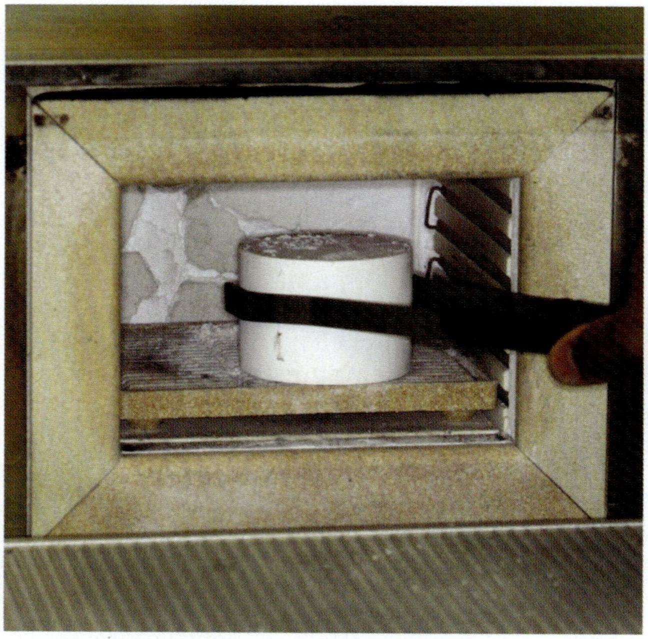

A

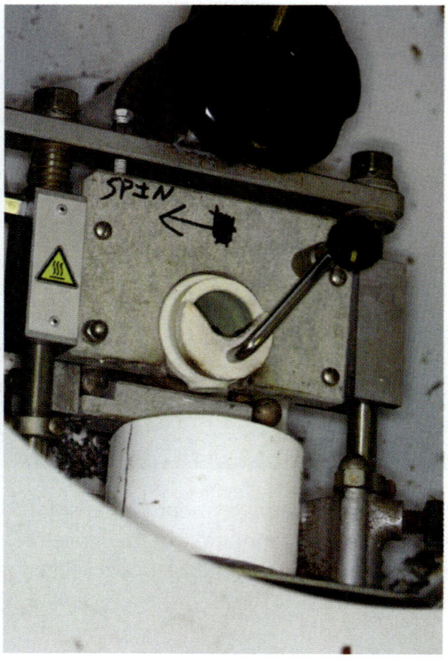

B

Figure 18-28 **A,** Invested pattern is removed from the burnout oven following complete elimination of the wax pattern. **B,** Investment mold is placed into the casting machine. Induction casting process provides consistency to the casting procedure.

should have been done in such a manner that a minimum of finishing is necessary and the intended relationship of the clasp to the abutment is maintained (Figure 18-33).

Actual polishing procedures may vary widely according to personal preference for certain abrasive shapes and sizes. However, the following several rules in finishing the casting are important:

1. High speeds are preferable to low speeds. Not only are they effective but also in experienced hands there is less danger of the casting being caught and thrown out of the hands by the rotating instrument.
2. The wheels or points and the speed of their rotation should do the cutting. Excessive pressure heats the work, crushes the abrasive particles, causes the wheels to clog and glaze, and slows the cutting.
3. A definite sequence for finishing should be adopted and followed for every framework.
4. Clean polishing wheels should be used. If contaminated wheels are used, foreign particles may become embedded in the surface, which will lead to later discoloration.
5. Be sure each finishing operation completely removes all scratches left by the preceding one. Remember that each successive finishing step uses a finer abrasive and therefore cuts more slowly and requires more time to accomplish.

MAKING RECORD BASES

Bases for jaw relation records should be made either of materials possessing accuracy or those that can be relined to provide such accuracy. Relining may be accomplished by seating the previously adapted base onto the tinfoil or lubricant in the cast with an intervening mix of zinc oxide–eugenol paste or with autopolymerizing acrylic resin. Some use has been made of the mercaptan and silicone impression materials for this purpose, but the wisdom of using an elastic lining material for jaw relation record bases is questionable. However, when rigid setting materials are used for this purpose, any undercuts on the cast must be blocked out with wax or clay to facilitate their removal without damage to the cast.

The ideal jaw relation record base is one that is processed (or cast) to the form of the master cast, becoming the permanent base of the completed prosthesis. Cast metal bases for either complete or removable partial dentures offer this advantage, as do acrylic resin bases that are processed directly to the master cast, thus becoming the permanent denture base. When undercuts are present, the master cast will be destroyed during removal of the base. Then existing undercuts must be blocked out inside the denture base before dental stone is poured into it to make a cast for articulator mounting. A second cast, which includes the undercuts, must be poured against the entire base to support it when

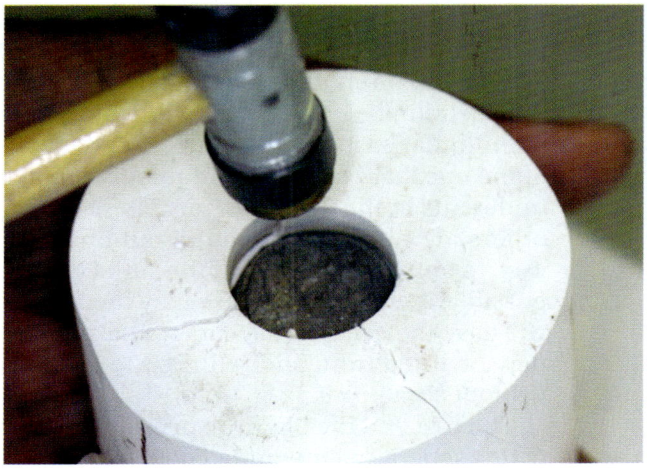

A

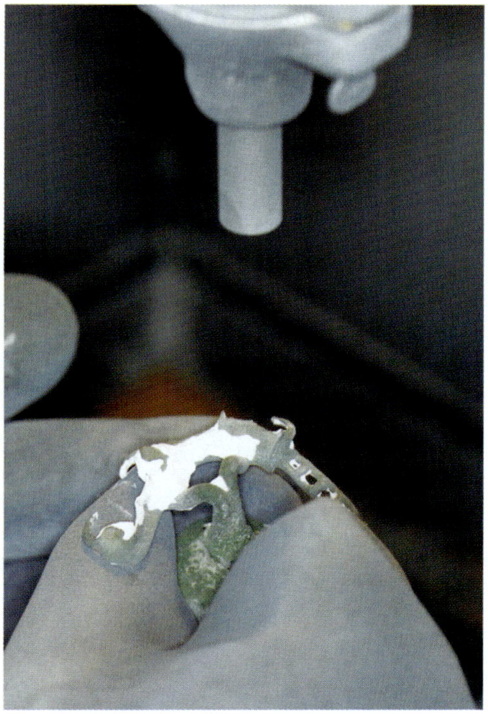

B

Figure 18-29 **A,** Divesting of the framework involves bulk removal of the investment. **B,** Framework is divested with aluminum oxide.

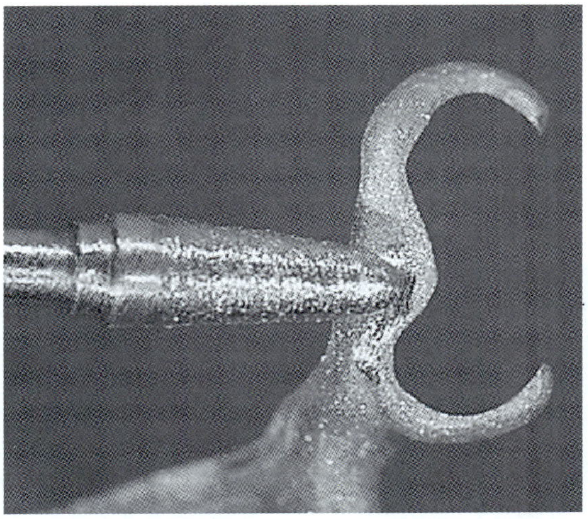

Figure 18-30 Gross finishing is accomplished with abrasive stones or sintered diamonds (except at contact areas). *(Courtesy Bego, Bremen, Germany.)*

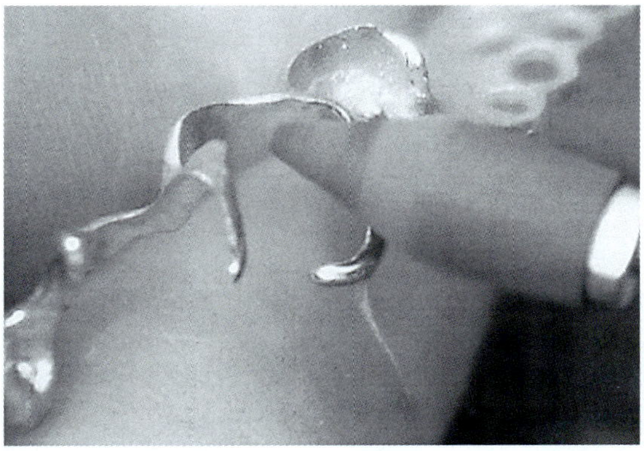

Figure 18-31 Polishing. Framework finished with a rubber polishing point prior to final "high-shine" polish. *(Courtesy Bego, Bremen, Germany.)*

processing the overlying acrylic resin. With both the processed base and the overlying acrylic resin, some care must be taken to prevent visible junction lines between the original acrylic resin base and the acrylic resin that supports the teeth and establishes facial contours.

Some autopolymerizing acrylic resin materials are sufficiently accurate for use as jaw relation bases. These are used with a sprinkling technique, which, when properly done, permits a base to be made that compares favorably with a processed base or a visible light polymerized base. A material must be selected that will polymerize in a reasonable time (usually a 12-minute monomer) and will retain its form during the sprinkling process. Because polymerization with typical shrinkage toward the cast begins immediately, alternate addition of monomer and polymer in small increments results in reduced overall shrinkage and greater accuracy. Another option is to use the visible light-cured (VLC) denture base materials, which employ a technique similar to that described for making custom impression trays in Chapter 15.

Technique for Making a Sprinkled Acrylic Resin Record Base

The technique for sprinkling a record base will be given here because the techniques for the VLC impression tray and record bases were presented in Chapter 15 and elsewhere in this chapter. Some blockout and lubrication of the cast is necessary (Figure 18-34). Relief of undercut areas on the cast is best accomplished with a water-soluble modeling clay or baseplate wax. Modeling clay is easily formed and shaped on the cast and is easily removed from either the cast or the base with a natural-bristle toothbrush under warm running water. Wax must be flushed off the cast with hot water and possibly removed from the inside of the base before use.

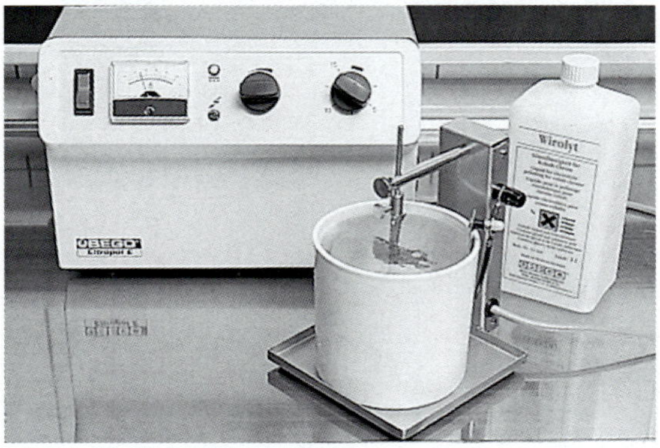

Figure 18-32 Removable partial denture framework being electropolished in heated polishing liquid. *(Courtesy Bego, Bremen, Germany.)*

Bases for jaw relation records must have maximum contact with the supporting tissue. The accuracy of the base will be in proportion to contact provided to the total area of intimate tissue. Those areas most often undercut and require blockout of the distolingual and retromylohyoid areas of the mandibular cast, the distobuccal and labial aspects of the maxillary cast, and, frequently, small multiple undercuts in the palatal rugae. These areas and any others are blocked out with a minimum of clay or wax, to obliterate as little of the surface of the cast as possible. A close-fitting base may then be made that will have the necessary accuracy and stability and yet may be lifted from and returned to the master cast without abrading it.

The cast and the blockout or relief are then coated with a separating medium. Following this the cast is wet with the monomer from a dropper bottle. After the surface is wetted with the monomer, the polymer is sprinkled or dusted onto the wet surface until all the monomer has been absorbed. Sprinkling is best accomplished with a large-mouthed bottle with a single hole in the lid near the rim. This facilitates the placement of the polymer without excess in any one area. A flexible bottle with suitable applicator tip also may be used. The objective should be the uniform application of polymer over the entire ridge rather

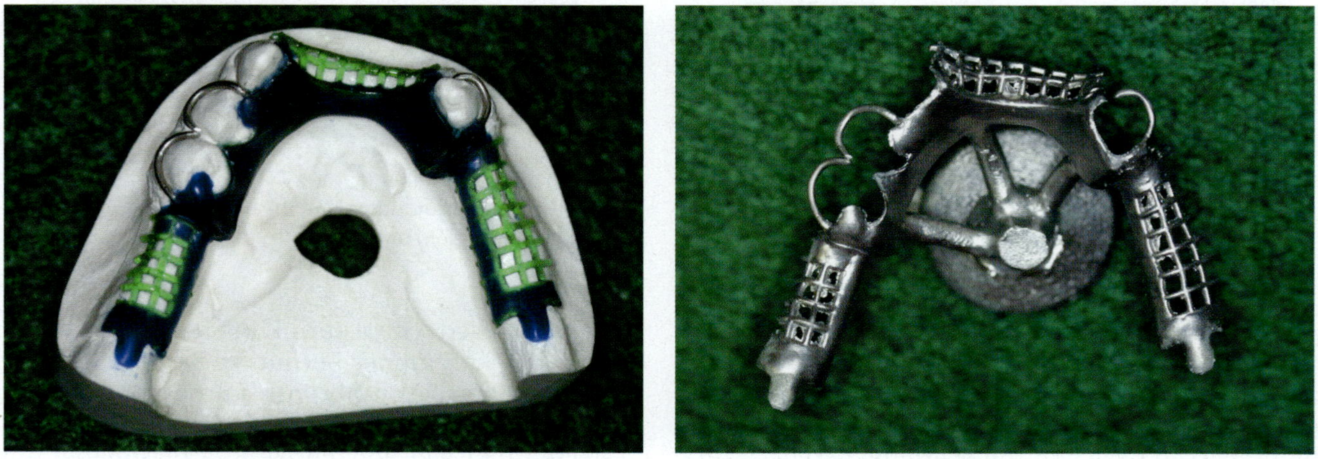

A B

Figure 18-33 Attention to detail in forming the wax pattern not only assures quality of the framework, but it also saves time in finishing and polishing the resultant casting. **A,** Wax pattern of mandibular framework that incorporates three wrought wire retainers. **B,** The same framework following casting showing smooth casting surface and attention to detail regarding casting completeness and clasp form.

than allowing excess to accumulate at the border to be trimmed later. An autopolymerizing acrylic resin material must be used that will retain its form during the sprinkling procedure without objectionable flow into low areas (Figures 18-35 and 18-36).

Once the polymer has been sprinkled in slight excess, the monomer is again added. Flooding must be prevented; therefore the monomer must be directed over the entire surface gradually until the polymer has just absorbed the monomer. A few seconds delay before the addition of excess monomer will allow the mass to reach a tacky consistency and prevent it from flowing when more monomer is added. Then the monomer may be added in excess, which is immediately absorbed by the application of more polymer as before. This process is repeated selectively until a uniform layer has been built up that is just thick enough so that none of the underlying cast or relief may be seen.

The final step in sprinkling is the addition of monomer sufficient to leave a wet surface. Immediately the cast should be placed in a covered glass

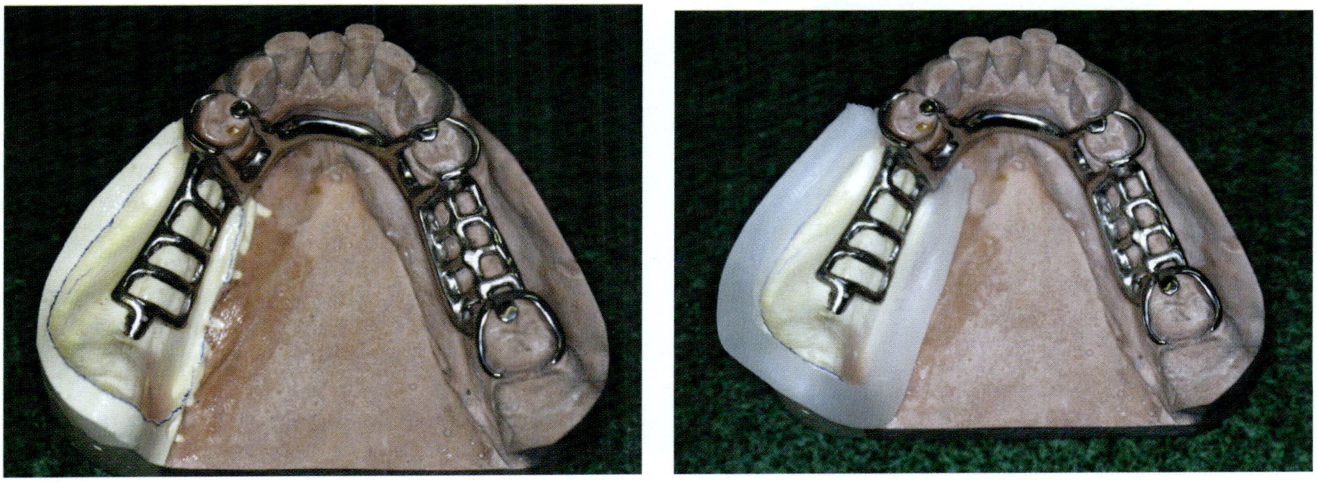

A B

Figure 18-34 **A,** Preparation of Kennedy Class I, mod 1 distal extension for sprinkle-on record base technique. Cast undercuts are blocked out with wax, and cast is coated with separator. **B,** Peripheral extent of base (the same as peripheral extent of prosthesis captured during border molding and impression making procedure for this altered cast) is outlined with rope wax to contain resin.

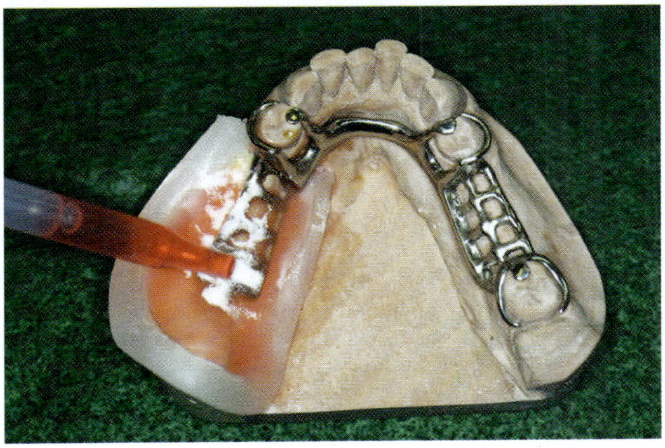

Figure 18-35 The cast is wetted with monomer and polymer resin is added in increments to uniformly control thickness. Use of typical eyedropper may be difficult if monomer addition cannot be controlled. Use of peripheral rope wax helps in this regard.

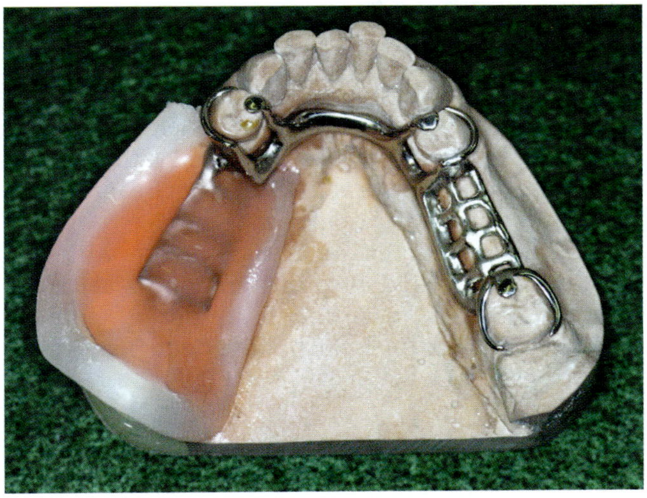

Figure 18-36 Record base is complete when a uniform thickness is created that provides strength and accuracy. The completed un-polymerized resin is covered to ensure polymerization without loss of surface monomer.

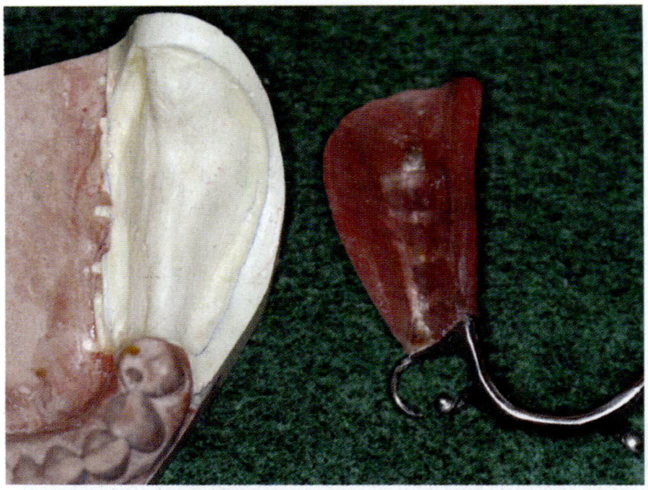

Figure 18-37 Once completely polymerized, the record base and framework can be removed from the cast, finished, and prepared for addition of the record base. The tissue side of the record base (intaglio) should possess similar accuracy and stability as seen with the completed prosthesis. Such a record base provides a significant advantage for jaw relation records when minimal teeth remain and ridge configurations along with extensive base areas place a premium on base accuracy and stability.

dish or covered with an inverted bowl. This permits final polymerization in a saturated atmosphere of monomer and prevents evaporation of surface monomer. The cast should not be placed in water nor any attempt made to accelerate polymerization. Slow polymerization is necessary so that shrinkage toward the cast will occur. Only then will overall shrinkage be negligible and accuracy of fit ensured. This is of little consequence in making an impression tray, but it is most essential in making a sprinkled acrylic resin base.

Although polymerization will be about 90% complete within an hour and an impression tray may even be lifted within a half-hour, it is critical that a sprinkled denture base be left overnight before being separated from the cast. It should then be lifted either dry or under lukewarm tap water. It should not be immersed in hot water, or some warping may occur.

A sprinkled acrylic resin base made with the precautions outlined above will retain its accuracy for days, or even for an indefinite period, comparable with that of a heat-polymerized resin base (Figure 18-37) or a VLC base.

OCCLUSION RIMS

It has been explained that jaw relation records for removable partial dentures always should be made on accurate bases that are either part of the denture casting itself or are attached to it in exactly the same relation as the final denture base will be. Further, it has been stated that although the use of the final denture base is best for jaw relation records, a sprinkled or corrected acrylic resin base may be used satisfactorily. In any case, accuracy of the base supporting a maxillomandibular record must be ensured before considering the function of occlusion rims.

Occlusion rims may be made of several materials. The material that is most commonly used to establish static occlusal relationships is the hard baseplate wax rim. However, use of a wax occlusion rim can be inaccurate when the occlusal portion of the rim is mishandled. When some soft material that sets to a rigid state, such as impression plaster or bite registration paste, is used in conjunction with wax rims to record static occlusal relations, many of the errors common to wax rims are eliminated—provided some space for the material exists between the occlusion rims, the opposing teeth, or both at the desired vertical dimension to be recorded. Registration made on wax occlusion rims using a wax registration material must be handled carefully and mounted immediately.

Occlusion rims for static jaw relation records should be so shaped that they represent the lost teeth and their supporting structures (Figure 18-38). An occlusion rim that is too broad and is extended beyond where prosthetic teeth will be located is inexcusable. Such rims will substantially alter the shape of the palatal vault and arch form of the mandibular arch, crowd the patient's tongue, have an unwelcome effect on the patient, and offer more resistance to jaw relation recording media than will a correctly shaped occlusion rim.

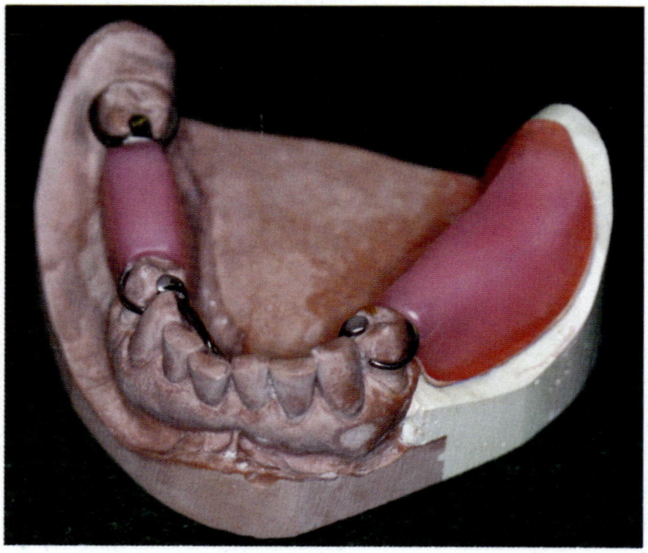

Figure 18-38 Occlusion rims are added to allow recording of jaw relation records. Placement of wax record is dictated by the opposing tooth position and the supporting ridge character. When possible, the occlusion rim should allow recording of the jaw position within the primary bearing area of the ridge.

Modeling plastic (compound) has several advantages and may be used rather than wax for occlusion rims. It may be softened uniformly by flaming, yet when chilled it becomes rigid and sufficiently accurate. It may be trimmed with a sharp knife to expose the tips of the opposing cusps to recheck or position an opposing cast into the record rim. Opposing occlusion rims of modeling plastic may be keyed with greater accuracy than opposing wax rims. Preferably, however, even those should be trimmed short of contact at the vertical dimension of occlusion, and bite registration paste should be interposed for the final record. As with wax rims, an adjustable frame also may be used to support the final record.

Occlusion rims made of either extra hard baseplate wax or modeling plastic may be used to support intraoral central bearing devices, intraoral tracing devices, or both. Because of its greater stability, modeling plastic is preferable for this purpose when the edentulous situation permits the use of flat plane tracings. An example of such a situation is when an opposing complete denture is being made concurrently with the removable partial denture. In such a situation, modeling plastic occlusion rims provide greater stability than wax rims, with corresponding improvement in the predictable accuracy of such a jaw relation record. Although sealing opposing occlusion rims or using clips for complete denture jaw relation records may be acceptable, particularly for an initial articulator mounting, the existence of a removable partial denture framework makes this practice hazardous. The framework and attached base should be seated accurately on its cast before the opposing cast is repositioned in occlusion to it, because it is necessary that the dentist be able to see that the removable partial denture framework is in its designed terminal relation to the supporting teeth before articulating the casts.

Occlusion rims for recording functional, or dynamic, occlusion must be made of a hard wax that can be carved by the opposing dentition. This method, outlined in Chapter 17, presumes that the opposing arch is intact or has been restored. Functional occlusion records by this method cannot be made when both arches are being restored simultaneously. Rather, an opposing arch must be as intact as the treatment plan calls for, or must be restored by whatever prosthetic means the situation dictates. Opposing removable partial dentures or an opposing complete denture may be carried concurrently up to the final occlusal record. One denture is then completed and the functional record is made in opposition to it. Often this necessitates that all opposing teeth be articulated first in wax to establish optimum ridge relations and the correct occlusal plane. One denture is then carried to completion, and the teeth that remain in wax on the opposing denture are removed while the functional occlusal record is being made.

While the laboratory steps required for establishing an occlusion using functional occlusal records were described in Chapter 17 the following provides more detail. Some inlay waxes are used for this purpose because they can be carved by the opposing dentition and because most of them are hard enough to support occlusion over a period of hours or days. A wax for recording functional crown and bridge occlusion, because it is established entirely in the dental office, is selected on the basis of how well it may be carved by the opposing dentition in a relatively short period of time. Therefore a softer wax may be used than is required for the recording of occlusal paths over a period of 24 hours or more. For this latter purpose, hard inlay wax seems to satisfy best the requirements for a wax that is durable yet capable of recording a functional occlusal pattern. This wax is packaged in the form of sticks. A layer of hard, sticky wax is first flowed onto the surface of the denture base. Two sticks of the inlay wax are then laid parallel along the longitudinal center of the denture base and secured to it with a hot spatula. This is the only preparation before the dental appointment. Because neither the height nor the width of the occlusion rim can be known in advance and because deep warming of a chilled wax rim is difficult, the rim is not completed before the appointment.

With the patient in the chair, a hot spatula is inserted into the crevice between the two sticks of wax, making the center portion fluid between two supporting walls. Some transfer of heat to the supporting walls occurs, resulting in the occlusion rims becoming uniformly softened. The patient is asked to close into this wax rim until the natural teeth are in contact, which establishes both the height and the width of the occlusion rim. Wax is then added or carved away as indicated, and the patient asked to make lateral excursions. Any excess wax is then removed, and any unsupported wax is supported by addition. Finally, wax is added to increase the occlusal vertical dimension sufficient to allow for (1) denture settling, (2) changes in jaw relation brought about by the reestablishment of posterior support, and (3) carving in all mandibular excursions. When sufficient height and width have been established to accommodate all excursive movements, the patient is given instructions for chewing in the functional record and is then dismissed.

Although this discussion has been included in this chapter on laboratory procedures, the entire procedure of establishing occlusion rims for recording functional occlusion should be considered a chair-side procedure rather than a laboratory procedure. It is necessary that the purpose of a functional occlusal record be clearly understood so that subsequent laboratory steps may be accomplished in a manner that the effect of such an occlusal record may be reproduced on the finished denture.

MAKING A STONE OCCLUSAL TEMPLATE FROM A FUNCTIONAL OCCLUSAL RECORD

After final acceptance of the occlusal record developed by the patient, the effectiveness of this method for establishing functional occlusion on the removable partial denture will depend on how accurately the following procedures are carried out. For this reason it will be given as a step-by-step procedure (see Figures 17-14 to 17-18). If the base of the master cast (or processing cast) has not been keyed previously, do this before proceeding. Reduce the thickness and width of the base if it is so large that difficulty will be encountered in flasking. The base may not be reduced after removal from the articulator because the mounting record would be lost.

Keying may be done in several ways, but a method whereby the keyed portions are visible on the articulator mounting eliminates some possibility of remounting error. According to the preferred method, form a 45° bevel on the base of the cast by hand or with the model trimmer, and then add three V-shaped grooves on the anterior and the posterior aspects of the base of the cast at the bevel. The bevel serves to facilitate reseating the cast on the articulator mounting, and the mounting surfaces are made still more definite by the triangular grooves. Being placed at the beveled margin, the triangular grooves are visible at all times, and any discrepancy may be clearly seen.

Inspect the underside of the cast framework and denture bases, removing any particles of wax or other debris. Similarly, inspect and clean the master cast of any particles of stone, wax, blockout material, or any other debris that might prevent the casting from being seated accurately on it.

Now seat the denture framework on the cast in its original terminal position. This is the position that is maintained by securing it with sticky wax with all the occlusal rests seated while making the trial denture base. It is also the position that the casting assumed in the mouth while the occlusal record was being made and that must be duplicated on returning the denture framework to the master cast. Holding the framework in this terminal position, secure it again with sticky wax. (If a processing cast is being used in place of the master cast, the denture base will have been made on that cast and the same precautions in returning the framework to its original position apply.)

With the denture framework and the occlusal record in position, form a matrix of clay around the occlusal record to confine the hard stone, which will form the stone occlusal template. The clay matrix is the same for a metal or electroplated surface as for the wax record. The clay matrix should rise at a 45° angle from the buccal and lingual limits of the occlusal registration. Then arch either clay or a sheet of wax across from one side to the other, forming a vault that will permit lingual access when articulating the teeth.

Leave the occlusal surfaces of a processing cast exposed so that they may act as vertical stops. This will serve to maintain the vertical relation in the articulator. Unless such stone-to-stone stops are used, the technician may alter the vertical relation in the articulator, either accidentally or otherwise. Any change in vertical relations is incompatible with a concept of dynamic conclusion because the occlusal pattern is directly related to the degree of jaw separation. Although it may be true that occlusal vertical dimension may be changed when casts are mounted in relation to the opening axis of the mandible, as long as natural cusps remain to influence mandibular movement, the occlusal vertical relation established with a functional occlusal record must not be changed in the articulator.

Cover the surfaces of the adjacent abutment teeth left exposed with sodium silicate, microfilm, or some other separating medium to ensure separation of the stone vertical stops. If the wax record has not been electroplated, use a hard dental stone to form the opposing template. This may be an improved stone, but the use of a stone die material is preferred. Only the occluding surface needs to be poured in the harder stone, a less costly laboratory stone being used to back it up. If this is done, add the second layer to the first before the former takes its initial set to prevent any possibility of accidental separation between the two materials.

Vibrate the stone only into the wax registration and against the stone stops. Pile on the rest of the stone and leave it uneven to facilitate attachment to the mounting stone. Attach the occlusal template to the articulator without provision for removal or remounting because only the working cast need be keyed for remounting.

After the stone template has set, attach the occluded casts to both arms of the articulator before separating the casts. The type of articulating instrument used is of little importance because all eccentric positions are recorded on the template, and whatever instrument is used acts purely as a simple hinge or a tripod. Therefore any laboratory articulator or tripod may be used.

Casts should be attached to the articulating instrument with stone rather than with plaster. Mounting stones are available that have been especially formulated and prepared to minimize the setting expansion inherent in most gypsum products. The least amount of setting expansion of the mounting medium is most desirable to maintain the intended relationship of the opposing casts.

One must remember which arch will be movable as a working cast, and the articulator mounting should be made accordingly. For example, for a mandibular denture, the template is attached to the upper arm of the articulator. For a maxillary denture, the template is mounted upside down on the lower arm. The keyed base of the working cast attached to the opposing arm must be coated with a light coat of microfilm, mineral oil, or petroleum jelly to facilitate its separation from the mounting stone.

After the mounting has been completed, separate the casts and remove the clay. The template, with its mounting, may be removed from the articulator if a mounting ring or mounting stud permits; otherwise trimming must be done on the articulator. With pencil, outline the limits of the occlusal registration and any excess stone around its borders. With a knife, trim the vertical stops to a sharp edge on the buccal surface where they contact the working cast.

Remove any overhanging stone, leaving the occluding template and vertical stops clearly visible and accessible. Remove the wax registration preparatory to arranging artificial teeth to the occluding template.

ARRANGING POSTERIOR TEETH TO AN OPPOSING CAST OR TEMPLATE

Whether posterior teeth are to be arranged to occlude with an opposing cast or an occlusal template, the denture base on which the jaw relation record has been made must first be removed and discarded unless metal bases are part of the denture framework, or heat-polymerized acrylic resin bases were used. This statement is based on the assumption that where an adjustable articulator has been used to develop the occlusion, the trial dentures have been evaluated, the articulator mounting has been proved, and the articulator has been programmed for eccentric positions. Because record bases that are entirely tissue supported have no place in recording occlusal relations for removable partial dentures, the bases must be attached to the denture framework. Metal bases that are a part of the prosthesis present no problem. The teeth may be arranged in wax or replaced on the metal base, depending on the type of posterior tooth used, and these must be occluded directly to the opposing cast or template.

Unless occlusal relations are recorded on final acrylic resin bases, autopolymerizing acrylic resin bases by the sprinkling method or VLC bases are the most accurate and stable of bases that may be used for this purpose. (An alternate method is the relining of the original impression bases, thus accomplishing the same purpose.) Although static relations may be recorded successfully on corrected bases, functional registrations are best accomplished on new acrylic resin bases made for that purpose. In either situation the denture cannot be completed on these bases; neither can the bases be removed conveniently from the retentive framework during the boil out after flasking. Therefore the metal framework must be lifted from the cast, and the original record base removed by flaming its underside. Care must be taken not to allow the acrylic resin to burn, or the cast framework will become discolored with carbon. The framework is repolished and is then returned to its original position on the master cast and secured there with sticky wax before arranging the artificial teeth.

Posterior Tooth Forms

Posterior tooth forms for removable partial dentures should not be selected arbitrarily. One should bear in mind that the objective in removable partial denture occlusion is harmony between natural and artificial dentition. Whether the teeth are arranged to occlude with an opposing cast or to an occlusal template, they should be modified to harmonize with the existing dentition. In this respect, removable partial denture occlusion may differ from complete denture occlusion. In the latter, posterior teeth may be selected and articulated according to the dentist's concept of what constitutes the most favorable complete denture occlusion, whereas removable partial denture occlusion must be made to harmonize with an existing occlusal pattern. Thus the occlusal surfaces on the finished removable partial denture may bear little resemblance to the original occlusal surfaces of the teeth as manufactured.

Artificial tooth forms should be selected to restore the space and fulfill the esthetic demands of the missing dentition. Manufactured tooth forms usually require modification to satisfactorily articulate with an opposing dentition. The original occlusal form, therefore, is of little importance in forming the posterior occlusion for the removable partial denture.

The posterior teeth may be made of porcelain or resin (including all resin forms—composite, interpolymer network, cross-link, double cross-link, etc.). An advantage of resin teeth is that they are more easily modified and subsequently reshaped for masticating efficiency by adding grooves and spillways. Resin teeth are also more easily narrowed buccolingually to reduce the size of the occlusal table without sacrificing strength or esthetics. They also may be more easily ground to fit minor connectors and irregular spaces and to avoid retentive elements of the removable partial denture framework. However, when resin teeth are used the occlusion must be evaluated periodically to make sure that the occlusal surfaces have not worn out of contact. It seems that the best combinations of opposing occlusal surfaces to maintain the established occlusion and to prevent deleterious abrasion are porcelain to porcelain surfaces, gold surfaces to natural or restored natural teeth, and gold surfaces to gold surfaces. A common method for making gold occlusal surfaces to conform to adjusted resin teeth occlusion is shown in Figure 18-39.

Arranging Teeth to an Occluding Surface

The procedure for arranging teeth to a static relationship with an opposing cast is essentially the same as for arranging teeth to an occluding template. On the other hand, articulation of artificial teeth on an adjustable instrument, which reproduces to some extent mandibular movement, will follow more closely the customary pattern for complete denture occlusion. The procedure for arranging posterior

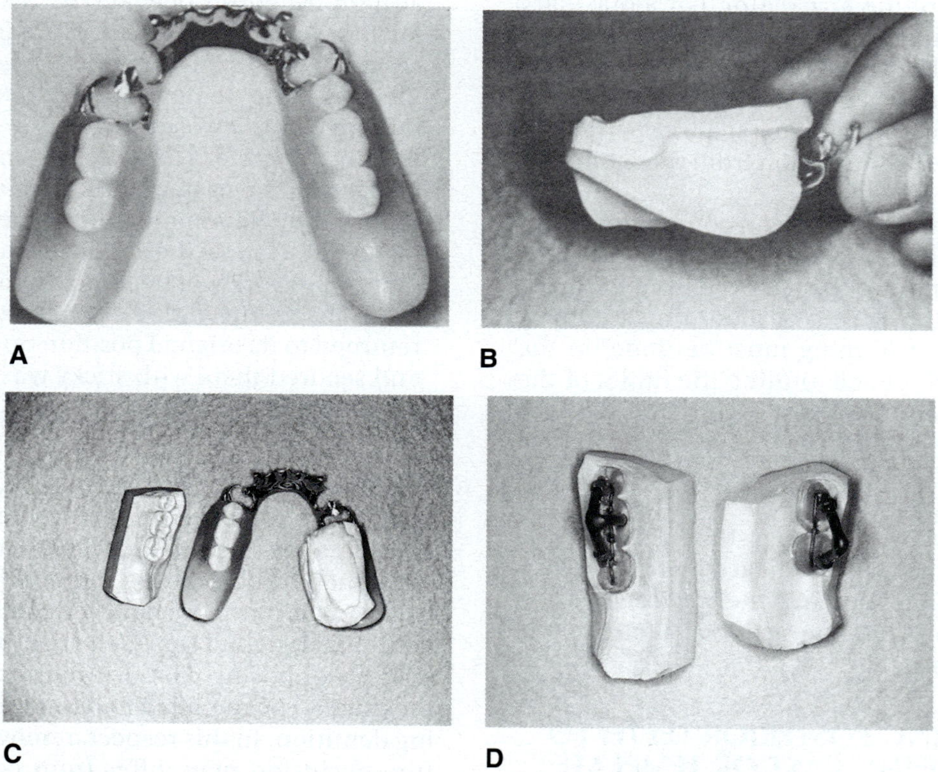

Figure 18-39 Gold occlusal surfaces, duplicating occlusal morphology of adjusted acrylic resin posterior teeth, are readily fabricated. **A,** Denture has been used by patient and all necessary occlusal adjustments have been accomplished on resin teeth in first 2 weeks of use. **B,** Stone matrix is poured over occlusal surfaces and extended over top one fourth of buccal surfaces. **C,** Stone matrix is extended to cover depth of lingual flange so that it can be positively relocated in same position after artificial teeth have been prepared for reception of gold occlusal surfaces. Buccal portion of matrix is trimmed so that wax patterns for gold surfaces will be about 1.5 mm thick. **D,** Stone matrices are painted with separating medium, and wax patterns of occlusal surfaces are formed by flowing inlay wax into occlusal portions of matrix. Small retention loops are placed—one in each individual occlusal pattern. Patterns are sprued and cast in Type III gold.

Continued

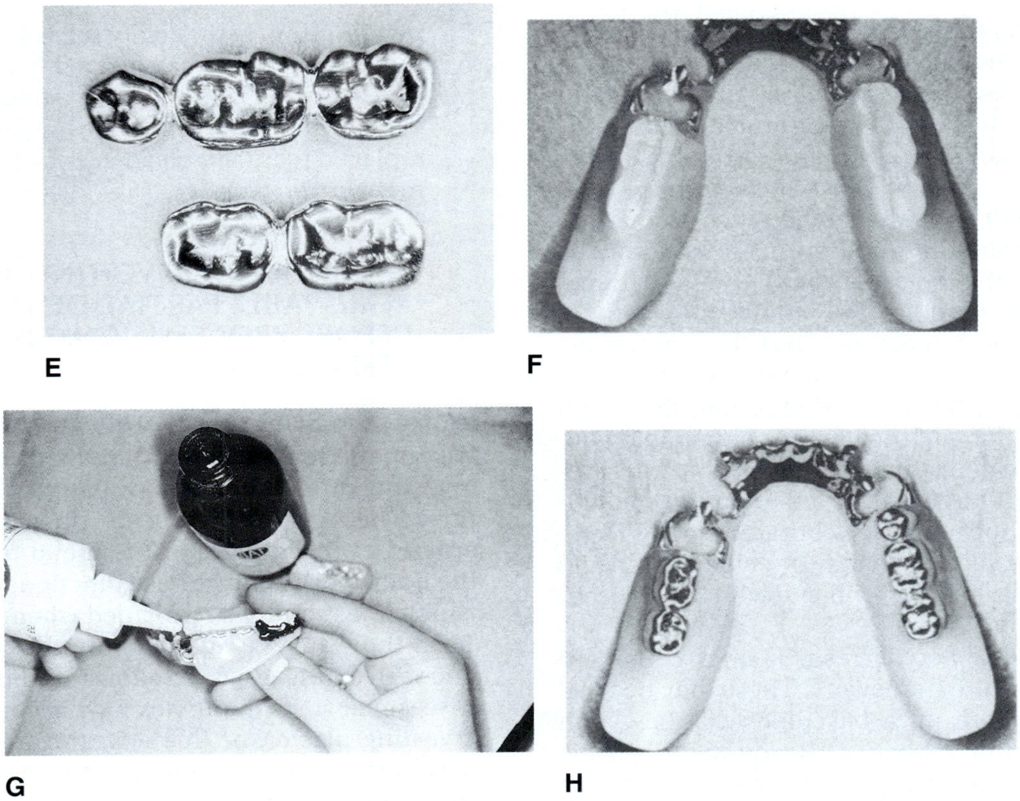

Figure 18-39 Cont'd E, Wax patterns have been cast and polished. F, Acrylic resin artificial teeth are prepared for reception of gold occlusal surfaces by reducing their occlusal portion about 2 mm and making undercut groove through central fossa of resin teeth. Groove should only be deep enough to accommodate retention loops on gold occlusal surfaces. G, Gold occlusals, stone matrix, and denture are assembled. Matrix is held in position with sticky wax. Tooth shade acrylic resin (autopolymerizing) is used to attach gold occlusal surfaces to denture by using the sprinkling method of application. H, Procedure is completed by finishing and polishing tooth shade resin. Although original occlusal surfaces have been duplicated in gold and now occupy same position as original resin surfaces, remounting cast should be made so that any possible resulting occlusal discrepancies can be corrected on articulator, using new interocclusal records to mount lower cast and denture. *(From Morris AL, Bohannon HM, eds: Dental specialties in general practice, Philadelphia, 1969, Saunders.)*

teeth to an occluding template was presented in Chapter 17.

TYPES OF ANTERIOR TEETH

Anterior teeth on removable partial dentures are concerned primarily with esthetics and the function of incising. These are best arranged when the patient is present because an added appointment for try-in would be necessary anyway. They may be arranged arbitrarily on the cast and then tried in, but a stone index of their labial surfaces should be made on the master cast after the final arrangement has been established to preserve the arrangement that the patient saw and approved.

From a purely mechanical standpoint, all missing anterior teeth are best replaced with fixed restorations rather than with the removable partial denture. However, for cosmetic or economic reasons, or in situations in which several missing anterior teeth are involved—such as in a Class IV partially edentulous arch—their replacement with the removable partial denture may be unavoidable.

Some types of anterior teeth used in removable partial dentures are as follows:

1. Porcelain or resin teeth, attached to the framework with acrylic resin.
2. Ready-made resin teeth processed directly to retentive elements on the metal framework with a matching resin. This is called a *pressed-on method* and has the advantage of permitting prior selection and evaluation of the anterior

teeth, plus the advantage of the use of ready-made resin teeth for labial surfaces. These are then hollowed out on the lingual surface to facilitate their permanent attachment to the denture framework with the resin of the same shade.

3. Resin teeth processed to a metal framework in the laboratory. Tooth forms of wax may be carved on the removable partial denture framework and tried in the mouth, adjusted for esthetics and occlusion, and then processed in an acrylic resin of a suitable shade. There is some question as to whether the shade and durability of such teeth are comparable with those of manufactured resin teeth, but improvements in materials have led to improved quality and appearance of laboratory-made teeth. Moreover, such teeth may often be shaped and characterized to better blend with the adjacent natural teeth.
4. Porcelain or acrylic resin facings cemented to the denture framework. These may be tried in the mouth on a baseplate wax base and adjusted for esthetics. Ready-made plastic backings may be used, which become part of the pattern for the removable partial denture framework. The teeth are then ultimately cemented to the framework. Esthetically, these are less satisfactory than other types of anterior teeth, but because the plastic backing is cast as part of the removable partial denture framework they have the advantage of greater strength and are replaced easily. A record of the mold and shade of each tooth should be kept, and only the ridge lap of the replacement teeth needs to be ground to fit. When replaceability is the main reason for its use, the stock facing should not be beveled or difficulty will be encountered in replacing it. Replacement also may be accomplished by waxing and processing a resin tooth that directly faces the metal backing. Stock tube or side-groove teeth are not ordinarily used for anterior teeth on removable partial dentures because of the horizontal forces that tend to dislodge them.
5. Anterior resin denture teeth can be modified to be used as resin veneers, the same as for veneer crowns and veneer pontics on fixed partial dentures. This is most applicable when the removable partial denture framework is to be cast in an alloy. Then labial surfaces may be waxed and the final carving for esthetics done in the mouth. A modification of this method is the waxing of the veneer coping on a previously cast metal base. These are then cast separately and attached to the framework by soldering. Esthetically the result is comparable with that obtained with resin veneer crowns. This method is particularly applicable when there is a desire to make the replaced teeth match adjacent veneered abutment crowns.

WAXING AND INVESTING THE REMOVABLE PARTIAL DENTURE BEFORE PROCESSING ACRYLIC RESIN BASES

Waxing the Removable Partial Denture Base

Waxing the removable partial denture base before investing differs little from waxing a complete denture. The only difference is the waxing of and around exposed parts of the metal framework. At the framework denture base junction, undercut finishing lines should be provided whenever possible. Then the waxing is merely butted to the finishing line with a little excess to allow for finishing. Otherwise, small voids in the wax may become filled with investing plaster, or fine edges of the investment may break off during boil out and packing. In either situation, small pieces of investment may become embedded in the acrylic resin at the finishing lines. This is prevented by slightly overwaxing and then finishing the acrylic resin back to the metal finishing line with finishing burs. Abrasive wheels and disks should not be used for this purpose, because they will cut into the metal and may burn the acrylic resin. Pumice and a rag wheel should be used sparingly for polishing, because they will abrade the acrylic resin more rapidly than the metal and leave the finishing line elevated above the adjacent acrylic resin.

When waxing to polished metal parts that do not possess a finishing line, it must be remembered that no attachment will exist and that over a period of time there inevitably will be some seepage, separation, and discoloration of the acrylic resin in this area. This may be prevented to some extent by roughening the metal whenever possible to effect some mechanical attachment by silicoating the attachment or by using one of the resin adhesives. The wax should be left 1.5 to 2.0 mm thick so that the acrylic resin will have some bulk at its junction with the polished metal. Thin films of acrylic resin over metal should be avoided. In finishing, these should be cut back to an area of bulk with finishing burs. Otherwise, any thin acrylic resin film will eventually separate and become discolored and unclean as a result of marginal seepage.

Gingival forms should be waxed in accordance with modern concepts of esthetics and should be made to prevent entrapment of food particles.

Dental students should become familiar with normal gingival architecture as found on diagnostic casts of natural dentitions, beginning in basic technique exercises with the casts of each other's mouths. In this manner they may have a better concept of gingival contours to be reproduced on prosthetic restorations.

Artificial teeth should be uncovered fully to expose the entire anatomic crown and beyond when simulating gingival recession. Adjacent or contralateral tooth-gingival relationships should be used as a guide to facilitate the harmonious esthetic presentation of the gingival contours. Relatively few prosthodontic patients are in an age bracket in which some gingival recession and exposed cementum would not normally be present, and this should be simulated on prosthodontic restorations in proportion to the patient's age. With removable partial dentures, gingival contours around the remaining natural teeth should be used as a guide to the gingival contours to be reproduced on the prosthesis. However, interproximal spaces are almost always filled, particularly between posterior artificial teeth.

Frush has listed the following rules for varying the height of the gingival tissue at the cervical portion of the teeth:

1. Slightly below the high lip line at the central incisors
2. Lower than the central incisor gingival margin at the lateral incisors
3. Higher than the central or lateral incisor gingival margin at the canine
4. Slightly lower than the canine at the premolar and variable for both premolars and molars*

The correctly formed papilla should be shaped so that it will be self-cleansing. It should be carved so that it is in harmony with the interpretation of age and will be the deciding factor in the visible outline form of the tooth. As Frush has pointed out, even a drop of wax properly placed can change the appearance of a square tooth to one of tapering or ovoid appearance. A properly formed papilla further enhances the natural appearance by increasing the color in this area.

The rules for forming the papilla were given by Frush as follows:

1. The papilla must extend to the point of tooth contact for cleanliness.
2. The papilla must be of various lengths.
3. The papilla must be convex in all directions.
4. The papilla must be shaped according to the age of the patient.

*From Frush JP: Dentogenic restorations and dynesthetics, Los Angeles, 1957, Swissdent Foundation.

5. The papilla must end near the labial face of the tooth and never slope inward to terminate toward the lingual portion of the interproximal surface.*

The denture should be waxed and carved as for a cast restoration, which it actually is, regardless of the material to be used or the method of processing. The fact that a split-mold technique is used for processing does not alter the fact that the form of the denture base is to be reproduced by a casting procedure. Therefore the denture pattern should be waxed with care in the same form as that desired for the finished restoration rather than attempting to shape facial contours on the prosthesis during the polishing phase (Figure 18-40). Polishing should consist primarily of trimming away the flash, stippling polished surfaces when desired, and polishing lightly with brush wheels and pumice, followed by final polishing with a soft brush wheel and a nonabrasive shining agent, such as whiting. Gross trimming and polishing with pumice should not be necessary if the denture has been properly waxed before investing.

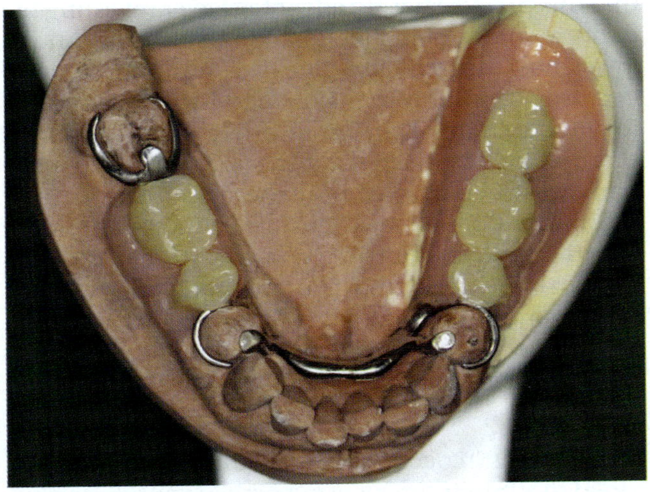

Figure 18-40 Waxing of removable partial denture base should reproduce anatomic contours normal for the specific patient's characteristics. This is especially important for regions where the junction of denture tooth and resin will be visible. Healthy interdental papillae are convex and extend to contact points of teeth. Root prominence can be carved in wax to create a natural appearance. Stippling is typically accomplished following processing using an eccentric round bur. All of these features should be considered against the specific oral environment in which the prosthesis will be placed. A finished and polished prosthesis that demonstrates esthetic features not found in the patient's mouth may be considered objectionable.

*From Frush JP: Dentogenic restorations and dynesthetics, Los Angeles, 1957, Swissdent Foundation.

Because the polished surfaces of any denture play an important part in both retention and the control of the food bolus, buccal and lingual contours generally should be made concave. In most situations border thickness of the denture should be left as recorded in the impression. The only exceptions are the distolingual aspect of the mandibular denture base to prevent interference with the tongue, and the distobuccal aspect of the maxillary denture base to prevent interference with the coronoid process of the mandible. These are the only areas that cannot ordinarily be waxed to final contour before investing and may need to be thinned by the dentist at the time of final polishing.

Investing the Removable Partial Denture

In investing a removable partial denture for processing an acrylic resin base, it must be remembered that the denture cast must be recovered from the flask intact for remounting. The practice of cutting the teeth off the cast to expose the connectors and retainers, which are then embedded in the upper half of the flask, is permissible only when an existing denture base is being relined and no provision has been made for remounting. (In such a situation, it seems that this practice has no advantage over investing the denture that is being so relined upside down in the lower half of the flask.) Because some increase in occlusal vertical dimension has in the past been inevitable in any split-mold processing technique, this method results in the removable partial denture framework being raised from the supporting teeth by the amount of increase. Occlusal adjustment in the mouth may temporarily reestablish a harmonious occlusal relation with the opposing teeth, whereas the removable partial denture framework will then settle into supporting contact with the abutment teeth at the expense of the underlying ridge.

Changes in occlusal vertical dimension may be held to a minimum by using acrylic denture resins that can be placed in the mold in a fluid rather than a doughy state or those that may be injected in a fluid state into a closed mold. Dimensional changes occurring during relining may also be held to a minimum by using autopolymerizing acrylic resins for this purpose, thus preventing the thermal expansion of a mold subjected to elevated temperatures.

When two opposing removable partial dentures are being made concurrently, one is sometimes processed and placed first and then the final occlusion established on the second denture to a fully restored arch. In such a situation, when there are no natural teeth in opposition, it is not necessary that the first denture be remounted after processing. In all other situations, remounting to correct for errors in occlusion is absolutely necessary. Flasking must be accomplished so that the cast may be recovered from the flask undamaged.

Minute voids in the base of the cast will have been reproduced in the stone mounting, and although the obvious larger blebs may be trimmed away, smaller blebs will remain. If the voids in the cast become filled with investing material, the effect is two particles trying to occupy the same space. Covering the base with tinfoil substitute before investing can prevent this. Coating the base and sides of the cast with petroleum jelly not only keeps the base of the cast isolated from investing material but also may allow the cast to be more easily recovered from the surrounding investment.

The entire cast, except for the wax and teeth, may then be invested in the lower half of the flask (Figure 18-41). As with a complete denture, only the supplied teeth and wax are left exposed to be invested in the upper half. Also, as with a complete denture, the investment in the lower half must be smooth and free of undercuts and must be coated with a separator to facilitate separation of the two halves of the flask.

An alternate and preferred procedure is to invest the cast only to the top of the tinfoil on the base, smoothing the investment and applying a reliable separator. Then a second layer of investment is placed around the anatomic portion of the cast and covers the natural teeth and the exposed parts of the denture framework. This is likewise smoothed and made free of undercuts and coated with a separator before pouring the top half of the flask. Recovery of the cast is thus made easier by having a shell of investment over the anatomic portion of the cast, which may be removed separately.

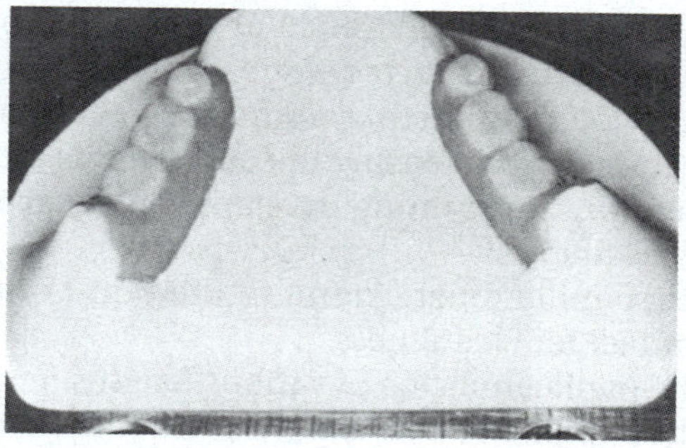

Figure 18-41 Prostheses invested in lower half of flasks. Master cast on which denture will be processed is completely covered with investing stone, exposing only artificial teeth and waxed denture bases. There are no undercuts in invested lower half of flask, thus ensuring separation of flask halves after investment procedure is completed.

When the denture base is to be characterized by applying tinted acrylic resins to the mold, care should be taken not to embed the wax border in the lower half of the flask. Bennett has pointed out the need for investing only to the border of the wax, leaving the entire surface that is to be tinted reproduced in the upper half of the flask. With this precaution, tinting may be carried all the way to the border, and later removal of the flask will not mar the tinted surface. If tinting is not to be done or is to be done only at the cervical margins of the teeth and the papillae, the wax border should be embedded in the lower half where it may be faithfully reproduced and preserved during polishing.

The use of acrylic resin materials that require trial packing is complicated by the presence of the retentive framework of the removable partial denture. With their use, trial packing must be done with two sheets of cellophane between two layers of the resin dough; otherwise the flask could not be opened without pulling the resin away from either the teeth in one half of the flask or the metal framework in the other. Acrylic resin dough is placed in each half of the flask, the sheets of cellophane are placed between them, and the flask is closed for trial packing. The flask is then opened, the cellophane is removed, and the excess flash is trimmed away. Trial packing should be repeated until no excess is visible. Final closure is accomplished without the intervening sheets of cellophane.

Acrylic resin materials have been developed that require no trial packing. These are mixed as usual but are either poured into the mold or placed into the mold in a soft state. They offer little or no resistance to closure of the flask, yet the finished product is comparable with acrylic resin materials packed in a doughy state. They must be used in some excess, with the excess escaping between the halves of the flask. Although they are soft enough to allow the escape of gross excess, the use of a land space is advisable to prevent a thin film from forming on the land area. Any film existing on the land area after deflasking may be interpreted as an opening of the flask by that amount, hence the need for some provision for an intervening space to accommodate the excess and to facilitate its escape as the flask is closed.

To provide such a land space, the land area on the lower half of the flask may be painted with melted baseplate wax before the top half is poured. After wax elimination, a space then remains to accommodate any excess acrylic resin remaining after the flask is completely closed. It is necessary that no plaster or wax be allowed to remain on the rim of the flask and that the flask makes metal-to-metal contact before the second half is poured. Only in this way is it possible to see that the flask is completely closed before it is placed in the curing unit.

The pouring of the top half of the flask follows the same procedure as with a complete denture. Although it is not absolutely necessary that the entire top half be poured in stone, it is necessary that a stone cap of some type be used to prevent tooth movement in an occlusal direction. This is because of the inability of plaster to withstand closing pressures. All plaster remaining on the occlusal surfaces of the teeth should be removed and a separator added before the stone cap is poured to facilitate its removal during deflasking. If the use of stone investment is preferred, a shell of improved stone or die stone may be painted or applied with the fingers onto the wax and teeth and allowed to harden before the remainder of the flask is filled with plaster. If a full stone investment is preferred, some provision should be made for easy separation during deflasking. Not only should a separator stone cap be used, but metal separators or knife cuts radiating out to the walls of the flask should also be placed on the partially set stone. Deflasking is then easily accomplished by removing the stone cap and inserting a knife blade between the sections of stone.

Boil out should be deferred until the investing material has set for several hours or preferably overnight. Boil out must effectively eliminate all wax residue; an adequate source of clean hot water must be available. Immersion of a flask containing the invested denture in boiling water for 5 minutes will adequately soften the wax supporting the artificial teeth so that flask halves may be separated and the remaining wax flushed out. After wax elimination with boiling water, the invested denture should be flushed with a solution of grease-dissolving detergent and again with clean boiling water.

Immediately after boil out, the warm mold should be painted with a thin film of tinfoil substitute, being careful not to allow it to collect around the cervical portions of the teeth. There should be no tinfoil substitute on any part of the denture teeth. A second coat should be applied after the first coat has reasonably dried, and packing of the mold should proceed immediately after this film has dried to the touch.

When the master cast for a distal extension removable partial denture has been repoured from a secondary impression, the supporting foot on the retention frame may not necessarily be in contact with the cast. Closing pressure within the flask may distort the unsupported extension of the metal framework, with subsequent rebound on deflasking. The finished denture base will then lack contact with the supporting tissue, resulting in denture rotation about the fulcrum line similar to that occurring after tissue resorption. To provide support for the distal extension of the metal framework during flask closure, autopolymerizing acrylic resin should be sprinkled or painted around the tissue stop at the distal end of the framework and allowed to harden before proceeding with packing the denture resin (see Figure 5-39).

PROCESSING THE DENTURE

Processing follows the same procedure as that for a complete denture. Denture base characterization tinting may be added just before packing. This is most desirable if denture base material will be visible when in the mouth. Posterior acrylic resin bases alone ordinarily do not require characterization, but the dentist should select a denture base material that closely resembles the color of the surrounding tissue. The ideal acrylic resin base material for removable partial dentures is therefore one that (1) may be used without trial packing; (2) possesses a shade that is compatible with surrounding tissue; (3) is dimensionally stable and accurate; (4) is dense and lends itself to polishing; and (5) polymerizes completely.

There has never been any question concerning the merits of placing tinfoil over the denture before investing, which results in a tinfoil-lined matrix and eliminates the need for a separating film. The fact remains, however, that the use of a tinfoil substitute has become universal.

At best, any tinfoil substitute creates an undesirable film at the gingival margins of the teeth, resulting in microscopic separation between the teeth and the surrounding acrylic resin. This may be shown by sectioning a finished denture and by observing the marginal discoloration around the cervical portions of the teeth after several months in the mouth. To some extent, injection molding obviates this objection to the use of a tinfoil substitute, which is one of the principal advantages of injection molding over compression molding.

Because the use of compression molding is widespread and is likely to continue, methods are needed that eliminate the use of a tinfoil substitute. The layered silicone rubber method results in more complete adaptation of the acrylic resin around the cervical portions of porcelain teeth and more complete bonding to acrylic resin teeth. In addition, denture base tints may be applied directly to the mold without first applying a separating film.

A room-temperature polymerizing silicone rubber, which has sufficient body and toughness for the purpose, is applied to the wax surface of the denture and over the teeth. To prevent movement of the teeth during processing, the occlusal surfaces should be exposed before pouring the upper half of the flask. The manufacturer's instructions must be followed as to mixing and time elapsed before the outer stone investment is added to ensure polymerization and bonding to the overlying investment. Boil out is then completed in the usual way.

A further advantage of the layered silicone rubber method is the ease in accomplishing deflasking. If the wax carving of the denture has been completed with care before flasking, denture tints remain unaltered by unnecessary trimming and polishing of the processed denture.

All resin base materials available up to the present time exhibit some dimensional change, both during processing and in the mouth. The fit of the denture is therefore dependent on the accuracy of the denture base material because impression and cast materials in use today are themselves reasonably accurate. In an attempt to minimize dimensional changes in the denture base, materials and techniques are being improved constantly.

Denture base materials that may be poured into the mold or placed into the mold in a soft state are also quite popular. This technique eliminates trial packing and excessive pressures, which lead to open flasks and altered occlusal vertical dimension as are sometimes experienced with compression molding acrylic resin base materials. Activated, or autopolymerizing, acrylic resins are commonly used to prevent mold expansions at higher temperatures. Materials other than acrylic resins are used with various techniques, some of these being styrene, vinyl, and experimentally epoxy resins. The main objectives behind the development of newer techniques and materials are greater dimensional accuracy and stability, combined with strength and better appearance.

The use of injection molding or poured materials to process removable partial denture base materials combines accuracy and efficiency to help create a well-fitting denture base. The Success Injection System by Dentsply Trubyte combines the accuracy of injection molding with Lucitone 199. The hardware consists of the injection unit, aluminum alloy flasks, and associated system flask components. The flasks are numbered; specifically, they are mated halves that need to be matched for more accurate results. The investment and processing techniques are as follows:

1. The cast with the completed wax up is embedded in the designated side "1" of the flask in the usual manner, placing the cast as close as possible to the back of the flask. After eliminating any undercuts on the cast, flattened wax sticks (approximately 7 mm in diameter) are used to build the injection sprues. For maxillary removable partial dentures, attach the sprue to the posterior border, ensuring that the sprue is sufficiently wide (Figure 18-42, *A*). For mandibular removable partial dentures, position one sprue for each base extension (Figure 18-42, *B*). Apply separator to the investment and place the top half of the flask on the bottom half, ensuring complete intimate metal contact and closure of the halves. Secure the flask's brackets to the flask and tighten (Figure 18-42, *C*). Place the flask on the leveler with side "2" up and complete the investing procedure in the usual manner (Figure 18-42, *D*).
2. When the investment has set, loosen the bolts and remove the metal flask brackets. Place the flask in boiling water (8 to 10 minutes) and complete the boil out procedure (Figure 18-43, *A*). Place the metal injection insert into the back of the flask (Figure 18-43, *B*) and slide the plastic injection socket into the metal insert as far as possible. The plastic injection socket lip should rest flush against the trim of the metal injection insert. Close the flask, position the metal flask brackets, and tighten the bolts.
3. Use the powder/liquid vials to measure sufficient resin for the removable partial denture. Note that the maximum powder and/or liquid that the injection cartridge can hold is 38 g (56 ml) powder and/or 17.5 ml liquid. Stir the powder and/or liquid approximately 15 seconds. Do not excessively mix. Cover the mixing jar until material reaches the "soft pack" stage

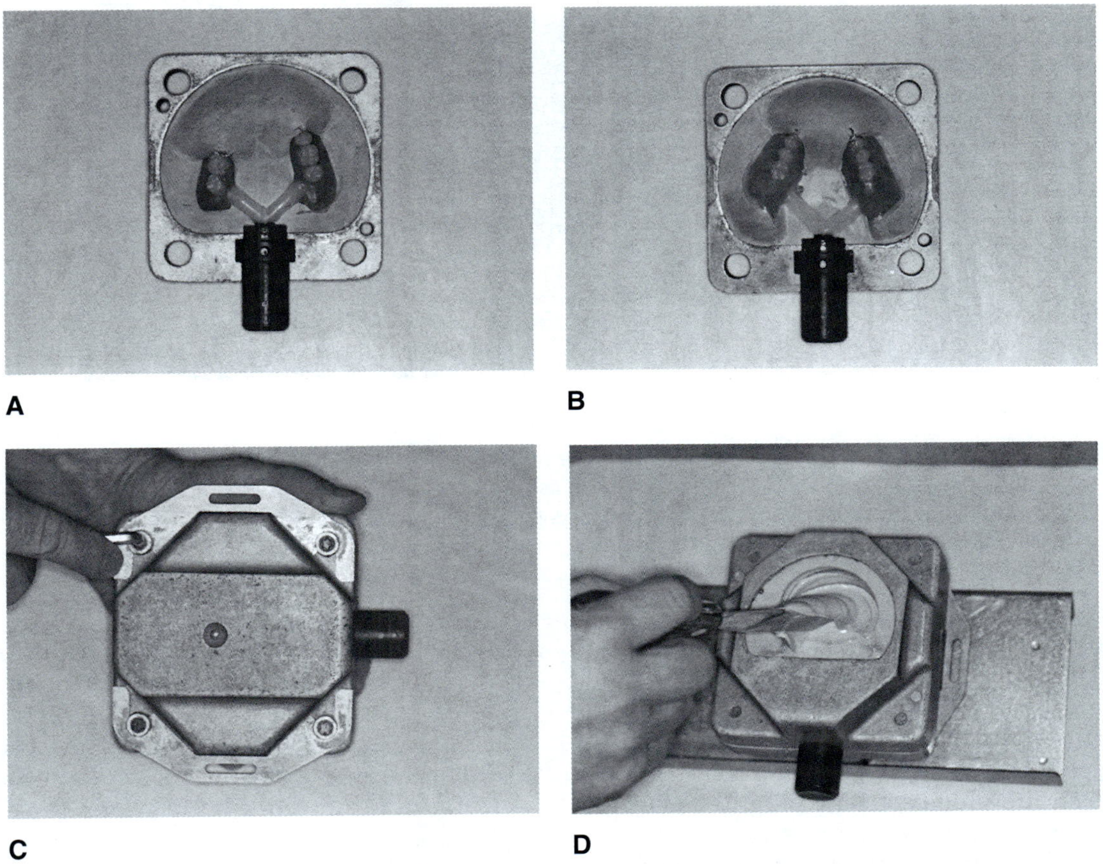

Figure 18-42 **A,** Maxillary prosthesis with sprue attached to posterior border ensuring that sprue is sufficiently wide to facilitate complete access for resin to fill mold. **B,** Mandibular sprue position with one sprue for each base extension. **C,** Flask brackets to flask are secured and tightened. **D,** Flask is placed on leveler with side "2" up, and investing procedure is completed.

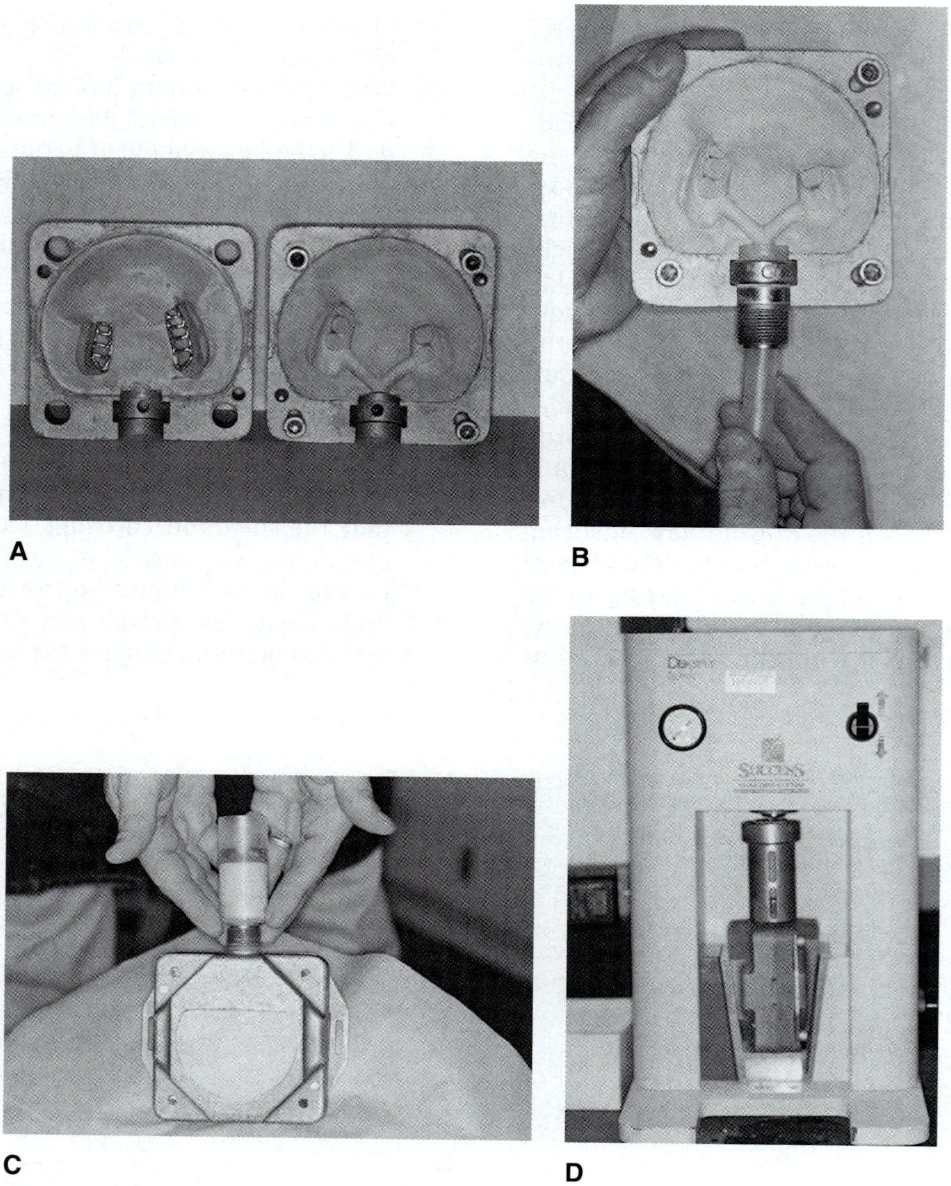

Figure 18-43 **A,** Completed boil-out. **B,** Place metal injection insert into back of flask and slide plastic injection socket into metal insert as far as possible. **C,** Insert plastic nozzle into plastic injection socket, and **D,** place metal protective sleeve over cartridge and place flask in injection unit.

(approximately 6 minutes). Do not allow material to reach the "snap set" stage.

4. Place the resin material into the plastic injection cartridge and insert the blue plastic cartridge plug into the large open end, ribbed side out. Push the blue cartridge plug in as far as possible to compress the material and insert the cartridge nozzle into the plastic injection socket until it seats on the injection socket's lip (Figure 18-43, *C*). Place the metal protective sleeve over the cartridge and place the flask in the injection unit, ensuring that the bolts and flask brackets face to the operator's right side (Figure 18-43, *D*). Position the open slots on the cartridge sleeve facing out, then push the sleeve up toward the unit's cross head, securing the sleeve around the blue rubber O ring. Tighten the unit's hand wheel to secure the flask.
5. Complete the injection process, ensuring that the mold is completely filled by viewing the blue cartridge plug through the sleeve slots until the plug stops moving. When completed, remove the flask from the unit, remove the

cartridge sleeve, and pull the plastic cartridge out of the flask with a slight twist. Keep the injection socket in place inside the metal injection insert. Fit the small, blue plastic piston cap onto the end of the pressing device piston (Figure 18-44, *A*). Place the piston of the processing device into the plastic injection socket at the back of the flask (Figure 18-44, *B*) and screw the pressing device onto the metal injection insert until the etched groove is visible on the pin at the top of the pressing device.

6. Allow the flask to sit for 30 minutes before heat polymerizing to ensure a good bond between the denture resin and the teeth. Submerge the closed flask in water at 163° ± 2° F for $1^1/_2$ hours. Follow with an additional 30-minute boil. An alternate polymerization method is 9 hours in a water bath of 163° ± 2° F with no boil. Remove the flask from the polymerization tank and allow to air cool for approximately 30 minutes. Place the flask in a lukewarm water bath to cool completely.
7. Unscrew the pressing device and loosen the bolts on the flask. Remove the flask brackets and separate the flask. Remove the investment and divest the removable partial denture and cast. Cut off the injection sprue(s) and finish and polish the removable partial denture in a conventional manner.

The use of VLC denture base materials is claimed to save considerable time in providing a processed base. The manufacturers recommend the use of a light-color cast to enhance the polymerization of the VLC material. A stone matrix must be fabricated so that the denture teeth can be positively relocated in the same position during the polymerizing process. Once the stone matrix is completed and verified, the wax and teeth can be removed from the framework, and it can be cleaned and silicoated or coated with the resin bonding agent.

The ideal thickness for the VLC material requires a 1.5-mm space between the edentulous ridge and the retentive component of the framework. The ridge lap of the denture teeth should also be 1.5 mm above the retentive component of the framework, and the tissue side finishing line of the framework should be even with or slightly higher than the palatal side finishing line. If VLC denture base material is to be used, these requirements need to be considered at the diagnosis and treatment planning stage.

Without the framework in place, a thin coat of model release agent (MRA) is applied to the denture base areas of the cast, and the VLC material is adapted to the edentulous denture base area and trimmed to the general outline with a sharp blade. The framework is then seated firmly, embedding it into the uncured VLC material. Make certain that the rests, tissue stops, and other components of the removable partial denture framework are correctly positioned in their designated terminal position on the cast. Remove any excess material that may interfere with articulation of the casts or positioning of the teeth, and check to be sure the VLC material is adapted into the tissue side finishing line of the framework on the cast. This will necessitate returning the cast with the framework to the articulator. Once this has been verified, remove the cast from the articulator and process in the light polymerizing unit for 2 minutes.

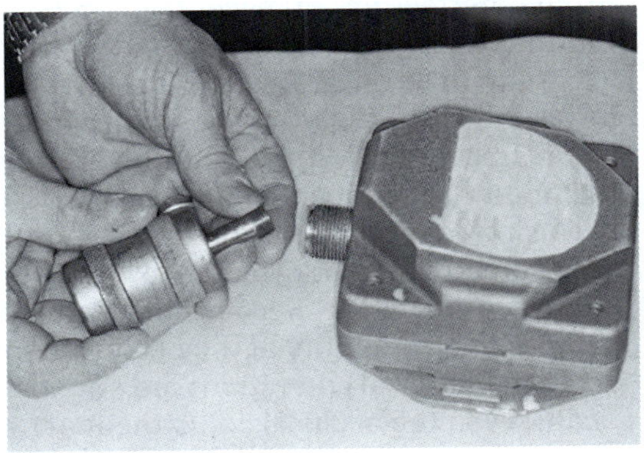

A

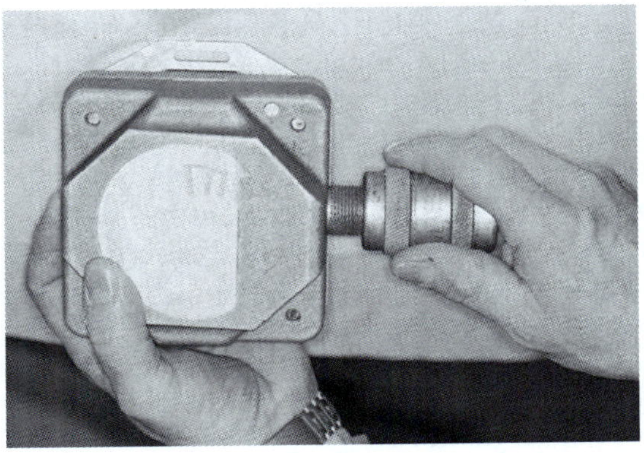

B

Figure 18-44 Injection process has been completed and flask removed from unit. **A,** Remove cartridge sleeve, pull plastic cartridge out of flask, and fit small blue plastic piston cap onto end of pressing device piston. **B,** Piston of processing device has been placed into plastic injection socket at back of flask.

The denture teeth can then be secured to the stone matrix and related to the cast with the framework and the removable partial denture base. The denture teeth may need to be adjusted to fit the removable partial denture base. To do this, trim the ridge lap areas of the teeth enough to provide the required 1.5 mm of space between the tooth and the denture base material. Remember that thin areas need to be avoided between the framework and the cast (minimum of 1.5 mm), and between the framework and the denture teeth (minimum of 1.5 mm).

The denture tooth surfaces that are to be bonded to the VLC denture base must be lightly ground and cleaned. The teeth may then be placed in modeling compound or putty to hold them while applying the bonding agent to all of the designated surfaces to be bonded to the VLC denture base. These coated surfaces should be allowed to sit for 2 minutes and then are processed in the light polymerization unit for 1 minute.

To secure the teeth into their designated position on the VLC denture base, apply a small piece of VLC material to each tooth with the modeling tool provided by the manufacturer. With the aid of the stone matrix and using a high-intensity light, tack each individual tooth into position on the VLC denture base.

After tacking the teeth to the VLC denture base, paint a narrow band of bonding agent on the junction line between the teeth and the denture base material. The bonding agent acts as a sealer to prevent leakage and aids the bonding of the teeth to the denture base material. Allow the bonding agent to set for 2 minutes and then process in the light unit for 1 minute. You can now complete the buccal and lingual contouring of the denture base with additional VLC material. Paint all of the exposed surfaces of the VLC denture base material with the air-barrier coating material and process in the light polymerization unit for 2 minutes. After processing, carefully remove the removable partial denture from the cast. Do not attempt to pry it off. Paint the tissue surfaces of the edentulous areas with the air-barrier coating material and place in the light polymerization unit for 6 minutes with the tissue side up. Clean the removable partial denture with water and a brush to remove all traces of the air-barrier coating. Trim and polish in a routine manner to complete the removable partial denture.

The study of the history of denture base materials is a most interesting one that has been covered elsewhere in dental literature. The future of denture base materials promises to be just as fascinating a study, but such a discussion cannot be included within the scope of this book. With newer materials, the future of methyl methacrylate as a denture base material is uncertain despite its acceptance as the best material available since its introduction in 1937. Although it has made possible the simulation of natural tissue color and contours combined with ease of manipulation, the fact remains that it leaves much to be desired as far as accuracy and dimensional stability are concerned. Whether other and newer materials will eventually supplant methyl methacrylate as a denture base material remains to be seen. The fact is that the denture base of the future (1) must be capable of accurately reproducing natural tissue tones faithfully through the use of characterizing stains and customizing procedures and (2) must not require elaborate processing procedures and equipment, which would make the cost prohibitive for general use.

REMOUNTING AND OCCLUSAL CORRECTION TO AN OCCLUSAL TEMPLATE

Even with improved denture base materials and processing techniques, some movement of artificial teeth will still occur because of the dimensional instability of the wax in which the artificial teeth were arranged. Until sources of error can be eliminated, remounting will continue to be necessary. How well the occlusion may be perfected by remounting will depend on the manner in which jaw relations were transferred to an instrument and how closely the instrument is capable of reproducing functional occlusion. But even though the articulator is capable of reproducing only a static centric relation, that relation at least should be reestablished before placement of the denture.

Although it is admitted that there are limitations to the perfection of eccentric occlusion in the mouth, some believe that it can be done with more accuracy than on an instrument that is incapable of reproducing eccentric positions. Correction for errors in centric occlusion, however, should not be included in a concept that presumes that centric occlusion may be established satisfactorily by intraoral adjustment, followed then by a perfecting of eccentric occlusion. Because of denture instability and the inaccessibility of the occlusion for analysis, accurate intraoral corrections are not possible. Practically, even the occlusal adjustment of natural dentition in which each tooth has its own support can best be done when preceded by an analysis of articulated diagnostic casts.

One cardinal premise must be accepted if prosthetic dentistry is to be anything more than a haphazard procedure. It is possible to transfer centric jaw relation to an instrument with accuracy and to maintain this relation throughout the fabrication of the prosthesis. If this is true, then centric occlusion, coinciding with centric jaw relation—with centric occlusion of the remaining natural teeth, or with both—must have been established before initial placement of the prosthesis. This means that occlusal correction to reestablish centric relation by remounting after final processing is an absolute necessity to the success of the restoration. Remounting after processing is accomplished by returning the cast to a keyed relationship with the articulator mounting.

Precautions to Be Taken in Remounting

The following precautions should be taken to ensure the accuracy of remounting to make final occlusal adjustment before the polishing and initial placement of the denture. These apply to all types of occlusal relationship records but are directed particularly at remounting an occlusal template when using stone vertical stops.

1. Make sure that the base of the cast has been reduced to fit the flask before keying and mounting, so it will not have to be altered later.
2. Bevel the margins of the base of the cast so that it will seat in a definite boxlike manner in the articulator mounting.
3. Notch the posterior and the anterior aspects of the base to ensure its return to its original position. Notches at the margins are preferable to depressions within the base because the former permit a visual check of the accuracy of the remounting.
4. Lubricate lightly the base and sides of the cast before it is mounted to facilitate its easy removal from the mounting stone.
5. Add tinfoil or lightly lubricate the base and sides of the cast before flasking it so that traces of investment will not be present to interfere with remounting.
6. When remounting the cast, secure it in the articulator with sticky wax, hot glue gun, or modeling plastic, followed by stone over both the mounting and the sides of the cast.
7. Before adjusting the occlusion, make certain that no traces of investment remain on the vertical stops.
8. Take care not to abrade the opposing occlusal surface during occlusal adjustment. The use of marking tape or inked ribbon is preferable to articulating paper. The artificial tooth is less likely to cut through and mar the opposing surface, and ink or dye will not build up a false opposing surface as will wax from articulating paper.
9. Occlusal readjustment to an occlusal template is complete when the stone vertical stops are again in contact. With other types of articulator mountings, readjustment is complete when the vertical pin is again in contact and any valid horizontal excursions are freed of interference.

Occlusal readjustment, as was the original articulation, is at the expense of the original tooth anatomy. Occlusal surfaces should be reshaped by adding grooves and spillways and by reducing the area of the occlusal table, thus improving the masticating efficiency of the artificial tooth. Although this may be done immediately after occlusal readjustment and before initial placement of the denture, it may be deferred until completion of the final adjustment. In any event, it is a necessary step in the completion of any removable prosthesis.

Porcelain teeth may be reshaped with abrasive or diamond-mounted points. Resin teeth lend themselves better to reshaping with small burs to restore functional anatomy. Either type should be repolished judiciously to prevent reduction of cuspal contacts. Although cusps may be narrowed, spillways added, and the total area of contact reduced to improve masticating efficiency, critical areas of contact, both vertical and horizontal, must always be preserved.

The term *remounting* is also applied to the mounting of a completed prosthetic restoration back into an instrument using some kind of interocclusal records. Discrepancies in occlusion resulting from processing of tooth-supported dentures may be corrected by reattaching the indexed processing cast and denture to the same instrument on which the occlusion was formulated. However, because of some instability inherent in distal extension removable partial dentures, such dentures should be retrieved from processing investment, finished, and polished and prepared for performing occlusal corrections by the use of new intraoral records. The dentist must make a remounting cast before occlusal corrections can be accomplished. This is simply done by first placing the denture in the mouth and making an irreversible hydrocolloid (alginate) impression of the denture and remaining teeth in the arch (Figure 18-45). When the impression is removed, the denture usually will remain in the impression or can be accurately replaced. Undercuts in the denture bases are blocked out, the retentive elements of the framework are covered with a thin layer of molten wax, and a remounting cast is poured in the impression. The remounting casts are then oriented in the articulator by the same type of interocclusal records that were used to orient the casts to formulate the occlusion. These procedures will be covered in Chapter 20 as an integral part of the initial placement appointment.

Occlusal harmony must exist before the patient is given possession of the dentures. Delaying the correction of occlusal discrepancies until the dentures have had a chance to settle is not justifiable.

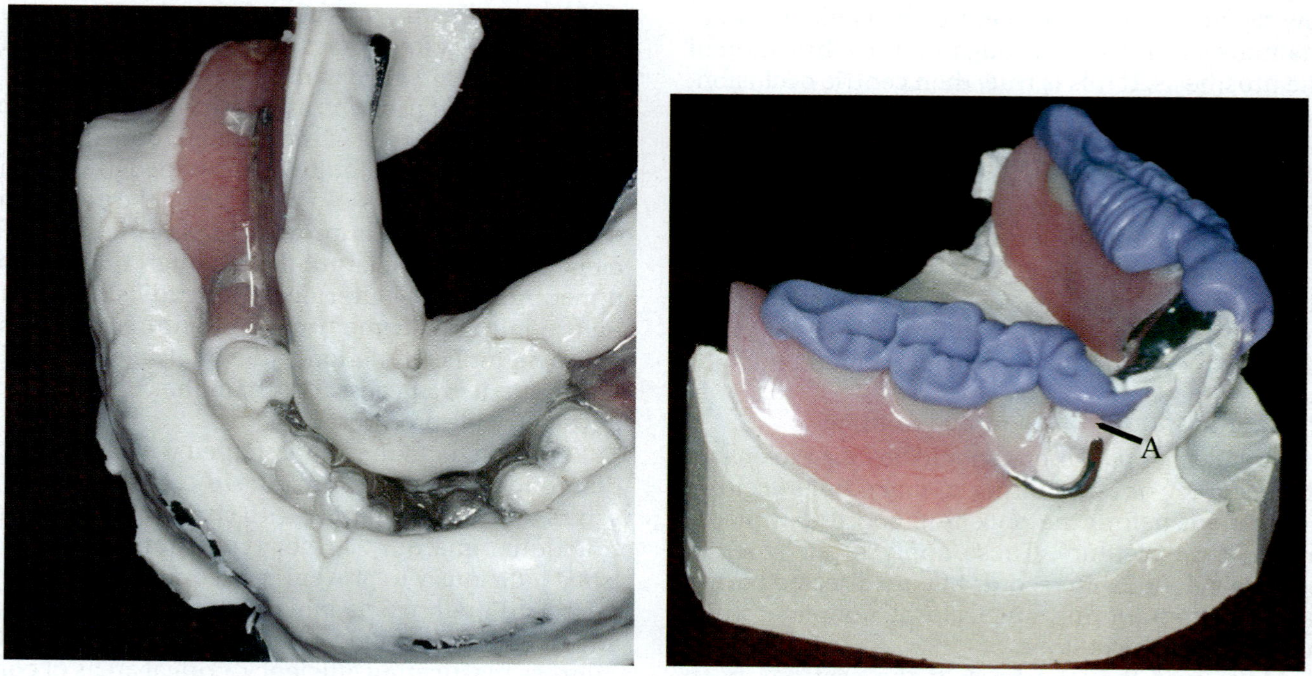

A **B**

Figure 18-45 **A,** Stock, perforated tray is used to make irreversible hydrocolloid (alginate) impression of denture and dental arch. Blockout of undercuts in denture base and of tips of direct retainers is necessary so that denture can be readily removed and replaced on resultant remounting cast, as illustrated in **B**. **B,** Remounting cast poured in stone with prosthesis in place and an interocclusal registration for mounting against a maxillary cast. Wax placed at retainer tip *(arrow)* allows the prosthesis to be readily removed and replaced on cast for occlusal correction procedures that use an articulator.

POLISHING THE DENTURE

The areas to be considered in the polishing of a removable partial denture are: (1) the borders of the denture bases, (2) the facial surfaces, and (3) the teeth and adjacent areas.

The borders on complete metal bases will have been established previously. On partial metal bases and complete acrylic resin bases, the accuracy with which the border may be finished will depend on the accuracy of the impression record and how well this was preserved on the stone cast. Edentulous areas recorded from impressions in stock trays generally lack the accuracy at the borders that is found on casts made from impressions in individualized trays and by secondary impression methods. Border accuracy is determined also by whether or not the impression recorded a functional or a static relationship of the bordering tissue attachments.

Denture Borders

The principal objectives to be considered in making an impression of edentulous areas of a partially edentulous arch are (1) maximal support for the edentulous removable partial denture base and (2) extension of the borders to obtain maximum coverage compatible with moving tissue. Although this second objective may be obtained with an adequate individualized impression tray, it is best accomplished with a secondary impression method. Not only should the extent of the border be recorded accurately but also its width. Both extent and width as recorded should be preserved on the stone cast. With the exception of certain areas that are arbitrarily thinned in polishing (mentioned previously in this chapter), finishing and polishing the denture borders should consist only of removing any flash and artifact blebs. Otherwise, borders should be left as recorded in the impression.

When the impression is made in a stock tray, the tray itself will have influenced both the extent and the width of the border. Some areas will be left short of the total area available for denture support, whereas others will be extended beyond functional limits by the overextension of the tray. Unfortunately the technician may attempt to interpret the anatomy of the mouth and arbitrarily trim the denture borders. This presumes that the technician has an intimate knowledge of the anatomy of the mouth of the patient for whom the restoration is being made, which is most unlikely. The dentist must correct any overextension remaining after arbitrarily trimming the border from cast landmarks in the mouth. It is preferable that the dentist finishes the borders of dentures, having painstakingly developed them during impression procedures.

Facial Surfaces

The facial surfaces of the denture base are those polished surfaces lying between the buccal borders and the supplied teeth. Methods have been proposed for making sectional impression records of buccal contours, thereby permitting the denture base to be made to conform to facial musculature. These have never received wide acceptance and may be considered impractical in removable partial prosthodontics.

Facial surfaces may be established in wax or may be carved into the denture base after processing. Generally, it is desirable that it be done in wax as part of the wax pattern because it is easier to do so and because contours can best be established at a time when modifications can be made if desired. Buccal surfaces should be contoured to aid in the retention of the denture by border molding, to preserve the border roll and thereby prevent food impaction, and to facilitate return of the food bolus back onto the masticating table. Lingual surfaces should be made concave to provide tongue room and to aid in the retention of the denture. Polishing of concave surfaces is always more difficult than polishing flat and convex surfaces. If such contours are established previously in wax, finishing is not only more easily accomplished but border and gingival areas are less likely to be inadvertently altered.

Finishing Gingival and Interproximal Areas

The contouring of gingival and interproximal areas after processing is difficult and generally unsatisfactory (Figure 18-46). The practice of doing so dates back to the days when vulcanite rubber was trimmed and shaped with Pearson-type chisels, and a trimming block was a necessary piece of equipment in any dental laboratory. Finishing was done with vulcanite burs and with brush wheels and pumice, creating the vertical interproximal grooves that for many years were typical of the denture look. Not only is this contrary to modern concepts of denture esthetics but also gingival and interproximal carving of the denture resin around plastic teeth may not be done without some damage to the teeth themselves.

Modern cosmetic considerations demand that gingival carving be done around each tooth individually, with variations in the height of the gingival curve and in the length of the papillae. Interproximally the papillae should be convex rather than concave. The gingival attachment should be free of grooves and

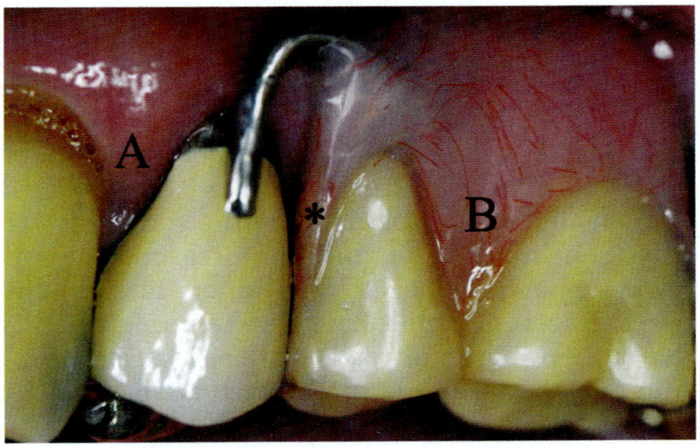

Figure 18-46 Attention to adjacent tooth-tissue contours can facilitate production of natural-appearing prostheses. The interproximal papilla at *A* demonstrates both a vertical and horizontal component. In general, the horizontal component increases with age. The prosthetic interproximal papilla at *B* only exhibits a vertical component and appears artificial. The anterior border (*) contour is blunted and provides an obvious and abrupt contour change. Contouring the border to bevel into the interproximal region will reduce its objectionable appearance.

ditches that would accumulate debris and stain and should be as free for cleansing as possible. All this precludes gross shaping and trimming of gingival areas after processing. Gingival carving should be done in wax, and investing should be done with care to prevent blebs and artifacts. Finishing should consist only of trimming around the teeth and the papillae with small round burs to create a more natural simulation of living tissue, plus light stippling with an off-center round bur for the same reason. Polishing should consist only of light buffing with brush wheels and pumice, and finally with a soft brush wheel and a nonabrasive polishing agent specially made for this purpose.

Pumicing of gingival areas can only serve to polish the high spots, and although it may be done lightly, its use should be limited to light buffing of areas already made as smooth as in the waxing phase. Heavy pumicing of the denture resin not only creates a typical denture look but also alters the delicately carved wax surface and any plastic teeth present. If pumicing must be done, plastic teeth should be protected with adhesive masking tape during the process.

Any polishing operation on a removable partial denture done on a lathe is made hazardous by the presence of direct retainers, which can easily become caught in the polishing wheel. Although the least damage that might occur is the distortion of a clasp arm, there is a greater possibility that the denture may be thrown forcibly into the lathe pan, with serious damage to the framework or other parts of the denture. The technician must ever be conscious of this possibility and must always cover any projecting clasp with the finger while it is near the polishing wheel. In addition, it is wise to keep a pumice pan well filled with wet pumice to cushion the shock should an accident occur. Any other lathe pan used in polishing should be lined with a towel or with a resilient material for the same reason. There is always a potential hazard of retainers catching the gloved fingers or hands that hold a removable partial denture. Serious injury can result, and extreme caution must be taken to prevent such an occurrence. The risk of infection is increased if the removable partial denture has been in place intraorally.

SELF-ASSESSMENT AIDS

1. Why should the dentist not only be familiar with laboratory procedures but also proficient in executing them?
2. Although certain laboratory procedures may be delegated to a dental laboratory technician, the dentist must be able to perform those procedures to troubleshoot, communicate, and instruct the technician. True or false?
3. An intimate knowledge of dental materials employed in the fabrication of removable partial dentures is a must for the dentist. Give three reasons why.
4. Duplicate casts are required in many instances in treating partially edentulous patients. Name one of these instances.
5. What armamentarium and materials are required to duplicate a cast?
6. What is the difference between a reversible and an irreversible hydrocolloid? Which one is most commonly used in duplicating a cast?
7. Is it critical that the duplicating material chosen be compatible with the material from which the duplicate cast will be made? Please explain why.
8. Describe a duplicating flask.
9. How is reversible hydrocolloid prepared for duplicating purposes? What temperature of the hydrocolloid is sufficient to duplicate a cast?
10. If a blocked-out master cast is being duplicated, what precautions must be exercised to prevent distortion of the blockout material?
11. Give a step-by-step procedure for duplicating a stone cast with reversible hydrocolloid.
12. What is the danger of soaking a stone cast in tap water? A cast must be wet before duplicating it with hydrocolloid. How is this wetting accomplished?
13. Describe the procedure for recovering an investment cast from a duplicating mold.
14. For what reasons should an investment cast not be trimmed on a cast trimmer?
15. An investment cast on which the pattern for the framework will be developed should be oven dried after it is removed from the duplicating material. True or false?
16. An investment cast should be lightly sprayed with a plastic model spray immediately after drying. True or false?
17. You should already know the specifications for all components of a removable partial denture framework. Describe a logical order of creating the wax or plastic pattern for a mandibular removable partial denture framework to which a wrought-wire retainer arm will be attached.
18. Describe the process of spruing a wax pattern for a removable partial denture framework.
19. There are three general rules that should be followed in spruing any wax or plastic pattern for casting. List and describe them.
20. After the pattern has been sprued, it must be covered with an investment (refractory) material to make a mold for casting. The outer investment must be the same material from which the investment cast was made. What are the purposes of the outer investment?
21. The casting shrinkage of gold alloys from the molten to the cold state is from __ % to __%. The casting shrinkage of chromium-cobalt alloys is approximately __%.
22. A casting ring, with a suitable liner, is used to confine the outer layer of investment around the pattern. The ring is not removed during burnout or casting procedures for gold alloys. What is the purpose of the liner in the ring?
23. After the investment material for a chromium-cobalt alloy casting has set, the ring is removed before burnout. Why?
24. Give a step-by-step procedure for investing a sprued pattern that will be cast in chromium-cobalt alloy.
25. The casting mold is prepared to receive the molten alloy by a process known as burnout. Burnout serves three purposes. State the three purposes.
26. What different methods are used to melt gold alloys for casting? Chromium-cobalt alloys for casting?
27. After the casting is completed, how long should the mold be allowed to bench cool before the mold and casting are plunged into water?
28. What is the purpose of pickling a casting? Describe a pickling procedure.
29. If the wax pattern for a casting was neatly and properly developed, and investing and casting procedures were correctly accomplished, finishing the casting should not be a time-consuming procedure. How would a chromium-cobalt alloy framework be finished?

30. Record bases, trial denture bases, and individual impression trays are conveniently made of autopolymerizing acrylic resin. What is an autopolymerizing acrylic resin, and how does it differ from a heat-cured acrylic resin?
31. Record bases or trial denture bases can be fabricated by a sprinkling technique using autopolymerizing acrylic resin, whereas individual or customized impression trays may be fabricated with adapted autopolymerizing acrylic resin. For what reason or reasons are the processes different?
32. Review the procedures for making individualized acrylic resin impression trays as given in Chapter 15.
33. If you use a secondary or altered cast impression tray for a mandibular distal extension denture, you will attach an individualized tray to the framework. Give a step-by-step procedure for making such a tray.
34. Record bases and occlusion rims are necessary to record maxillomandibular relations for Class I and II arches and in Class III arches with long edentulous spans. Describe a step-by-step procedure for making record bases by the VLC method and by the sprinkle on method.
35. A record base is attached to the framework for a distal extension mandibular denture and is fabricated after the secondary impression has been made and the master cast has been recovered. How is such a record base made and attached?
36. What purpose does an occlusion rim serve?
37. If an occlusion rim represents the missing teeth and supporting structures in a partially edentulous arch, should the occlusion rims be wider than the occlusal surfaces of the teeth they are replacing? Should occlusion rims occupy the same position (buccolingually) of the missing teeth? There are several advantages to correctly proportioned occlusion rims as opposed to badly proportioned occlusion rims. What are these advantages?
38. Artificial posterior teeth were arranged on mandibular and maxillary trial bases made of acrylic resin and attached to the respective frameworks. The arrangement was acceptable and approved. What procedures must now take place before the final arrangement of teeth and development of the external forms of the bases for processing?
39. Except around metal portions of the framework, should there be any difference in developing gingival contours, root indices, interdental papillae, lingual contours of individual teeth, and so on for removable partial denture bases and complete denture bases? What are they?
40. A removable partial denture must be so invested for processing acrylic resin bases that the processed denture and its cast can be recovered intact and unmarred from the flask. This procedure will facilitate and simplify correction of occlusal discrepancies resulting from processing. True or false?
41. Before investing the master cast and waxed denture in the lower half of the flask, what should be done to the base of the cast to facilitate recovery of the cast and remounting procedures?
42. After the processing flask containing the invested denture has been separated, the residual wax flushed out, and a tinfoil substitute correctly applied, there is one observation that must be made and dealt with in regard to the minor connector for attaching the acrylic resin distal extension base and its relation to the residual ridge. What is this observation, and how is it dealt with before acrylic resin is packed in the mold?
43. Describe the pour technique of processing finished denture bases.
44. Describe the VLC technique of processing finished denture bases.
45. Discrepancies in occlusion as a result of processing may be corrected by returning the processed denture and cast (intact) directly to the instrument on which the occlusion was developed—provided the dentures are tooth supported or the occlusion was developed using an occlusal template. Describe this type of process for correcting occlusal discrepancies.
46. Correction of occlusal discrepancies for distal extension dentures should be accomplished by an entirely different procedure than the above procedure. This procedure is described in Chapter 20. Review and state how this differs.
47. Finishing and polishing the removable partial denture may be accomplished in the same manner as for a complete denture. However, polishing the removable partial denture on a lathe is made more hazardous and requires more attention because of the presence of ________.

19

WORK AUTHORIZATIONS FOR REMOVABLE PARTIAL DENTURES

WORK AUTHORIZATION

A work authorization contains the written directions for laboratory procedures to be performed for fabrication of dental restorations. The responsibility of a dentist to the public and to the dental profession to safeguard the quality of prosthodontic services is controlled in part through meaningful work authorizations. If the work authorizations are properly completed, they provide a means for increased professional quality assurance and satisfaction in a removable partial denture service.

A work authorization by a dentist is similar to granting power of attorney. It grants authority for others to act in the dentist's behalf and specifically prescribes what is authorized.

When properly executed, work authorizations are effective channels of communication. They enhance the quality of the completed restorations by providing instruction for individually and scientifically considered prostheses.

Content

The information contained in a work authorization should include: (1) the name and address of the dental laboratory; (2) the name and address of the dentist who initiates the work authorization; (3) the identification of the patient; (4) the date of work authorization; (5) the desired completion date of the request; (6) specific instructions; (7) the signature of the dentist; and (8) the registered license number of the dentist. All these requirements can be accommodated in a simply designed form (Figure 19-1).

Function

The following four important functions are performed by a work authorization:

1. It furnishes definite instructions for the laboratory procedures to be accomplished and implies an expectation of a level of acceptable quality for the services rendered.
2. It provides a means of protecting the public from the illegal practice of dentistry.
3. It is a protective legal document for both the dentist and dental laboratory technician.
4. It completely delineates the responsibilities of the dentist and the dental laboratory technician.

Characteristics

A work authorization must be legible, clear, concise, and readily understood. It is unreasonable to assume that laboratory technicians are decoding experts. Sufficient information must be included in a work authorization to enable the technician to understand and execute the request. Many dentists are overly presumptive in assuming that a request can be acceptably fulfilled without proper directions.

It is sound practice to provide the dental laboratory technician with adequate written instructions

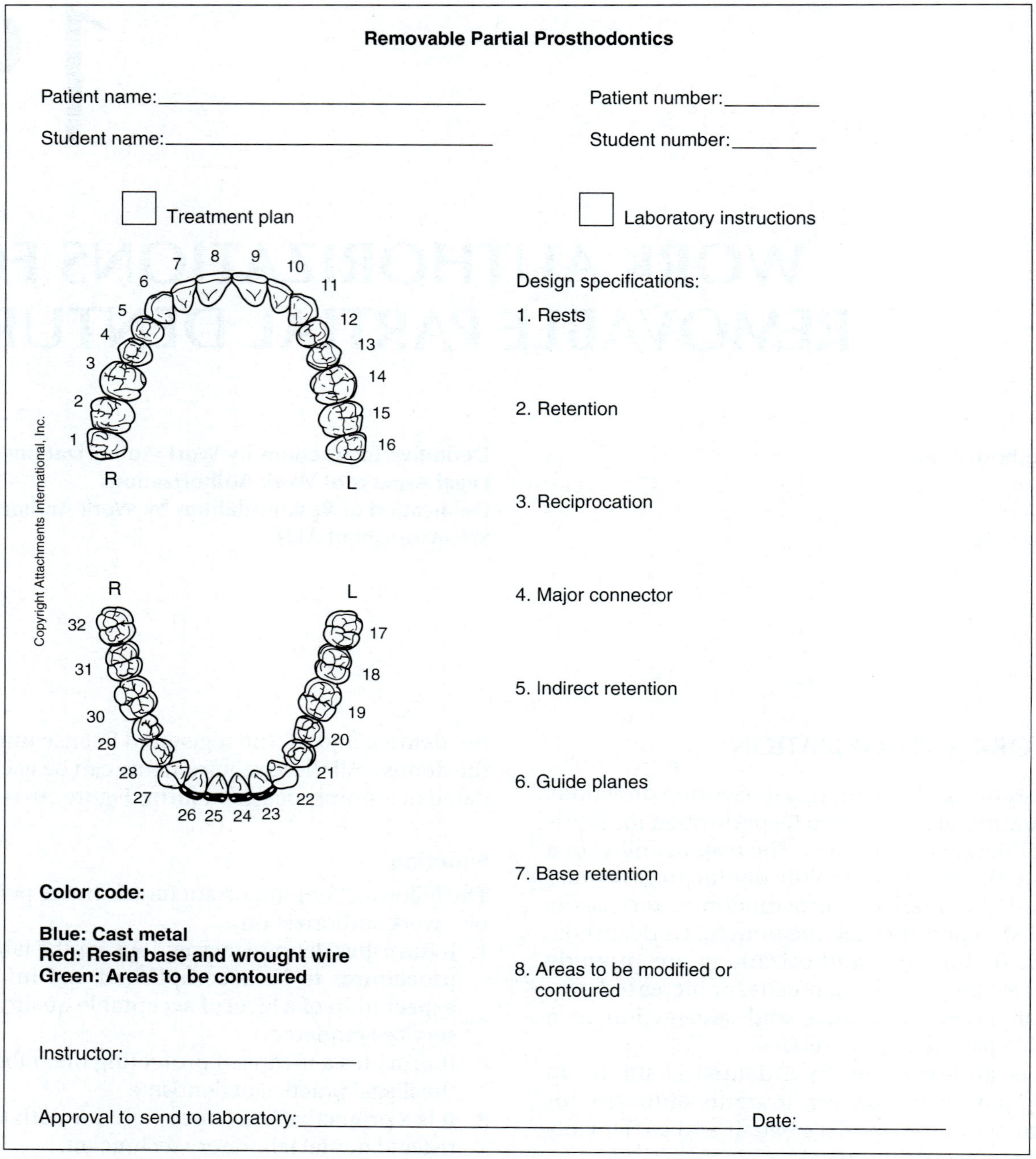

Removable Partial Prosthodontics

Patient name:____________________ Patient number:__________

Student name:____________________ Student number:__________

☐ Treatment plan ☐ Laboratory instructions

Design specifications:

1. Rests
2. Retention
3. Reciprocation
4. Major connector
5. Indirect retention
6. Guide planes
7. Base retention
8. Areas to be modified or contoured

Color code:

Blue: Cast metal
Red: Resin base and wrought wire
Green: Areas to be contoured

Instructor:________________

Approval to send to laboratory:________________________ Date:__________

Figure 19-1 Work authorization form used in undergraduate clinic, designed specifically for removable partial dentures, to furnish detailed information to laboratory technician. Form initially used for student to specifically plan framework design and to designate mouth alterations and preparations.

for each required laboratory service in the fabrication of a restoration. Therefore a new work authorization should accompany the material returned to the laboratory for continuing progress to complete the restoration. In a modern dental practice, it is highly improbable that a one-trip laboratory service is adequate to provide a truly professional removable restoration.

No single work authorization form is adequate to furnish detailed instructions for accomplishing the laboratory phases in the fabrication of removable partial dentures, crowns, and fixed partial dentures, or complete dentures or for accomplishing orthodontic laboratory procedures. Inherent differences in the many types of restorations themselves and differences in the laboratory phases necessary for their fabrication establish a requirement for individual work authorization forms.

DEFINITIVE INSTRUCTIONS BY WORK AUTHORIZATIONS

Work authorization forms may be designed so that only a minimum of writing is necessary to provide thorough instructions (Figure 19-2). The form can contain printed listings of materials and specifications that require either a check mark or a fill-in for authorization of their use.

A reminder space to designate the choice of metal for the framework is included. Frameworks for removable partial dentures are usually cast in type VII gold, chromium-cobalt alloy, or a titanium alloy. The nature of the material of the denture base may also be indicated by a check mark. It is difficult

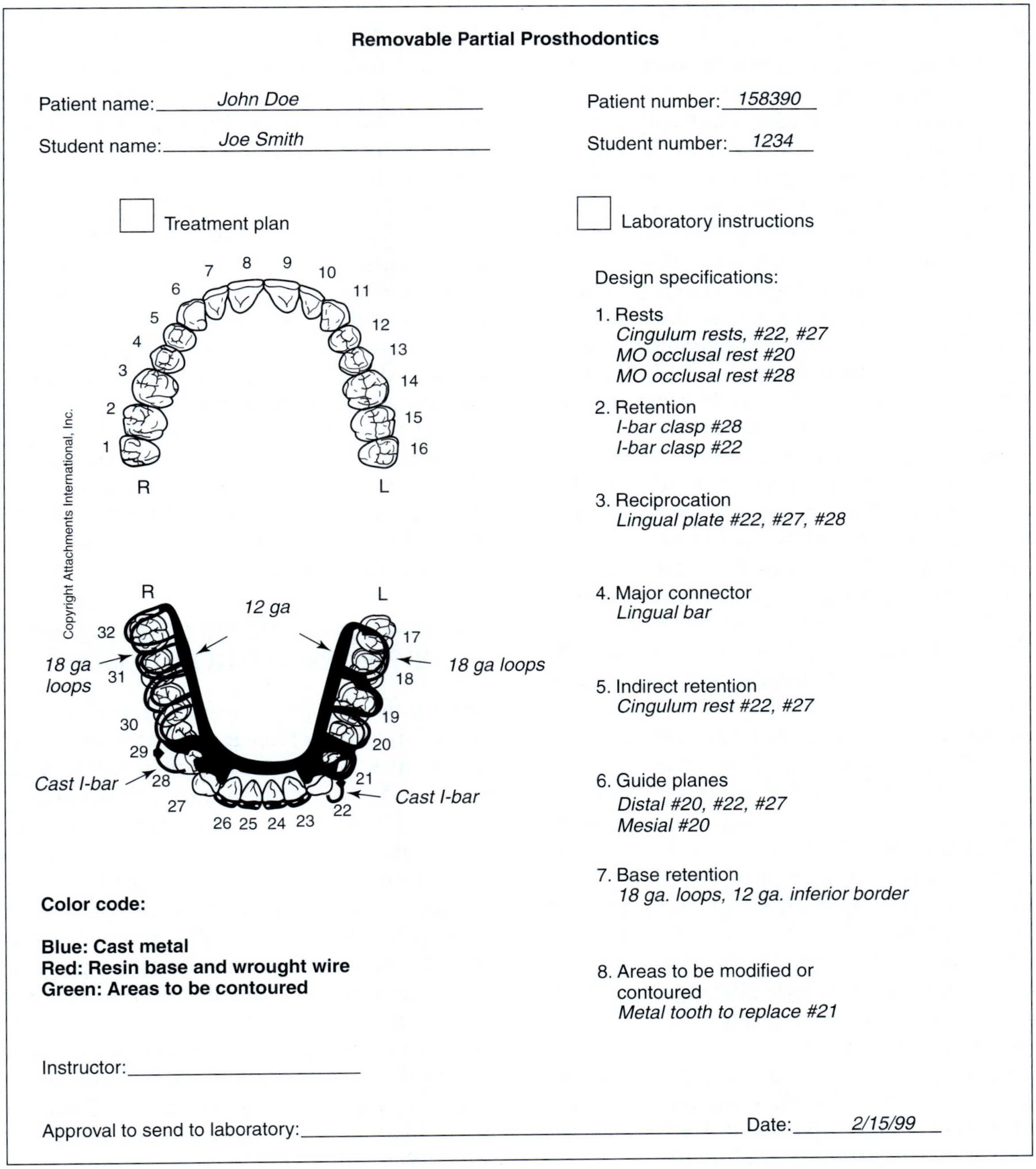
Removable Partial Prosthodontics

Patient name: *John Doe* Patient number: *158390*

Student name: *Joe Smith* Student number: *1234*

☐ Treatment plan ☐ Laboratory instructions

Design specifications:

1. Rests
   Cingulum rests, #22, #27
   MO occlusal rest #20
   MO occlusal rest #28
2. Retention
   I-bar clasp #28
   I-bar clasp #22
3. Reciprocation
   Lingual plate #22, #27, #28
4. Major connector
   Lingual bar
5. Indirect retention
   Cingulum rest #22, #27
6. Guide planes
   Distal #20, #22, #27
   Mesial #20
7. Base retention
   18 ga. loops, 12 ga. inferior border
8. Areas to be modified or contoured
   Metal tooth to replace #21

Color code:

Blue: Cast metal
Red: Resin base and wrought wire
Green: Areas to be contoured

Instructor:__________

Approval to send to laboratory:__________ Date: *2/15/99*

Figure 19-2 This work authorization accompanies master cast on which dentist has designed and drawn outline for removable partial denture framework. It is simple and is not time consuming to execute, yet it furnishes detailed information so that the request can be properly fulfilled.

to elicit this information from the markings on master casts.

Space is reserved on the work authorization form to furnish the technician with information on the dentist's selection of teeth. The responsibility for tooth selection must remain with the dentist. Success of the removable partial denture partly depends on the consideration given to the size, number, and placement of the artificial teeth, and to the material from which they are made.

A display of courtesy deserved by and a demonstration of respect for the laboratory technician are indicated. The general request is prefaced by *please* and the specific instructions are ended with *thank you.* Do any other three words promote better relations?

A good work authorization form not only ensures clarity but also simplifies correct execution. Figures can be provided on which diagrams may be drawn to enhance written descriptions when necessary. These diagrams may show the occlusal and lingual surfaces of the posterior teeth and the lingual surfaces of the anterior teeth. The palatal region of the maxillary arch and the lingual slopes of the mandibular alveolar ridge can also be included. These features allow a clear, diagrammatic representation of the location of major connectors, which will complement the outline of the framework on the master cast.

A color-code index can be used to explain the markings on the master cast when it is submitted to the laboratory for the fabrication of a framework. For example, a green pencil can be used to outline the framework; red to designate the desired location of finishing lines on the framework; and black lines to denote the height of contour on teeth and soft tissue created during the survey of the cast. The color code eliminates confusion in interpreting the markings on the master cast.

Specifications for waxing the framework components for gold, chromium-cobalt, or titanium alloy castings must be furnished for the technician and are an integral part of the work authorization form. Specifications that are adequate for most removable partial denture frameworks may be listed. This feature alone saves time and effort in preparing the work authorization and is also a handy reference for the laboratory technician. The listing of average specifications does not preclude altering a specification when the situation necessitates other characteristics in a given component.

The specific instructions in a work authorization must be so constructed that they will be a constant source of direction and supervision for the laboratory phases of a removable partial denture service. Instructions should leave no doubt of the dentist's requirements in a request for laboratory services. It is foolish to use undercut dimensions of 0.01 or 0.02 inches when a master cast is surveyed, unless directions are included to incorporate these dimensions in the finished framework.

Work authorization blanks should be available in tablet form so that a carbon duplicate can be conveniently made and thus will supply a copy for both the dentist and the dental laboratory technician. The original may be a different color than the carbon copy for ready identification.

LEGAL ASPECTS OF WORK AUTHORIZATIONS

While the National Association of Dental Laboratories (NADL) provides guidelines for statutory regulation, it is the inherent right of each state to implement their own regulation. Fortunately, all states exercise this control. Interpretations of acts that constitute the practice of dentistry are moderately uniform. However, statutory restrictions on dental laboratory operations vary from state to state. Properly executed work authorizations serve to document communication and protect the professional relationship between the dentist and dental laboratory.

Many states require that work authorizations be made in duplicate and that both the dentist and dental laboratory technician retain a copy for a specified period from the date of work authorization. Thus documents are available to substantiate or refute claims and counterclaims that concern the illegal practice of dentistry or to aid in the settlement of misunderstandings between a dentist and a dental laboratory technician.

DELINEATION OF RESPONSIBILITIES BY WORK AUTHORIZATIONS

The dentist is responsible for all phases of a removable partial denture service in the strict sense of the word, although the dental laboratory technician may be requested to perform certain technical phases of the service. However, the laboratory technician is responsible only to the dentist and never to the patient. A dentist who relegates the design of a removable partial denture to a less qualified individual accepts the possibility of an inferior removable partial denture service.

A dentist who imposes on auxiliary personnel those responsibilities that legally and morally belong with the dentist does a great injustice to the patients, the technicians, and the dental profession. There is little doubt that the illegal practice of dentistry and the presently existing impasse between dentist and some dental laboratory technicians are partly a result of many individual dentists who impose unrealistic responsibility on the laboratory technicians. Furthermore, this unwelcome relationship may have been caused by the submission of poor impressions, casts, records, and instructions to the laboratory technician, with the demand of impossible quality in the returned restoration under threat of economic boycott.

Most dental laboratory technicians are ethical and earnestly desire to contribute their talents to the dental profession. The dental profession is vitally interested in increasing the number of serious-minded dental auxiliary personnel to share in providing oral health. However, until the dental profession elevates itself in the eyes of laboratory technicians and also elevates the stature of dental laboratory technology, greater availability of responsible auxiliary personnel is more fancied than real.

The dental laboratory technician is a member of a team whose objectives are the prevention of oral disease and the maintenance of oral health as adjuncts to the physical and mental well-being of the public. A good dental laboratory technician is a valuable team member with the dentist and contributes much to the team effort in providing oral health for patients. The degree and quality of the team effort are the responsibility of the dentist and depend on the knowledge, experience, technical skill, administrative ability, integrity, and ability of the dentist to communicate effectively.

A dentist may delegate much of the laboratory phase of a removable partial denture service. Work authorizations help fulfill the moral obligation to supervise and direct those technical phases that can be accomplished by dental laboratory technicians. There are substantial indications that many members of the dental profession either are not cognizant of the rewards of writing good work authorizations or are not proficient in their execution. It is not a secret that some dentists do not submit instructions when availing themselves of commercial dental laboratory services.

If the practice of prosthodontics is to remain in the control of dentists, each member of the dental profession must avoid delegating responsibility to those who are less qualified to accept the responsibility. Movements to allow denturism are seemingly becoming more prevalent and possibly are related to poor laboratory communication regarding removable prosthodontics.

SELF-ASSESSMENT AIDS

1. What is a work authorization?
2. What are the national statutory regulations regarding work authorizations?
3. Work authorizations go by different names in various parts of the country, such as work order or work order form. What is it called in your state?
4. Do state dental practice acts in your state include a requirement for work authorizations from dentists to dental laboratory technicians?
5. Are work authorizations legal documents?
6. Properly executed work authorizations are effective channels of communication between a dentist and a dental laboratory technician. What accrues to a dentist who always furnishes the dental laboratory or dental laboratory technician a clear work authorization?
7. The contents of a properly executed work authorization will include eight categories of transmitted data. What information do these eight areas include?
8. A dental work authorization performs four distinct functions. What are they?
9. If you were a dental laboratory technician, what specific characteristics would you like to see in a work authorization from the dentist?
10. A dentist has a responsibility to the patient and to the dental laboratory technician. A dental laboratory technician has a responsibility to the dentist, never to a patient. Are both statements true? Please explain your answer.
11. If clear instructions and other information are clearly presented to a good dental laboratory technician, should quality laboratory services be received? What can be expected from vague instructions?
12. Whose responsibility is it to select artificial teeth, denture base materials, and metal alloys for frameworks—the dentist or the technician?
13. If the definitive instructions contained on a work authorization form have been reduced to "Make partial," is that document legal?
14. Should a dentist be responsible for the physical characteristics of framework components? How does the dentist relate requirements or specifications to the dental laboratory technician?
15. A work authorization, properly executed, will delineate responsibilities. Expand this statement in your own words.
16. Why is a dental laboratory technician a dental health team member?
17. Why do states require that the dentist and dental laboratory technician retain a copy of work authorizations for certain lengths of time?
18. Do the words *please* and *thank you* have a place in writing authorizations?
19. After carefully studying the work authorization forms illustrated in this chapter, are there any suggestions for their improvement?

20

INITIAL PLACEMENT, ADJUSTMENT, AND SERVICING OF THE REMOVABLE PARTIAL DENTURE

Initial placement of the completed removable partial denture, the fifth of six essential phases of removable partial denture service mentioned in Chapter 2, should be a routinely scheduled appointment. All too often the prosthesis is quickly placed and the patient dismissed with instructions to return when soreness or discomfort develops. Patients should not be given possession of removable prostheses until denture bases have been initially adjusted as required, occlusal discrepancies have been eliminated, and patient education procedures have been continued.

Although it is true that some accommodation is a necessary part of adjusting to new dentures, many other factors are also pertinent. Among these are how well the patient has been informed of the mechanical and biological problems involved in the fabrication and wearing of a removable prosthetic restoration and how much confidence the patient has acquired in the excellence of the finished product. Knowing in advance that every step has been carefully planned and executed with skill, and having acquired confidence in both the dentist and the excellence of the prosthesis, the patient is better able to accept the adjustment period as a necessary but transient step in learning to wear the prosthesis. This confidence could be lost if the dentist does not approach the insertion and postinsertion phases as equally important to the success of the treatment.

The term *adjustment* has two connotations, each of which must be considered separately. First is adjustment of the denture bearing and occlusal surfaces of the denture made by the dentist at the time of initial placement and thereafter. Second is the adjustment or accommodation by the patient, both psychologically and biologically, to the new prosthesis.

After the resin bases are processed and before dentures are separated from the casts, the occluding teeth must be altered to perfect the occlusal relationship between opposing artificial dentition or between artificial dentition and an opposing cast or template. Denture bases must be finished to eliminate excess and perfect the contours of polished surfaces for the best functional and esthetic result. This is made necessary by the inadequacies of casting procedures, because both the metal and resin parts of a prosthetic restoration are produced by casting methods. Unfortunately, such procedures in the laboratory rarely eliminate the need for final adjustment in the mouth to perfect the fit of the restoration to the oral tissue.

Included in this final step in a long sequence of finishing procedures necessary to produce a biologically acceptable prosthetic restoration are: (1) the adjustment of the bearing surfaces of the denture bases to be in harmony with the supporting soft tissue; (2) the adjustment of the occlusion to accommodate the occlusal rests and other metal parts of the denture; and (3) the final adjustment of occlusion on the artificial dentition to harmonize with natural occlusion in all mandibular positions.

ADJUSTMENTS TO BEARING SURFACES OF DENTURE BASES

Altering bearing surfaces to perfect the fit of the denture to the supporting tissue should be accomplished by use of some kind of indicator paste (Figure 20-1). The paste must be one that will be readily displaced by positive tissue contact and will not adhere to the tissue of the mouth. Several pressure indicator pastes are commercially available. However, combining equal parts of a vegetable shortening and USP zinc oxide powder can make an acceptable paste. The components must be thoroughly spatulated to a homogeneous mixture. A quantity sufficient to fill several small ointment jars may be mixed at one time.

Rather than dismiss the patient with instructions to return when soreness develops and then overrelieve the denture for a traumatized area to restore patient comfort, use a pressure indicator paste with any tissue-bearing prosthetic restoration. The paste should be applied by the dentist in a thin layer over the bearing surfaces. The material should be rinsed in water so it will not stick to the soft tissue, and then digital pressure should be applied to the denture in a tissueward direction. The patient cannot be expected to apply a heavy enough force to the new denture bases to register all of the pressure areas present. The dentist should apply both vertical and horizontal forces with the fingers in excess of what might be expected of the patient. The denture is then removed and inspected. Any areas where pressure has been heavy enough to displace a thin film of indicator paste should be relieved and the procedure repeated with a new film of indicator until excessive pressure areas have been eliminated. This is particularly difficult to interpret when patients exhibit xerostomia. An area of the denture base that shows through the film of indicator paste may be erroneously interpreted as a pressure spot, when actually the paste had adhered to the tissue in that area. Therefore only those areas showing through an intact film of indicator paste should be interpreted as pressure areas and relieved accordingly. The decision to relieve an area of pressure must consider whether the pressure is in a primary, secondary, or nonsupportive denture-bearing area. The primary denture-bearing areas should be expected to show greater contact than other areas.

Pressure areas most commonly encountered are as follows: in the mandibular arch—(1) the lingual slope of the mandibular ridge in the premolar area, (2) the mylohyoid ridge, (3) the border extension into the retromylohyoid space, and (4) the distobuccal border in the vicinity of the ascending ramus and the external oblique ridge; in the maxillary arch—(1) the inside of the buccal flange of the denture over the tuberosities, (2) the border of the denture lying at the malar prominence, and (3) at the pterygomaxillary notch where the denture may impinge on the pterygomandibular raphe or the pterygoid hamulus. In addition, in either arch there may be bony spicules or irregularities in the denture base that will require specific relief.

The amount of relief necessary will depend on the accuracy of the impression registration, the master cast, and the denture base. Despite the accuracy of modern impression and cast materials, many denture base materials leave much to be desired in this regard, and the element of technical error is always present. It is therefore essential that discrepancies in the denture base be detected and corrected before the tissues of the mouth are subjected to the stress of supporting a prosthetic restoration. One of our major responsibilities to the patient is that trauma always be held to a minimum. Therefore the appointment time for the initial placement of the denture must be adequate to permit such adjustment.

OCCLUSAL INTERFERENCE FROM DENTURE FRAMEWORK

Any occlusal interference from occlusal rests and other parts of the denture framework should have been eliminated before or during the establishment of occlusal relations. The denture framework should have been tried in the mouth before a final jaw relation is established, and any such interference should have been detected and eliminated. Much of this need not exist if mouth preparations and the design of the removable partial denture framework are carried out with a specific treatment plan in mind. In any event occlusal interference from the framework should not ordinarily require further adjustment at the time the finished denture is initially placed. For the dentist to have sent an impression or casts of the patient's mouth to the laboratory and to receive a finished removable partial denture prosthesis without having tried the cast framework in the mouth is a dereliction of responsibility to the patient and the profession.

ADJUSTMENT OF OCCLUSION IN HARMONY WITH NATURAL AND ARTIFICIAL DENTITION

The final step in the adjustment of the removable partial denture at the time of initial placement is the adjustment of the occlusion to harmonize with the natural occlusion in all mandibular excursions. When opposing removable partial dentures are

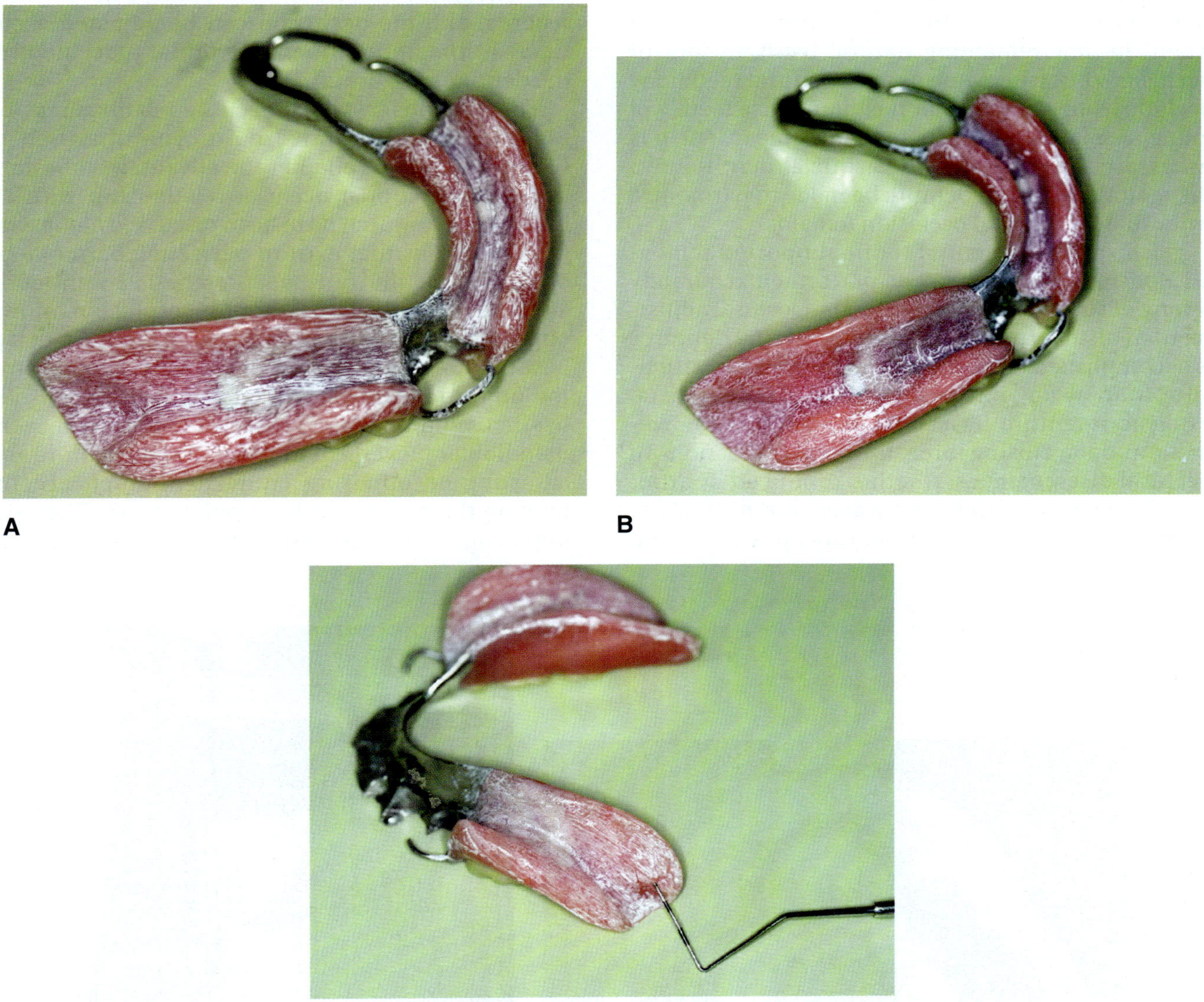

A B C

Figure 20-1 **A,** Tissue side of finished bases of a Kennedy Class I, mod 1 removable partial denture where pressure indicating paste has been applied. Paste was applied following careful inspection of the tissue surface for irregularities or sharp projections, which must be eliminated prior to fitting in the mouth. The entire tissue surface of the bases was dried prior to coating with a thin coat of pressure indicator paste using stiff-bristle brush. Brush marks are evident, and it is the change in pattern of brush marks that guides adjustment. It is important to avoid thick application of indicator paste, which can hide the presence of significant pressure. **B,** The prosthesis can be dipped in cold water or sprayed with a provided release agent before placement in the patient's mouth to prevent paste from sticking to oral tissues. After careful seating of denture, the patient can either close firmly on cotton rolls for a few seconds or the dentist can alternately apply a tissue-ward pressure over the bases to simulate functional movement. The presence of tissue contact is evident in the pattern of the paste, which is different from the brushed pattern. There is no suggestion of excessive pressure in this tissue contact pattern. However, it is not uncommon to relieve the area adjacent to abutment sparingly. Several placements of the denture with indicator paste are usually necessary to evaluate accuracy of bases. **C,** A different denture base recovered from the mouth after manipulation simulating function. The tissue contact reveals excessive pressure at the region lingual to the retromolar pad.

placed concurrently, the adjustment of the occlusion will parallel to some extent the adjustment of occlusion on complete dentures. This is particularly true when the few remaining natural teeth are out of occlusion. But where one or more natural teeth may occlude in any mandibular position, those teeth will influence mandibular movement to some extent. It is necessary therefore that the artificial dentition on the removable partial denture be made to harmonize with whatever natural occlusion remains.

Occlusal adjustment of tooth-supported removable partial dentures may be performed accurately by any of several intraoral methods. Occlusal adjustment of distal extension removable partial dentures is accomplished more accurately by use of an articulator than by any intraoral method. Because distal extension denture bases will exhibit some movement under a closing force, intraoral indications of occlusal discrepancies, whether produced by articulating paper or disclosing waxes, are difficult to interpret. Distal extension dentures positioned on remounting casts can conveniently be related in the articulator with new, nonpressure interocclusal records, and the occlusion can be adjusted accurately at the appointment for initial placement of the dentures (Figure 20-2).

The methods by which occlusal relations may be established and recorded have been discussed in Chapter 17. In this chapter the advantages of establishing a functional occlusal relationship with an intact opposing arch have been discussed along with the limitations that exist to perfecting harmonious occlusion on the finished prosthesis by intraoral adjustment alone. Even when the occlusion on two opposing removable partial dentures is adjusted, it is best that one arch be considered an intact arch and the other one adjusted to it. This is accomplished by first eliminating any occlusal interference to mandibular movement imposed by one denture and adjusting any opposing natural dentition to accommodate the prosthetically supplied teeth. Then the opposing removable partial denture is placed, and

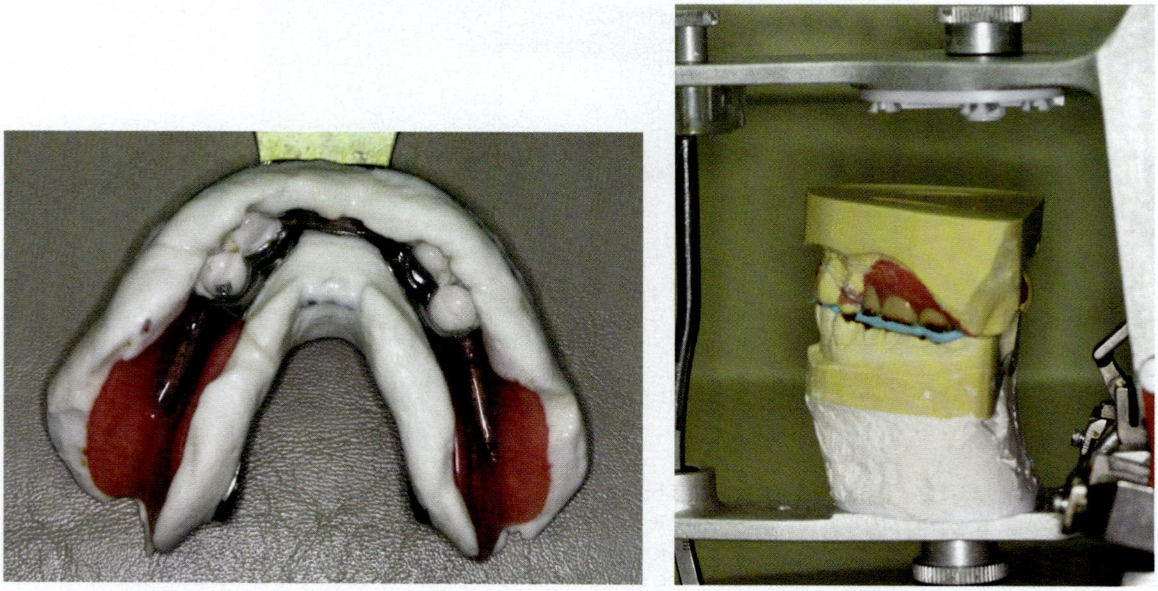

A B

Figure 20-2 Sequence of laboratory and clinical procedures for correction of occlusal discrepancies as a result of processing removable partial dentures. The arch with the prosthesis will require a new cast and record to provide occlusal correction. If it is a maxillary prosthesis, this involves either preserving the facebow record by replacing the processed maxillary removable partial denture and cast on the articulator and indexing the occlusal surfaces using a remount jig, or making another facebow record at the try-in appointment. If a mandibular prosthesis, the opposing arch can be prepared prior to insertion. **A,** In this example the opposing arch is a complete denture that is not to be altered. To produce a cast to use for correcting the occlusion on the articulator, a pick-up impression of the mandibular prosthesis is made. The prosthesis stays within the irreversible hydrocolloid impression; the clasps, proximal plates, and any undercut or parallel surface are carefully blocked out with wax prior to forming the remount cast. **B,** The remount cast that is formed is then inverted and positioned using an interocclusal record.

Continued

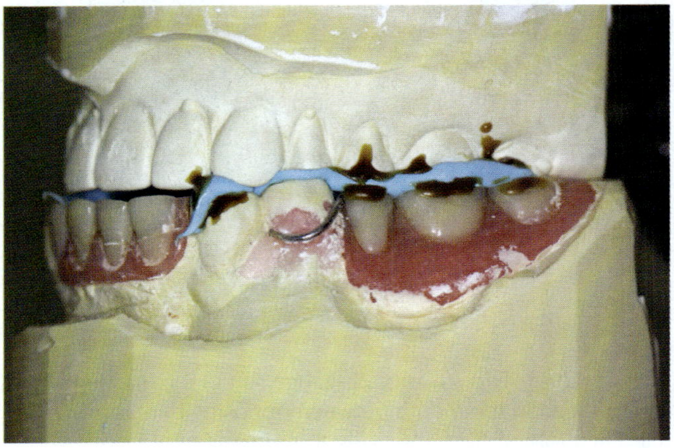

C

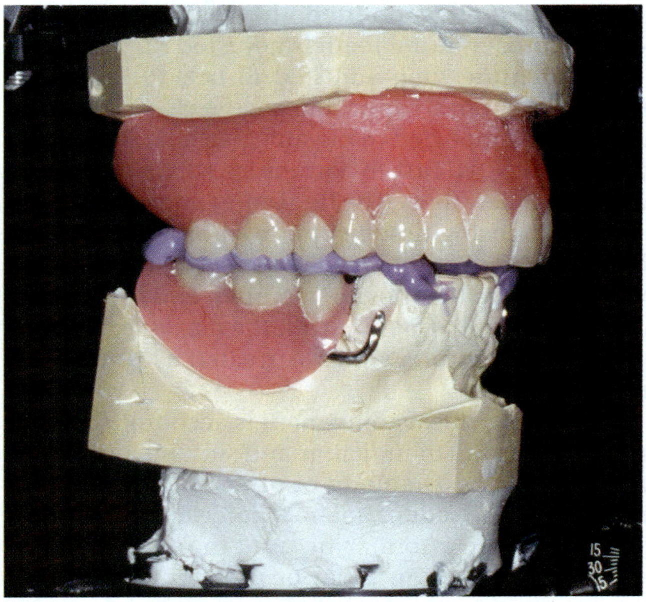

D

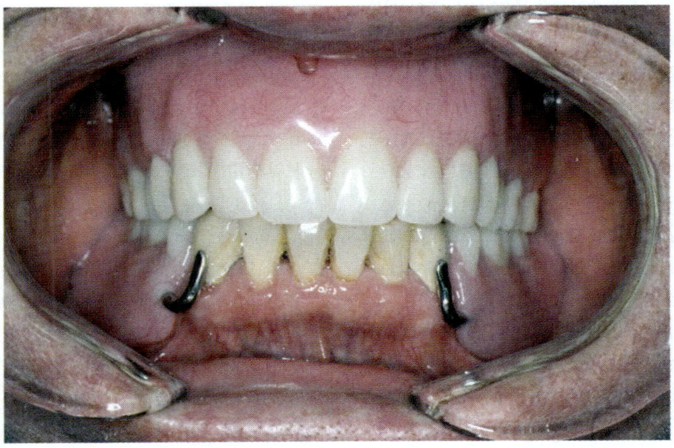

E

Figure 20-2 Cont'd C, The mounted mandibular cast and interocclusal record showing that the record was made without tooth contact. This allows the position recorded to not be influenced by the teeth, which could alter the closure path and introduce error. **D,** This example shows a maxillary complete denture, that was mounted before the patient visit by using a remount index (preserved facebow by indexing before recovery from the processed cast), and the mandibular remount cast and interocclusal record (as in **C**). The record is removed and occlusal correction accomplished to control the post-processed occlusion. Use of the completed prostheses provides the best chance to obtain an accurate and reliable interocclusal record given the fact that the bases are very accurate and stable. **E,** The goal of the remounting procedure is to provide the occlusal position prescribed by the arrangement of prosthesis teeth. It would be inappropriate to allow the patient to attempt to accommodate to new prostheses in which the occlusion is not optimized.

occlusal adjustments are made to harmonize with both the natural dentition and the opposing denture, which is now considered part of an intact dental arch. Which removable partial denture is adjusted first, and which one is made to occlude with it is somewhat arbitrary, with the following exceptions: If one removable partial denture is entirely tooth supported and the other has a tissue-supported base, the tooth-supported denture is adjusted to final occlusion with any opposing natural teeth. That arch is then treated as an intact arch and the opposing denture adjusted to occlude with it. If both removable partial dentures are entirely tooth supported, the one that occludes with the most natural teeth is adjusted first and the second denture then adjusted to occlude with an intact arch. Tooth-supported segments of a tooth- and tissue-supported removable partial denture are likewise adjusted first to harmonize with any opposing natural dentition. The final adjustment of occlusion on opposing tissue-supported bases is usually done on the mandibular removable partial denture because this is the moving member, and the occlusion is made to harmonize with the maxillary removable partial denture, which is treated as part of an intact arch.

Intraoral occlusal adjustment is accomplished by use of some kind of indicator and suitable mounted points and burs. Diamond or other abrasive points must be used to reduce enamel, porcelain, and metal contacts. These also may be used to reduce plastic tooth surfaces, but burs may be used for plastic with greater effectiveness. Articulation paper may be used as an indicator if one recognizes that heavy interocclusal contacts may become perforated, leaving only a light mark. Secondary contacts, which are lighter and frequently sliding, may make a heavier mark. Although articulation ribbon does not become perforated, it is not easy to use in the mouth, and the differentiation between primary and secondary contacts is difficult, if not impossible, to ascertain.

In general, occlusal adjustment of multiple contacts between natural and artificial dentition when tooth-supported removable partial dentures are involved follows the same principles as those for natural dentition alone. This is because the removable partial dentures are retained by devices attached to the abutment teeth, whereas no mechanical retainers are present with complete dentures. The use of more than one color of articulation paper or ribbon to record and differentiate between centric and eccentric contacts is just as helpful in adjusting removable partial denture occlusion as natural occlusion, and this method may be used for the initial adjustment.

For final adjustment, because one denture will be adjusted to occlude with a predetermined arch, the use of an occlusal wax may be necessary to establish points of excessive contact and interference. This cannot be done by articulation paper alone. An occlusal indicating wax that is adhesive on one side, or strips of 28-gauge casting wax or other similar soft wax, may be used. It should always be used bilaterally, with two strips folded together at the midline. Thus the patient is not as likely to deviate to one side as when wax is introduced unilaterally (Figure 20-3).

For centric contacts, the patient is guided to tap into the wax. Then the wax is removed and inspected for perforations under transillumination. Premature contacts or excessive contacts appear as perforated areas and must be adjusted. One of two methods may be used to locate specific areas to be relieved. Articulation ribbon may be used to mark the occlusion, and then those marks that represent areas of excessive contact are identified by referring to the wax record and are relieved accordingly. A second method is to introduce the wax strips a second time, this time adapting them to the buccal and lingual surfaces for retention. After having the patient tap into the wax, perforated areas are marked with waterproof pencil. The wax is then stripped off and the penciled areas are relieved.

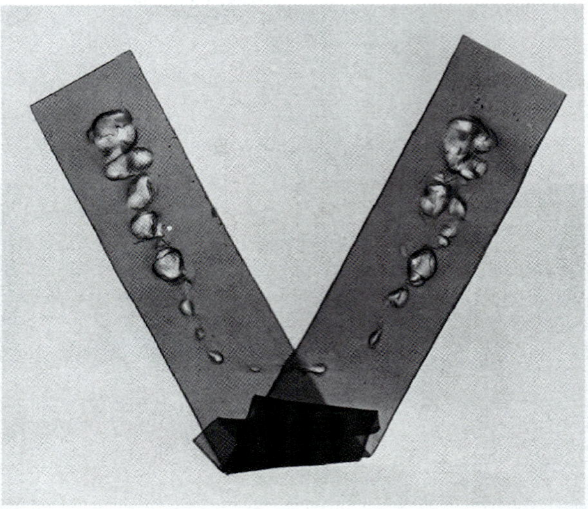

Figure 20-3 Two strips of 28-gauge soft green (casting) wax are placed in the mouth between opposing dentition. These are first folded over anteriorly to unite the two halves, and patient is guided to tap in centric occlusion two or three times. Viewed out of the mouth, against source of light, uniform contacts free of perforations may be considered simultaneous contacts. Perforations in wax represent occlusal prematurities that should be relieved. Accuracy of this method or any other intraoral method depends not only on dentist's interpretation of marks (perforations) but also on the stability of the denture bases.

Whichever method is used, it must be repeated until occlusal balance in the planned intercuspal position has been established and uniform contacts without perforations are evident from a final interocclusal wax record. After adjustment has been completed, any remaining areas of interference are then reduced, thus ensuring that there is no interference during the chewing stroke. Adjustments to relieve interference during the chewing stroke should be confined to buccal surfaces of mandibular teeth and lingual surfaces of maxillary teeth. This serves to narrow the cusps so that they will go all the way into the opposing sulci without wedging as they travel into the planned intercuspal contact. Skinner proposed giving a small bite of soft banana to chew rather than to expect the patient to chew without food actually being present. The small bolus of banana promotes normal functional activity of the chewing mechanism, yet by its soft consistency does not in itself cause indentations in the soft wax. Any interfering contacts encountered during the chewing stroke are thus detected as perforations in the wax, which are marked with pencil and relieved accordingly.

After the adjustment of occlusion, the anatomy of the artificial teeth should be restored to maximal efficiency by restoring grooves and spillways (food escapeways) and by narrowing the teeth buccolingually to increase the sharpness of the cusps and reduce the width of the food table. Mandibular buccal and maxillary lingual surfaces in particular should be narrowed to ensure that these areas will not interfere with closure into the opposing sulci. Because artificial teeth used on removable partial dentures that oppose natural or restored dentition should always be considered material out of which a harmonious occlusal surface is created, final adjustment of the occlusion should always be followed by the meticulous restoration of the most functional occlusal anatomy possible. Although this may be done after a subsequent occlusal adjustment at a later date, the possibility that the patient may fail to return on schedule is always present, and in the meantime, broad and inefficient occlusal surfaces may cause an overloading of the supporting structures, which would be traumatogenic. Therefore the restoration of an efficient occlusal anatomy is an essential part of the denture adjustment at the time of placement. Again, this necessitates that sufficient time be allotted for the initial placement of the removable partial denture to permit accomplishment of all necessary occlusal corrections.

Adjustments to occlusion should be repeated at a reasonable interval after the dentures have reached a point of equilibrium and the musculature has become adjusted to the changes brought about by restoration of occlusal contacts. This second occlusal adjustment usually may be considered sufficient until such time as tissue-supported denture bases no longer support the occlusion, and corrective measures, either reoccluding the teeth or relining the denture, must be used. However, a periodic recheck of occlusion at intervals of 6 months is advisable to prevent traumatic interference resulting from changes in denture support or tooth migration.

INSTRUCTIONS TO THE PATIENT

Finally, before the patient is dismissed, the difficulties that may be encountered and the care that must be given the prosthesis and the abutment teeth must be reviewed with the patient.

The patient should be instructed in the proper placement and removal of the removable partial denture. They should demonstrate that they can place and remove the prosthesis themselves. Clasp breakage can be avoided by instructing the patient to remove the removable partial denture by the bases and not by repeated lifting of the clasp arms away from the teeth with the fingernails.

The patient should be advised that some discomfort or minor annoyance might be experienced initially. To some extent, this may be caused by the bulk of the prosthesis to which the tongue must become accustomed.

The patient must be advised of the possibility of the development of soreness despite every attempt on the part of the dentist to prevent its occurrence. Because patients vary widely in their ability to tolerate discomfort, it is best to advise every patient that needed adjustments will be made. On the other hand, the dentist should be aware that some patients are unable to accommodate the presence of a removable prosthesis. Fortunately, these are few in any practice. However, the dentist must avoid any statements that might be interpreted or construed by the patient to be positive assurance tantamount to a guarantee that the patient will be able to use the prosthesis with comfort and acceptance. Too much depends on the patient's ability to accept a foreign object and to tolerate reasonable pressures to make such assurance possible.

Discussing phonetics with the patient in regard to the new dentures may indicate that this is a unique problem to be overcome because of the influence of the prosthesis on speech. With few exceptions, which usually result from excessive and preventable bulk in the denture design, contour of denture bases, or improper placement of teeth, the average patient will experience little difficulty in wearing the removable partial denture. Most of the hindrances to normal speech will disappear in a few days.

Similarly, perhaps little or nothing should be said to the patient about the possibility of gagging or the tongue's reaction to a foreign object. Most patients will experience little or no difficulty in this regard, and the tongue will normally accept smooth, nonbulky contours without objection. Contours that are too thick, too bulky, or improperly placed should be avoided in the construction of the denture, but if present, these should be detected and eliminated at the time of placement of the denture. The dentist should palpate the prosthesis in the mouth and reduce excessive bulk accordingly before the patient has an opportunity to object to it. The area that most often needs thinning is the distolingual flange of the mandibular denture. Here the denture flange should always be thinned during the finishing and polishing of the denture base. Sublingually the denture flange should be reproduced as recorded in the impression, but distal to the second molar the flange should be trimmed somewhat thinner. Then, when the denture is placed, the dentist should palpate this area to ascertain that a minimum of bulk exists that might be encountered by the side and base of the tongue. If this needs further reduction, it should be done and the denture repolished before the patient is dismissed.

The patient should be advised of the need to keep the dentures and the abutment teeth meticulously clean. If cariogenic processes are to be prevented, the accumulation of debris should be avoided as much as possible, particularly around abutment teeth and beneath minor connectors. Furthermore, inflammation of gingival tissue is prevented by removing accumulated debris and substituting toothbrush massage for the normal stimulation of tongue and food contact with areas that will be covered by the denture framework.

The mouth and removable partial denture should be cleaned after eating and before retiring. Brushing before breakfast also may be effective in the reduction of the bacterial count, which may help to lessen acid formation after eating in the caries-susceptible individual. A removable partial denture may be effectively cleaned by use of a small, soft-bristle brush. Debris may be effectively removed through the use of nonabrasive dentifrices, because they contain the essential elements for cleaning. Household cleaners and toothpastes should not be used, because they are too abrasive for use on acrylic resin surfaces. The patient, and the elderly or the handicapped patient in particular, should be advised to clean the denture over a basin partially filled with water so that the denture impact will be less if the denture is dropped accidentally during cleaning.

In addition to brushing with a dentifrice, additional cleaning may be accomplished by use of a proprietary denture cleaning solution. The patient should be advised to soak the dentures in the solution for 15 minutes once daily, followed by a thorough brushing with a dentifrice. Although hypochlorite solutions are effective denture cleansers, they have a tendency to tarnish chromium-cobalt frameworks and should be avoided.

In some mouths the precipitation of salivary calculus on the removable partial denture necessitates taking extra measures for its removal. Thorough daily brushing of the denture will prevent deposits of calculus for many patients. However, any buildup of calculus noted by the patient between scheduled recall appointments should be removed in the dental office. This can be quickly and readily accomplished with an ultrasonic cleaner.

Because many patients may dine away from home, the informed patient should provide some means of carrying out midday oral hygiene. Simply rinsing the removable partial denture and the mouth with water after eating is beneficial if brushing is not possible.

Opinion is divided on the question of whether or not a removable partial denture should be worn during sleep. Conditions should determine the advice given the patient, although generally the tissue should be allowed to rest by removing the denture at night. The denture should be placed in a container and covered with water to prevent its dehydration and subsequent dimensional change. About the only situation that possibly justifies wearing removable partial dentures at night is when stresses generated by bruxism would be more destructive because they would be concentrated on fewer teeth. Broader distribution of the stress load, plus the splinting effect of the removable partial denture, may make wearing the denture at night advisable. However, an individual mouth protector should be worn at night until the cause of the bruxism is eliminated.

Often the question arises whether an opposing complete denture should be worn when a removable partial denture in the other arch is out of the mouth. The answer is that if the removable partial denture is to be removed at night, the opposing complete denture should not be left in the mouth. There is no more certain way of destroying the alveolar ridge, which supports a maxillary complete denture, than to have it occlude with a few remaining anterior mandibular teeth.

The removable partial denture patient should not be dismissed as completed without at least one subsequent appointment for evaluation of the response of oral structures to the restorations and minor adjustment if needed. This should be made at an interval of 24 hours after initial placement of the denture. It need not be a lengthy appointment but should be made as a definite rather than a drop-in appointment. This not only gives the patient assurance that any necessary adjustments will be made and provides the dentist with an opportunity to check on the patient's acceptance of the prosthesis but also avoids giving the patient any idea that the dentist's schedule may be interrupted at will and serves to give notice that an appointment is necessary for future adjustments.

FOLLOW-UP SERVICES

The patient must understand the sixth and final phase of removable partial denture service (periodic recall) and its rationale. Patients need to understand that the support for a prosthesis (Kennedy Class I and II) may change with time. Patients may experience only limited success with the treatment and prostheses, so meticulously accomplished by the dentist, unless they return for periodic oral evaluations.

After all necessary adjustments to the removable partial denture have been made and the patient has been instructed on the proper care of the denture, they must also be advised as to the future care of the mouth to ensure health and longevity of the remaining structures. How often the dentist should examine the mouth and denture depends on the oral and physical condition of the patient. Patients who are caries susceptible or who have tendencies toward periodontal disease or alveolar atrophy should be examined more often. Every 6 months should be the rule if conditions are normal.

The need to increase retention on clasp arms to make the denture more secure will depend on the type of clasp that has been used. Increasing retention should be accomplished by contouring the clasp arm to engage a deeper part of the retentive undercut rather than by forcing the clasp in toward the tooth. The latter creates only frictional retention, which violates the principle of clasp retention. An active force, such retention contributes to tooth or restoration movement, or both, in a horizontal direction, disappearing only when either the tooth has been moved or the clasp arm returns to a passive relationship with the abutment tooth. Unfortunately, this is almost the only adjustment that can be made to a half-round cast clasp arm. On the other hand, the round wrought-wire clasp arm may be cervically adjusted and brought into a deeper part of the retentive undercut. Thus the passivity of the clasp arm in its terminal position is maintained, but retention is increased because it is forced to flex more to withdraw from the deeper undercut. The patient should be advised that the abutment tooth and the clasp will serve longer if the retention is held minimally, which is only that amount necessary to resist reasonable dislodging forces.

Development of denture rocking or looseness in the future may be the result of a change in the form of the supporting ridges rather than lack of retention. This should be detected as early as possible after it occurs and corrected by relining or rebasing. The loss of tissue support is usually so gradual that the patient may be unable to detect the need for relining. This usually must be determined by the dentist at subsequent examinations as evidenced by rotation of the distal extension denture about the fulcrum line. If the removable partial denture is opposed by natural dentition, the loss of base support causes a loss of occlusal contact, which may be detected by having the patient close on wax or Mylar strips placed bilaterally. If, however, a complete denture or distal extension removable partial denture opposes the removable partial denture, the interocclusal wax test is not dependable because posterior closure, changes in the temporomandibular joint, or migration of the opposing denture may have maintained occlusal contact. In such cases evidence of loss of ridge support is determined solely by the indirect retainer leaving its seat as the distal extension denture rotates about the fulcrum.

No assurance can be given to the patient that crowned or uncrowned abutment teeth will not decay at some future time. The patient can be assured, however, that prophylactic measures in the form of meticulous oral hygiene, coupled with routine care by the dentist, will be rewarded by greater health and longevity of the remaining teeth.

The patient should be advised that maximal service may be expected from the removable partial denture if the following rules are observed:

1. Avoid careless handling of the denture, which may lead to distortion or breakage. Damage to the removable partial denture occurs while it is out of the mouth, as a result of dropping it during cleaning, or an accident occurring when the denture is not worn. Fractured teeth, denture bases, and broken clasp arms can be repaired, but a distorted framework can rarely if ever be satisfactorily readapted or repaired.
2. Protect teeth from caries with proper oral hygiene, proper diet, and frequent dental care. The teeth will be no less susceptible to caries when a removable partial denture is being worn but may be more so because of the retention of debris. At the same time, the remaining teeth have become all the more important because of oral rehabilitation, and abutment teeth have become even more valuable because of their importance to the success of the removable partial denture. Therefore the need for a rigid regimen of oral hygiene, diet control, and periodic clinical observation and treatment is essential to the future health of the entire mouth. Also the patient must be more conscientious about returning periodically for examination and necessary treatment at intervals stated by the dentist.
3. Prevent periodontal damage to the abutment teeth by maintaining tissue support of any distal extension bases. As a result of periodic evaluation, this can be detected and corrected by relining or whatever procedure is indicated.
4. Accept removable partial denture treatment as something that cannot be considered permanent but must receive regular and continuous care by both the patient and the dentist. The obligations for maintaining caries control and for returning at stated intervals for treatment must be clearly understood along with the fact that regular charges will be made by the dentist for whatever treatment is rendered.

SELF-ASSESSMENT AIDS

1. The term *adjustment* has two connotations in relation to removable partial dentures. What are they?
2. At what stage of treatment should any occlusal interference by a framework have been corrected?

3. What is meant by adjustments to the bearing surfaces of denture bases?
4. How are areas of the denture base that may contribute to soreness detected?
5. What is a pressure indicator paste? Give a detailed procedure for the use of a pressure indicator paste. How are prospective pressure spots interpreted when a pressure indicator paste is used?
6. How does one interpret overextension or underextension of borders of the denture base with the use of a pressure indicator paste?
7. What happens if the borders of either maxillary or mandibular distal extension bases impinge the pterygomandibular raphe?
8. Some occlusal discrepancies are bound to occur in dentures as a result of the processing of acrylic resin. True or false?
9. The dentist must correct any and all occlusal discrepancies as completely as possible before the patient is given possession of the restorations. True or false?
10. In placing a tooth-supported removable partial denture, how are occlusal discrepancies corrected and how is the existence of occlusal harmony ensured?
11. What is the danger in trying to correct occlusal discrepancies of distal extension dentures by an intraoral technique?
12. What is a remount cast? How is it made?
13. Give a detailed procedure for correcting occlusal discrepancies by remounting distal extension removable partial dentures on an articulator.
14. What are several advantages of the use of an articulator to correct occlusal discrepancies?
15. After correction of occlusal discrepancies, should the occlusal anatomy of prosthetically supplied teeth be restored by ensuring that adequate grooves and spillways are present? How do you determine where and where not to recontour?
16. What procedures are used to restore the glaze on occlusal surfaces of vacuum-fired porcelain artificial teeth attached to an acrylic resin denture base?
17. An informed patient will adjust to new restorations better than an uninformed patient. At what phase of treatment should patient education begin?
18. What instructions are reviewed with the patient before ending the initial placement appointment?
19. Why should an appointment be made for 24 hours after the initial placement of restorations?
20. When does responsibility in the treatment of a patient end?
21. Should the dentist provide the patient with printed suggestions relative to the care and use of restorations before the initial placement appointment?
22. What length of time should be scheduled for the initial placement of distal extension removable partial dentures?
23. How would the following clasp arms be safely adjusted to make them more retentive and to remain passive? A cast circumferential clasp, a combination clasp.

III

Maintenance

Temporary and Maxillofacial Prostheses

21

RELINING AND REBASING THE REMOVABLE PARTIAL DENTURE

Differentiation between relining and rebasing the removable partial denture has been discussed previously in Chapter 1. Briefly, *relining* is the resurfacing of the tissue of a denture base with new material to make it fit the underlying tissue more accurately. *Rebasing* is the replacement of the entire denture base with new material. The artificial teeth may need to be replaced in a rebase procedure. Relining removable partial dentures is a common occurrence in many dental practices; however, rebasing is not indicated as often.

In either situation a new impression is necessary and uses the existing denture base with modifications (Figure 21-1) as an impression tray for either a closed-mouth or an open-mouth impression procedure. One of several types of impression materials may be used, such as metallic oxide impression paste, rubber-base or silicone elastomers, tissue conditioning materials, or mouth-temperature wax. With a tooth-supported prosthesis, the impression method (open- or closed-mouth) is not as critical. In deciding between a closed-mouth and an open-mouth impression method for relining a distal extension removable partial denture, a major consideration is the resiliency of the mucosa covering the residual ridge. As with secondary impression techniques, a firm mucosal foundation can likely accommodate either a closed-mouth functional impression technique or an open-mouth selective pressure technique. However, when the mucosa is easily displaced, the open-mouth selective pressure technique is preferable. Both techniques should guard against framework movement during the impression procedure.

Before relining or rebasing is undertaken, the oral tissue must be returned to an acceptable state of health (Figure 21-2). For more information refer to the Chapter 13 discussion about conditioning abused and irritated tissue.

RELINING TOOTH-SUPPORTED DENTURE BASES

When total abutment support is available but for one reason or another a removable partial denture has been the restoration of choice, support for that restoration is derived entirely from the abutment teeth at each end of each edentulous span. This support may be effective through the use of occlusal rests, boxlike internal rests, internal attachments, or supporting ledges on abutment restorations. Except for intrusion of abutment teeth under functional stress, the supporting abutments prevent settling of the restoration toward the tissue of the residual ridge. Tissue changes that occur beneath tooth-supported denture bases do not affect the support of the denture, and therefore relining or rebasing is usually done for reasons that include: (1) unhygienic conditions and the trapping of debris between the denture base and the residual ridge; (2) an unsightly condition that results from the space that has developed; or (3) patient discomfort associated with lack of tissue contact that arises from open spaces between

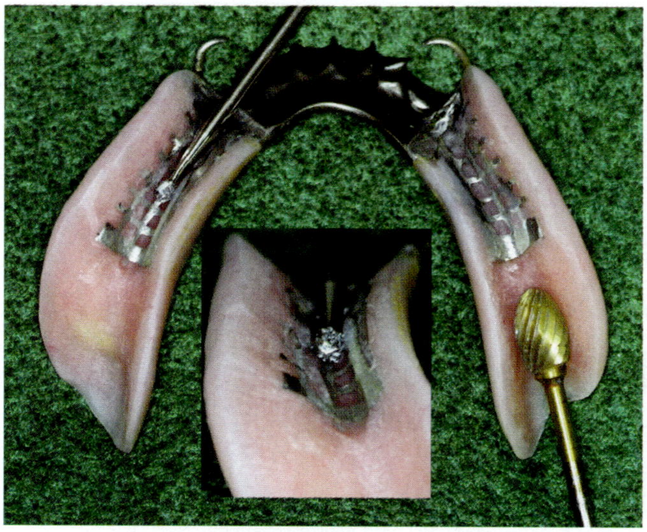

Figure 21-1 Use of an existing Kennedy Class I removable partial denture base as a tray during reline impression. The selective pressure impression philosophy requires space for the impression material that is greater over the ridge crest (secondary stress-bearing area) than at the buccal shelf region (primary stress bearing area). A pear-shaped lab bur is used to provide general relief (0.5–1 mm) of the denture base with additional relief (1 mm) over the ridge crest obtained using a number 8 round straight shank lab bur. Care must be taken to assure tissue surface is relieved of all undercuts, which could cause cast fracture when recovering the cast from the impression.

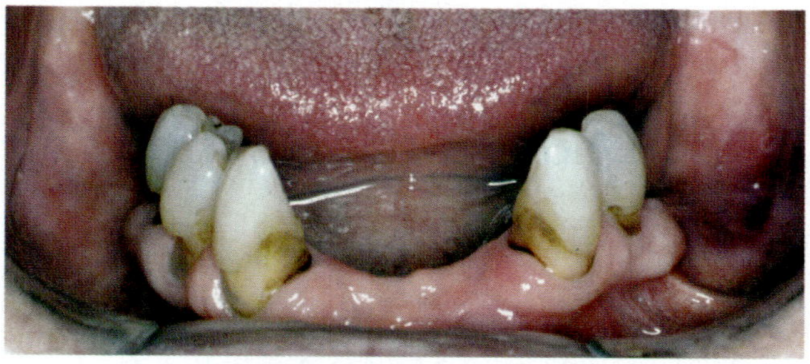

Figure 21-2 Kennedy Class I, mod 1 arch with a removable partial denture that requires relining. Tissue abuse evident at the left buccal shelf region must be corrected prior to making the reline impression. Management requires either a period of function without the prosthesis or relief of the prosthesis in the affected region along with placement of a tissue resilient liner in an effort to reduce the traumatic effect of pressure.

the denture base and the tissue. Anteriorly, loss of support beneath a denture base may lead to some denture movement, despite occlusal support and direct retainers located posteriorly. Rebasing would be the treatment of choice if the artificial teeth are to be replaced or rearranged, or if the denture base needs to be replaced for esthetic reasons or because it has become defective.

To accomplish either relining or rebasing, the original denture base must have been made of a resin material that can be relined or replaced. Commonly, tooth-supported removable partial denture bases are made of metal as part of the cast framework. These generally cannot be satisfactorily relined, although they may sometimes be altered by drastic grinding to provide mechanical retention for the attachment of an entirely new resin base, or some of the new resin bonding agent may be used. Ordinarily a metal base, with its several advantages, is not used in a tooth-supported area in which early tissue changes are anticipated. A metal base should not be used after recent extractions or other surgery or for a long span when relining is anticipated to provide secondary tissue support. A distal extension metal base is ordinarily used only when a removable partial denture is made over tissue that has become conditioned to supporting a previous denture base.

Because the tooth-supported denture base cannot be depressed beyond its terminal position with the occlusal rests seated and the teeth in occlusion, and because it cannot rotate about a fulcrum, a closed-mouth impression method is used. Virtually any impression material may be used, provided sufficient space is allowed beneath the denture base to permit the excess material to flow to the borders—where it is either turned by the bordering tissue or, as in the palate, allowed to escape through venting holes without unduly displacing the underlying tissue. The qualities of each type of impression material must be kept in mind when selecting the material to be used. Ordinarily an impression material is used that will record the anatomic form of the oral tissue.

A word of caution should be mentioned when relining a tooth-supported resin base with autopolymerizing resin as an intraoral procedure. When one or more relatively short spans are to be relined, making an impression for relining purposes necessitates that the denture be flasked and processed. The possibilities that the vertical dimension of occlusion may be increased and that the denture may be distorted during laboratory procedures must be weighed against the disadvantages of the use of a direct reline material. Fortunately these materials are constantly improved with greater predictability and color stability. The possibility that the original denture base will become crazed or distorted by the action of the activated monomer is minimal when the base is made of modern cross-linked resin. However, caution should be exercised to ensure that the older types of resin bases are compatible when relining with direct reline resins.

When relining in the mouth with a resin reline material is done with an appropriate technique, the results can be quite satisfactory, with complete bonding to the existing denture base, good color stability, permanence, and accuracy. The procedure for applying a direct reline of an existing resin base is as follows:

1. Generously relieve the tissue side of the denture base. Lightly relieve the borders. This not only provides space for an adequate thickness of new material but also eliminates the possibility of tissue impingement because of confinement of the material.
2. Apply lubricant or tape over the polished surfaces from the relieved border to the occlusal surfaces of the teeth to prevent new resin from adhering to the preserved bases and teeth.
3. Mix the powder and liquid in a suitable container according to the proportions recommended by the manufacturer.
4. While the material is reaching the desired consistency, have the patient rinse the mouth with cold water. At the same time, wipe the fresh surfaces of the dried denture base with a cotton pellet or small brush saturated with some of the reline resin monomer. This facilitates bonding and ensures that the surface is free of any contamination.
5. When the material has first begun to thicken, but while it is still quite fluid, apply it to the tissue side of the denture base and over the borders. Immediately place the removable partial denture in the mouth in its terminal position, and have the patient lightly close into occlusion. Be sure no material flows over the occlusal surfaces or alters the established vertical dimension of occlusion. Then, with the patient's mouth open, manipulate the cheeks to turn the excess at the border and establish harmony with bordering attachments. If a mandibular removable partial denture is being relined, have the patient move the tongue into each cheek and then against the anterior teeth to establish a functional lingual border. It is necessary that the direct retainers be effective to prevent displacement of the denture while molding of the borders is accomplished. Otherwise the denture must be held in its terminal position with finger pressure on the occlusal surfaces while border molding is in progress.
6. Immediately remove the denture from the mouth and with fine curved iris scissors, trim away gross excess material and any material that has flowed onto proximal tooth surfaces and other components of the removable partial denture framework. While doing this, have the patient again rinse the mouth with cold water. Then replace the denture in its terminal position to bring the teeth into occlusion. Then repeat the border movements with the patient's mouth open. By this time, or soon thereafter, the material will have become firm enough to maintain its form out of the mouth.
7. Remove the denture, quickly rinse it in water, and dry the relined surface with compressed air. Apply a generous coat of glycerin with a brush or cotton pellet to prevent frosting of the surface caused by evaporation of monomer. Allow the material to polymerize in a container of cold water. This will eliminate any patient discomfort and tissue damage that could have resulted from exothermic heat or prolonged contact of the tissue with unreacted monomer. Although it is preferable that 20 to 30 minutes elapse before trimming and polishing, it may be done as soon as the material hardens. Polymerization may be expedited and made denser by placing the denture in warm water in a pressure pot for 15 minutes at 20 psi. The masking tape must be removed before trimming is done but should be replaced over the teeth and polished surfaces below the junction of the new and old materials to protect those surfaces during final polishing.

Properly done, a direct reline is entirely acceptable for most tooth-supported removable partial denture bases made of a resin material, except when some tissue support may be obtained for long spans between abutment teeth. In the latter situation, a reline impression in tissue-conditioning material or other suitable elastic impression material may be accomplished. The denture may then be flasked, and a processed reline may be added for optimal tissue contact and support.

RELINING DISTAL EXTENSION DENTURE BASES

A distal extension removable partial denture, which derives its major support from the tissue of the residual ridge, requires relining much more often than does a tooth-supported denture. Because of this, distal extension bases are usually made of a resin material that can be relined to compensate for loss of support caused by tissue changes. Although tooth-supported areas are relined for other reasons, the primary reason for relining a distal extension base is to reestablish tissue support for that base.

The need for relining a distal extension base is determined by evaluating the stability and occlusion at reasonable intervals after initial placement of the denture. Before initial placement of the denture, the patient must be advised that: (1) periodic examination and also relining, when it becomes necessary, are imperative; (2) the success of the removable partial denture and the health of the remaining tissue and abutment teeth depend on periodic examination and servicing of both the denture and the abutment teeth; and (3) a charge will be made for these visits in proportion to the required treatment.

There are two indications of the need for relining a distal extension removable partial denture base. First, a loss of occlusal contact between opposing dentures or between the denture and opposing natural dentition may be evident (see Figures 9-13 and 9-14). This is determined by having the patient close on two strips of 28-gauge, soft green or blue (casting) wax or Mylar matrix strips. If occlusal contact between artificial dentition is weak or lacking while the remaining natural teeth in opposition are making firm contact, the distal extension denture needs to have occlusion reestablished on the present base by altering the occlusion, reestablishing the original position of the denture framework and base, or sometimes both. In most instances, reestablishing the original relationship of the denture is necessary, and the occlusion will automatically be reestablished.

Second, a loss of tissue support that causes rotation and settling of the distal extension base or bases is obvious when alternate finger pressure is applied on either side of the fulcrum line. Although checking for occlusal contact alone may be misleading, such rotation is positive proof that relining is necessary. If occlusal inadequacy is detected without any evidence of denture rotation toward the residual ridge, all that needs to be done is to reestablish occlusal contact by rearranging the teeth or by adding to the occlusal surfaces with resin or cast gold onlays. On the other hand, if occlusal contact is adequate but denture rotation can be demonstrated, it is usually a result of migration or extrusion of opposing teeth or a shift in position of an opposing maxillary denture, thus maintaining occlusal contact at the expense of the stability and tissue support of that denture. This is often the situation when a maxillary complete denture opposes a removable partial denture. It is not unusual for a patient to complain of looseness of the maxillary complete denture and request relining of that denture when actually it is the removable partial denture that needs relining. Relining and thus repositioning the removable partial denture results in repositioning of the maxillary complete denture with a return of stability and retention in that denture. Therefore evidence of rotation of a distal extension removable partial denture about the fulcrum line must be the deciding factor as to whether relining needs to be done.

Rotation tissueward about the fulcrum line always results in a lifting of the indirect retainer(s). The framework of any distal extension removable partial denture must be in its original terminal position with indirect retainers fully seated during and at the end of any relining procedure. Any possibility of rotation about the fulcrum line because of occlusal influence must be prevented, and therefore the framework must be held in its original terminal position during the time the impression is being made. This all but eliminates the use of a closed-mouth impression procedure when relining unilateral or bilateral distal extension bases.

Therefore the best way to ensure framework orientation throughout the impression procedure for a distal extension removable partial denture is with an open-mouth procedure done in exactly the same manner as the original secondary impression (see Figure 16-11). The denture to be relined is first relieved generously on the tissue side (see Fig. 21-1) and then is treated the same as the original impression base for a functional impression. The step-by-step procedure is the same, with the dentist's three fingers placed on the two principal occlusal rests and at a third point between, preferably at an indirect retainer farthest from the axis of rotation. The framework is thus returned to its original terminal position, with all tooth-supported components fully seated. The tissue beneath the distal extension base is then registered in a relationship to the original position of the denture that will ensure (1) the denture framework will be returned to its intended relationship with the supporting teeth; (2) the reestablishment of optimum tissue support for the distal extension base; and (3) the restoration of the original occlusal relationship with the opposing teeth.

Although it is true that the teeth are not allowed to come into occlusion during an open-mouth impression procedure, the original position of the denture is positively determined by its relationship with the supporting abutment teeth. Because this is the relationship on which the original occlusion was established, returning the denture to that position should bring about a return to the original occlusal relationship if two conditions are satisfied. The first condition is that laboratory procedures during relining must be done accurately without any increase in vertical dimension of occlusion. This is essential to any reline procedure, but it is a particular necessity with a removable partial denture because any change in occlusal vertical dimension will prevent occlusal rests from seating and will result in overloading and trauma to the underlying tissue. The second condition is that the opposing teeth have not extruded or migrated or that the position of an opposing denture has not become altered irreversibly. In the latter situation, some adjustment of the occlusion will be necessary, but this should be deferred until the opposing teeth or denture and the structures associated with the temporomandibular joint have had a chance to return to their original position before denture settling occurred. One of the greatest satisfactions of a job well done is in the execution of an open-mouth reline procedure as described previously (Figure 21-3), which results in the restoration not only of the original denture relationship and

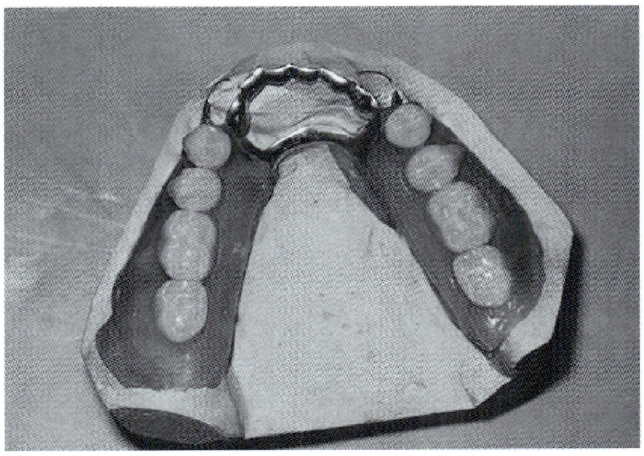

A

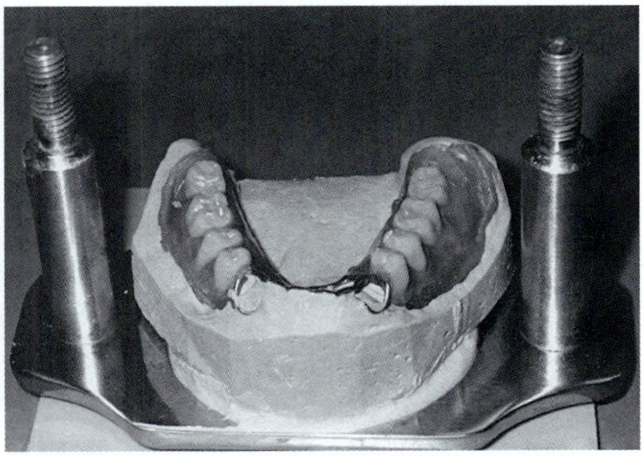

B

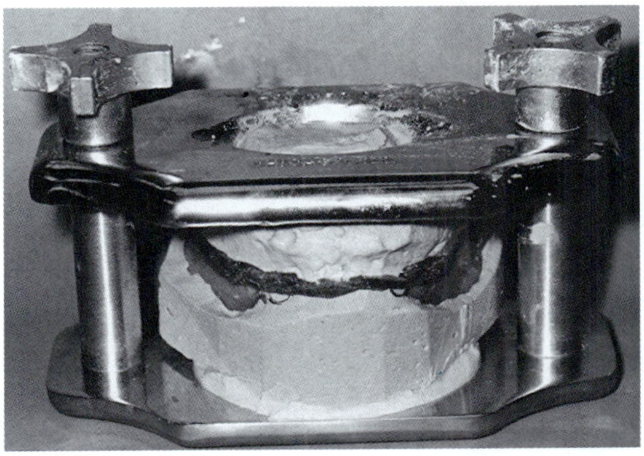

C

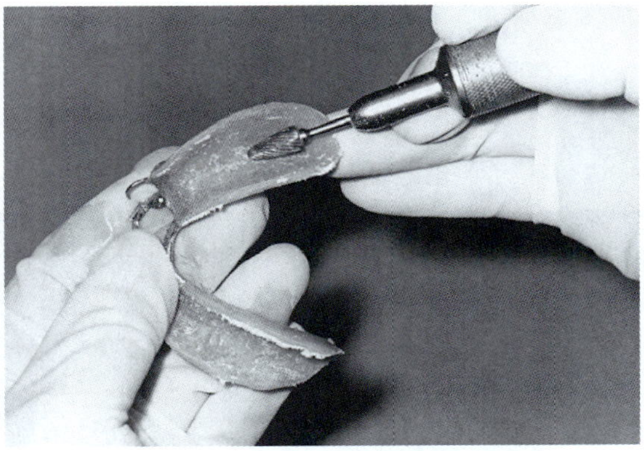

D

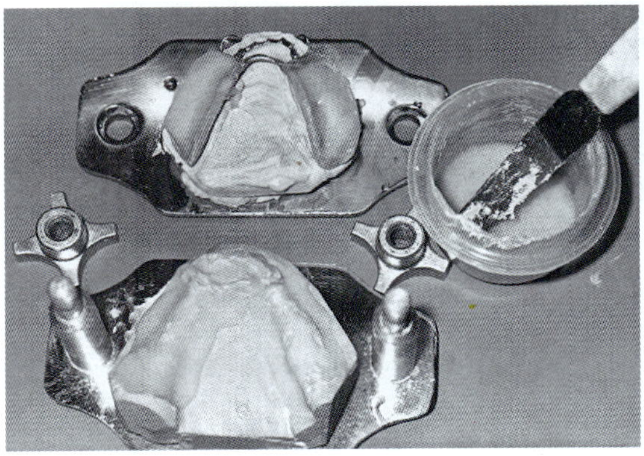

E

Figure 21-3 Because of potential for occlusal distortion, alternative procedure for relining should be considered. Metal reline jig may be used effectively to preserve vertical and occlusal relationships of partial denture. Procedure first requires that suitable impression be accomplished, following guidelines discussed in text. **A,** Stone cast is made to record impression portion and also to contact, but not entrap, sufficient parts of framework to ensure stable cast base. **B,** Cast is then affixed to upper or lower member of reline jig. **C,** Occlusal surfaces are isolated in blockout, and stone opposing cast is poured and secured to other member of jig. **D,** When stone has thoroughly set, jig is separated, partial denture is removed from cast, and tissue surface(s) and borders are relieved. **E,** Autopolymerizing acrylic resin is mixed to thick, runny consistency and carefully placed into base and into any deep areas of cast.

Continued

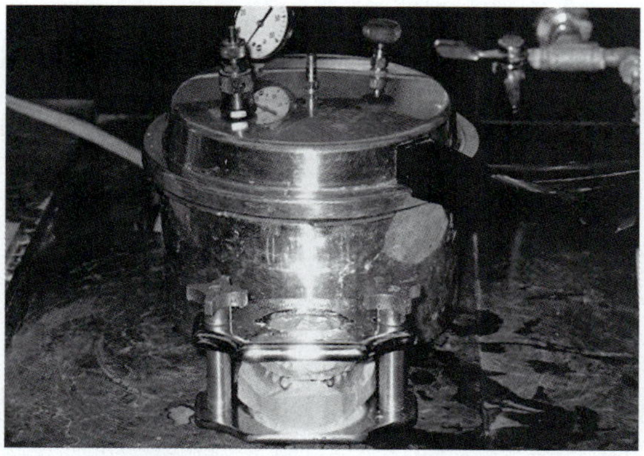

F

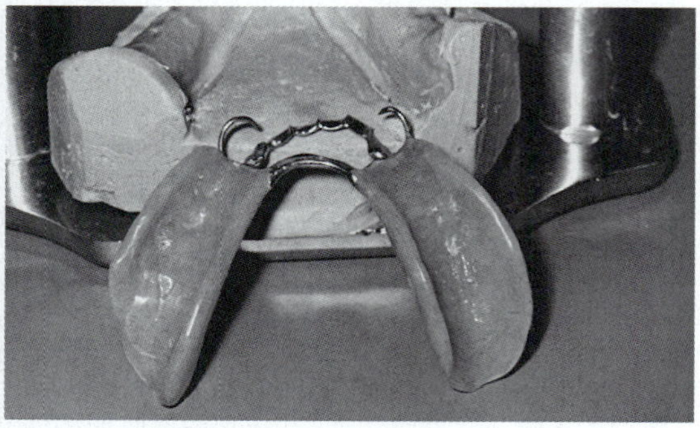

G

Figure 21-3 Cont'd F, Framework is replaced on cast, and members of jig are realigned and tightened to complete closure, covered with warm water, and placed in a pressure pot at 20 psi for 15 minutes. **G,** Restoration is finished and polished. Because of secure positioning of base to cast, this method virtually ensures that no changes will occur in occlusal vertical dimension or in occlusal relationship.

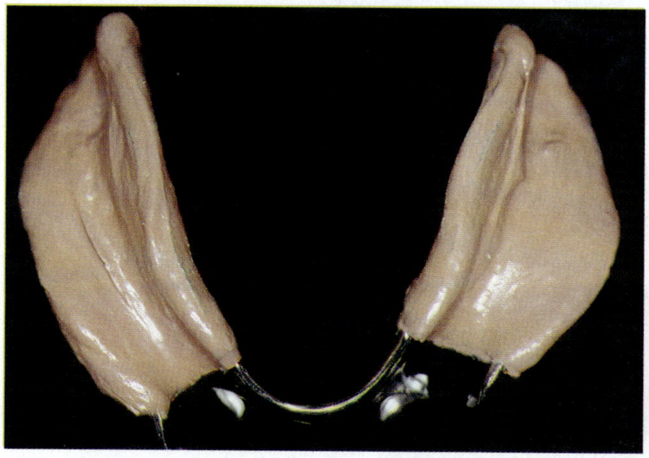

A

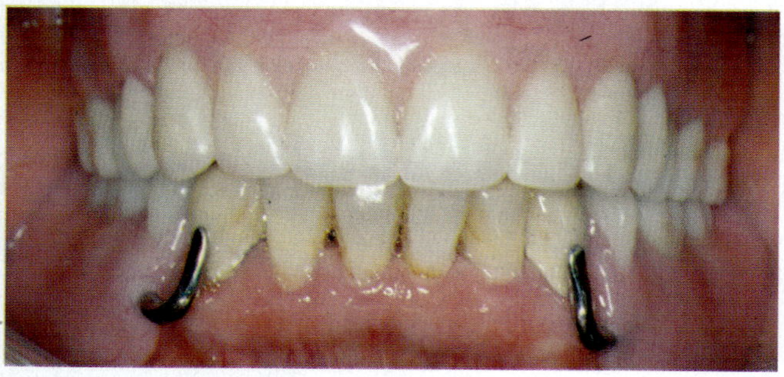

B

Figure 21-4 A, Mandibular reline impression accomplished with an open-mouth impression technique. **B,** Following processing of the reline and occlusal correction using a clinical remount procedure (see Chapter 20), the occlusion is restored to the original relationship.

tissue support but also of the original occlusal relationship (Figure 21-4).

METHODS OF REESTABLISHING OCCLUSION ON A RELINED REMOVABLE PARTIAL DENTURE

Occlusion on a relined removable partial denture may be reestablished by several methods depending on whether the relining results in an increase in the vertical dimension of occlusion or in a lack of opposing occlusal contacts. In either instance, it is usually necessary to make a remounting cast for the relined removable partial denture so that the denture can be correctly related to an opposing cast or prosthesis in an articulator (Figure 21-5).

In rare instances, after the relining of a distal extension removable partial denture by the method previously described, the occlusion is found to be negative rather than positive, or the same as it was before relining. This may be a result of wear of occlusal surfaces over a period of time, the original occlusion being high with resulting depression of opposing teeth, or other reasons. In such a situation, occlusion on the denture must be restored to reestablish an even distribution of occlusal loading over both natural and artificial dentition. Otherwise the natural dentition must carry the burden of

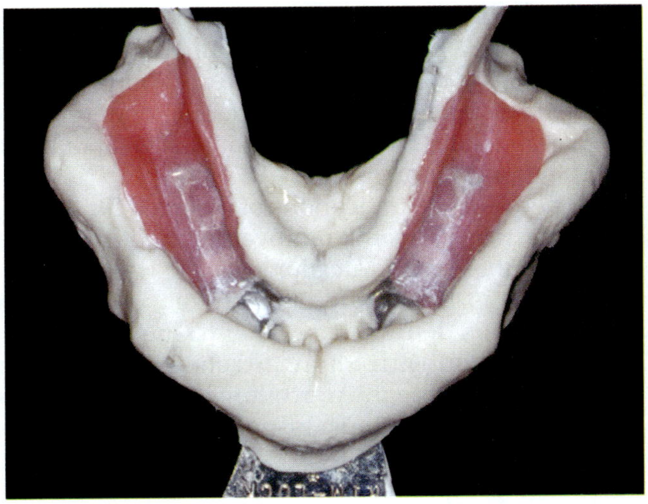

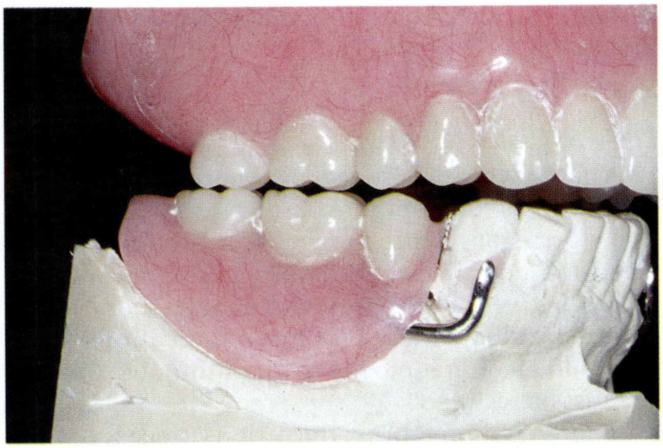

A B

Figure 21-5 **A,** An irreversible hydrocolloid pick-up impression made following reline of the mandibular removable partial denture. All regions in the framework that are below the height of contour will be coated with a thin layer of baseplate wax to allow recovery of the prosthesis from the remount cast without damage to the cast. This allows replacement of the prosthesis in the mouth for an interocclusal registration. **B,** Mounted mandibular prosthesis against a maxillary complete denture. The maxillary prosthesis was mounted using a remount cast made after finishing and polishing the prosthesis. It is not uncommon to see a significant occlusal problem when relining a mandibular distal extension removable partial denture when the residual ridge resorption has been left unchecked for a long period of time. The maxillary prosthesis can often assume a more inferior position, and when the mandibular prosthesis is reoriented to the natural dentition, this raises the mandibular occlusal plane, resulting in an occlusal relationship as shown. The best resolution of this requires addressing the maxillary arch at the same time, and requires a repositioning of the maxillary occlusal plane.

mastication unaided, and the denture becomes only a space-filling or cosmetic device.

If the artificial teeth to be corrected are resin, the occlusion can be reestablished either by adding autopolymerizing or light-activated resin to occlusal surfaces or by fabricating gold occlusal surfaces, which can be attached to the original replaced teeth. The original teeth may also be removed from the denture base and replaced by new teeth arranged to harmonize with the opposing occlusal surfaces. Baseplate wax may be used to support the teeth as they are arranged. The wax should be carved to restore the lingual anatomy of the teeth and the portion of the denture base that was eliminated when the original teeth were removed. A stone matrix is made that covers the occlusal and lingual surfaces of the teeth and denture flange. Then wax may be removed from the denture base and teeth and the tissue-bearing surface coated with a bonding agent. Those areas on the stone matrix, intimate to the new resin to be added, should be painted with a tinfoil substitute or an air- barrier coating material if a visible light-cured (VLC) material is to be used. The new teeth are placed in the stone matrix, and the matrix is accurately attached to the denture base with sticky wax or a hot glue gun. VLC material or an autopolymerizing resin is then used to attach the teeth. If an autopolymerizing material is used, it can be conveniently sprinkled on by a buccal approach. The buccal surface of the denture base adjacent to the teeth should be slightly overfilled so the correct shape may be restored to this portion of the base during finishing and polishing procedures. Occlusal discrepancies caused by this procedure should be corrected in the articulator by new jaw relation records if the denture has a distal extension base.

A second method is to remove the original teeth and replace them with a hard inlay wax occlusion rim on which a functional registration of occlusal pathways is then established (see Chapter 17). Either the original teeth or new teeth may then be arranged to occlude with the template thus obtained and subsequently attached to the denture base with processed VLC material or autopolymerizing resin. If the latter is used, the need for flasking may be eliminated by securing the teeth to a stone matrix while the resin attachment is applied with a brush technique. Regardless of the method used for reattaching the teeth, the occlusion thus established should require little adjustment in the mouth and should exhibit the occlusal harmony that is possible by this method.

SELF-ASSESSMENT AIDS

1. What is the difference between relining and rebasing a resin denture base?
2. On occasion, tissue changes beneath tooth-supported denture bases require correction of the bases to reestablish intimate contact of the base and residual ridge. List three indications that would lead one to believe that intimate contact must be restored.
3. In any relining procedure, it is necessary to relieve the borders and tissue surface of the denture base before making an impression. Why is this required?
4. Tooth-supported removable partial denture bases may often be relined with a color-matching, autopolymerizing, or VLC resin as a chair-side procedure. Describe such a procedure, and include preparation of the bases and the precautions that must be observed for patient comfort.
5. When relining a tooth-supported base, why should the anatomical or functional form of the ridge be used?
6. Suppose that rests are not correctly seated in their prepared seats when a chair-side reline procedure is accomplished. What must be done?
7. Suppose a Kennedy Class III, modification 1 type of removable restoration must be relined. The edentulous areas of the residual ridge are from canine to third molar on each side, and some support of the bases by the residual ridges is desired. What procedure should be undertaken to acceptably reline the restoration? Include impression procedure, impression material, processing, and correction of any occlusal discrepancies encountered.
8. There are two indications of the need for relining a distal extension removable partial denture. State these two indications.
9. There is little difference in relining a distal extension denture base and making a secondary impression with a tray attached to the framework. Describe the procedures, both clinical and laboratory, that must be performed in relining a distal extension base.
10. After completion of the reline procedure and finishing of the restoration, occlusal discrepancies invariably occur. They must be corrected before the patient is given possession of the restoration. How are occlusal discrepancies for a relined distal extension denture corrected?
11. Should the same adjustment procedures of the denture base to residual ridge be undertaken for a relined base as was performed for initial placement of a new denture? Why or why not?
12. Does adjustment of the denture base to the basal seat precede or follow correction of occlusal discrepancies? Why?
13. Suppose that after relining a distal extension denture base one finds occlusal contacts of opposing posterior artificial teeth are minimal or nonexistent. What then?
14. Before relining or rebasing is undertaken, the oral tissue should be returned to a state of health. True or false? Rationalize your answer.

22

REPAIRS AND ADDITIONS TO REMOVABLE PARTIAL DENTURES

The need for repairing or adding to a removable partial denture will occasionally arise. However, the frequency of this occurrence should be held to a minimum by careful diagnosis, intelligent treatment planning, adequate mouth preparations, and the carrying out of an effective removable partial denture design with proper fabrication of all component parts. Any need for repairs or additions will then be the result of unforeseen complications that arise in abutment or other teeth in the arch, breakage or distortion of the denture through accident, or careless handling by the patient rather than to faulty design or fabrication.

It is important that the patient be instructed in the proper placement and removal of the prosthesis so that undue strain is not placed on clasp arms, on other parts of the denture, or on contacted abutment teeth. The patient also should be advised that care must be given to the prosthesis when it is out of the mouth and that any distortion may be irreparable. It should be made clear that there can be no guarantee against breakage or distortion from causes other than obvious structural defects.

BROKEN CLASP ARMS

The following are several reasons for breakage of clasp arms:

1. Breakage may result from repeated flexure into and out of too severe an undercut. If the periodontal support is greater than the fatigue limit of the clasp arm, failure of the metal occurs first. Otherwise the abutment tooth is loosened and eventually lost because of the persistent strain that is placed on it. Locating clasp arms only where an acceptable minimum of retention exists, as determined by an accurate survey of the master cast, can prevent this type of breakage.
2. Breakage may occur as a result of structural failure of the clasp arm itself. A cast clasp arm that is not properly formed or is subject to careless finishing and polishing will eventually break at its weakest point. This can be prevented by providing the appropriate taper to flexible retentive clasp arms and uniform bulk to all rigid nonretentive clasp arms. Wrought-wire clasp arms may eventually fail because of repeated flexure at the region where it exits from the resin base (Figure 22-1), or at a point at which a nick or constriction occurred as a result of careless use of contouring pliers. They also may break at the point of origin from the casting as a result of excessive manipulation during initial adaptation to the tooth or subsequent readaptation. Clasp breakage can best be prevented by cautioning the patient against removing the removable partial denture by sliding the clasp arm away from the tooth with the fingernails. A wrought-wire clasp arm can normally be adjusted several times over a period of years without failure. It is only when the number of

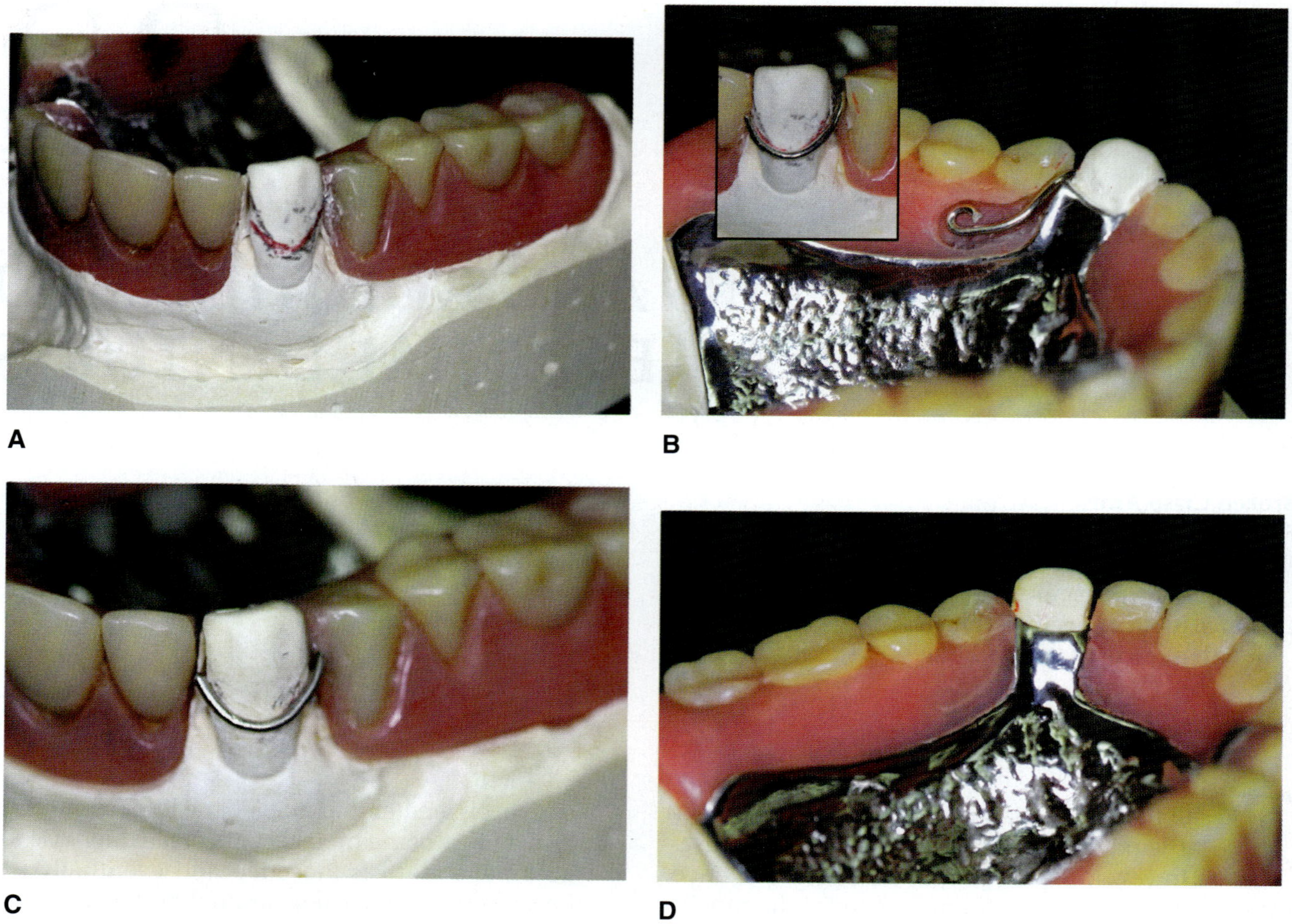

Figure 22-1 Fractured direct retainer on canine abutment. Reason for breakage is likely the long-term repeated flexure from movement associated with this 8-year-old distal extension prosthesis. Denture must be evaluated for prospective serviceability if retainer arm is repaired. Often, patient will best be served by replacing denture with new restoration. **A,** Cast produced from a irreversible hydrocolloid pick-up impression. Height of contour is shown in pencil with red line illustrating to lab the location of repair wire (18 gauge). **B,** Clasp adapted to designated line on canine and fitted into resin trough distal to canine and palatal to first and second premolars. Note the curvature placed at the end of the wire to prevent movement within polymerized resin. **C,** Finished and polished wire repair from the buccal and, **D,** palatal view.

adjustments is excessive that breakage is likely to occur. Wrought-wire clasp arms also may break at the point of origin because of recrystallization of the metal. This can be prevented by proper selection of wrought wire, avoiding burnout temperatures exceeding 1300° F, and avoiding excessive casting temperatures when a cast-to method is used. When wrought wire is attached to the framework by soldering, the soldering technique must avoid recrystallization of the wire. For this reason, it is best that soldering be done electrically to prevent the wrought wire from overheating. A low-fusing (1420° to 1500° F), triple-thick, color-matching gold solder should be used rather than a solder that possesses a higher fusing temperature.

3. Breakage may occur because of careless handling by the patient. Any clasp arm will become distorted or will break if subjected to excessive abuse by the patient. The most common cause of failure of a cast clasp arm is distortion caused by accidentally dropping the removable partial denture. A broken retentive clasp arm, regardless of its type, may be replaced with a wrought-wire retentive arm embedded in a resin base (see Figure 22-1, *C* and *D*) or attached to a metal base by electric soldering. Often this avoids the necessity of fabricating an entirely new clasp arm.

FRACTURED OCCLUSAL RESTS

Breakage of an occlusal rest almost always occurs where it crosses the marginal ridge. Improperly prepared occlusal rest seats are the usual cause of such weakness: an occlusal rest that crosses a marginal ridge that was not lowered sufficiently during mouth preparations either is made too thin or is thinned by adjustment in the mouth to prevent occlusal interference. Failure of an occlusal rest rarely results from a structural defect in the metal and rarely if ever is caused by accidental distortion. Therefore the blame for such failure must often be assumed by the dentist for not having provided sufficient space for the rest during mouth preparations.

Soldering may repair broken occlusal rests, as illustrated in Figure 22-2. In preparation for the repair, it may be necessary to alter the rest seat of the broken rest or to relieve occlusal interferences. With the removable partial denture in its terminal position, an impression is made in irreversible hydrocolloid and then removed, with the removable partial denture remaining in the impression. The dental stone is poured into the impression and allowed to set. The removable partial denture is then removed from the cast, and platinum foil is adapted to the rest seat and the marginal ridge and overlaps the guiding plane. The removable partial denture is returned to the cast and, with a fluoride flux, gold solder is electrically fused to the platinum foil and minor connector in sufficient bulk to form an occlusal rest. An alternative solder to use is an industrial brazing alloy, which is higher fusing but responds excellently to electric soldering and does not tarnish.

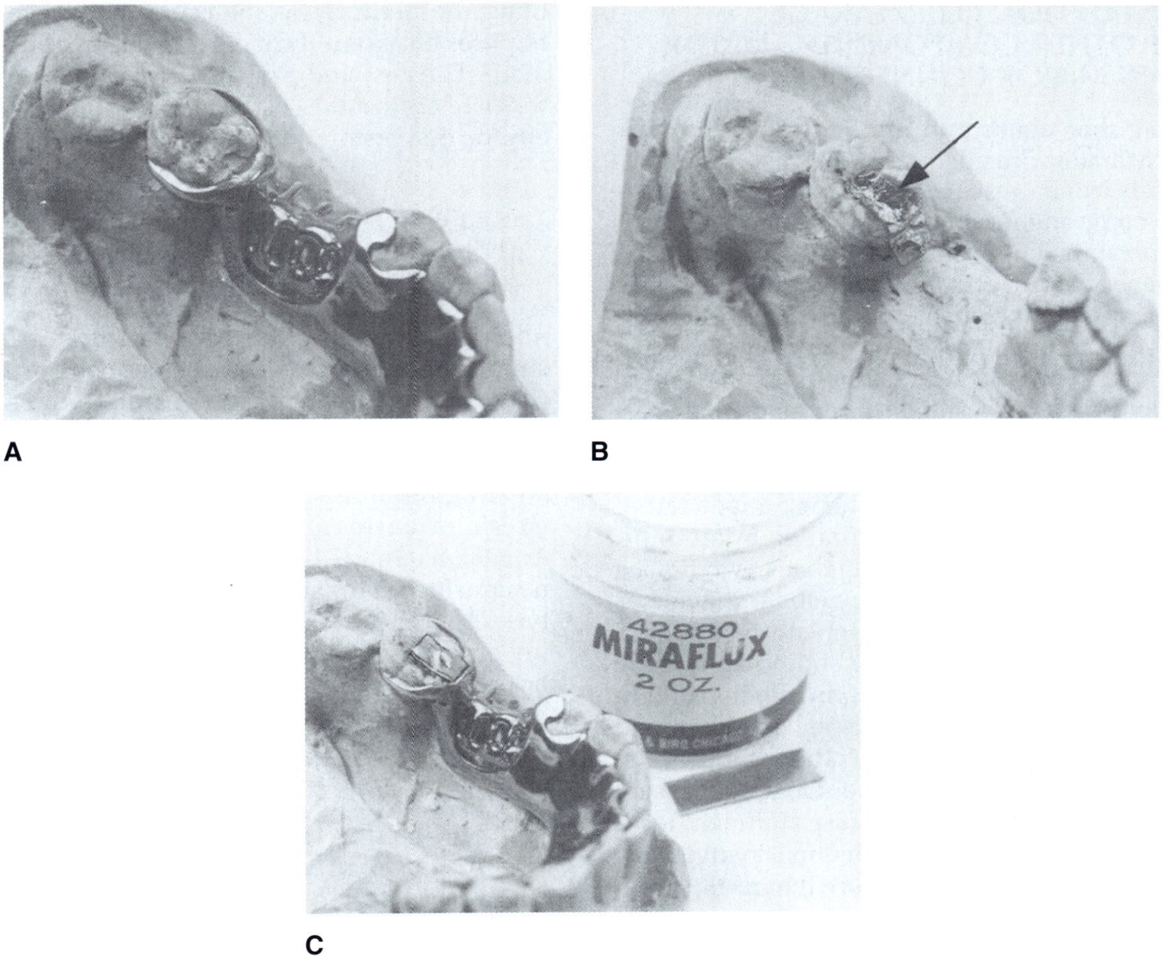

Figure 22-2 **A,** Occlusal rest on molar fractured and was lost. Adequacy of present rest seat must be evaluated as well as interocclusal space available for rest before repair procedure is undertaken. **B,** Denture is removed from cast, and platinum foil *(arrow)* is adapted to rest seat area and over marginal ridge of abutment. **C,** Flux is applied sparingly to areas involved, and solder is placed in position.

Continued

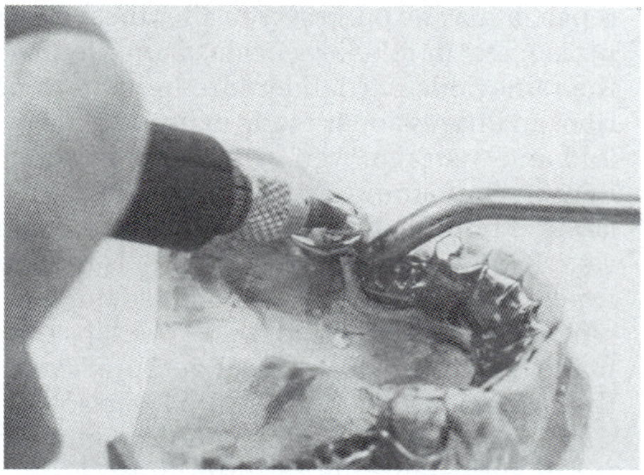

D

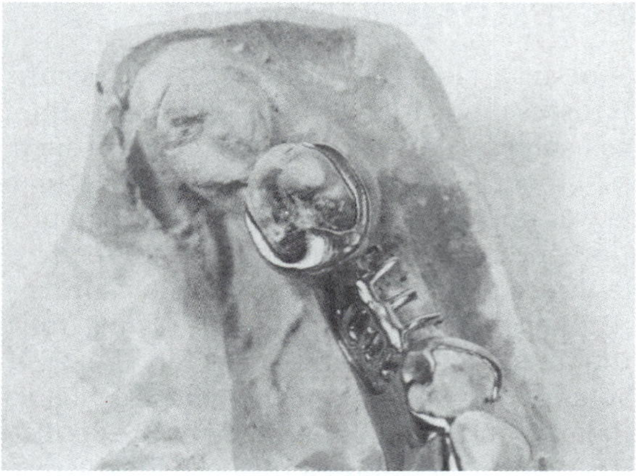

E

Figure 22-2 Cont'd D, Electric soldering is used to repair rest. **E,** Rest is shaped to conform to rest seat outline. Framework is tried in patient's mouth for any necessary adjustment, and rest is polished.

DISTORTION OR BREAKAGE OF OTHER COMPONENTS—MAJOR AND MINOR CONNECTORS

Assuming that major and minor connectors were originally made with adequate bulk, distortion usually occurs from abuse by the patient (Figure 22-3). All such components should be designed and fabricated with sufficient bulk to ensure their rigidity and permanence of form under normal circumstances.

Major and minor connectors occasionally become weakened by adjustment to prevent or eliminate tissue impingement. Such adjustment at the time of initial placement is a result of either inadequate survey of the master cast or faulty design or fabrication of the casting. This is inexcusable and reflects on the dentist. Such a restoration should be remade rather than further weakening the restoration by attempting to compensate for its inadequacies by relieving the metal. Similarly, tissue impingement that arises from inadequately relieved components results from faulty planning, and the casting should be remade with enough relief to prevent impingement. Failure of any component that was weakened by adjustment at the time of initial placement is the responsibility of the dentist. However, adjustment made necessary by settling of the restoration because abutment teeth have become intruded under functional loading may be unavoidable. Subsequent failure that results from the weakening effect of such adjustment may necessitate making a new restoration as a consequence of tissue changes. Commonly, repeated adjustment to a major or minor connector results in a loss of rigidity to the point that the connector can no longer function effectively. In such situations, either a new restoration must be made or that part must be replaced by casting a new section and then reassembling the denture by soldering. This occasionally requires disassembly of denture bases and artificial teeth. The cost and probable success must then be weighed against the cost of a new restoration. Generally the new restoration is advisable.

LOSS OF A TOOTH OR TEETH NOT INVOLVED IN THE SUPPORT OR RETENTION OF THE RESTORATION

Additions to a removable partial denture are usually simply made when the bases are made of resin (Figure 22-4). The addition of teeth to metal bases is more complex and necessitates either casting a new component and attaching it by soldering or creating retentive elements for the attachment of a resin extension. In most instances when a distal extension denture base is extended, the need should be considered for subsequent relining of the entire base. After the extension of the denture base, a relining procedure of both the new and old base should be carried out to provide optimal tissue support for the restoration.

LOSS OF AN ABUTMENT TOOTH NECESSITATING ITS REPLACEMENT AND MAKING A NEW DIRECT RETAINER

In the event of a lost abutment, the next adjacent tooth is usually selected as a retaining abutment, and it generally will require modification or a restoration. Any new restoration should be made to conform to the original path of placement, with proximal guiding plane, rest seat, and suitable retentive area. Otherwise modifications to the existing tooth should be

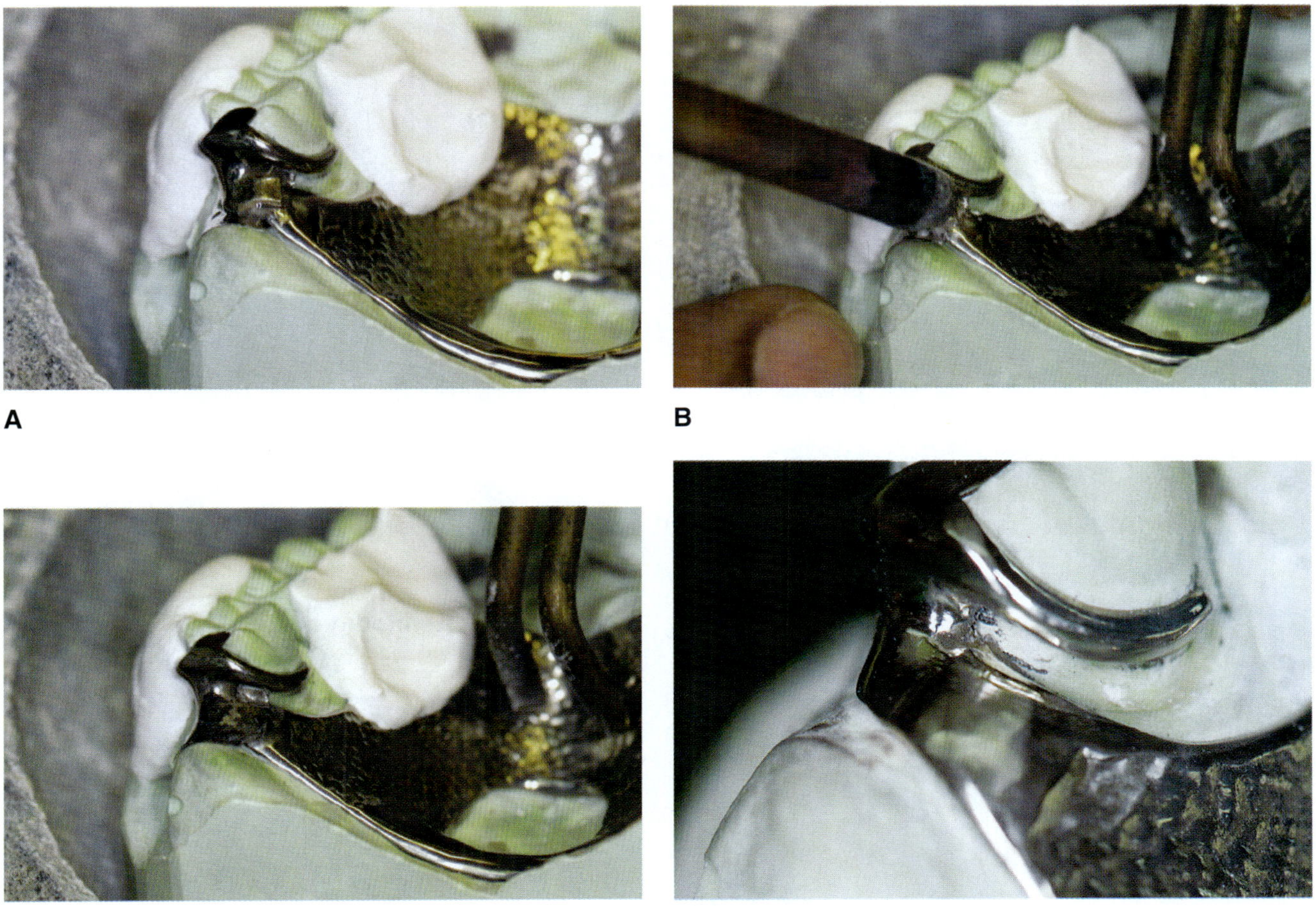

A B C D

Figure 22-3 **A,** Maxillary juncture between major and minor connector at the distal of most posterior molar has fractured. Thin platinum foil has been adapted to the cast beneath the fracture, the clasp assembly has been stabilized on the cast with fast-set plaster, the remainder of the prosthesis has been positioned on the cast in full contact with teeth and tissues, and the solder has been positioned for the electric tip to be placed. **B,** The electric soldering tip and ground are in place. **C,** Immediately following solder flow, the fracture has been eliminated by the solder connecting the two segments. **D,** The polished solder repair is ready to be cleaned and returned to the patient. The patient is told that this repair is not as strong as the original and, while it is difficult to know how long it could serve the patient, careful handling of the prosthesis is mandatory.

done the same as during any other mouth preparations, with proximal recontouring, preparation of an adequate occlusal rest seat, and any reduction in tooth contours necessary to accommodate retentive and stabilizing components. A new clasp assembly may then be cast for this tooth and the denture reassembled with the new replacement tooth added.

OTHER TYPES OF REPAIRS

Other types of repairs may include the replacement of a broken or lost prosthetic tooth, the repair of a broken resin base, or the reattachment of a loosened resin base to the metal framework. Breakage is sometimes the result of poor design, faulty fabrication, or use of the wrong material for a given situation. Other times it results from an accident that will not necessarily repeat itself. If the latter occurs, repair or replacement usually suffices. On the other hand, if fracture has occurred because of structural defects or if it occurs a second time after the denture has been repaired once before, then some change in the design—either by modification of the original denture or with a new denture—may be necessary.

REPAIR BY SOLDERING

Approximately 80% of all soldering in dentistry can be done electrically. Electric soldering units are available for this purpose and most dental laboratories

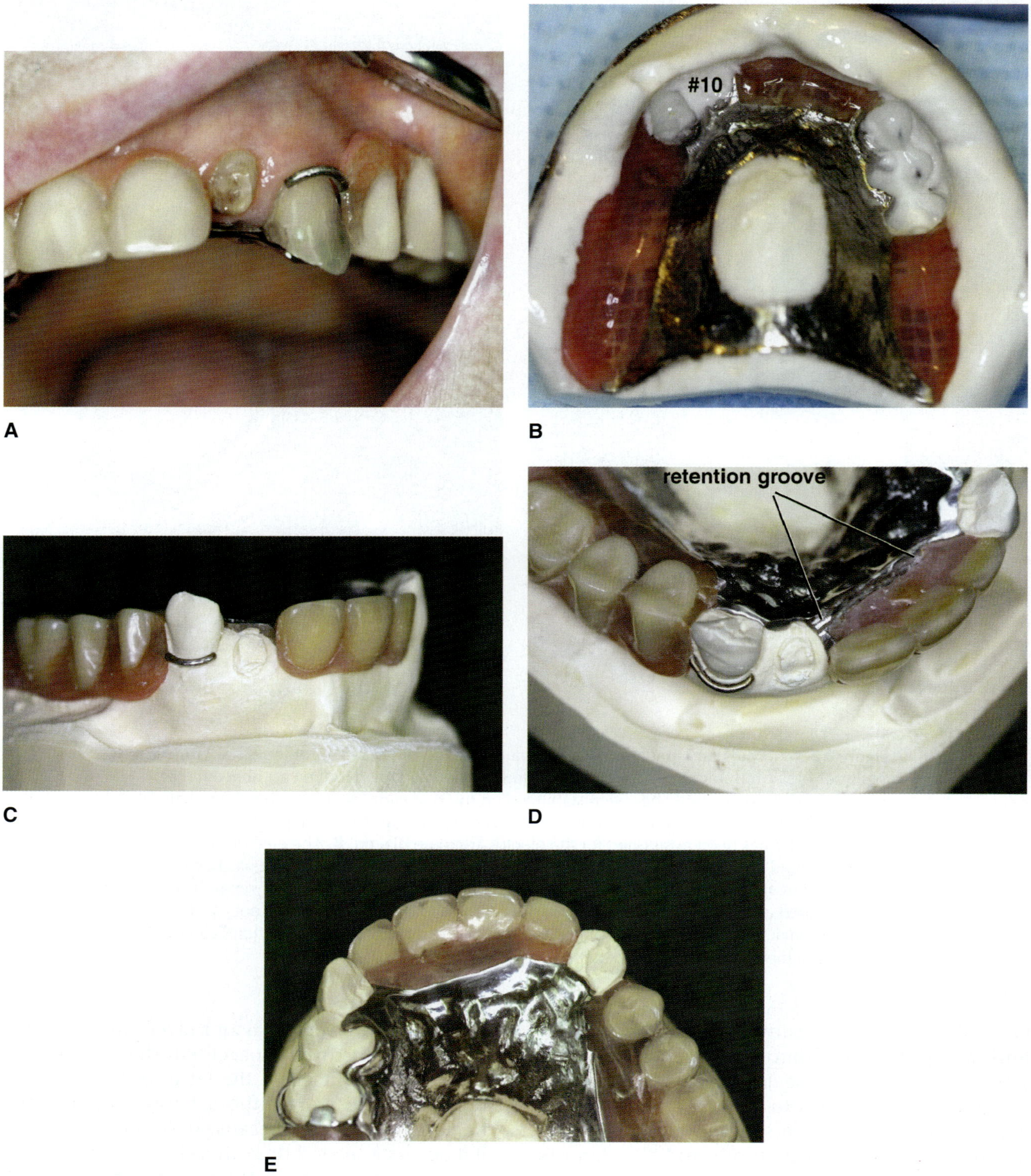

Figure 22-4 This patient presented with an asymptomatic fractured lateral incisor. **A,** Clinical presentation of fractured tooth and prosthesis. Evaluation of the prosthesis revealed it to be adequately fitting, stable, and retentive. **B,** Pick-up impression of prosthesis. **C,** Cast formed from pick-up impression, showing a fully seated prosthesis. **D,** Preparation of the prosthesis included mechanical means for retention (which was provided by creating a recess in the resin adjacent to the missing tooth), and creating a trough at the external finishing line to repair an area of marginal breakdown. **E,** Finished repair that will be taken to the mouth and checked for occlusal clearance lingual to the maxillary anterior teeth.

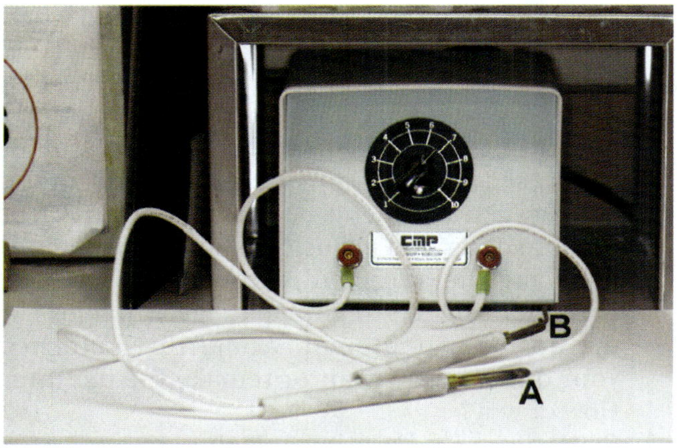

Figure 22-5 Electric soldering machine with variable adjustment (1-10) for low to high heat. Carbon electrode that furnishes heat for soldering is at *A*. Electrode at *B* completes electric circuit when touched to framework being soldered. Carbon electrode should be placed first on framework and removed last when soldering.

are so equipped (Figure 22-5). Electric soldering permits soldering close to a resin base without removing that base because of the rapid localization of heat at the electrode. The resin base needs only to be protected with a wet casting ring liner during soldering.

Color-matching gold solder may be used for soldering both gold and chromium-cobalt alloys. A solder for gold alloys that melts between 1420° and 1500° F is entirely adequate to solder gold alloys to chromium-cobalt alloys, thereby lessening the chance of recrystallizing gold wrought wire by excessive and prolonged heat. For electric soldering, triple-thick solder should be used so that the additional bulk of the solder will retard melting momentarily, while the carbon electrode conducts heat to the area to be soldered. For soldering chromium-cobalt alloys, a color-matching white 19 K gold solder—which melts at about 1676° F—is used. An application of flux is essential to the success of any soldering operation to prevent oxidation of the parts to be joined and the solder itself. A borax-type flux is used when soldering gold alloys. Fluoride-type flux must be used when soldering chromium-cobalt alloys. When a gold alloy is to be soldered to a chromium-cobalt alloy, a fluoride-type flux should be chosen.

The following is a procedure for electric soldering:

1. Roughen both sections to be joined.
2. Adapt platinum foil to the master cast beneath the framework to serve as a backing on which the solder will flow. Lift the edges of the foil to form a trough to confine the flow of the solder.
3. Seat the pieces to be soldered onto the master cast and secure them temporarily with sticky wax. Over each piece, add enough soldering investment to secure them after the sticky wax is eliminated, but leave as much metal exposed as possible.
4. After flushing off the sticky wax with hot water, secure the cast to the soldering stand. Cut sufficient solder and place conveniently nearby.
5. Flux both sections. Put sufficient triple-thick solder on or in the joint to complete the soldering in one operation, always starting with enough solder to complete the job.
6. Wet the carbon tip with water to aid conduction of the current and then touch the carbon tip to the solder (be sure the solder is held firmly in place). Place the other electrode on any portion of the framework to complete the electric circuit and heat the carbon electrode. Do not push the solder with the carbon tip, but let the heat alone make the solder flow. Do not remove the carbon tip from the solder while the soldering operation is in progress; this will cause surface pitting because of arcing. After the solder has flowed, remove the electrodes, removing the carbon tip electrode last, and proceed to remove the work from the cast for finishing.

Torch soldering requires an entirely different approach. It is used when the solder joint is long or unusually bulky and when a larger quantity of solder has to be used. Torch soldering cannot be undertaken to repair a removable partial denture framework that has resin denture bases or artificial teeth supported by resin. The procedure for torch soldering is as follows:

1. Roughen both sections to be joined.
2. Adapt platinum foil to the master cast so that it extends under both sections.
3. Seat the sections on the master cast in the correct relationship and secure them temporarily with sticky wax. Also flow sticky wax into the joint to be soldered.
4. Attach a dental bur or nail over the two sections with a liberal amount of sticky wax. Attach a second and even a third nail or bur across other areas to lend additional support. Never use pieces of wood for this purpose because the wood will swell if it gets wet, thus distorting the relationship of the two sections.
5. Remove the assembled casting from the master cast carefully. Adapt a stock of utility wax directly under each section on either side of the platinum foil. After boil out is done, investment will remain in the center to support the platinum foil.

6. Invest the casting in sufficient soldering investment to secure it, and expose as much of the area to be soldered as possible. When the investment has set, boil out the sticky and utility waxes. Then place the investment in a drying oven at a temperature not exceeding 200° F until elimination of the contained moisture. Do not dry or preheat the investment with a torch because oxides then will be formed that will interfere with the flow of the solder.
7. Use the reducing part of the flame, which is that feathery part just outside the blue inner cone. Flux the joint thoroughly and dry out the flux with the outer part of the flame until it has a powdery appearance. Heat the casting until it is dull red and then, holding a strip of solder in the soldering tweezers, dip it into the flux and feed it into the joint, while the casting is being held at a dull-red heat with the torch. Once the soldering operation has begun, do not remove the flame, because any cooling will cause oxides to form. The heat from the casting should be sufficient to melt the solder; therefore do not put the flame directly on the solder because it will become overheated and pitting will result.
8. After the soldering has been completed, allow the investment to cool slowly before quenching and proceeding with finishing. Remember that any soldering operation that heats the entire casting is in effect a softening heat-treating operation, and heat-hardening of a repaired gold alloy casting is desirable to restore its optimal physical properties.

SELF-ASSESSMENT AIDS

1. The need for repairing a component of a removable partial denture may arise occasionally. How may the frequency of breakage of components be minimized?
2. For what three reasons may breakage of a direct retainer arm occur?
3. An occlusal or incisal rest may fracture in use and invariably occurs at marginal ridge or incisal areas. What is the predominant reason for lack of strength at the junction of the rest and minor connector?
4. What problems if any can be encountered when one tries to adjust a distorted minor connector?
5. Other than by accident, for what reasons could a major connector become distorted?
6. An abutment with a guarded prognosis is sometimes used to prevent an extension-type denture. Loss of such abutments necessitates extension of denture bases and inclusion of an artificial tooth replacing the abutment. Suppose the denture was not designed to anticipate eventual loss of the posterior abutment. Would this influence your decision to repair or remake the denture? How or why?
7. Extension of a base in replacing an abutment tooth usually necessitates relining of the entire base. True or false?
8. When a terminal abutment for a distal extension removable partial denture is lost, can the existing denture be modified with a new clasp assembly on another abutment? How?
9. Porcelain artificial teeth that have been excessively ground or that were not arranged in occlusal harmony sometimes fracture in use and have to be replaced. To perform this procedure, is an impression necessary? If the replaced tooth is on an extension base, is the occlusion adjusted?
10. What is a distinct advantage of electric soldering over torch soldering for the repair of a metallic element of a removable partial denture?
11. Suppose a rest broke at its junction with the minor connector. How does soldering create a new rest? Would a clinical procedure on the old rest seat preparation be performed first? Why? What kind of procedure?
12. When soldering a chromium-cobalt alloy, what solder should be used? Is any special type of flux required?
13. When an electric soldering unit is used, why must the carbon electrode be removed from the work last?
14. What is the purpose of using a flux when performing soldering operations?
15. Should torch soldering be attempted on a restoration with acrylic resin bases?
16. After either electric or torch soldering has repaired a framework, should a heat-hardening treatment be performed? Why or why not?

23

TEMPORARY REMOVABLE PARTIAL DENTURES

Tooth replacement is required for a variety of reasons. Sometimes replacement is necessary for shorter periods of time that serve alternative purposes than permanent replacement, such as while tissue is healing or related treatment is being provided. When such applications require the temporary use of removable partial dentures, their fabrication and use must be incorporated into a total prosthodontic treatment plan.

These various uses of temporary prostheses for the partially edentulous mouth strive to achieve the temporary goals with minimum time and expense. The prostheses are typically resin with wire retention and may include components to provide tooth support. The difficulty in achieving and maintaining strategic tooth support and stability with such prostheses makes it important that patients be made aware that such prostheses are temporary and may jeopardize the integrity of adjacent teeth and health of supporting tissue if worn for extended periods without supportive care.

Temporary prostheses may be indicated as a part of total treatment for:

1. Sake of appearance
2. Maintenance of a space
3. Reestablishment of occlusal relationships
4. To condition teeth and residual ridges
5. Interim restoration during treatment
6. To condition the patient for wearing a prosthesis

APPEARANCE

For the sake of appearance, a temporary removable partial denture may replace one or more missing anterior teeth or it may replace several teeth, both anterior and posterior. Such a restoration is usually made of resin, which is produced either by a sprinkling method, by the visible light-cured (VLC) method, or by waxing, flasking, and processing with either autopolymerizing or heat polymerizing resin (Figure 23-1). It may be retained by circumferential wrought-wire clasps, Crozat-type clasps, interproximal spurs, or wire loops.

SPACE MAINTENANCE

When a space results from recent extractions or traumatic loss of teeth, it is usually prudent to maintain the space while tissue heals. In younger patients the space should be maintained until the adjacent teeth have reached sufficient maturity to be used as abutments for fixed restorations or so that an implant can be placed. In adult patients the maintenance of the space can prevent undesirable migration and extrusion of adjacent or opposing teeth until definitive treatment can be accomplished (Figure 23-2).

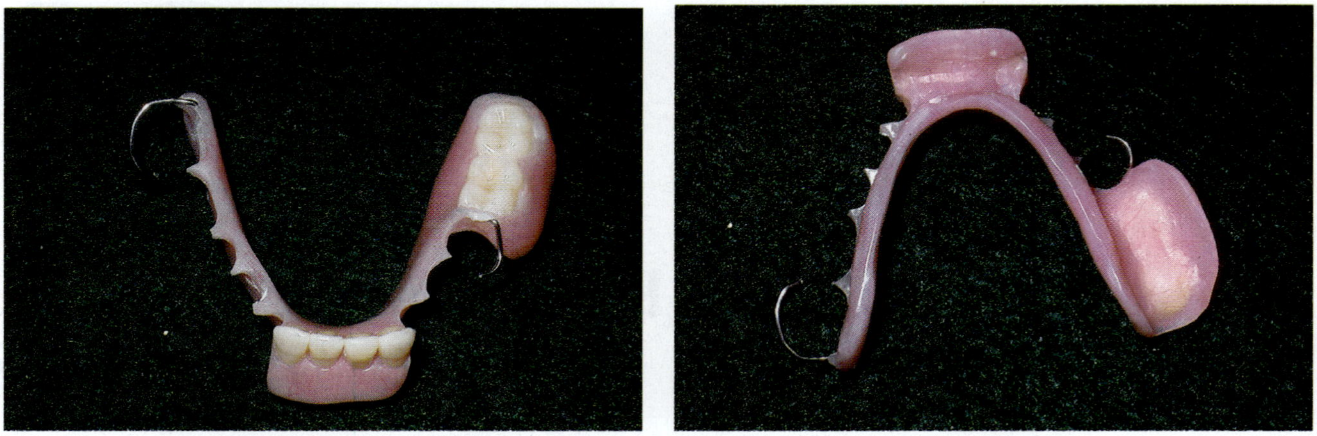

A B

Figure 23-1 **A,** While loss of mandibular teeth does not always carry a significant esthetic impact, this temporary removable partial denture was needed because of the visibility of the mandibular incisors. Provision of the mandibular left molars allowed early accommodation of the residual ridge during the temporary prosthesis period. **B,** Tissue surface of temporary prosthesis revealing rounded lingual flange and tapered labial flange. The latter was needed to improve lip movement and reduce the feeling of bulk, both enhancing normal lip activity.

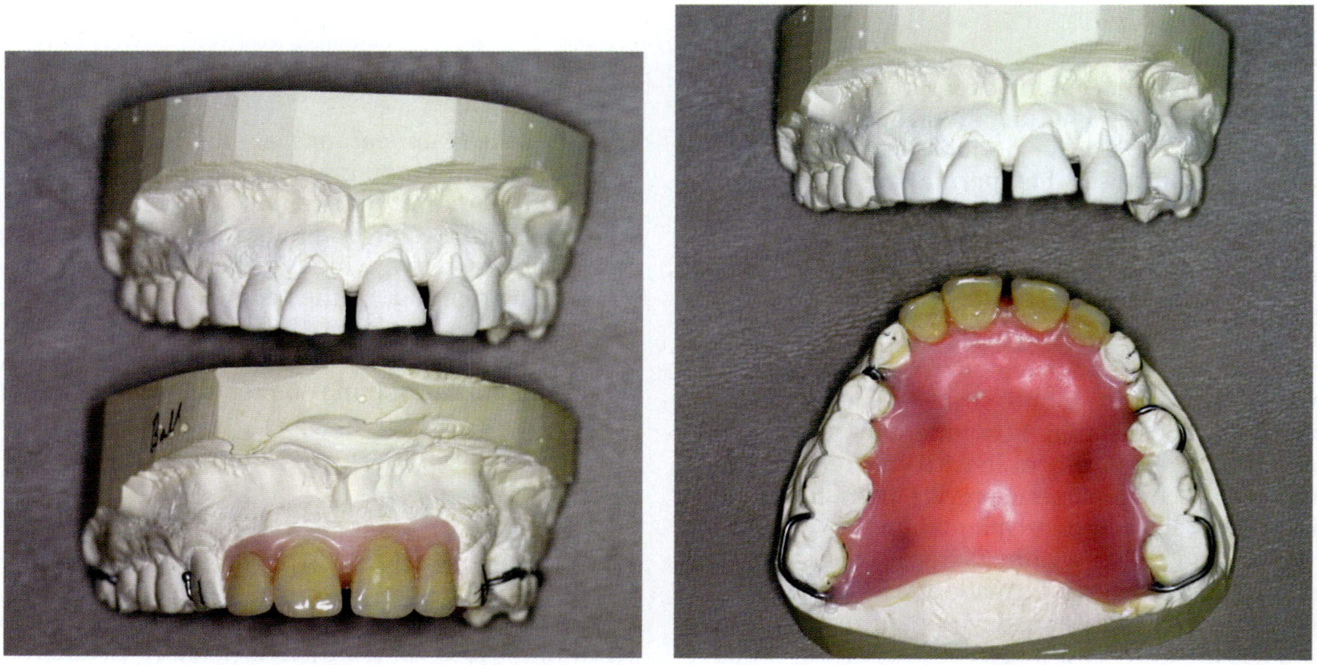

A B

Figure 23-2 **A,** Malpositioned maxillary anterior teeth require extraction. Following a period of healing the patient will decide a definitive treatment option, which could include a removable partial denture or an implant-supported prosthesis. Because the period of time until definitive care will be provided is not known, a temporary prosthesis not only replaces esthetically important teeth but provides stabilization of adjacent and opposing dentition as well. **B,** Occlusal view of temporary prosthesis showing clasp placement at the most posterior locations without crossing the occlusion and anterior positions bilaterally. Full palatal coverage allows less stress to the remaining maxillary dentition and may prevent prosthesis-induced gingival trauma and tooth movement.

REESTABLISHING OCCLUSAL RELATIONSHIPS

Temporary removable partial dentures are used for the following reasons: (1) to establish a new occlusal relationship or occlusal vertical dimension and (2) to condition teeth and ridge tissue for optimum support of the definitive removable partial denture that will follow.

Temporary removable partial dentures may be used as occlusal splints in much the same manner as cast or resin occlusal splints are used on natural teeth. When total tooth support is available, there is little difference between a fixed and a removable occlusal splint, except that a removable splint is likely to be left out of the mouth unless the patient is actually made more comfortable by its presence. This is usually true when the wearing of an occlusal splint alleviates a temporomandibular joint condition. In other situations it may be advisable to cement the removable restoration to the teeth until such time as the patient has become accustomed to, and dependent on, the jaw relationship provided by the splint.

Both fixed and removable tooth-supported occlusal splints have much in common. Either of them may be eliminated in sections as restorative treatment is being done, thus maintaining the established jaw relation until all restorative treatment has been completed. The dentist decides whether these are to be fixed or removable and whether they are made of a cast alloy, composite, or a resin material.

When one or more distal extension bases exist on an occlusal splint, a different situation exists. The establishment of a new occlusal relation depends on the quality of support and stability the splint receives from the denture support. Both broad coverage and functional basing of tissue-supported bases are desirable, along with some type of occlusal rest on the nearest abutments. Any tissue-supported occlusal splint should be at least relined in the mouth with an autopolymerizing reline resin to afford optimal coverage and support for the distal extension base.

CONDITIONING TEETH AND RESIDUAL RIDGES

O.C. Applegate, in an article on the choice of partial or complete denture treatment, has emphasized the advantages of conditioning edentulous areas to provide stable support for distal extension removable partial dentures. This is accomplished by having the patient wear a temporary removable partial denture for a period of time before fabrication of the final base. In the absence of opposing occlusion, stimulation of the underlying tissue by applying intermittent finger pressure to the denture base is advised. Whether the stimulation is from occlusal or finger pressure, there seems to be little doubt that the tissue of the residual ridge becomes more capable of supporting a distal extension removable partial denture when they have been previously conditioned by wearing a restoration.

Abutment teeth also benefit from wearing a temporary restoration when such a restoration applies an occlusal load to those teeth, either through occlusal coverage or through occlusal rests. Commonly a tooth that is to be used as an abutment for a removable partial denture has been out of occlusion for some time. Immediately on applying an occlusal load to that tooth sufficient to support any type of removable prosthesis, some intrusion of the tooth will occur. If such intrusion is allowed to occur after initial placement of the final prosthesis, the occlusal relationship of the prosthesis and its relation to the adjacent gingival tissue will be altered. Perhaps this is one reason for gingival impingement, which occurs after the prosthesis has been worn for some time, even though seemingly adequate relief had been provided initially. When a temporary removable partial denture is worn, such abutment teeth have an opportunity to become stabilized under the loading of the temporary restoration, and intrusion will have occurred before making the impression for the master cast. There is sufficient reason to believe that both abutment teeth and supporting ridge tissue are more capable of providing continued support for the removable partial denture when they have been previously conditioned by the wearing of a temporary restoration.

INTERIM RESTORATION DURING TREATMENT

In some instances an existing removable partial denture can be used with modifications as an interim removable partial denture. Such modifications may include relining and adding teeth and clasps to an existing denture. In other instances an existing removable partial denture may be converted to a transitional complete denture for immediate placement while tissue heals and an opposing arch is prepared to receive a removable partial denture. Sometimes a temporary removable partial denture must be made to replace missing anterior teeth in a partially edentulous arch, which are ultimately to be replaced with fixed restorations. On occasion, the anterior portion of the restoration is cut away when the fixed restorations are placed, and leaves the remainder of the denture to be worn while posterior abutment teeth are prepared. Still another type of temporary denture is one in which missing posterior teeth are replaced temporarily with a resin occlusion rim rather than with occluding teeth.

CONDITIONING THE PATIENT FOR WEARING A PROSTHESIS

A temporary restoration may be made to aid the patient in making a transition to complete dentures when the total loss of teeth is inevitable. Such a removable partial denture also may be considered a valid part of the treatment, because the patient is at the same time being conditioned to wear a removable prosthesis. It should be considered strictly a temporary measure that provides the patient with a restoration for the remaining life of the natural teeth when further restorative treatment of those teeth is impractical or economically or technically impossible.

This type of a removable partial denture may be worn for prolonged periods, in the meantime undergoing revision, modification to include additional teeth lost, or relining when such becomes necessary or advisable. The dentist should agree to provide such a removable partial denture only under the following conditions: (1) that a definite fee for the treatment is appropriate and that the fee will depend on the servicing necessary; and (2) that when further wearing of the transitional denture is unwise and jeopardizes the health of the remaining tissue, the transition to complete dentures will proceed.

It is imperative that a distinction is made between temporary restorations and a true removable partial denture service and that the patient be advised of the purposes and limitations of such restorations.

CLINICAL PROCEDURE FOR PLACEMENT

It is important to consider proper fitting of the prosthesis to assure comfortable use during the temporary phase of treatment. Careful attention to a planned use of the teeth for support, stability, and retention without undue stress from gingival tissue contact or improper occlusal loading will help assure more comfortable use.

To assure proper use of the remaining natural teeth, the prosthesis must be completely seated in the arch. Common areas requiring adjustment to ensure complete seating include interproximal extensions, regions where clasps exit from the acrylic-resin base, tissue undercuts (labial undercuts from recent extractions or lingual/retromylohyoid region), and any portion of the prosthesis that lies inferior to the height of contour, especially if bilaterally opposed (Figure 23-3).

Once seated it is important to check that no undue pressure to the marginal gingival region is present. To facilitate this step, and to help with the complete seating requirement, it is possible to have the laboratory block out the marginal gingival region and infrabulge regions to reduce seating problems (Figure 23-4). Infrabulge regions can include lingual and palatal

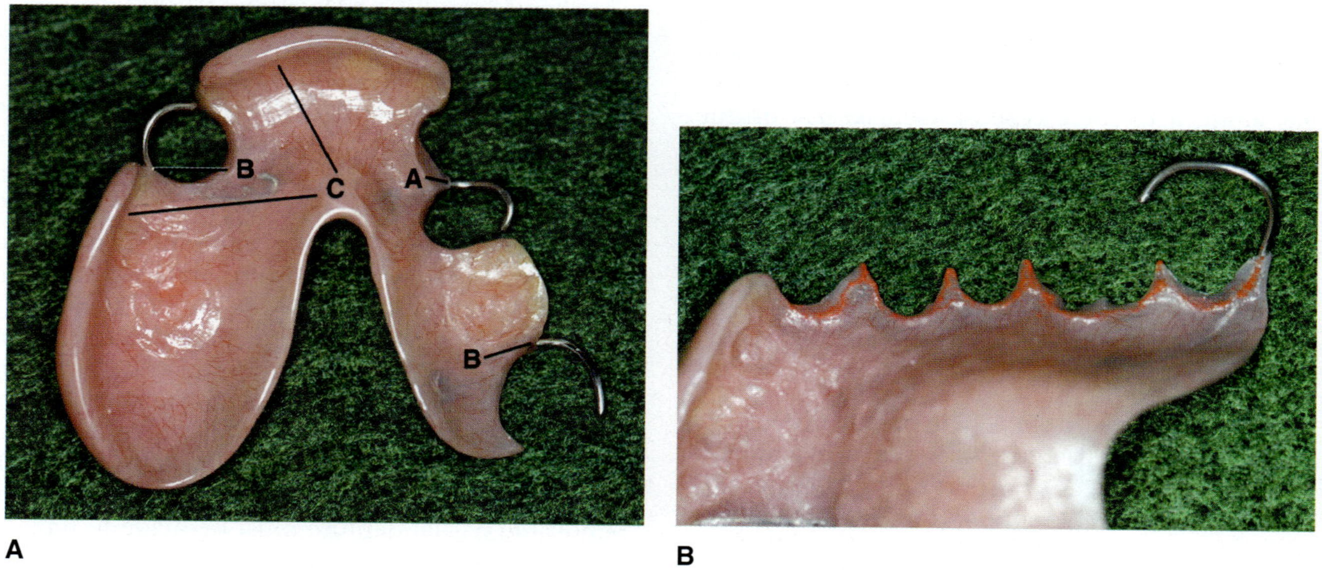

Figure 23-3 **A,** Maxillary temporary removable partial denture. Areas that require adjustment commonly include interproximal extensions *(A)*, region where clasp exits from resin *(B)*, and tissue undercuts of prosthesis extensions *(C)*. **B,** Interproximal tooth extensions and regions where marginal gingiva is crossed by the prosthesis should be carefully adjusted *(outlined in red)*.

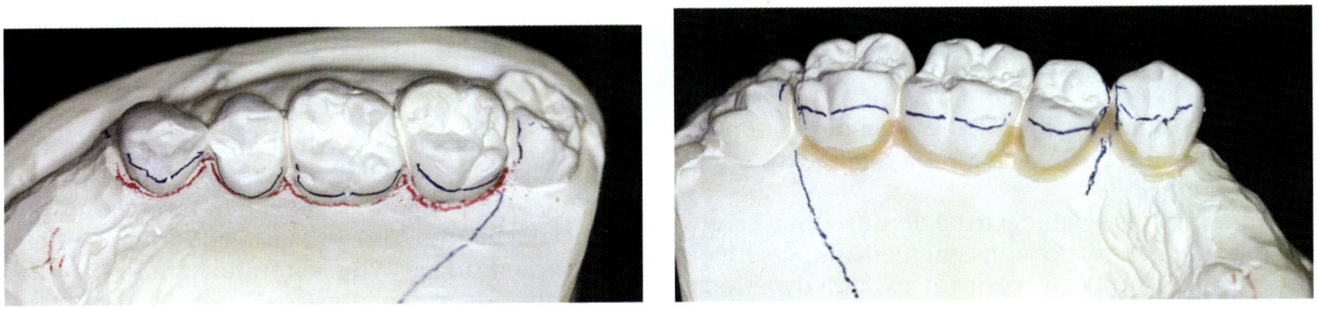

A B

Figure 23-4 A, Maxillary cast with outline of prosthesis design and region at marginal gingival crossing outlined. If the cast is not relieved at the marginal gingiva, the prosthesis should be corrected prior to insertion. B, Cast showing gingival regions relieved with baseplate wax. A duplicate of this cast will provide the necessary relief for use as a processing cast. If interproximal regions have undercuts, these can also be blocked out to allow easier insertion of temporary prosthesis.

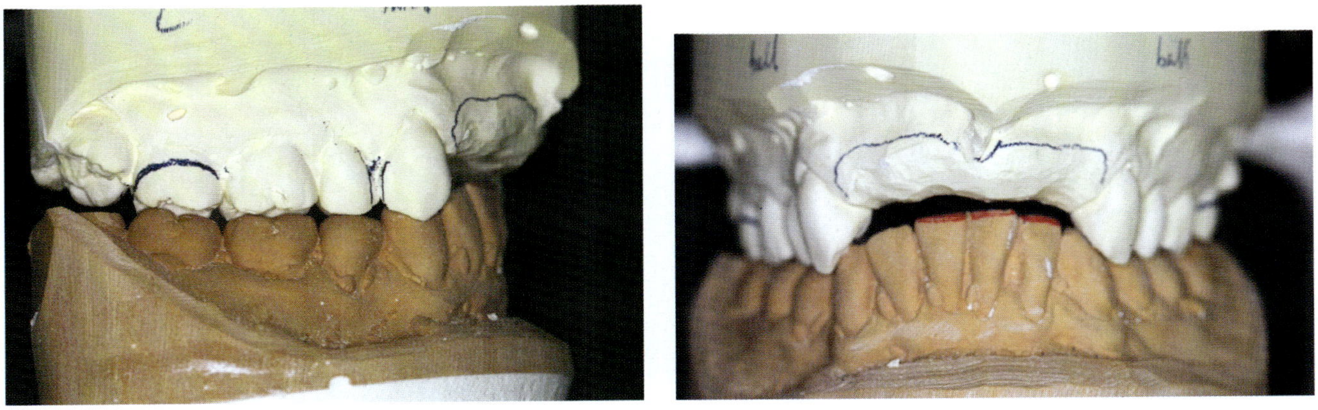

A B

Figure 23-5 A, Evaluation of mounted casts allows a determination of the occlusal impact on maxillary temporary prosthesis clasp selection and placement. Interocclusal space allows placement of a ball clasp distal to the canine and a circumferential clasp from the distal of the second molar, both without occlusal interference if the clasps are carefully contoured. B, Anterior cast modification in anticipation of post-extraction ridge contours for this immediate temporary prosthesis. Diagnosis of the limited space at the anterior region before surgery allows presurgical discussion of the possible need for mandibular incisor modification to improve the temporary and final prosthesis occlusion.

tooth surfaces, and modification space regions. Since temporary prostheses are generally fabricated on unprepared teeth, these regions often require correction. However, if the blockout is not accomplished carefully, the prosthesis may seat easily but it may not be as stable as possible because of insufficient tooth contact. Stability and retention are improved when it is possible to have the prosthesis contact portions of the teeth superior to the height of contour because of the tooth-dictated control of movement.

It is possible to create occlusal imbalance if the lingual/palatal portion of the prosthesis is too bulky. Consequently an opposing cast should be provided to allow placement of clasps and acrylic-resin contours to be provided that do not cause occlusal interference (Figure 23-5). Once fully seated and relieved appropriately, the occlusion should contribute to the remaining natural dentition (as in a definitive prosthesis) and harmonize with natural tooth-dictated function. Typically the prosthesis should not be the sole source of occlusal contact. In such situations the functional forces are concentrated at the acrylic resin to tooth junction and, predictably, a change in orientation occurs allowing tissueward movement and both a change in occlusion and an increase in soft tissue contact.

SELF-ASSESSMENT AIDS

1. Removable partial dentures designed to be used for short intervals are temporary restorations and serve definite purposes. They must not be represented to the patient as other than temporary. True or false?
2. Temporary removable partial dentures may jeopardize the integrity of adjacent teeth and health of supporting tissue if worn for extended periods without supportive care. True or false? Rationalize your answer.
3. Temporary removable partial dentures serve many useful purposes. Two of these are (1) to maintain appearance and (2) to reestablish occlusal relationships. Name the other four purposes.
4. In adult patients the placement of a temporary removable partial denture to maintain a space can prevent undesirable migration and extrusion of adjacent or opposing teeth until definitive treatment can be accomplished. True or false?
5. The use of a temporary removable partial denture as an occlusal splint to reestablish the occlusal relationship for a Kennedy Class I removable partial denture requires broad coverage and functional basing of the tissue-supported bases. What is the best method to achieve functional basing?
6. One of the functions that a temporary removable partial denture provides is to condition teeth and residual ridges. Why is it important to condition teeth and residual ridges?
7. The fabrication of temporary removable partial dentures necessitates that prosthodontic principles not be violated and that procedures be meticulously executed. True or false?
8. Temporary removable partial dentures should, or should not, have occlusal rests provided. Defend your answer.
9. Periodic recalls and assessments are essential during the use of temporary removable partial dentures. Why is this true?

24

REMOVABLE PARTIAL DENTURE CONSIDERATIONS IN MAXILLOFACIAL PROSTHETICS

MAXILLOFACIAL PROSTHETICS

The preceding chapters have dealt with prosthesis considerations for partially edentulous individuals. In these patients the extent of loss includes teeth and a varying degree of residual ridge bone, yet the remaining anatomy of the jaws and adjacent regions is both functionally and physically intact. For these patients the major distinguishing feature impacting removable partial denture design is whether the prosthesis will be tooth-supported or tooth- and tissue-supported.

The maxillofacial patient can experience unique alterations in the normal oral/craniofacial environment, which are the results of surgical resections (Figure 24-1), maxillofacial trauma, congenital defects, developmental anomalies, or neuromuscular disease. In contrast to the above, when removable partial dentures are considered for these individuals, not only are tooth and tissue support considerations important, but the design must also take into account what impact the altered environment will have on prosthesis support, stability, and retention. In general, environmental changes reduce the capacity for residual teeth and tissue to provide optimal cross-arch support, stability, and retention.

As a subspecialty of prosthodontics, maxillofacial prosthetics is concerned with the restoration and/or replacement of the stomatognathic system and associated facial structures with prostheses that may or may not be removed on a regular or elective basis. This chapter discusses important background information related to maxillofacial prostheses and the principles involved in removable partial denture design for the maxillofacial patient.

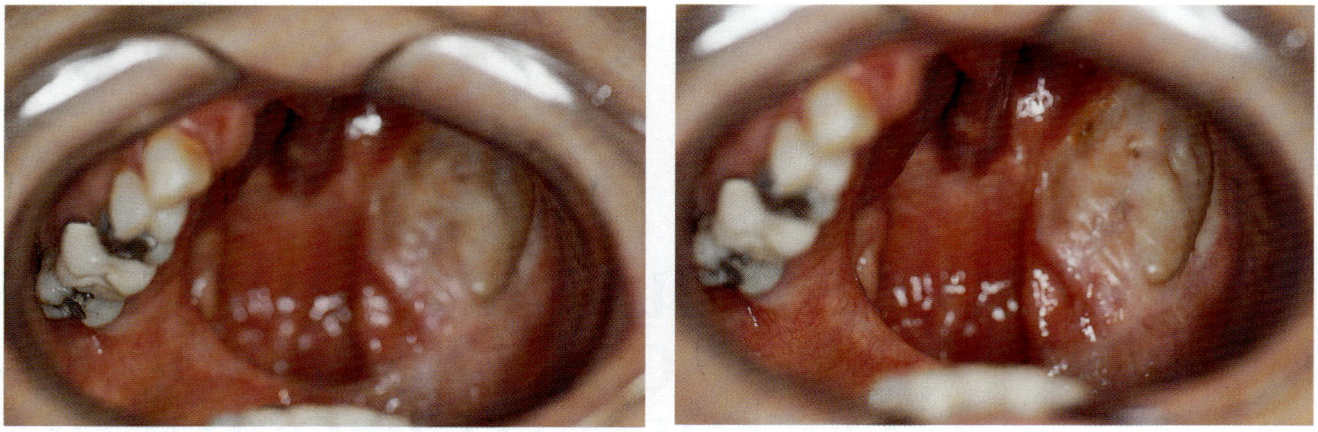

A B

Figure 24-1 A unilateral arrangement of maxillary teeth (**A**), no remaining horizontal hard palate, and a surgical defect, which includes nasal and sinus cavities (**B**). This unique environment, which is the result of a surgical resection, requires careful application of removable prosthodontic principles modified for maxillofacial needs.

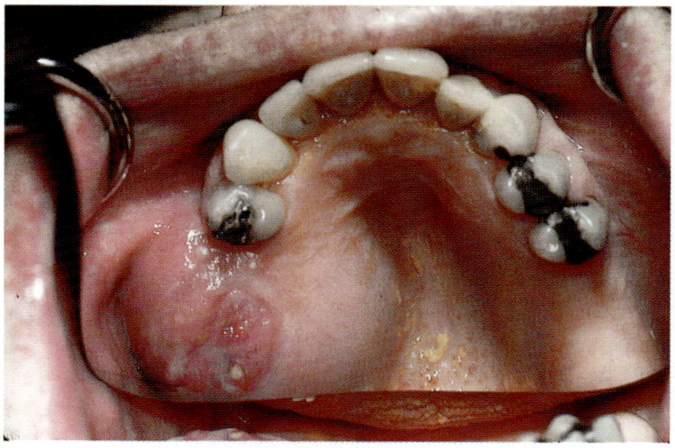

Figure 24-2 Large squamous cell carcinoma involving the maxillary tuberosity region, which will result in an acquired defect following surgical removal.

Maxillofacial Classification

Patients can be categorized by maxillofacial defects that are acquired, congenital, or developmental. Acquired defects include those that are the result of trauma, or disease and its treatment. This could include a soft and/or hard palate defect resulting from removal of a squamous cell carcinoma of the region (Figure 24-2). Congenital defects are typically craniofacial defects present from birth. The most common of these include cleft defects of the palate that can include the premaxillary alveolus. Developmental defects are those defects that occur because of some genetic predisposition that is expressed during growth and development (Figure 24-3). Such a classification order is helpful as patients within each category share similar characteristics (beyond those features specifically related to the prosthesis design), which become part of the total management plan. For example, prosthetic management of an adult who has experienced a maxillectomy procedure can be quite different from management of a patient with an unrepaired cleft palate.

Another helpful way to classify maxillofacial patients is by the type of prosthesis under consideration. Consequently, prostheses are said to be extraoral (cranial or facial replacement) or intraoral (involving the oral cavity); interim (for short periods of time, often perioperative) or definitive (more permanent); and treatment (used as a component of management, such as a splint or stent) prostheses.

TIMING OF DENTAL AND MAXILLOFACIAL PROSTHETIC CARE FOR ACQUIRED DEFECTS

Acquired defects are the most common maxillofacial defects managed by using removable prostheses. A conceptual framework for the timing of dental/oral care that best emphasizes the initial important surgical requirements, followed later by the important prosthetic requirements, is helpful to consider regarding the coordination of care for patients with acquired defects. Such a framework considers preoperative and intraoperative interim care and definitive care. Though it may initially seem unrelated, it is included in this discussion of removable partial dentures for maxillofacial applications because of the important impact decisions made at all stages of management can have on prosthesis function and patient outcomes.

Preoperative and Intraoperative Care

The planning of prosthetic treatment for acquired oral defects should begin before surgery. For the

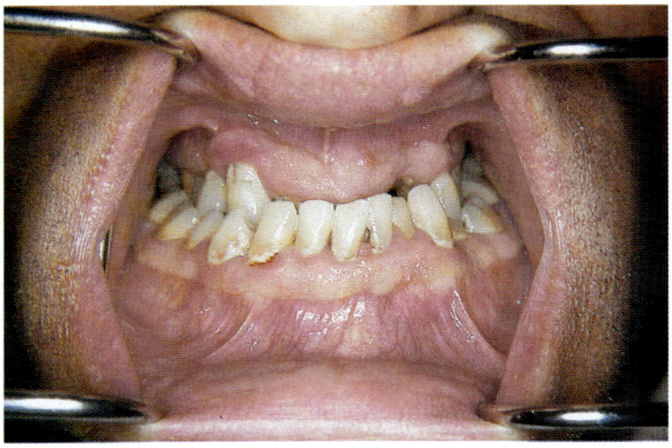

A

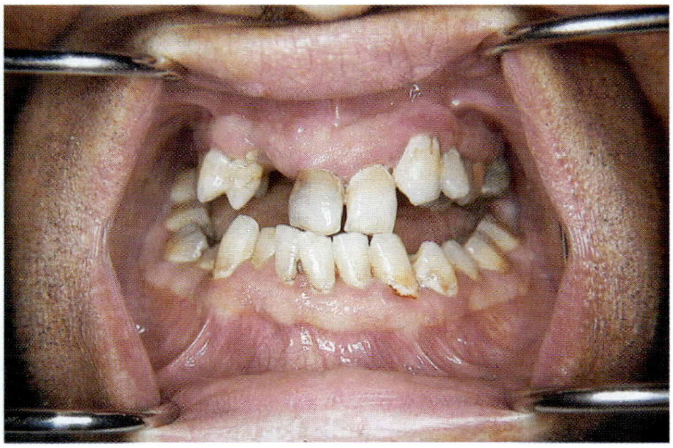

B

Figure 24-3 A functional jaw position developed because of a combination of tooth loss and growth discrepancy. This developmental defect is illustrated by a protruded and overclosed mandibular position (**A**), which has created a significantly irregular maxillary occlusal plane (**B**).

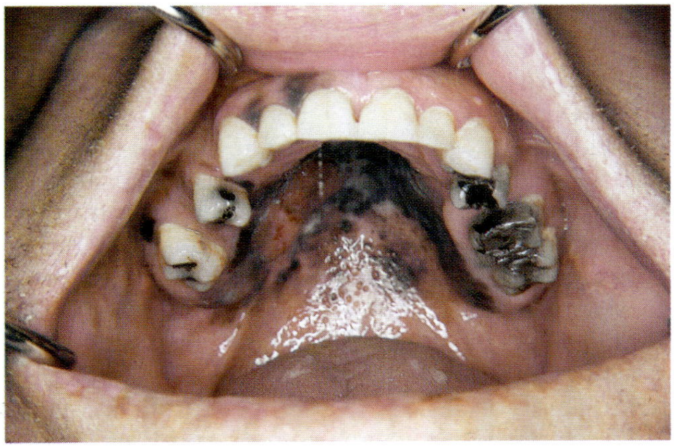

Figure 24-4 Presurgical presentation of a patient with a maxillary malignant melanoma. The benefits of having such a visit before surgery are both psychological and functional. The psychological benefits include the chance to discuss the functional deficits associated with the anticipated surgical procedure and to describe how and to what extent the stages of prosthetic management will address them. The functional benefit from a prosthesis standpoint is that strategically important teeth, for either definitive and/or interim prosthesis use, can be discussed with the surgical team and treatment planned for preservation.

patient facing head and neck surgery, consideration should be given to dental needs that will improve the immediate postoperative course. Consequently the prosthodontist who will help with management of the patient's care should see the patient before surgery (Figure 24-4). The dental objectives of the preoperative and intraoperative care stage are to remove potential dental postoperative complications, to plan for the subsequent prosthetic treatment, and to make recommendations for surgical site preparation that improve structural integrity. Important patient benefits of such a preoperative consultation include the opportunity to develop the patient-clinician relationship, to discuss the functional deficits associated with the anticipated surgical procedure, and to describe how and to what extent the stages of prosthetic management will address them. The benefit from a prosthesis standpoint is that strategically important teeth, for either definitive and/or interim prosthesis use, can be discussed with the surgical team and treatment planned for preservation.

The immediate postoperative period will be significantly challenging to the patient. If preexisting dental disease is severe enough to potentially create symptoms during the immediate postoperative period, treatment should be provided to remove such a complication. Large carious lesions, which could create pain, can be temporarily restored by endodontic therapy if they offer some advantage to postoperative prosthetic function. Teeth exhibiting acute periodontal disease (such as acute necrotizing ulcerative gingivitis) should be treated, as should any periodontal condition that could potentially cause postoperative pain because of excessive mobility or oral infection. Any tooth deemed nonrestorable because of advanced caries or periodontal disease, and not critical for temporary use during the interim care period following temporary treatment, should be removed before, or at the time of, surgical resection. Teeth that may appear to have a limited long-term prognosis may significantly enhance prosthetic service during the initial postsurgical period and should be maintained until the initiation of definitive care.

Impressions are made of the maxillary and mandibular arches to provide a record of existing conditions and occlusion to allow fabrication of immediate or interim prostheses (Figure 24-5) and

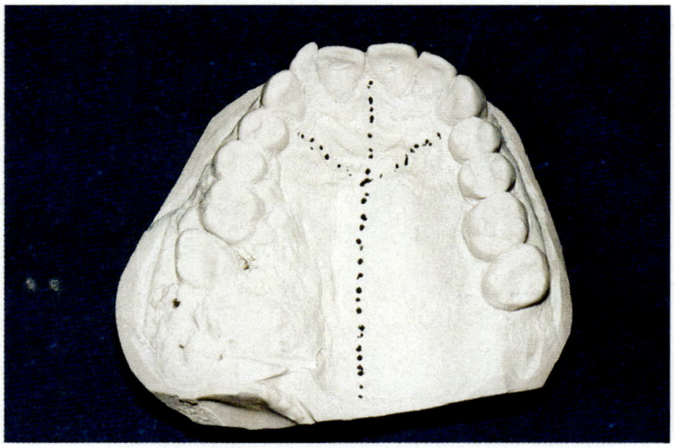

A

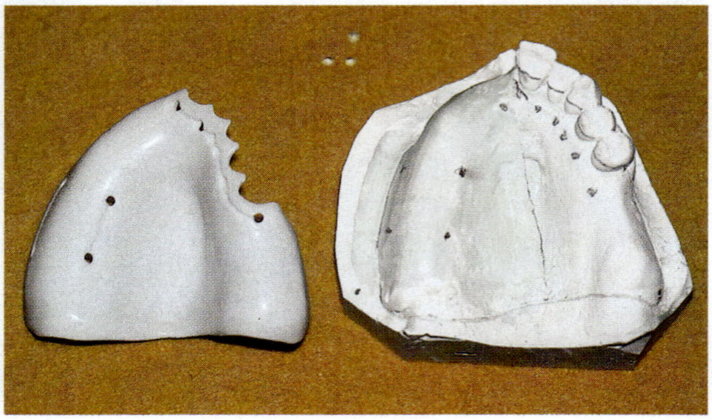

B

Figure 24-5 **A,** A maxillary cast of the presurgical oral condition, which allows consultation with the surgeon regarding resection margins and the benefit of preservation of teeth. **B,** Another maxillary cast altered, following consultation with the head and neck surgeon, to allow fabrication of a surgical stent. Perforations are made to allow fixation to both the remaining teeth and superior anatomic regions using wires.

to assess the need for both immediate and delayed modification of the teeth or adjacent structures to optimize prosthetic care. It is important at this stage to begin planning for the definitive prosthesis because the greatest impact on the success of the maxillofacial prosthesis stems from the integrity of the remaining teeth and surrounding structures.

Interim Care

The major emphasis during this stage of care is the surgical (and adjunctive) management needs of the patient. In today's environment of appropriately aggressive mandibular surgical reconstruction, mandibular discontinuity defects are seldom a surgical outcome. When discontinuity defects in the mandible result following surgery, interim prosthetic care is not indicated and the discussion will be directed to the maxillary defect.

The typical maxillary acquired defect results in oral communication with the nose and/or maxillary sinus, though the composition of the surgical defect may vary widely (Figure 24-6). This creates physiological and functional deficiencies in mastication, deglutition, and speech. Such defects have a negative impact on the psychological disposition of patients, especially if the defect also affects cosmetic appearance. The major deficiencies directly addressed by prosthetic management at this interim care time are deglutition and speech. This immediate postsurgical time is very challenging for the patient, and it is important that they have been mentally prepared for it during the preoperative period. However, even with preliminary discussion, the impact of the surgery is often very distressing. An initial focus on improvement in swallowing and speech with the interim prosthesis can help boost the rehabilitation process significantly.

The patient is counseled that chewing on the defect side is not allowed because of the effect on prosthesis movement. The objective of this interim obturator prosthesis is to separate the oral and nasal cavities by obturating the communication. Such obturator prostheses most commonly refer to obturation of a hard palatal defect but conceptually can be considered the same for soft palatal defects at this stage of management. This is because both attempt to artificially block the free transfer of speech sounds and food/liquids between the oral and nasal cavities. The advantages of having the ability to take nourishment by mouth without nasal reflux (allowing for nasogastric tube removal) and to communicate with family members are a significant component of early prosthetic management. How immediately such care should be provided is dependent on a number of factors.

A prosthesis can be provided at surgery (see Figure 24-5, *B*). Such a surgical obturator prosthesis is placed at the time of surgical access closure and serves to control the surgical dressing and split-thickness skin graft during the immediate postsurgical period. Such prostheses are best stabilized by appropriate wiring to remaining teeth, alveolar bone, or suspended from superior skeletal structures. For some patients who have teeth remaining, such an immediate surgical prosthesis could be retained by wires in the prosthesis that engage undercuts on the teeth and would be removable; however, the ability to control the surgical dressing may be less predictable with such an approach. Immediate placement of a prosthesis has been suggested to improve patient acceptance of the surgical defect, though

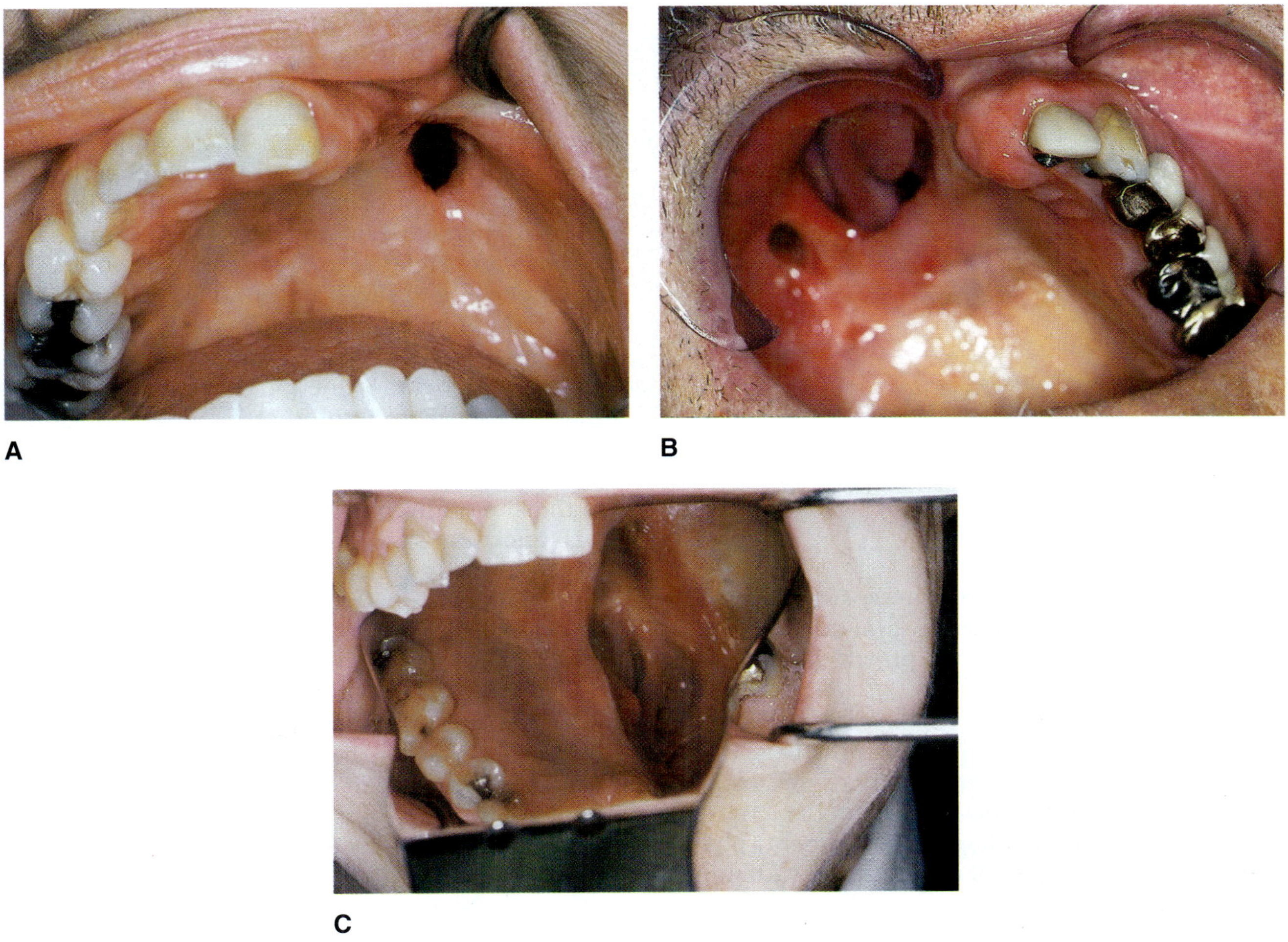

Figure 24-6 Maxillary defects. **A,** A resection that resulted in a small communication with the sinus, some hard palate remaining, and adjacent mucosa typical of the oral cavity. **B,** A resection that did not follow classic maxillectomy technique; however, the midline resection was made through the socket of tooth No. 9, preserving its alveolar housing. **C,** A resection along the palatal midline that did not preserve oral mucosa at the resection margin, which allows chronic ulceration at this point of prosthesis fulcrum. Notice the split-thickness skin graft in the superior-lateral region. Engagement of this region can provide support to the obturator extension, minimizing movement with function.

no measure of this psychological impact has been shown, and offers greater assurance of adequate nourishment by mouth—potentially precluding the use of a nasogastric tube.

It may be preferable to stabilize the surgical dressing by suturing a sponge bolster to provide stabilization to the split-thickness skin graft. Following the primary healing stage, the sponge and packing (or the immediate prosthesis if used) are removed by the surgeon and an interim obturator prosthesis can be placed (Figure 24-7). For the patient who has been provided with bolster obturation, the presurgical prosthodontic evaluation is very important to ensure that the patient is prepared for the transition from bolster to prosthesis and to ensure that plans for the prosthesis are made, especially if an interim prosthesis is to be fabricated. Interim prostheses are wire-retained resin prostheses that generally do not have teeth initially but may be modified with the addition of teeth after an initial period of accommodation (Figure 24-8).

When surgical defects become large, as in a near total maxillectomy defect, prosthesis support, stability, and retention are not likely to be satisfactory unless extension into the defect can be accomplished. When teeth remain, the impact of the defect size is somewhat lessened. But when the remaining teeth are few or located unilaterally in a straight line (see Figure 24-1), the mechanical advantage for prosthesis stability is less. The ability of the defect tissue to offer the needed mechanical characteristics to the interim prosthesis is unpredictable at best.

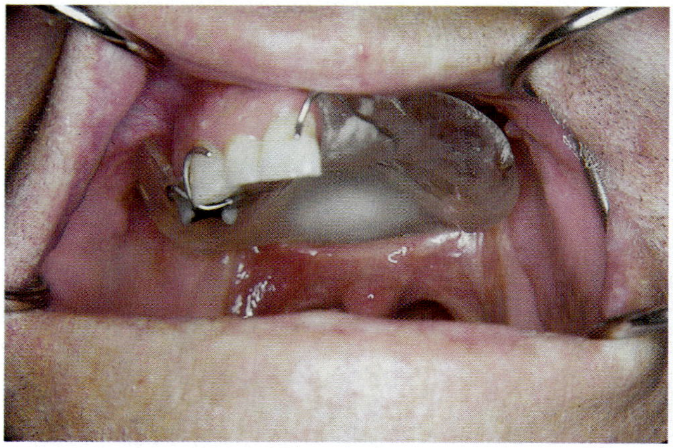

Figure 24-7 An interim obturator prosthesis fabricated of resin, retained by wires, and provided following surgical pack removal.

It is this patient that benefits the most from a well-planned surgery that preserves oral and defective anatomy to the advantage of the prosthesis.

Potential Complications

The duration for the interim phase of prosthetic management can be a period of three or more months. The primary objective is to allow the patient to pass from an active surgical (and adjunctive treatment) phase to an observational phase of management with minimal complications. During the transition, the patient recovers from the systemic effects of the treatment, deals with the psychological impact of the defect using his or her own coping strategy, and becomes more aware of the functional deficits associated with the surgical defect (s). Minimizing potential complications during the transition, which includes preparing the patient for those anticipated to occur, facilitates the process for the patient and family. Common interim prosthetic complications relate to tissue trauma and the associated discomfort; inadequate retention (looseness) of the maxillary prosthesis; incomplete obturation with leakage of air, food, and liquid around the obturator portion of the prosthesis; and the tissue effects of chemotherapy and radiation therapy.

Discomfort related to the use of interim prostheses can be due to surgical wound healing dynamics, defect conditions, mucosal effects of adjunctive treatment, and/or prosthetic fit. Common areas of surgical wound pain include junctions of oral and lip/cheek mucosa, especially at the anterior alveolar region for maxillectomy patients. The lateral scar band produced when the skin graft heals to the oral mucosa can also be the site of discomfort in some patients. When a split-thickness skin graft is not placed, discomfort caused by the prosthesis fit within the defect can be a consistent and long-term problem. The hard palate surgical margin when not covered with surgically reflected oral mucosa will most often be covered by nasal epithelium, which is also very prone to discomfort. Alveolar bone cuts that have not been rounded will perforate the oral mucosa and be painful whether a prosthesis is worn or not. This is most frequently a finding for mandibular resection superior alveolar margins when the reconstruction has restored the lower and labial contour to the mandible, but the intraoral mucosa at the superior surface is under tension because of a difference in height.

The prosthesis can create discomfort from excessive static pressure from the internal surfaces or from overextension into the vestibular tissue. The prosthesis can also create discomfort caused by functional movement associated with swallowing and speech.

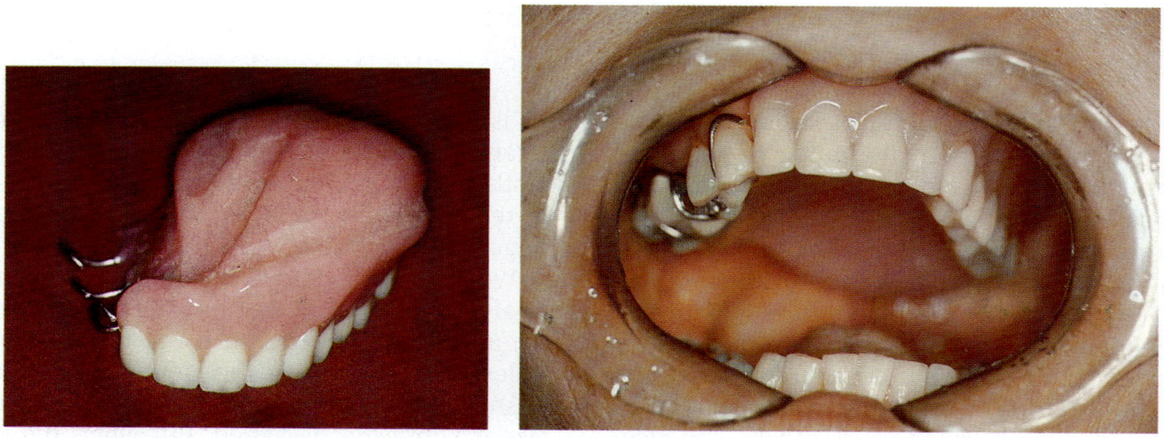

A B

Figure 24-8 **A** and **B,** An interim obturator prosthesis fabricated of resin, retained by wires, and including artificial teeth for cosmesis during an extended period of recovery. The superior and lateral surfaces may need modification to improve stability and retention as the surgical site matures and allows more aggressive engagement.

As discussed previously, prosthesis movement is dependent on the quality of the supporting structures. Teeth offer the best support followed by firm edentulous ridges and lastly, surgical defect structures. The tongue, opposing dentition, and cheek/lips place force on the prosthesis that must be resisted over a large area to prevent movement. Since the defect is least likely to be able to resist movement, the relative size and structural integrity of the defect compared with the remaining teeth and/or edentulous ridge determine the potential prosthesis movement and most impact the discomfort related with such movement.

When teeth are available (and especially if located both close to and far away from the defect), retention is enhanced by engaging them with prosthetic clasps. Clasp retention is the most efficient means for effectively resisting dislodgment. The clasps will require periodic adjustment to maintain their effectiveness as the movement of the prosthesis flexes the clasps beyond their elastic recovery capacity. For edentulous patients, since the surgical defect allows communication between cavities, the fitting surface of the prosthesis can no longer create a closed environment to develop a seal for resisting dislodgment. Consequently, during the interim phase when complete engagement of the defect is not possible because of tissue sensitivity, the careful use of denture adhesives is required to facilitate retention. The patient should be instructed that adhesives can alter the prosthesis fit and disrupt the close adaptation of the prosthesis to the remaining tissue. Also, used adhesive must be removed before reapplying new adhesive to maintain fit and hygiene. Also related to retention is the inability to completely place the prosthesis, which for maxillectomy patients can be due to contracture of the scar band. When the maxillary resection leaves the cheek unsupported by bone, the prosthesis provides the necessary support for wound maturation. If the patient removes the interim obturator prosthesis for a period sufficient to allow contraction, the prosthesis will be more difficult to place. Once placed, however, the scar band will relax and subsequent removal and placement will be more easily accomplished. The discomfort associated with this phenomenon is mostly due to patient anxiety and can be effectively addressed by reassuring the patient that this is an easily handled complication.

During the immediate postoperative healing stage, the surgical defect will undergo a change in dimension that impacts the prosthesis fit and seal. If space is created with the change, speech will be altered (increase in nasality) and nasal reflux with swallowing will occur. The interim prosthesis is made of easily adjustable material to allow accommodation for such changes. The most common manner of adjustment is through the use of temporary resilient denture lining materials, which offer the ability to mold to the tissue directly and reduce the mechanical effects of movement by virtue of its viscoelastic nature. Leakage can occur quite easily when swallowing unless the patient follows certain instructions. Since the prosthesis cannot offer a water-tight seal that matches the presurgical state, patients will be instructed not to swallow large quantities at one time and to hold their heads horizontal when swallowing. When the head posture is forward, as in taking soup from a spoon, leakage easily occurs around the obturator component of a prosthesis. Another condition that presents difficulty in controlling leakage on swallowing is the midline soft palatal resection. The functional movement of the remaining soft palate is often very difficult to retain with a prosthesis. It is also difficult to provide an adequate seal during the interim prosthesis stage.

When combination treatment is prescribed for the patient, it is commonly provided during the postsurgical phase when the patient is using an interim prosthesis. The major intraoral complication associated with both radiation therapy and chemotherapy, and that impacts interim prosthetic service, is mucositis. A careful balance between comfort and adequate fit for speech and swallowing needs must be determined with input from the patient. If prosthesis adjustment can offer relief to ensure completion of treatment and the patient understands the impact adjustment may have on speech and swallowing, then it should be accomplished.

The long-term effects of radiation therapy, especially radiation-induced xerostomia and capillary bed changes (obliterative endarteritis) within the mandible, present a potentially significant threat to any remaining dentition and to the development of osteoradionecrosis. During the interim prosthesis stage, the patient will begin to notice the xerostomic effects, which include development of thick, ropy saliva that makes swallowing more difficult, and an increase in discomfort associated with removable prostheses.

Defect and Oral Hygiene

Following surgical pack removal, the defect site will mature with time and exposure to the external environment. Initial loss of incompletely consolidated skin graft, mucous secretions mixed with blood, and residual food debris within the cavity are common oral findings for the patient with a maxillary defect. These cause concern for patients who are unprepared and unfamiliar with these new oral findings. As they become more familiar with the surgical defect, they should be encouraged to clean the defect of food debris and mucous secretions routinely. Defect hygiene will allow timelier healing and improve the ability to adequately fit a prosthesis. Common defect hygiene practices are either lavage procedures, which include rinsing of the defect during normal showering, rinsing of the defect using a bulb syringe or a modified oral irrigating device (modified to provide a multiple orifice "shower" effect), or manual cleaning procedures, such as the use of a sponge-handled cleaning aid. Frequently, dried mucous secretions are difficult to remove and require adequate hydration before mechanical removal.

Following surgical pack removal, the patient may be reluctant to begin oral hygiene practices because of oral discomfort. As the patient uses the interim prosthesis, which requires daily removal and cleaning at a minimum, they will realize the need for and benefit to normal oral hygiene practices because of improved prosthesis fit and tolerance. When teeth are remaining, it is important to the success of long-term prosthetic care to maintain a high level of oral hygiene. This is more critical for patients who exhibit xerostomia and have an increased risk of caries. For these patients a daily application of fluoride in custom-formed carriers is prescribed along with frequent professional cleanings. The successful use of maxillofacial prostheses is enhanced greatly by the support provided by natural teeth. Consequently, during the interim prosthetic period, periodontal management procedures are begun in anticipation of the definitive treatment to allow a smooth transition from the interim to definitive prosthetic stages.

Definitive Care

Definitive prosthetic management can be initiated when the active treatment phase has been completed and continue until the defect tissue has matured sufficiently to tolerate more aggressive manipulation and obturation. This phase can be considered a transition for the patient-physician relationship, where the primary emphasis shifts from active treatment to observation. The primary emphasis from the patient's standpoint shifts to the prosthetic management, and the goals and design of the prosthesis differ from the interim prosthesis (Figure 24-9). However, for some patients, more definitive prostheses are delayed because of general health concerns, questionable tumor prognosis or control, or when the patient has failed to reach a level of oral and/or defect hygiene that warrants more sophisticated treatment. Though this phase of management can be considered elective, without definitive prostheses patients are not afforded the opportunity for complete rehabilitation. It is the extended use of temporary prostheses beyond their serviceable life span that has given a poor impression of prosthetic service to many surgeons and patients. Every opportunity should be provided to the patient for the most complete rehabilitation possible, and this necessitates consideration of more definitive prostheses.

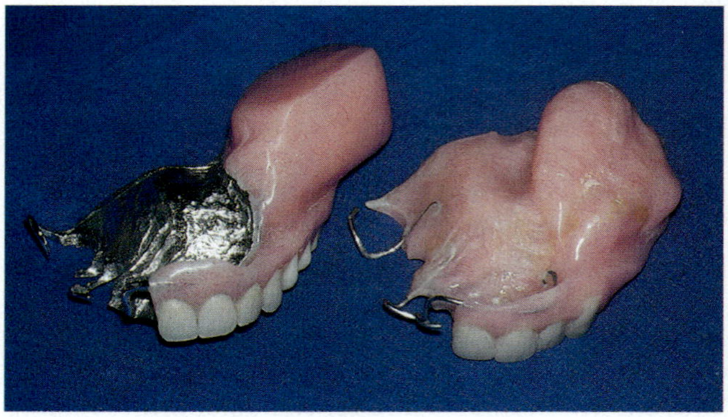

Figure 24-9 A definitive *(left)* and interim *(right)* obturator prosthesis contrasting the materials used and the obturator bulb contour. Clasp retention is more stabilizing with the definitive prosthesis because of the cast half-round clasp configuration, the use of embrasure clasps, and the opportunity for guide plane use. Also, since the surgical site is more mature, prosthesis extension into this region to augment support, stability, and retention when necessary is possible.

From the previous discussion regarding removable prosthetic physiology, the inability of these static artificial replacements to mimic their natural counterparts results in less than ideal functional measures. Factors related to the structural integrity of the surgical defect and associated reconstructions as they impact this already compromised functional capacity are important considerations, especially when few teeth remain. As stated previously, the fact that control of removable maxillofacial prostheses has a large skilled performance requirement of patients suggests that oral and defect structures adjacent to the prostheses are important for successful performance. This is crucial to the understanding of the impact postsurgical defect characteristics and soft tissue reconstructions have on maxillofacial prosthesis management. The reason for this is twofold: (1) the opportunity for maximal prosthetic benefit necessitates consideration of surgical site characteristics that are separate from classic tumor control approaches, and (2) the ability of the patient to biomechanically control large removable prostheses following surgery may be notably hindered by surgical closure/reconstruction options. Surgical outcomes that can improve prosthetic function without adversely effecting tumor control should be considered and will be described for the more common surgical defects and associated prostheses.

INTRAORAL PROSTHESES DESIGN CONSIDERATIONS

Maxillofacial prosthetics is largely a removable prosthetic discipline, with the exception of dental implant retained–prostheses for some applications.

For maxillofacial reconstruction with removable partial denture prostheses, typical goals of treatment are a well-supported, stable, retentive prosthesis that is acceptable in appearance and exhibits minimal movement under function, thereby preserving the maximum amount of supporting tissue. A strategy for achieving these goals includes maximum coverage of the edentulous ridge within the movement capacity of the muscular attachments, maximal engagement of the remaining teeth to help control retention and movement under function, and placement of artificial teeth to facilitate maintenance of this prescribed tooth/tissue contact during normal functional contacts. Maintaining these basic concepts within an otherwise normal anatomic environment (relative to food control and deglutition) has provided reasonable success for patients requiring replacement of missing teeth. The challenges faced in doing so for removable maxillofacial prostheses are quite different.

Normal resistance to functional loads is achieved by the highly sophisticated periodontal attachment of the natural dentition, which provides support and stability to teeth. When the dentition is partially depleted and replaced by prostheses that are tooth-supported, the support and stability of the replacement teeth remain to be provided by the natural attachment. When tooth loss includes several posterior teeth, replacements are placed over the residual edentulous ridge and the prosthesis receives support and stability from both teeth and mucosa. When all the teeth are lost, the support and stability are totally provided by the mucosa covering the residual edentulous ridges. Finally, when surgical removal of tumors results in tooth and supporting structure loss, the support and stability are provided by combinations of remaining teeth and/or residual ridges and areas within the surgical defect. For both partial and complete tissue-supported prostheses, the mechanism of functional load support—as provided by the mucosa—is unsuited to the task from a biological standpoint. Given this understanding, when a maxillofacial prosthesis is required to involve a surgical defect for support and stability, it is obvious that the environment within the surgical defect is even less suited to the task.

SURGICAL PRESERVATION FOR PROSTHESIS BENEFIT

Maxillary Defects

Surgical outcomes that impact prosthetic success can be considered as either those that impact the amount of maxillary structures removed (Figure 24-10) and/or those that impact the structural integrity and quality of the defect. For surgical defects of the hard and/or soft palate, the primary prosthetic objectives are restoration of the physical separation of the oral and nasal cavities in a manner that restores mastication, deglutition, speech, and facial contour to as near a normal state as possible. The typical prostheses used to achieve these objectives include the obturator prosthesis (Figure 24-11, *A* and *B*), typically referring to prostheses that obturate defects within the bony palate, and the speech aid prosthesis (Figure 24-11, *C* and *D*), which typically refers to prostheses that restore palatopharyngeal function for defects of the soft palate.

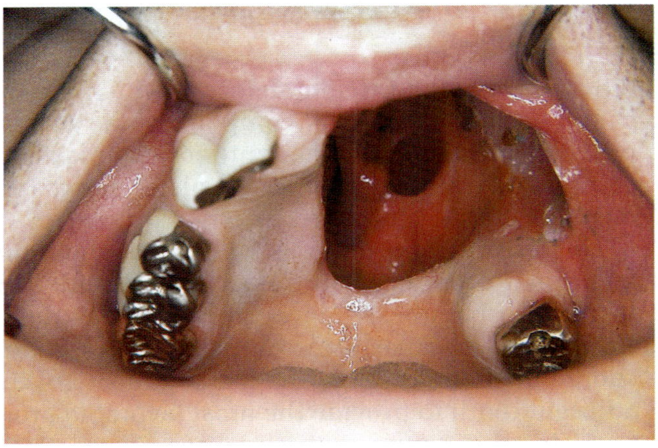

A

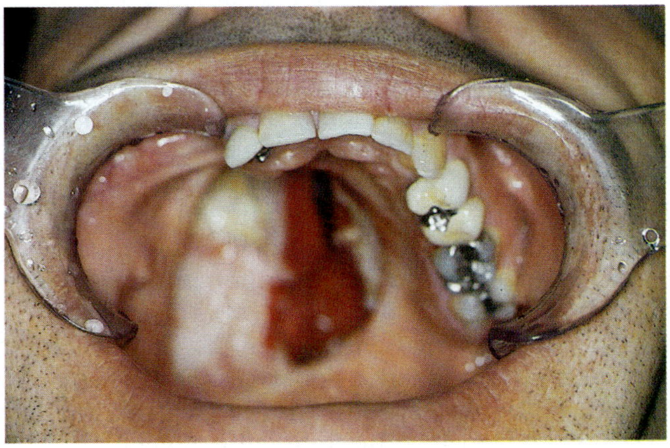

B

Figure 24-10 **A,** A maxillary defect in which a tooth distal to the resection was maintained. The tooth will significantly stabilize the prosthesis by preventing movement of the obturator bulb into the defect at the distal resection margin. **B,** A maxillary defect that demonstrates preservation of the anterior arch curvature, providing increased stability through a tripod effect. Also evident is the use of a split-thickness skin graft in the superior-lateral region, which improves the opportunity for useful support.

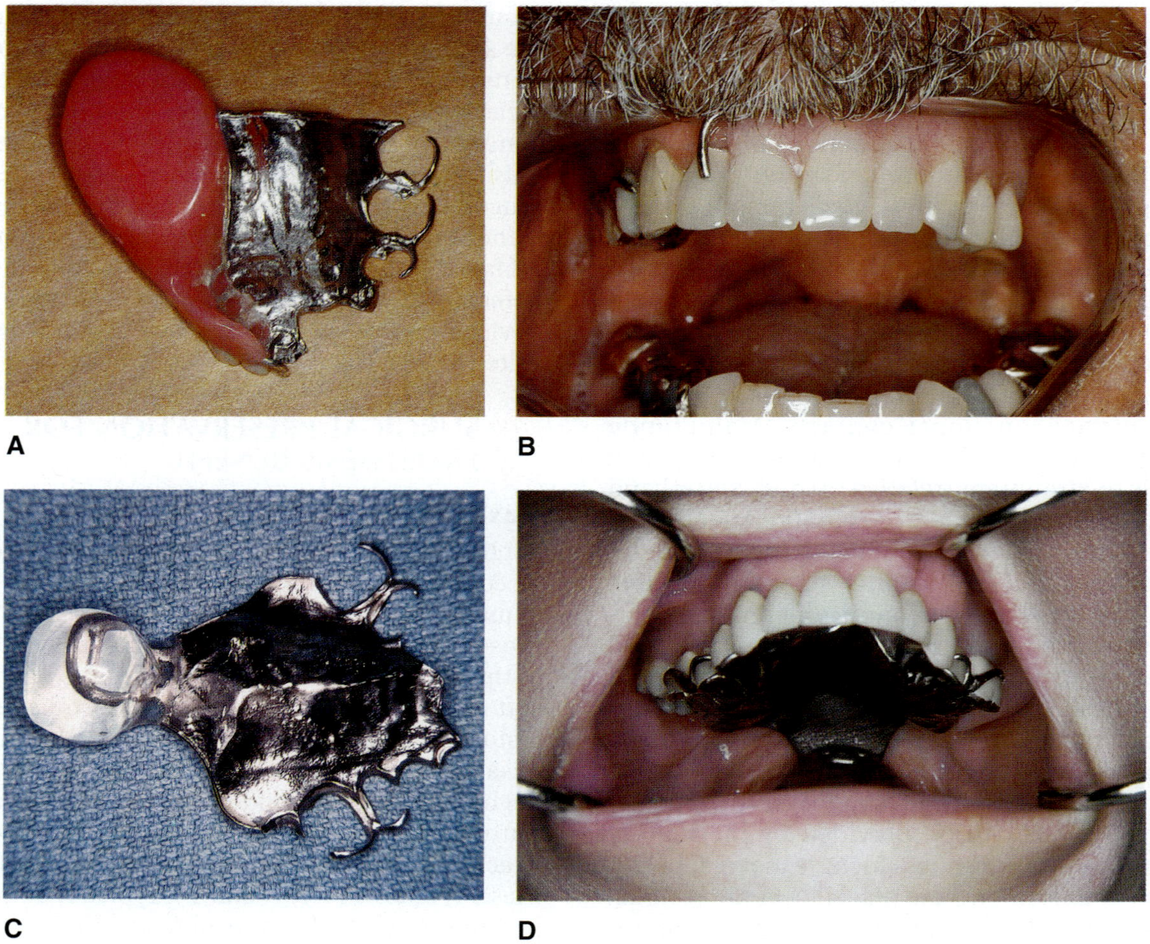

Figure 24-11 **A,** Superior view of an obturator prosthesis demonstrating the cast framework, three posterior cast half-round clasps and an anterior I-bar clasp, and a superior obturator surface contoured to encourage secretions to flow posteriorly. **B,** The same prosthesis seated intraorally. **C,** A speech aid prosthesis with posterior retention and anterior indirect retention, and a resin speech bulb. **D,** The same prosthesis showing bilateral embrasure clasps and obturation of the palatopharyngeal defect.

Current preoperative diagnostic procedures have improved the ability to discern the location and regional bone involvement of tumors of the maxilla and associated paranasal sinuses. Relative to prosthetically important surgical modifications, if it can be determined that tumor control does not require a classic radical maxillectomy approach or that the inferior sinus floor, hard palate, and alveolus are uninvolved, preservation of as much hard palate, alveolar bone, and teeth as possible should be considered. Tooth preservation has the greatest impact on success because of the stabilizing effect on prosthetic movement. When teeth can be retained in the premaxilla for more posterior tumors, or in the posterior molar region for more anterior tumors, control of prosthesis movement is more easily accomplished and prosthetic success can be considerably improved (see Figure 24-10). Since the classic midline maxillectomy defect is significantly more debilitating for the average patient than a defect in which preservation of the premaxillary component was accomplished, inclusion of the anterior premaxillary component should be an individual decision based on tumor control and classic resection technique.

For resections in patients with teeth, the tooth adjacent to the defect is subjected to significant force from prosthesis movement. When planning the surgical alveolar ostectomy cut, the resection should be made through the extraction site of the adjacent tooth to provide the most favorable prognosis for this supportive tooth (see Figure 24-6). This procedure ensures adequate alveolar support to the adjacent tooth, which is a critical tooth for prosthesis success, and improves the tooth's prognosis for long-term survival. The midline of the hard palate is a common area of removable prosthesis pressure because of the movement of the prosthesis into the defect under functional forces of swallowing and mastication. To provide the best surgical preparation for this area, when the hard palate is resected, the vertical surface of the bone cut should be covered with an advancement flap of palatal mucosa to provide a firm and resistant mucosal covering to this region, where the prosthesis can notably act as a fulcrum.

The soft palate owes its normal function to the bilateral sling nature of the musculature, which provides the shape and movement capacity specific for speech and deglutition requirements. When this is altered because of surgery, there appears to be a variable response in the ability to continue to provide palatopharyngeal competence based on the amount of continuous band of posterior tissue remaining. Often an insufficient band of palatal tissue fails to provide palatopharyngeal competence and hinders the ability of prosthetic management for the problem. To serve as a guide for decision making in surgery, it has been suggested that if the required resection leaves less than one third of the posterior aspect of the soft palate, the entire soft palate should be removed. The exception to this would be the edentulous patient who is undergoing a radical maxillectomy. Without teeth to provide the necessary retention to one side of a prosthesis, the patient benefits from the ability to place the prosthesis above the posterior soft tissue band for retention (Figure 24-12).

The preparation of the maxillary surgical site can improve prosthesis tolerance through the use of a split-thickness skin graft (see Figure 24-1). Lining the reflected cheek flap and posterior denuded structures with a graft improves the tissue response by decreasing the pain associated with functional contact often seen when this surface is left to heal secondarily. If the posterior structures, pterygoid plates, or anterior temporal bone can provide a firm supportive base for the prosthesis, a skin graft covering is extremely helpful. Laterally the junction of the skin and oral mucosa creates a scar contracture, which provides a natural retentive region for the obturator portion of the prosthesis. Careful attention is given to this region in fabricating a prosthesis to maximize the support, stability, and retention of the prosthesis.

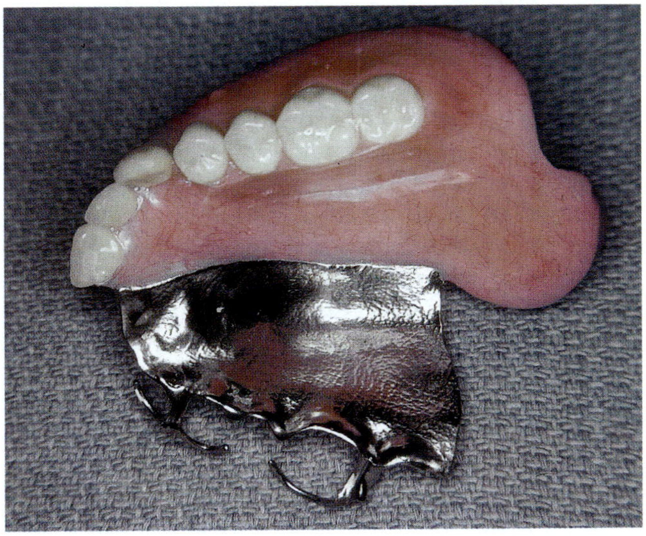

Figure 24-12 A maxillary obturator prosthesis demonstrating a distal extension, which engages a soft palatal remnant for added retention.

In general the need to extend a prosthesis into the defect is greater for edentulous patients than for patients with teeth. When teeth remain, they are used to a greater extent to stabilize and retain the obturator component of the prosthesis, and the defect region is not required for such objectives. However, all patients with maxillary defects should have access to the lateral-posterior region of the defect sufficient to seal the defect at a minimum. In the edentulous patient, for maximal ability to obturate a maxillary defect there must be access to the regions superior to the defect opening. Nasal turbinates and mucosal connections that do not allow full extension into the necessary retentive and supportive areas of the defect compromise function. The function of turbinates in the newly externalized environment is not beneficial to breathed air humidification or warming, and consequently may not warrant preservation.

Surgical reconstruction of maxillary defects should be undertaken when restoration of the functional goals of speech, deglutition, and mastication are better served by such procedures. To surgically reconstruct a maxillary hard palatal defect in a manner that provides separation of the oral and nasal cavities without consideration for oral space requirements for speech, or for the supportive requirements of replacement teeth, is not only incomplete management but can preclude subsequent prosthetic management. When surgical defects are 3 cm or less and can be reconstructed to normal contours without compromising adjacent tissue function, surgical management is an appropriate consideration. Larger defects are very difficult to surgically reconstruct, and without careful planning for subsequent functional needs, could create an environment incapable of supporting a prosthesis. For partial soft palatal reconstructions, it is very difficult to provide for functional tissue replacement without compromising palatal function. In light of this unpredictability, the predictable prosthetic management of such defects is most often the treatment of choice.

Mandibular Defects

The functions of mastication, deglutition, speech, and oral competence (saliva control) are possible through coordinated efforts of separate anatomic regions, which include the oral sphincter, alveololingual and buccal sulci, alveolar ridges, floor of mouth, mobile tongue, base of tongue, tonsillar pillars, soft palate, hard palate, and buccal mucosa. The more regions that are involved in a surgical procedure, the greater the demand on the surgical reconstructive efforts. When the mandible is also involved, the complexity of the reconstructive procedure is dependent on the location and amount of mandible to be included in the resection and the decision to maintain continuity with normal mandibular position and contour (Figure 24-13). For disease involving the functional anatomy around the mandible, surgical outcomes that impact prosthetic success are based on the decisions to take mandibular portions or segments and the decisions regarding reconstruction.

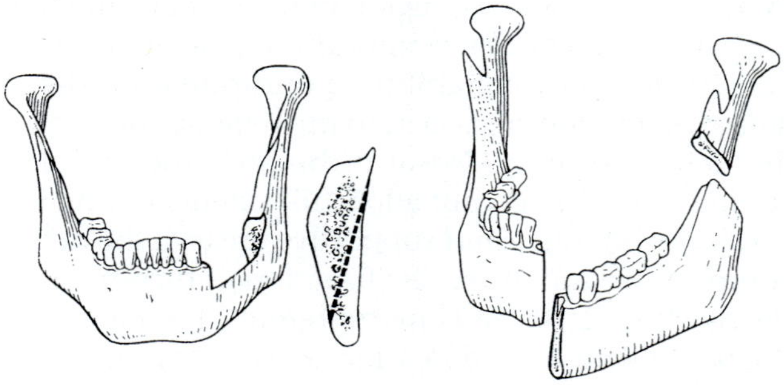

A

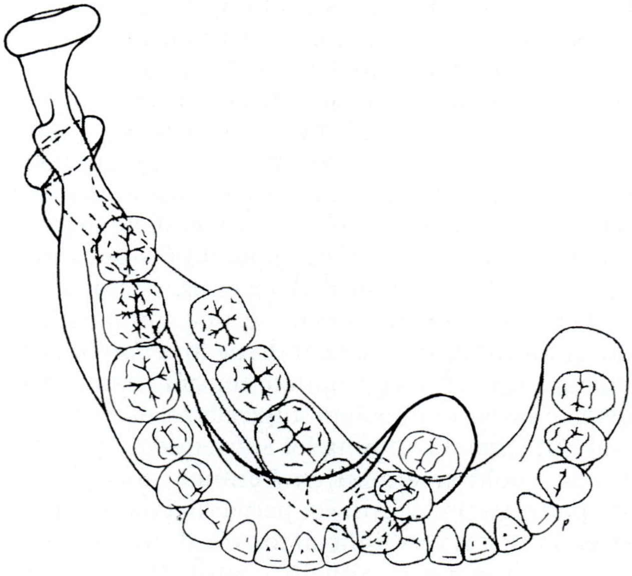

B

Figure 24-13 **A,** Marginal *(left)* and segmental *(right)* resections of the mandible. When a segmental resection is not stabilized with a reconstruction bar or bone graft, the continuity of the mandible is lost. Such a defect is a discontinuity defect of the mandible. **B,** When not stabilized, the discontinuous mandible deviates toward the defect and presents significant problems with mastication restoration.

The primary prosthetic objectives for mandibular defects are to restore mastication and cosmesis by the replacement of teeth. Achieving the mastication goal requires an understanding that regardless of the manner of prosthesis support (natural teeth, reconstructed soft tissue, or implants) the impact of the prosthetic device on success is dependent on the appropriate surgical management of both soft tissue and bone.

Disease involving soft tissue structures adjacent to and enveloping the mandible necessitates consideration of a mandibular resection to ensure control. When the soft tissue disease is clearly separate from the mandible and does not require bone removal, surgical defects involving these structures should be surgically reconstructed and therefore do not require prosthetic management. The exception to this is the large tongue resection that may require augmentation of the palatal contours to facilitate speech production. Such a palatal augmentation prosthesis is most beneficial when coordinated speech therapy can guide the optimal prosthesis configuration. Other resections may appear to require palatal augmentation for speech, yet the functional problem is tongue immobility secondary to tension created by the reconstructive tissue. Consideration should be given to soft tissue reconstructions that are of sufficient size and mobility, are less prone to contracture tension, and can produce a more normal alveololingual sulcus because these characteristics have been shown to have a significant influence on tongue mobility. Other desirable characteristics, such as sensation and lubrication, are also possible but necessitate a choice of which one is most required given the goals desired.

When tumors are primary to the mandible, such as an ameloblastoma, or involve the mandible from adjacent regions, surgical resection of segments of the mandible is required for tumor control. It may be difficult to always predict the functional deficit and the exact plan of reconstruction because the surgeon determines the extent of the resection based on presurgical and surgical findings. However, the common anatomically based mandibular resections seen include the lateral mandibular resection, the anterior mandibular resection, and the hemimandibular resection. From the standpoint of the surviving mandibular resection patient, the most significant decision regarding his or her management is the decision to maintain mandibular continuity, which allows maintenance of position for adjacent intraoral and extraoral soft tissue.

Surgical evolution of procedures that maintain continuity for the mandible has significantly improved the opportunity for functional restoration of mastication, deglutition, and speech. The debilitating effects of the discontinuity defect include a significant cosmetic deformity to the lower third of the face, decreased masticatory function secondary to unilateral closure, a compromised coordination of tongue and teeth, altered speech ability, and impaired deglutition (Figure 24-14). Given an appreciation of the decreased performance seen with conventional mucosal-borne denture prostheses, it should be obvious that masticatory rehabilitation for the resection patient without mandibular continuity is unpredictable at best and never achieved for most patients. Even for patients with remaining teeth, the altered mandibular position created in time presents a significant functional and cosmetic handicap. From a prosthetic rehabilitation standpoint, the most significantly handicapped post surgical head and neck condition is the discontinuous mandible. Consequently, such a post surgical condition should be the rare exception (typically because of reconstruction plate failure) and should not be the planned surgical outcome.

The cosmetic deformity associated with mandibular resection is improved through the use of reconstruction plates to maintain the presurgical contour to the lower jaw. This form of mandibular contour and position maintenance should be considered the minimal standard of care for mandibular resection patients from a functional standpoint. Use of reconstruction plates can maintain cosmetic appearance and preserve the bilateral nature of mandibular movement. However, the use of reconstruction plates alone precludes replacement of teeth in the region of resection. Prosthetic replacement of teeth cannot be provided for regions superior to the reconstruction bar because of the potential for mucosal perforation and exposure of the bar from functional loading of the soft tissue. From a masticatory function standpoint, this may not be a significant negative impact for some patients because of the maintenance of sufficient numbers of occlusal contacts postsurgically.

Mandibular Reconstruction—Bone Grafts

The evolution of head and neck reconstructive surgery has been dramatic over the past three decades. The vascularized tissue options of the forehead and deltopectoral regions gave way to the more popular pedicled myocutaneous flaps from the 1960s to the 1970s. By the 1980s, numerous osteomyocutaneous free-flap donor sites were identified and being used for mandibular reconstruction and particulate cancellous bone marrow in formed allogeneic frames. Equally important to the functional outcome of mastication was the development of the science and clinical application of the osseointegration phenomenon in the area of dental implants.

The ideal prosthetic characteristics of the replacement mandible include a stable union to proximal and distal segments, restoration of contour to the lower third of the face, a rounded ridge contour with attached mucosa of 2 to 3 mm thickness, and adjacent sulci providing free movement of buccal and lingual soft tissues for food control. Regardless of the type of prosthesis to be used, the appropriate placement of the bone relative to the opposing arch is vital to the intended functional use. If a removable prosthesis is planned and expected to cover the bone reconstruction, the contour of the developed ridge should provide a surface covered with firm, thin soft tissue, and a rounded superior contour with buccal and lingual slopes approaching parallel to each other and with sufficient vestibular depth to provide horizontal stability. Such a ridge condition is the surgical analog of a minimally resorbed edentulous ridge. With adequate cheek and tongue movement, it should

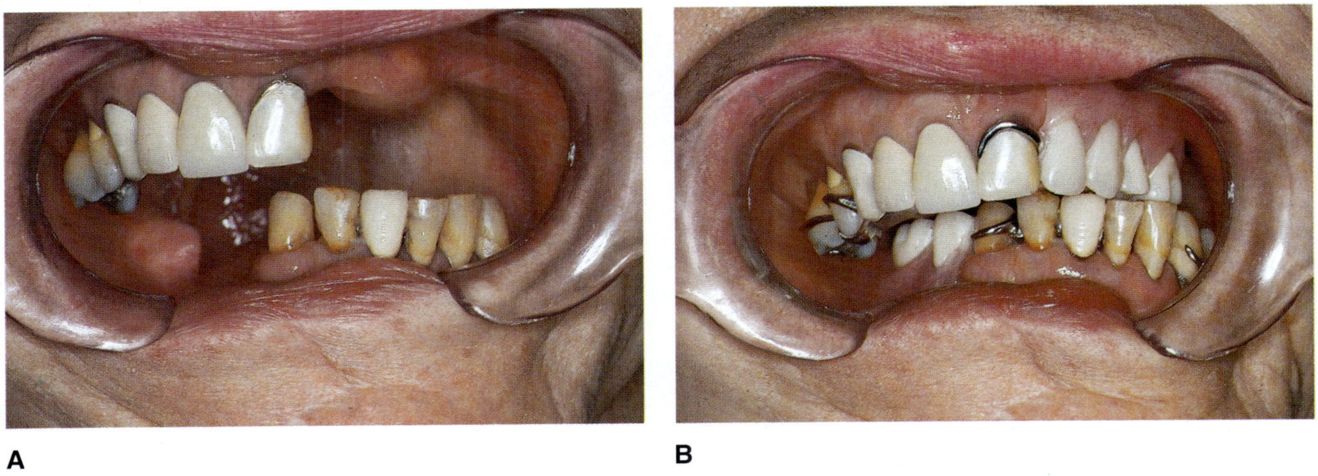

Figure 24-14 **A,** A deviated mandibular position following segmental resection without reconstruction. The mandibular midline is left of the maxillary midline by two teeth. **B,** With mandibular and maxillary prostheses in place, the patient closes to a functional position that is unique to the unilateral closure pattern.

provide a reasonable prognosis for prosthetic success provided sufficient numbers of teeth remain on the nonresected side. For the optimal chance of prosthetic function, dental implants should be considered, and with sufficient bulk of bone and the same characteristics listed for the removable prosthesis the prognosis for success is the greatest. To reiterate, the major determining factor for improved function will be the quality of the soft tissue reconstruction.

The major complications seen with mandibular reconstructions relate to the bulk of the soft tissue component and lack of mobility of the tongue. When these factors are controlled for, complications are mostly caused by bone placement and size. The common use of free flaps, including bone from other regions of the body that do not possess the native mandibular shape, presents a significant degree of technical difficulty associated with the procedure. The fibula, which is a popular choice for mandibular replacement, presents some challenges in meeting the ideal requirements mentioned above. Because of the straight nature of the bone, it is easy to err in both the horizontal and vertical positioning, especially for reconstructions that span to the midline. Lingual positioning requires prosthetic placement at a position that may be functionally unstable with time. Such a location requires implant positions that create a mechanical cantilever that can be detrimental to the long-term success of the implant-supported prosthesis. Posteriorly the inability to recreate the natural ascending curve of the mandible can restrict placement of teeth and preclude restoring complete occlusion on the resected side. It is common to have a mismatch in height at the anterior junction of the graft with the resident mandible. For implant-supported prostheses, this area can present significant challenges to adequate hygiene of the implants, and with time can compromise implant health. For removable prostheses, this can become a source of irritation if fulcrumlike action occurs with movement.

MAXILLARY PROSTHESES

Obturator Prostheses

The defining characteristic of an obturator prosthesis is that it serves to restore separation of the oral and adjacent cavities following surgical resection of tumors of the nasal and paranasal regions (Figure 24-15). Aramany developed a classification for partially edentulous maxillectomy dental arches (Figure 24-16). The various defects resulting from resection contain and are bounded by anatomic structures and an epithelial lining (either transplanted skin and/or native mucosa) that is quite different from normal partially edentulous arch anatomic features. The expectation for this altered region to contribute significantly to prosthesis support, stability, or retention is infrequently met. Consequently, prosthesis support and stabilization are largely dependent on the ability to aggressively engage the remaining teeth and residual ridge structures.

In comparison with partially edentulous arches, the movement potential for the prosthesis extension into the defect can be significant. When engagement of the distobuccal temporal bone is possible, upward movement of the obturator bulb can be greatly minimized. Movement potential increases as the remaining tooth number decreases and their arrangement becomes more linear (Figure 24-17). This illustrates the importance of maintaining teeth when possible, which allows for more prosthesis stabilization through direct tooth engagement and through cross-arch stabilization that increases with nonlinear tooth configurations (Figure 24-18).

To help control potential movement, various suggestions have been made relative to prosthesis design. The basic principle of placing support, stabilization, and retention immediately adjacent to and as far from the defect as possible acts to distribute the tooth effect on prosthesis performance to the greatest mechanical advantage. Because the teeth adjacent to the anterior resection margin are often incisors, it may be necessary to consider splinting them to improve the long-term prognosis. This region is critical for prosthesis performance, and the requirement for a cingulum rest and labial retention is often difficult to optimize without crowns. Distally, it is often necessary to incorporate an embrasure clasp to provide maximal retention and stabilization. Such a clasp assembly must have sufficient room for occlusal clearance, and it is not uncommon for the opposing occlusion to need adjustment to accommodate such a rest complex. When possible the palatal surfaces of the maxillary teeth should be surveyed to determine if guide plane surfaces can be produced to impart a stabilizing effect. When accomplished, the prosthesis benefits from improved movement resistance, and it does so with more teeth contributing to the effect, thereby distributing the stress more appropriately. Brown described how the vertical height of the lateral portion of the obturator above the buccal scar band can contribute to prosthesis movement control by helping prevent vertical displacement (see Figure 24-15).

Speech Aid Prostheses

The defining characteristics of speech aid prostheses are that they are functionally shaped to the palatopharyngeal musculature to restore or compensate for areas of the soft palate that are deficient because of surgery or congenital anomaly (see Figure 24-11). Such a prosthesis consists of a palatal component, which contacts the teeth to provide stability and

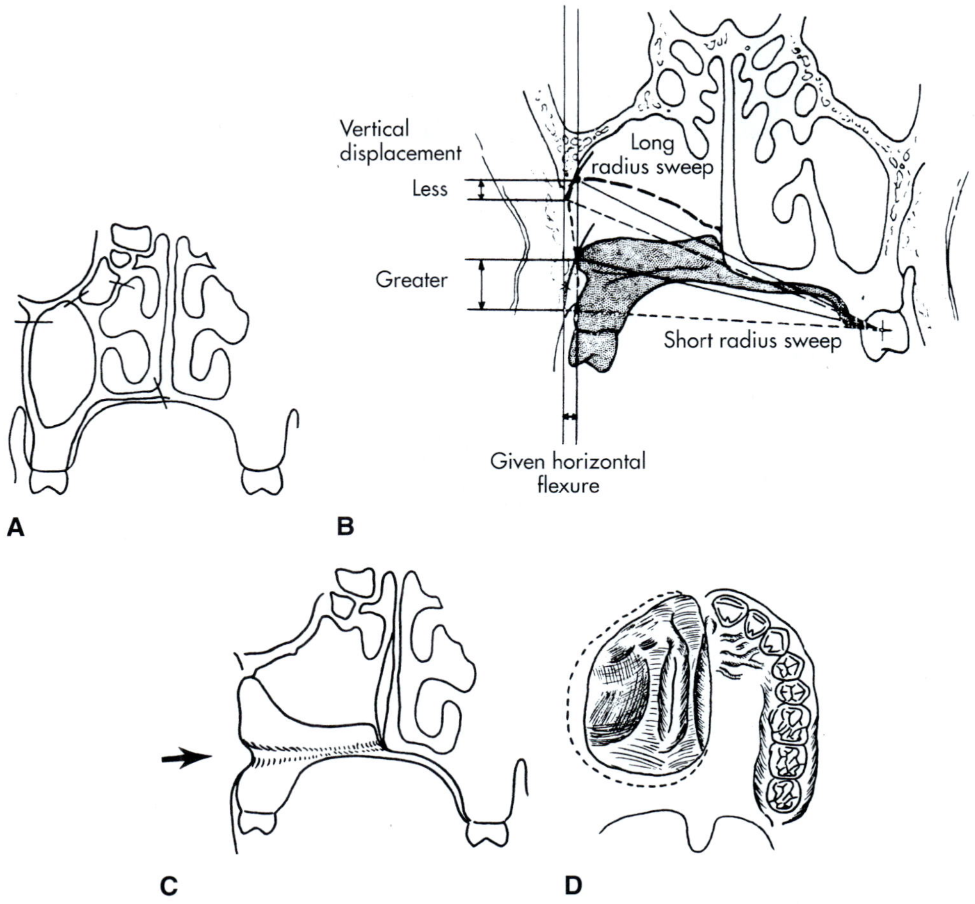

Figure 24-15 **A,** Coronal view of proposed maxillary resection. *Bold lines* designate typical area to be resected. **B,** Demonstrates value of lateral wall height in design of removable partial denture obturator. As defect side of prosthesis is displaced, lateral wall of obturator will engage scar band and aid in retaining the prosthesis. **C,** Coronal section with surgical obturator in place. With prosthesis in place, relation of scar band *(arrow)* to lateral portion of the obturator can be seen. Buccal scar band will develop at height of previous vestibule where buccal mucosa and skin graft in surgical defect join. **D,** Axial view of resected area illustrates defect. *Dotted lines* indicate areas available for intraoral retention.

anchorage for retention; a palatal extension, which crosses the residual soft palate; and a pharyngeal component, which fills the palatopharyngeal port during muscular function, serving to restore the speech valve of the palatopharyngeal region.

Because the typical speech aid prosthesis does not provide tooth replacement, the patient should expect only minimal functional movement. Movement of the pharyngeal extension imposed by the residual palatopharyngeal musculature is generally undesired and a sign of required modification. Common reasons for such movement include a low position, causing tongue encroachment; superior extension that does not account for head flexure; or impression procedures that do not accurately record residual soft palatal position or movement.

A pediatric speech aid is a temporary prosthesis used to improve voice quality during the growing years. It is made of materials that are easily modified as growth or orthodontic treatment progresses. Because a speech aid has a significant posterior extension into the pharyngeal region, torque is evident from the long moment arm. A basic principle of posterior retention with anterior indirect retention must be applied to the design of such a maxillary prosthesis. Posterior retention is gained by the use of wrought-wire clasps around the most distal maxillary molars, whereas the anterior extension of the prosthesis onto the hard palate provides the indirect retention. If there is inadequate clinical crown length and undercut to provide retention, orthodontic bands with buccal tie wings can be used in conjunction with the wrought wires. This design facilitates the maintenance of the pharyngeal part of the pediatric speech aid in the proper position in the palatopharyngeal opening.

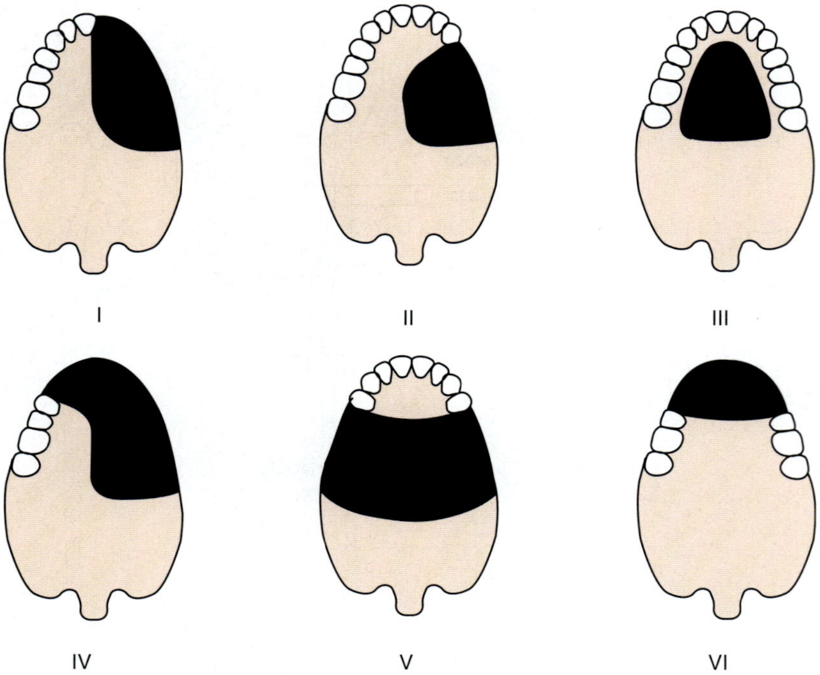

Figure 24-16 Aramany's classification for partially edentulous maxillectomy dental arches: Class I—Midline resection. Class II—Unilateral resection. Class III—Central resection. Class IV—Bilateral anteroposterior resection. Class V—Posterior resection. Class VI—Anterior resection.

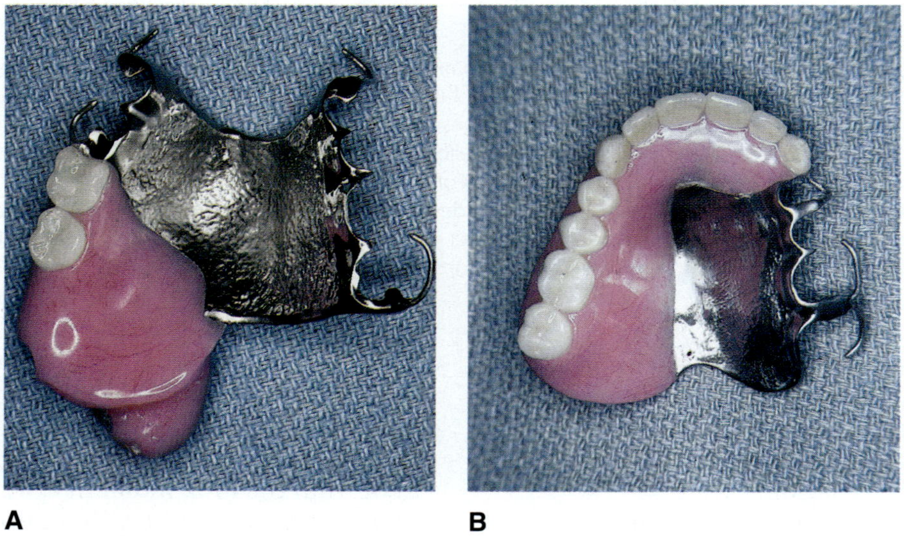

Figure 24-17 **A,** A maxillary obturator prosthesis in which remaining teeth provide significant stabilization to the obturator extension because of their number and location, which allows cross-arch prosthesis engagement. **B,** An obturator prosthesis, which benefits from teeth in a linear arrangement and therefore does not have any cross-arch tooth stabilization. Obturator movement in **B** is likely to be significantly greater than in **A**. The requirement for using the defect to provide support where possible is therefore greater in **B** than in **A**.

In the adult whose palatopharyngeal insufficiency is a result of a cleft palate or palatal surgery, an adult speech aid prosthesis can be constructed of more definitive materials because growth changes will not have to be accommodated. If teeth are missing, the prosthesis will incorporate a retentive partial denture framework. The basic design should include posterior retention and anterior indirect retention.

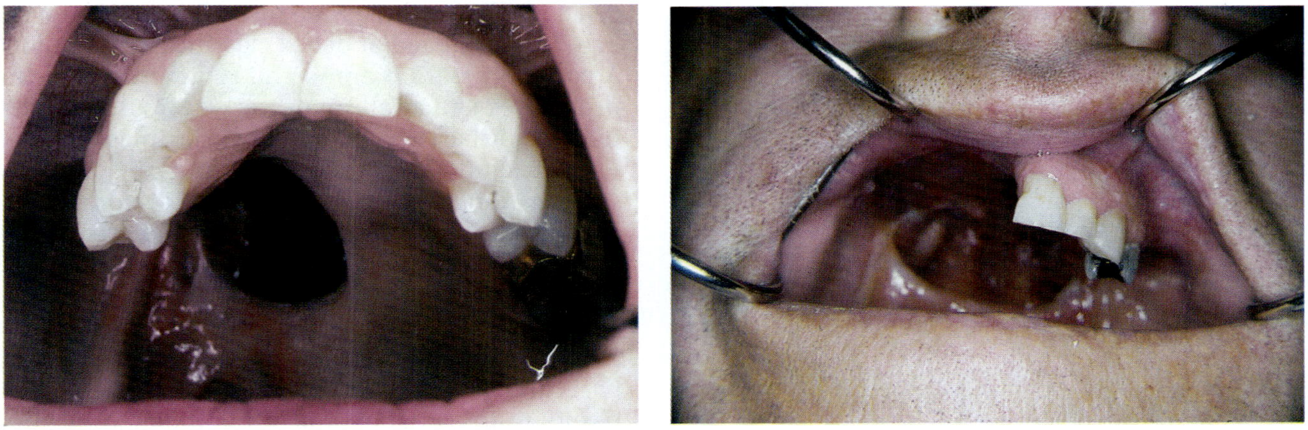

A B

Figure 24-18 **A,** Tooth arrangement that offers cross-arch stability (as in Figure 24-17, *A*) because of the arch curvature of the remaining tooth distribution and the tripod effect it allows. **B,** More linear arrangement of teeth does not provide cross-arch stability and places greater demand on the defect integrity for prosthesis performance.

Palatal Lift Prostheses

The defining characteristic of a palatal lift is that it positions a flaccid soft palate posteriorly and superiorly to narrow the palatopharyngeal opening for the purpose of improving oral air pressure and therefore speech. Patients who exhibit a structurally normal soft palate and pharyngeal port can demonstrate hypernasal speech caused by a paralysis of the regional musculature. This condition is referred to as *palatopharyngeal incompetence* since the failure lies in function, not anatomic deficiency. The paralysis can result from a variety of neuromuscular conditions (flaccid paralysis of the soft palate from closed head injuries, cerebral palsy, muscular dystrophy, or myasthenia gravis) that have varying clinical courses. The palatal lift prosthesis must physically position the soft palate to redirect air pressure orally. In placing the soft palate, any tissue resistance met acts as a dislodging force on the prosthesis. This dislodging force must be resisted by adequate direct and indirect retention.

To efficiently maintain prosthesis position, the dislodging force is best resisted by bilateral direct retainers placed close to the posterior lift and anteriorly placed indirect retention. Success with a palatal lift prosthesis depends upon the presence of a number of maxillary posterior teeth, which can provide retention for the prosthesis, coupled with an easily placed flaccid soft palate.

Palatal Augmentation Prostheses

When surgical resection involving the tongue and/or floor of the mouth limits tongue mobility, it affects both speech and deglutition. With tongue mobility limitations, the contour of the palate can be augmented by a prosthesis to modify the space of Donder to allow food manipulation to be more easily transferred posteriorly into the oropharynx.

Prosthesis movement potential is low since the functional forces involved are those imparted by the tongue during deglutition and speech, neither of which creates force similar to mastication. It is common to use a diagnostic resin augmentation prosthesis retained with wire clasps to plan the necessary contour needs. Once the appropriate palatal contour has been determined, a definitive augmentation prosthesis can be constructed of cast metal with appropriately placed minor connectors for attaching the resin augmentation. Bilateral rests and direct retainers should be positioned to facilitate the design for the acrylic retention, since stability needs related to functional force are not a significant design concern.

MANDIBULAR PROSTHESES

Resection prostheses are those prostheses provided to patients who have acquired mandibular defects that result in loss of teeth and significant portions of the mandible. Mandibular resections result in defects that either preserve mandibular continuity or result in discontinuity defects. These are further subclassified by Cantor and Curtis (Figure 24-19) and provide a meaningful foundation for discussing removable prosthesis design considerations.

Evolution of Mandibular Surgical Resection

When mandibular continuity is preserved, as in a marginal resection (type I mandibular defect, see Figure 24-13), function is the least affected and the major prosthesis concern relates to the soft tissue

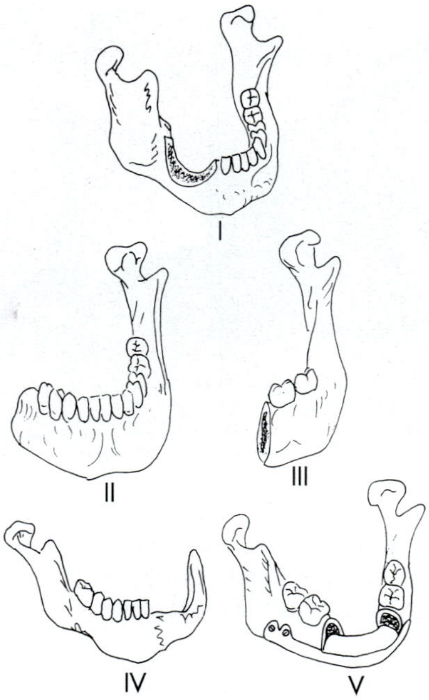

Figure 24-19 Cantor and Curtis classification of partial mandibulectomy. *(Redrawn from Cantor R, Curtis TA: J Prosthet Dent 25:446–457, 1971.)*

potential for support. With good remaining dental support, near-normal function can often be achieved with prosthodontic rehabilitation.

Although not as common an outcome as in the past, when continuity of the mandible is lost because of a segmental resection that was not reconstructed, the bilateral joint complex no longer controls the remaining mandibular segment. Consequently the function of the remaining mandibular segment is severely compromised because of the loss of the coordinated bilateral muscular action functioning across a bilateral joint. The resulting segmental movement is an uncoordinated action dictated by the remaining unilateral muscular activity within a surgical environment that changes with healing dynamics and patient rehabilitation efforts. Successful removable prosthodontic intervention for these situations necessitated a combination of knowledge of the functional movements of the remaining residual mandible and patient concerted effort and persistence.

Historically, mandibular stabilization by bone grafts or reconstruction bars was not always a surgical goal. The major exception was the anterior defect (type V), which was recognized to pose significant airway risks if not managed. Currently, most lateral segmental mandibulectomies are also reconstructed surgically. When the mandible is not stabilized following resection and a discontinuity defect results, a mandibular resection prosthesis should be provided to restore mastication within the unique movement capabilities of the residual functioning mandible.

The following discussion highlights design considerations for the major defect classifications outlined. A common feature among all removable resection prostheses is that all framework designs should be dictated by basic prosthodontic principles of design. Those include broad stress distribution, cross-arch stabilization using a rigid major connector, stabilizing and retaining components at locations within the arch to best minimize dislodging functional forces, and replacement tooth positions that optimize prosthesis stability and functional needs. Modifications to these principles are determined on an individual basis and are greatly influenced by unique residual tissue characteristics and mandibular movement dynamics.

Type I Resection

In a type I resection of the mandible, the inferior border is intact and normal movements can be expected to occur. The major difference between this situation and a typical edentulous span is the nature of the soft tissue foundation. For type I resections, the denture-bearing area may be compromised because of the closure of the defect using adjacent lining mucosa (which can reduce the buccolingual width), or because of the presence of a split-thickness skin graft.

Ideally, one would like to see a firm, nonmovable tissue bed with normal buccal and lingual vestibular extension. If the defect is unilateral and posterior, the framework would be typical of a Kennedy Class II design, taking into account whatever modification spaces may be present. When the marginal resection is in the anterior area, the design may be more typical of a Kennedy Class IV design (Figure 24-20).

Anterior marginal resections sometimes include part of the anterior tongue and floor of the mouth. With the loss of the normal tongue function, the remaining teeth are no longer retained in a neutral zone, and as a result they often collapse lingually because of lip pressure. If this occurs, it may necessitate the use of a labial bar major connector.

Corrected cast impression procedures provide a major advantage for fabrication of removable partial dentures in partial mandibulectomy patients. Capture of the unique buccal, lingual, and labial functional contours in the final prosthesis can contribute significantly to stabilization of the prosthesis, especially in discontinuity defects.

Type II Resection

In the type II resection, the mandible is often resected in the region of the second premolar and first molar. If there are no other missing teeth in the arch, a prosthesis is usually not indicated. There are situations, however, in which a prosthesis may need to be fabricated to support the buccal tissue and to help fill the

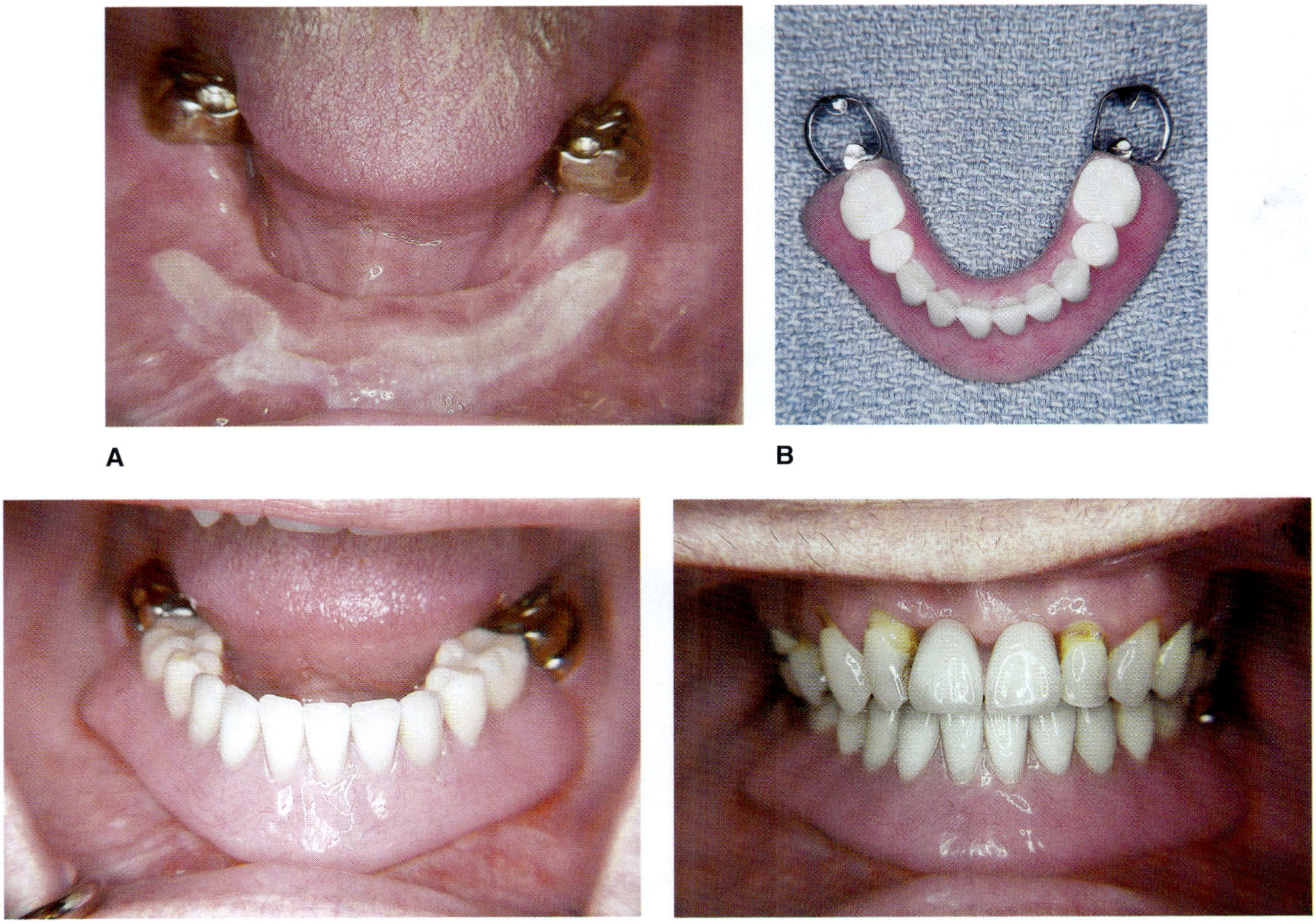

A B C D

Figure 24-20 A type I resection of the anterior mandible. **A,** Bilateral molars remain to stabilize an anterior extension removable partial denture. Split-thickness skin graft has been used to reconstruct the denture-bearing area. **B,** The prosthesis showing cast clasps and anterior extension base. **C,** The prosthesis in place and covering the skin graft with a configuration produced through a corrective cast impression technique. **D,** The resection prosthesis in occlusion. It is critical to have the remaining natural teeth occlude at the same vertical dimension as the prosthetic teeth to ensure comfortable function.

space between the tongue and cheek to prevent food and saliva from collecting in the region.

Framework design should be similar to a Kennedy Class II design, with extension into the vestibular areas of the resection. This area would be considered nonfunctional and should not be required to support mastication. It must be remembered that extension into the defect area can place significant stress on the remaining abutment teeth, therefore occlusal rests should be placed near the defect, along with an attempt to gain tripod support from remaining teeth and tissue where possible.

An example of a framework design for a type II mandibular resection with missing molars on the nonsurgical side is illustrated in Figure 24-21. The choice of major connector depends on the height of the floor of the mouth as it relates to the position of the attached gingival margins during function. An extension base with artificial teeth can be used on the surgical side if space is available. The extent of this base is determined by a functional impression and should be cautious of the potential for bone exposure at the superior margin of the resection.

Retention can be achieved through the use of various types of clasp assemblies on the distal abutments. Indirect retention can be derived from rests prepared in the mesial fossae of the first premolars and/or the lingual surfaces of the canines. Unlike the result in Figure 24-21, use of an infrabulge retainer on the surgical side may be difficult if a shallow vestibule results from surgical closure. Location of minor connectors should be physiologically determined to minimize the stress on the abutment teeth and to enhance resistance to reasonable dislodging

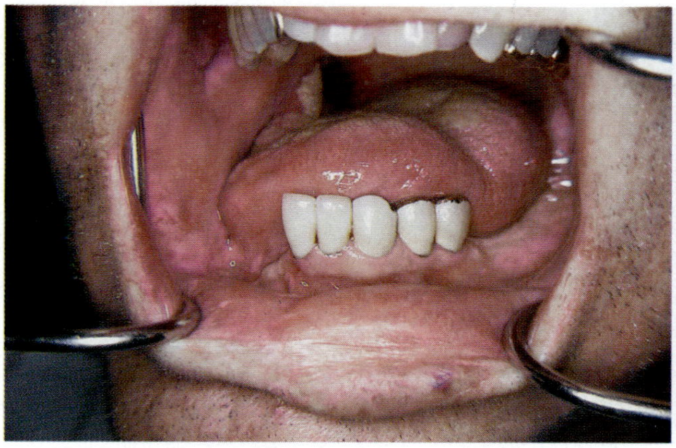

A

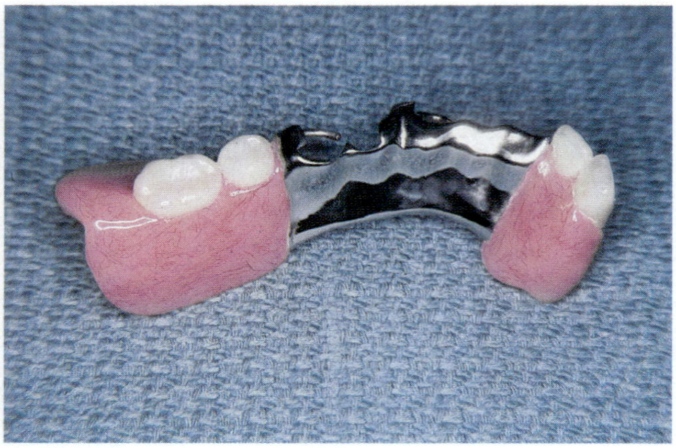

B

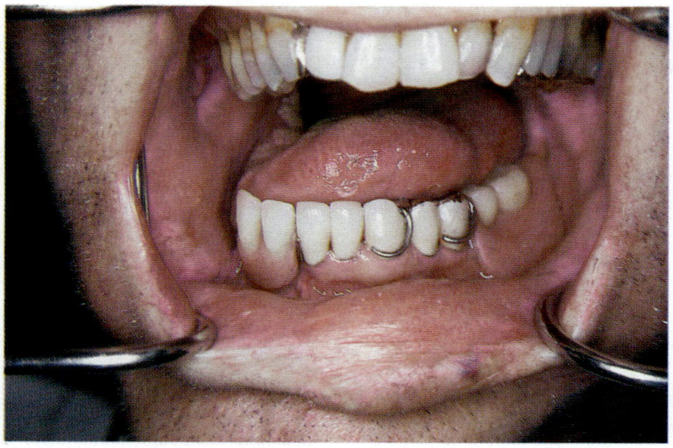

C

Figure 24-21 A type II resection and prosthesis. **A,** Clinical presentation of mandibular right resection and missing mandibular left molars. **B,** Resection prosthesis with cast lingual plate major connector and wrought-wire clasps. **C,** Resection prosthesis in place demonstrating the two-tooth extension on the defect side *(patient's right). (Courtesy of Dr. Ron Desjardins, Rochester, Minn.)*

forces. Wrought-wire circumferential retainers are acceptable alternatives.

In a type II mandibular resection, in which posterior and anterior teeth are missing on the defect side, the remaining teeth on the intact side of the arch are often present in a straight-line configuration. Embrasure clasps may be used on the posterior teeth, with an infrabulge retainer on the anterior abutment. In some situations, a rotational path design may be used to engage the natural undercuts on the mesial proximal surfaces of the anterior abutments. Lingual retention with buccal reciprocation on the remaining posterior teeth should also be considered. The longitudinal axis of rotation in this design should be considered to be a straight line through the remaining teeth. Depression of the prosthesis on the edentulous side will have less of a chance to dislodge the prosthesis if retention is on the lingual surfaces than if on the buccal. Suggested framework designs for this patient group are illustrated in Figure 24-22.

Physiological relief of minor connectors is always recommended. Where the remaining teeth are in a straight line, a Swing-Lock major connector design may be used to take advantage of as many buccal and/or labial undercuts as possible. Because elderly patients often complain of difficulty manipulating Swing-Lock mechanisms, in straight-line situations it may be possible to use alternate buccal and lingual retention effectively (Figure 24-23).

In the type II resection with anterior and posterior missing teeth on the resected side and posterior missing teeth on the nonresected side, the prosthesis will have three denture base regions. This prosthesis may have a straight-line longitudinal axis of rotation as previously discussed. Rests should be placed on as many teeth as possible, minor connectors should be

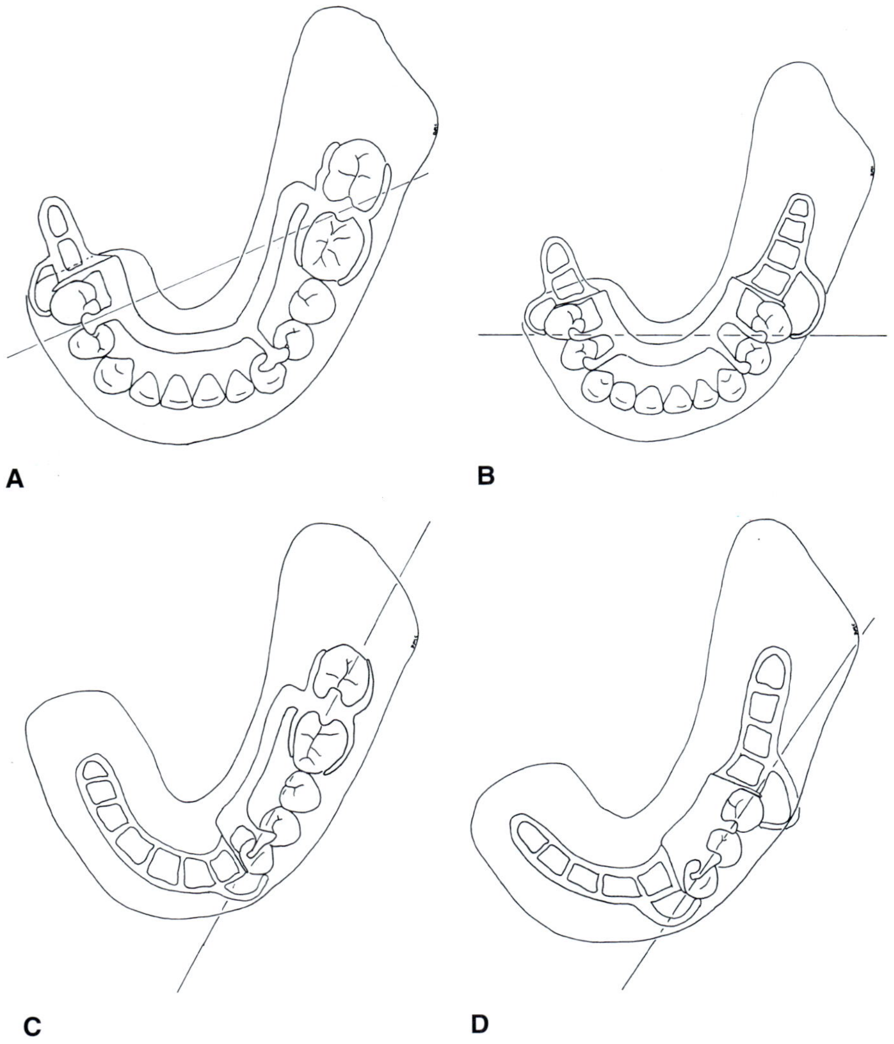

Figure 24-22 **A,** Frame design for type II resection, no teeth missing on the nonresected side. Note provision for extension into resection space between tongue and cheek. **B,** Type II design, with missing posterior teeth on nonresected side. **C,** Type II design, with missing anterior teeth. **D,** Type II design, with missing anterior and posterior teeth.

placed to enhance stability, and wrought-wire retainers are an acceptable alternative to the bar clasps.

Type III Resection

A type III resection (see Figure 24-19) produces a defect to the midline or farther toward the intact side, leaving half or less of the mandible remaining.

The importance of retaining as many teeth as possible in this situation cannot be overemphasized. The design of a framework for this situation would be similar to the type II resection. The longitudinal axis of rotation is again considered to be a straight line through the remaining teeth. In this resection there is a greater chance of prosthesis dislodgment caused by a lack of support under the anterior extension.

Alternating buccal and lingual retention in a rigid design or the Swing-Lock design should be considered.

Type IV Resection

A type IV resection (see Figure 24-19) would use the same design concepts as the type II or III resections with the corresponding edentulous areas.

If the graft does not provide an articulation and the soft tissue covering the graft is not firmly attached to the bone graft, the movement potential will be dictated by the functional forces of movement coupled with the soft tissue supportive capacities.

If a type IV resection extends to the midline with the extension of a graft into the defect area, but does not include temporomandibular joint reconstruction on the surgical side, the design would be similar to the type III resection with an extension base on the surgical side.

If the type IV resection extends beyond the midline, with less than half of the mandible remaining,

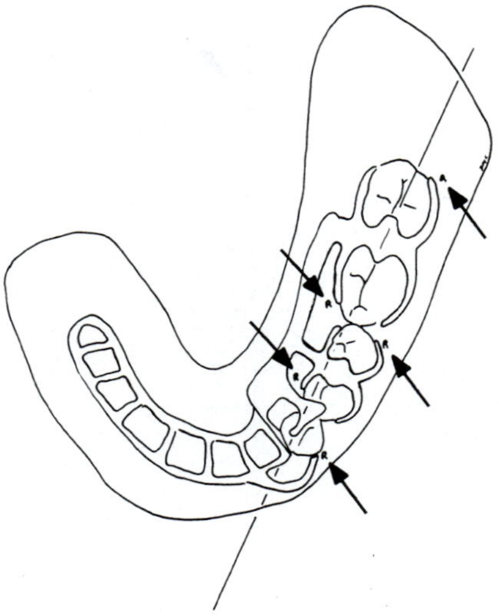

Figure 24-23 Conventional clasping by use of alternating buccal and lingual retention *(arrows)*.

the design will be similar to the type II resection that has an extension base into the surgical defect area.

Type V Resection

In the type V resected mandible, when the anterior or posterior denture-bearing area of the mandible has been surgically reconstructed, the removable partial denture design is similar to the type I resection design.

The principle difference between a type V resected mandible and the intact mandible with the same tooth loss pattern is in the management of the soft tissue at the graft site. For design purposes, one should consider the residual mandibles of the type I and V resections to be similar to nonsurgical mandibles with the same tooth-loss pattern.

Mandibular Guide Flange Prosthesis

As mentioned earlier, in a discontinuity defect, the movement of the residual mandibular segment is an uncoordinated action dictated by two features unique to the specific defect and patient. The first is the remaining unilateral muscular activity that will be specific to the surgical resection and will have a characteristic resting posture to the defect side with a diagonal movement on "closure." The second is that the surgical environment will change as healing progresses, and patient efforts to train movement during this healing period will help maintain both position and movement range. To facilitate training of the mandibular segment to maintain a more midline closure pattern, clinicians have used a guide flange prosthesis.

The mandibular guide flange prosthesis is used primarily as an interim training device. When no missing teeth are supplied, it may be considered a training appliance rather than a prosthesis. This appliance is used in dentulous patients with nonreconstructed lateral discontinuity defects who have severe deviation of the mandible toward the surgical side and are unable to achieve unassisted intercuspation on the nonsurgical side (Figure 24-24). Generally these patients have had a significant amount of soft tissue removed along with the resected mandibular segment and have had surgical closure by suturing the lateral surface of the tongue to the buccal mucosa, which causes a deviation toward the defect side. Scarring also occurs and is worse for patients who have not been placed on an exercise program during the healing period. The guide flange prosthesis is designed to restrict the patient to vertical opening and closing movements into maximum occlusal contacts. Over a period of time, this guided function should promote scar relaxation, allowing the patient to make unassisted masticatory contact.

The components of the guide flange prosthesis include the major and minor connectors needed to support, stabilize, and retain the prosthesis and the guiding mechanism. This can include a cast buccal guide bar and guide flange, or simply a resin flange, which engages the opposing arch buccal tooth surfaces. In either case the opposing arch must provide a stable foundation to resist any forces needed to guide the deviated mandibular segment into maximum occlusal contact.

The buccal guide bar is placed as close as possible to the buccal occlusal line angle of the remaining natural teeth to allow maximal opening. The lateral position of the bar must be adequate to prevent the guide from contacting the buccal mucosa of the maxillary alveolus. The length of the bar should overlie the premolars and first molar where possible. Retention of the maxillary frame should not be problematic because the force directed on the bar is in a palatal direction. The guide flange is attached to the mandibular major connector by two generous interproximal minor connectors. As with the maxillary frame, significant interproximal tooth structure must be cleared to provide the necessary bulk for the minor connectors. The height of the guide flange is determined by the depth of the buccal vestibule. A small hook is placed on the middle of the top of the guide to prevent disengagement on wide opening. Because the mandibular segment has a constant medial force, the flange acts as a powerful lever with a strong lateral force on the teeth. Therefore extra rests and additional stabilization and retention on multiple teeth must be considered to prevent overstressing individual teeth. Retention on the tooth adjacent to the defect is critical for resistance to the lifting of the frame. Lingual retention in the premolar area may be considered as an aid in resistance to

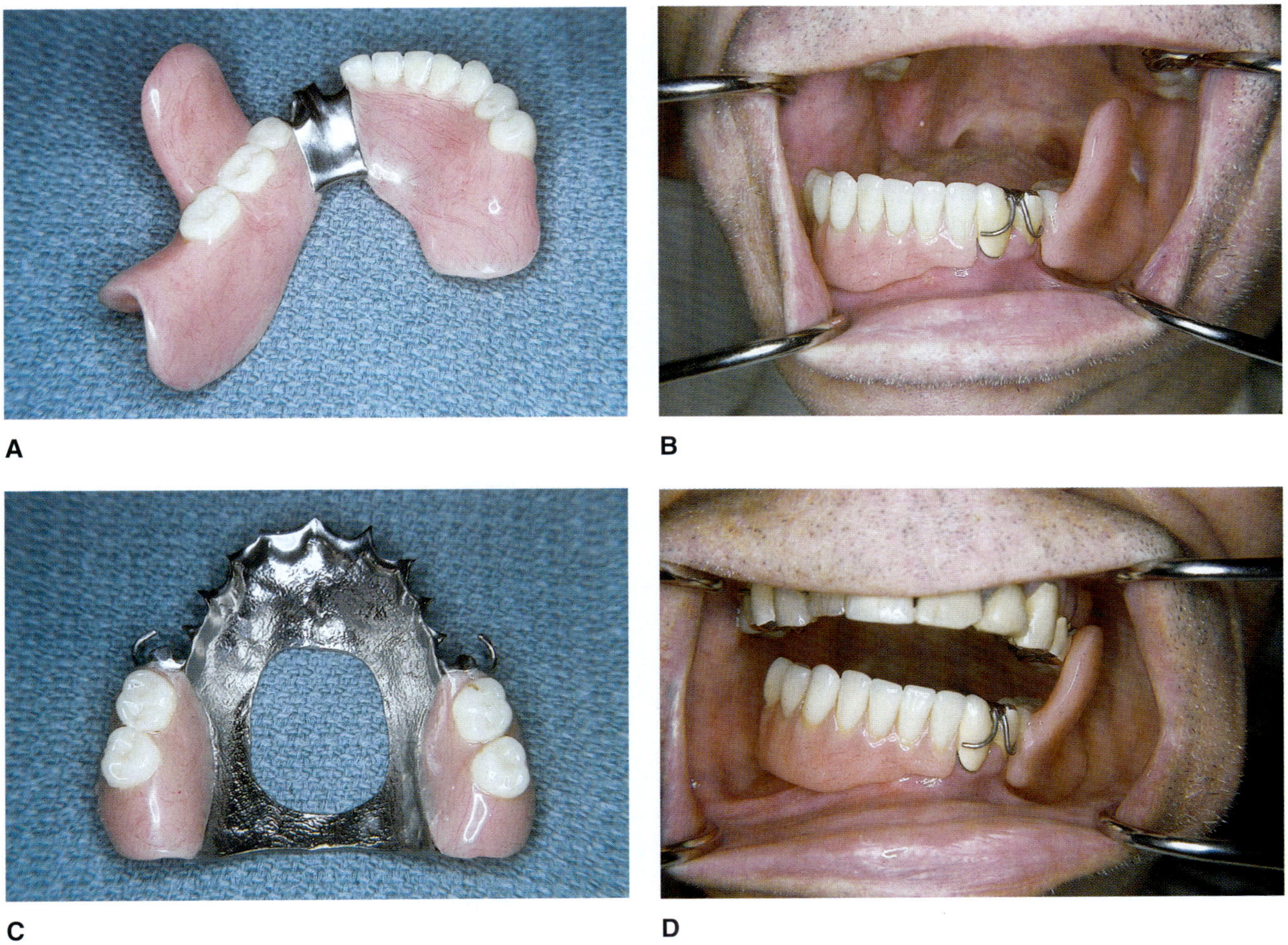

Figure 24-24 A mandibular guide flange prosthesis. **A,** Flange extension is incorporated into a mandibular type II resection prosthesis using a resin extension. **B,** Resection prosthesis inserted. **C,** Opposing maxillary prosthesis designed to engage palatal surfaces of all remaining teeth for maximal stability against flange-induced forces. **D,** Flange extending to the buccal region of the opposing prosthesis and teeth. Upon closure the flange will guide the mandible to maximal intercuspation at which time the flange extension will reside in the maxillary left buccal vestibule. *(Courtesy Dr. Ron Desjardins, Rochester, Minn.)*

displacement. When necessary, missing teeth can be added to a guide flange prosthesis. Flange prostheses can be provisionally designed for modification into definitive removable partial dentures after guidance is no longer necessary. This is accomplished by removal of the buccal flange and buccal guide bar components after the patient is able to make occlusal contacts without the use of the guide. However, many patients with mandibular resections have difficulty making repeated occlusal contacts, a fact described in several studies. Occlusal considerations in mandibulectomy patients have been discussed extensively by Desjardins.

Palatal occlusal ramps have been used to guide those patients with less severe deviation than those who require a guide flange into a more stable intercuspal contact position. These prostheses incorporate a palatal ramp that simulates the function of the guide flange prosthesis. This inclination of the palatal ramp is determined by the severity of the deviation of the remaining mandible. Some patients have the ability to move laterally into occlusion but have a tendency to close medially and palatally rather than close into an acceptable cuspal relationship. These patients can benefit from a palatal ramp, which can be functionally generated in wax at the try-in stage. This provides a platform for occlusal contact in the entire buccolingual range of movement. A supplemental row of prosthetic teeth may be arranged, then removed at the boil out stage, and processed in pink acrylic resin for esthetics. Patients who have experienced both smooth and tooth-form ramps usually prefer the tooth form if the width is adequate.

JAW RELATION RECORDS FOR MANDIBULAR RESECTION PATIENTS

Interocclusal records must be made using verbal guidance only for resection patients with discontinuity defects. A hands-on approach, like that used for conventional edentulous jaw relation records, will lead to unnatural rotation of the mandible and an inaccurate record. The patient should be instructed to move the mandible toward the nonsurgical side and close into a nonresistant recording medium at the preestablished occlusal vertical dimension, which will be the occlusal contact position. If the surgical side is significantly deficient, an occlusion rim may have to be extended into the defect area to support the recording medium. Head position is of extreme importance during registration of jaw relation records. If the patient is in a semirecumbent position in the dental chair during the recording procedure, the mandible may be retracted and deviated toward the surgical side, preventing movement toward the intact side. To minimize this problem, the recording should be made with the patient seated in a normal upright postural position.

Most patients with lateral discontinuity defects can make lateral movements toward the nonsurgical side, even without the presence of a lateral pterygoid muscle functioning on the balancing (surgical) side. This is due to the compensatory effects of the horizontal fibers of the temporalis and the lateral pterygoid muscle on the normal side, causing a rotational effect on the remaining condyle.

SUMMARY

Maxillofacial prosthetic treatment of the patient with an oral defect is among the most challenging in dentistry. Defects are highly individual and require the clinician to call upon all knowledge and experience to fabricate a functional prosthesis. The basic principles and concepts described throughout this text will help to successfully design maxillofacial removable partial dentures. The interested reader is encouraged to pursue maxillofacial texts for more information regarding prosthesis design for this patient group.

SELF-ASSESSMENT AIDS

1. In planning the surgical and restorative treatment for a patient with malignant oral disease, the dentist should see the patient before surgery to coordinate definitive care. To solicit the surgeon's cooperation in this regard, what rationale would you give for seeing the patient at this time?
2. What is the primary purpose for placement of a surgical obturator?
3. Speech aids and palatal lifts often require significant posterior extension into the pharyngeal region. This necessitates the clinician to use what basic principles of design?
4. Other than natural teeth, what structures associated with the resultant defect from maxillectomy can be used to augment prosthetic stability and retention?
5. How do natural tooth crown contour and palatal configuration influence the retention and stability of a maxillary obturator prosthesis?
6. Clinical methods used to stabilize the residual mandible after surgery that results in discontinuity depend on at least three criteria. Identify these and suggest methods used for postoperative stabilization.
7. To eliminate potential sources of posttreatment complication, all irradiated teeth should be removed before the initiation of restorative care. True or false?
8. The positioning of a palatopharyngeal obturator for a cleft palate patient with palatopharyngeal inadequacy is determined by several anatomic and functional criteria. What are the most significant factors?
9. To be effective, the cast framework must be:
   a. Rigid
   b. Made of chrome-cobalt alloy
   c. Thin
   d. Retained by wire clasps
   e. None of the above
   f. *a* and *c*
   g. *c* and *d*
10. The palatopharyngeal muscles that produce the sphincteric action required to provide palatopharyngeal competence include ____________.
11. Patients wearing metal obturators require extensive speech therapy. True or false?
12. Describe the patient postural head positions required to assist in border molding a palatopharyngeal obturator during the impression phase of treatment.
13. Palatal occlusal ramps can be used to guide mandibulectomy patients with less severe deviation than those who require a guide flange into a more stable intercuspal contact position. True or false?
14. Interocclusal jaw relation records for mandibulectomy patients must be made using verbal guidance only. A hands-on approach, similar to that used for conventional edentulous jaw relation records, will lead to unnatural rotation of the mandible and an inaccurate record. True or false?
15. What is the recommended position of the head for a mandibulectomy patient during the registration of jaw relation records? Why is this position important?

SELECTED READING RESOURCES

Rarely, if ever, is a textbook found to be all-inclusive in subject matter related to a dental clinical discipline or subdiscipline. Therefore this section, listing other textbooks and articles from dental periodical literature, may assist in broadening a student's perspectives in principles and concepts of removable partial prosthodontics.

Some of the articles have historic significance and are considered classics. Contemporary selections are included, and many of the articles are current to the submission of the manuscript for this 11th edition. The serious student of dentistry may extract background and progress of removable partial prosthodontics over the years from this section.

We do not imply that sources have been exhausted in compiling the lists of either textbooks or articles. We have attempted to correctly classify listed articles for ready reference; however, the length of the Miscellaneous section attests to the difficulties encountered.

TEXTBOOKS

Alberktsson T, Zarb GA: The Branemark osseointegrated implant, 1989, Chicago, Quintessence.

Anusavice KJ: Phillips' science of dental materials, ed 11, St Louis, 2003, WB Saunders.

Applegate OC: Essentials of removable partial denture prosthesis, Philadelphia, 1965, WB Saunders.

Ash MM, Nelson SJ: Wheeler's dental anatomy, physiology, and occlusion, ed 8, St Louis, 2003, WB Saunders.

Beumer J, Curtis TA, Firtell DN: Maxillofacial prosthetics, St Louis, 1979, Mosby.

Brand RW, Isselhard DE: Anatomy of orofacial structures, ed 7, St Louis, 2003, Mosby.

Brewer AA, Morrow RM: Overdentures, ed 2, St Louis, 1980, Mosby.

Brunette DM: Critical thinking: understanding and evaluating dental research, Chicago, 1996, Quintessence.

Craig RG, Powers JM: Restorative dental materials, ed 11, St Louis, 2002, Mosby.

Craig RG, Powers JM, Wataha JC: Dental materials: properties and manipulation, ed 8, St Louis, 2004, Mosby.

Dawson PE: Evaluation, diagnosis, and treatment of occlusal problems, ed 2, St Louis, 1989, Mosby.

Dolder EJ, Durrer GT: The bar-joint denture, Chicago, 1978, Quintessence.

Dubrul EL: Sicher's oral anatomy, ed 7, St Louis, 1980, Mosby.

Dykema RW, Cunningham DM, Johnston JF: Modern practice in removable partial prosthodontics, Philadelphia, 1969, WB Saunders.

Fonseca RJ, Davis WH: Reconstructive preprosthetic oral and maxillofacial surgery, ed 2, Philadelphia, 1995, WB Saunders.

Graber G: Removable partial dentures, Stuttgart, Germany, 1988, Thieme Medical.

Graber DA, Goldstein RE, Feinman RA: Porcelain laminate veneers, Chicago, 1988, Quintessence.

Grasso JE, Miller EL: Partial prosthodontics, ed 3, St Louis, 1991, Mosby.

Hoag PM, Pawlak EA: Essentials of periodontics, ed 4, St Louis, 1990, Mosby.

Johnson DL, Stratton RJ: Fundamentals of removable prosthodontics, Chicago, 1980, Quintessence.

Johnston JF et al: Modern practice in crown and bridge prosthodontics, ed 4, Philadelphia, 1986, WB Saunders.

Jordon RE: Esthetic composite bonding, ed 2, St Louis, 1993, Mosby.

Kratochvil FJ: Partial removable prosthodontics, Philadelphia, 1988, WB Saunders.

Krol AJ: Removable partial denture design outline syllabus, ed 4, San Francisco, 1990, University of the Pacific School of Dentistry.

Laney WR et al: Maxillofacial prosthetics, Littleton, Mass, 1979, PSG.

Laney WR, Gibilisco JA: Diagnosis and treatment in prosthodontics, Philadelphia, 1983, Lea & Febiger.

Little JW, Falace DA, Miller C, Rhodus NL: Dental management of the medically compromised patient, ed 6, St Louis, 2002, Mosby.

Malamed SF: Medical emergencies in the dental office, ed 5, St Louis, 1999, Mosby.

Malone WPF, Koth DC: Tylman's theory and practice of fixed prosthodontics, ed 8, Tokyo, 1989, IEA.

Miller CH, Palenik CJ: Infection control and management of hazardous materials for the dental team, ed 3, St Louis, in press, Mosby.

Morrow RM, Rudd KD, Rhoads JE: Dental laboratory procedures: complete dentures, vol 1, St Louis, 1985, Mosby.

Mosby's dental dictionary, St Louis, 2004, Mosby.

Nevins M, Mellonig JT: Periodontal therapy: clinical approaches and evidence of success, vol 1, Chicago, 1989, Quintessence.

O'Brien WJ: Dental materials and their selection, ed 2, Chicago, 1989, Quintessence.

Okeson JP: Management of temporomandibular disorders and occlusion, ed 5, St Louis, 2003, Mosby.

Okeson JP: Orofacial pain: guidelines for assessment, diagnosis, and management, Chicago, 1996, Quintessence.

Osborne J: Osborne and Lammie's partial dentures, ed 5, Oxford, 1986, Blackwell Scientific.

Preiskel HW: Precision attachments in prosthodontics, Chicago, 1996, Quintessence.

Rahn AO, Hartwell CM: Textbook of complete dentures, ed 5, Baltimore, 1993, Waverly.

Ramfjord SP, Ash MM Jr: Occlusion, ed 4, Philadelphia, 1995, WB Saunders.

Renner RP, Boucher LJ: Removable partial prosthodontics, Chicago, 1987, Quintessence.

Rosenstiel SF, Land MF, Fujimoto J: Contemporary fixed prosthodontics, ed 3, St Louis, 2001, Mosby.

Rudd KD, Rhoads JE, Morrow RM: Dental laboratory procedures, vol 3, ed 2, St Louis, 1986, Mosby.

Sarnat BG, Laskin DM: The temporomandibular joint: a biological basis for clinical practice, ed 4, Philadelphia, 1992, WB Saunders.

Shillingberg HT et al: Fundamentals of fixed prosthodontics, ed 3, Chicago, 1997, Quintessence.

Stewart KL, Kueliker WA, Rudd KD: Clinical removable partial prosthodontics, Tokyo, 1992, IEA.

Stratton RP, Wiebelt FJ: An atlas of removable partial denture design, Chicago, 1988, Quintessence.

Watt DM, MacGregor AR: Designing partial dentures, Littleton, Mass, 1985, PSG.

Winkler S: Essentials of complete denture prosthodontics, ed 2, Littleton, Mass, 1988, PSG.

Wood NK: Review of diagnosis, oral medicine, radiology, and treatment planning, ed 4, St Louis, 1999, Mosby.

Wood NK: Differential diagnosis of oral and maxillofacial lesions, ed 5, St Louis, 1997, Mosby.

Yalisove IL, Dietz JB Jr: Telescopic prosthetic therapy, Philadelphia, 1979, George F Stickley.

Zarb GA: Temporomandibular joint and masticatory muscle disorders, St Louis, 1995, Mosby.

Zarb GA et al: Prosthodontic treatment for edentulous patients: complete dentures and implant-supported prostheses, ed 12, St Louis, 2004, Mosby.

ABUTMENT RETAINERS: EXTERNAL AND INTERNAL ATTACHMENTS

Adisman IK: The internal clip attachment in fixed removable partial denture prosthesis, N Y J Dent 32:125-129, 1962.

Ainamo J: Precision removable partial dentures with pontic abutments, J Prosthet Dent 23:289-295, 1970.

Augsburger RH: The Gilmore attachment, J Prosthet Dent 16:1090-1102, 1966.

Becker CM, Campbell MC, Williams DL: The Thompson dowel-rest system modified for chrome-cobalt removable partial denture frameworks, J Prosthet Dent 39:384-391, 1978.

Ben-Ur Z, Aviv I, Cardash HS: A modified direct retainer design for distal extension removable partial dentures, J Prosthet Dent 70:342-344, 1988.

Benson D, Spolsky VW: A clinical evaluation of removable partial dentures with I-bar retainers. Part I, J Prosthet Dent 41:246, 1979.

Berg T Jr: I-bar: myth and counter myth, Dent Clin North Am 23:1, 65-75, 1979.

Blatterfein L: Study of partial denture clasping, J Am Dent Assoc 43:169-185, 1951.

Blatterfein L: Design and positional arrangement of clasps for partial dentures, N Y J Dent 22:305-306, 1952.

Brodbelt RHW: A simple paralleling template for precision attachments, J Prosthet Dent 27:285-288, 1972.

Brudvik JS, Morris HF: Stress-relaxation testing. Part III: influence of wire alloys, gauges, and lengths on clasp behavior, J Prosthet Dent 46:374, 1981.

Brudvik JS, Wormley JH: Construction techniques for wrought-wire retentive clasp arms as related to clasp flexibility, J Prosthet Dent 30:769-774, 1973.

Chandler JA, Brudvik JS: Clinical evaluation of patients eight to nine years after placement of removable partial dentures, J Prosthet Dent 51:736, 1984.

Chou TM et al: Photoelastic analysis and comparison of force-transmission characteristics of intracoronal attachments with clasp distal-extension removable partial dentures, J Prosthet Dent 62:313-319, 1989.

Chou TM et al: Stereophotogrammetric analysis of abutment tooth movement in distal-extension removable partial dentures with intracoronal attachments and clasps, J Prosthet Dent 66:343-349, 1991.

Clayton JA: A stable base precision attachment removable partial denture (PARPD): theories and principles, Dent Clin North Am 24:3-29, 1980.

Cooper H: Practice management related to precision attachment prostheses, Dent Clin North Am 24:45-61, 1980.

DeVan MM: Preserving natural teeth through the use of clasps, J Prosthet Dent 5:208-214, 1955.

Dietz WH: Modified abutments for removable and fixed prosthodontics, J Prosthet Dent 11:1112-1116, 1961.

Dixon DL et al: Wear of I-bar clasps and porcelain laminate restorations, Int J Prosthet 5:28-33, 1992.

Dolder EJ: The bar joint mandibular denture, J Prosthet Dent 11:689-707, 1961.

Eliason CM: RPA clasp design for distal-extension removable partial dentures, J Prosthet Dent 49:25-27, 1983.

Frank RP, Brudvik JS, Nicholls JI: A comparison of the flexibility of wrought-wire and cast circumferential clasps, J Prosthet Dent 49:471-476, 1983.

Getz II: Making a full-coverage restoration on an abutment to fit an existing removable partial denture, J Prosthet Dent 54:335-336, 1985.
Gilson TD: A fixable-removable prosthetic attachment, J Prosthet Dent 9:247-255, 1959.
Gindea AE: A retentive device for removable dentures, J Prosthet Dent 27:501-508, 1972.
Grasso JE: A new removable partial denture clasp assembly, J Prosthet Dent 43:618-621, 1980.
Green JH: The hinge-lock abutment attachment, J Am Dent Assoc 47:175-180, 1953.
Hebel KS, Graser GN, Featherstone JD: Abrasion of enamel and composite resin by removable partial denture clasps, J Prosthet Dent 52:389, 1984.
Highton R, Caputo AA, Matyas J: Retention and stress characteristics for a magnetically retained partial denture, J Dent Res (IADR. abstract 279) 62:entire issue, 1982.
Isaacson GO: Telescope crown retainers for removable partial dentures, J Prosthet Dent 22:436-448, 1969.
Ivanhoe JR: Alternative cingulum rest seat, J Prosthet Dent 54:395-396, 1985.
James AG: Self-locking posterior attachment for removable tooth-supported partial dentures, J Prosthet Dent 5: 200-205, 1955.
Johnson DL, Stratton RJ, Duncanson MG Jr: The effect of single plane curvature on half-round cast clasps, J Dent Res 62:833-836, 1983.
Johnson JF: The application and construction of the pinledge retainer, J Prosthet Dent 3:559-567, 1953.
Kapur KK et al: A randomized clinical trial of two basic removable partial denture designs. Part I: comparisons of five-year success rates and periodontal health, J Prosthet Dent 72(3):268-282, 1994.
Knodle JM: Experimental overlay and pin partial denture, J Prosthet Dent 17:472-478, 1967.
Knowles LE: A dowel attachment removable partial denture, J Prosthet Dent 13:679-687, 1963.
Koper A: Retainer for removable partial dentures: the Thompson dowel, J Prosthet Dent 30:759-768, 1973.
Kotowicz WE: Clinical procedures in precision attachment removable partial denture construction, Dent Clin North Am 24:143-164, 1980.
Kotowicz WE et al: The combination clasp and the distal extension removable partial denture, Dent Clin North Am 17:651-660, 1973.
Kratochvil FJ, Davidson PN, Tandarts JG: Five-year study of treatment with removable partial dentures. Part I, J Prosthet Dent 48:237, 1982.
Krol AJ: Clasp design for extension base removable partial dentures, J Prosthet Dent 29:408-415, 1973.
Krol AJ: RPI clasp retainer and its modifications, Dent Clin North Am 17:631-649, 1973.
Langer A: Combinations of diverse retainers in removable partial dentures, J Prosthet Dent 40:378-384, 1978.
LaVere AM: Analysis of facial surface undercuts to determine use of RPI or RPA clasps, J Prosthet Dent 56:741-743, 1986.
Leupold RJ, Faraone KL: Etched castings as an adjunct to mouth preparation for removable partial dentures, J Prosthet Dent 53:655-658, 1985.
Lubovich RP, Peterson T: The fabrication of a ceramic-metal crown to fit an existing removable partial denture clasp, J Prosthet Dent 37:610-614, 1977.
Marinello CP et al: Resin-bonded etched castings with extracoronal attachments for removable partial dentures, J Prosthet Dent 66:52-55, 1991.
Maroso DJ, Schmidt JR, Blustein R: A preliminary study of wear of porcelain when subjected to functional movements of retentive clasp arms, J Prosthet Dent 45:14, 1981.
McLeod NS: A theoretical analysis of the mechanics of the Thompson dowel semiprecision intracoronal retainer, J Prosthet Dent 37:19-27, 1977.
McLeod NS: Improved design for the Thompson dowel rest semiprecision intracoronal retainer, J Prosthet Dent 40:513-516, 1978.
Mensor MC Jr: Attachment fixation for overdentures. Part I, J Prosthet Dent 37:366-373, 1977.
Mensor MC Jr: Attachment fixation of the overdentures. Part II, J Prosthet Dent 39:16-20, 1978.
Morris HF et al: Stress distribution within circumferential clasp arms, J Oral Rehabil 3:387-391, 1976.
Morris HF et al: Stress-relaxation testing. Part II: Comparison of bending profiles, microstructures, microhardness, and surface characteristics of several wrought-wires, J Prosthet Dent 46:256, 1981.
Morris HF et al: Stress-relaxation testing. Part IV. Clasp pattern dimensions and their influence on clasp behavior, J Prosthet Dent 50:319, 1983.
Morrison ML: Internal precision attachment retainers for partial dentures, J Am Dent Assoc 64:209-215, 1962.
Morrow RM: Tooth-supported complete dentures: an approach to preventive prosthodontics, J Prosthet Dent 21:513-522, 1969.
Oddo VJ Jr: The movable-arm clasp for complete passivity in partial denture construction, J Am Dent Assoc 74:1009-1015, 1967.
Plotnik IJ: Internal attachment for fixed removable partial dentures, J Prosthet Dent 8:85-93, 1958.
Pound E: Cross-arch splinting vs. premature extractions, J Prosthet Dent 16:1058-1068, 1966.
Preiskel H: Precision attachments for free-end saddle prostheses, Br Dent J 127:462, 468, 1969.
Preiskel H: Screw retained telescopic prosthesis, Br Dent J 130:107-112, 1971.
Prince IB: Conservation of the supportive mechanism, J Prosthet Dent 15:327-338, 1965.
Sato Y et al: Effect of friction coefficient on Akers clasp retention, J Prosthet Dent 78(1):22-27, 1997.
Seto BG, Avera S, Kagawa T: Resin bonded etched cast cingulum rest retainers for removable partial dentures, Quintessence Int 16:757-760, 1985.
Singer F: Improvements in precision: attached removable partial dentures, J Prosthet Dent 17:69-72, 1967.
Smith RA, Rymarz FP: Cast clasp transitional removable partial dentures, J Prosthet Dent 22:381-385, 1969.
Snyder HA, Duncanson MG, Johnson D: Effect of clasp flexure on a 4-meta adhered light-polymerized composite resin, Int J Prosthodont 4:364-370, 1991.
Soderfeldt B et al: A multilevel analysis of factors affecting the longevity of fixed partial dentures, retainers and abutments, J Oral Rehabil 25(4):245-252, 1998.
Spielberger MC et al: Effect of retentive clasp design on gingival health: a feasibility study, J Prosthet Dent 52:397, 1984.

Stankewitz CG, Gardner FM, Butler GV: Adjustment of cast clasps for direct retention, J Prosthet Dent 45:344, 1981.
Stansbury BE: A retentive attachment for overdentures, J Prosthet Dent 35:228-230, 1976.
Stern MA, Brudvik JS, Frank RP: Clinical evaluation of removable partial denture rest seat adaptation, J Prosthet Dent 53:658-662, 1985.
Stewart BL, Edwards RO: Retention and wear of precision-type attachments, J Prosthet Dent 49:28-34, 1983.
Strohaver RA, Trovillion HM: Removable partial overdentures, J Prosthet Dent 35:624-629, 1976.
Symposium on semiprecision attachments in removable partial dentures, Dent Clin North Am 29:1-237, 1985.
Tautin FS: Abutment stabilization using a nonresilient gingival bar connector, J Am Dent Assoc 99:988-989, 1979.
Tietge JD et al: Wear of composite resins and cast direct retainers, Int J Prosthet 5:145-153, 1992.
Vig RG: Splinting bars and maxillary indirect retainers for removable partial dentures, J Prosthet Dent 13:125-129, 1963.
Walter JD: Anchor attachments used as locking devices in two-part removable prostheses, J Prosthet Dent 33:628-632, 1975.
Waltz ME: Ceka extracoronal attachments, J Prosthet Dent 29:167-171, 1973.
White JT: Visualization of stress and strain related to removable partial denture abutments, J Prosthet Dent 40:143-151, 1978.
Wiebelt FJ, Shillingburg HT Jr: Abutment preparation modifications for removable partial denture rest seats, Quintessence Dent Technol 9:449-451, 1985.
Williams AG: Technique for provisional splint with attachment, J Prosthet Dent 21:555-559, 1969.
Willis LM, Swoope CC: Precision attachment partial dentures. In Clark JW, ed: Clinical dentistry, vol 5, New York, 1976, Harper & Row.
Wright SM: Use of spring-loaded attachments for retention of removable partial dentures, J Prosthet Dent 51:605-610, 1984.
Zakler JM: Intracoronal precision attachments, Dent Clin North Am 24:131-141, 1980.
Zinner ID, Miller RD, Panno FV: Semiprecision rest system for distal extension removable partial denture design, J Prosthet Dent 42:131-134, 1979.
Zinner ID, Miller RD, Panno FV: Precision attachments, Dent Clin North Am 31:395-416, 1987.
Zinner ID, Miller RD, Panno FV: Clinical management of abutments with intracoronal attachments, J Prosthet Dent 67:761-767, 1992.

ANATOMY

Bennett NG: A contribution to the study of the movements of the mandible, J Prosthet Dent 8:41-54, 1958.
Boucher CO: Complete denture impressions based upon the anatomy of the mouth, J Am Dent Assoc 31:1174-1181, 1944.
Brodie AG: Anatomy and physiology of head and neck musculature, Am J Orthod 36:831-844, 1950.
Casey DM: Palatopharyngeal anatomy and physiology, J Prosthet Dent 49:371-378, 1983.
Craddock FW: Retromolar region of the mandible, J Am Dent Assoc 47:453-455, 1953.
Haines RW, Barnett SG: The structure of the mouth in the mandibular molar region, J Prosthet Dent 9:962-974, 1959.
Martone AL et al: Anatomy of the mouth and related structures: I. J Prosthet Dent 11:1009-1018, 1961; II, 12:4-27, 1962; III, 12:206-219, 1962; IV, 12:409-419, 1962; V, 12:629-636, 1962; VI, 12:817-834, 1962; VII, 13:4-33, 1963; VIII, 13:204-228, 1963.
Merkeley HJ: The labial and buccal accessory muscles of mastication, J Prosthet Dent 4:327-334, 1954.
Merkeley HJ: Mandibular rearmament. I. Anatomic considerations, J Prosthet Dent 9:559-566, 1959.
Monteith BD: Management of loading forces on the mandibular extension prosthesis. Part II: Classification for matching modalities to clinical situations, J Prosthet Dent 52:832-835, 1984.
Pendleton EC: Anatomy of the face and mouth from the standpoint of the denture prosthetist, J Am Dent Assoc 33:219-234, 1946.
Pendleton EC: Changes in the denture supporting tissues, J Am Dent Assoc 42:1-15, 1951.
Pietrokovski J: The bony residual ridge in man, J Prosthet Dent 34:456-462, 1975.
Pietrokovski J, Sorin S, Zvia H: The residual ridge in partially edentulous patients, J Prosthet Dent 36:150-158, 1976.
Preti G, Bruscagin C, Fava C: Anatomic and statistical study to determine the inclination of the condylar long axis, J Prosthet Dent 49:572-575, 1983.
Roche AF: Functional anatomy of the muscles of mastication, J Prosthet Dent 13:548-570, 1963.
Silverman SI: Denture prosthesis and the functional anatomy of the maxillofacial structures, J Prosthet Dent 6:305-331, 1956.

BIOMECHANICS

Asher ML: Application of the rotational path design concept to a removable partial denture with a distal-extension base, J Prosthet Dent 68:641-643, 1992.
Augthun M et al: The influence of spruing technique on the development of tension in a cast partial denture framework, Int J Prosthodont 7(1):72-76, 1994.
Avant WE: Factors that influence retention of removable partial dentures, J Prosthet Dent 25:265-270, 1971.
Avant WE: Fulcrum and retention lines in planning removable partial dentures, J Prosthet Dent 25:162-166, 1971.
Aviv I, Ben-Ur Z, Cardash HS: An analysis of rotational movement of asymmetrical distal-extension removable partial dentures, J Prosthet Dent 61:211-214, 1989.
Aydinlik E, Akay HU: Effect of a resilient layer in a removable partial denture base on stress distribution to the mandible, J Prosthet Dent 44:17-20, 1980.
Ben-Ur Z et al: Designing clasps for the asymmetric distal extension removable partial denture, Int J Prosthodont 9(4):374-378, 1996.
Berg TE, Caputo AA: Comparison of load transfer by maxillary distal extension removable partial dentures with a spring-loaded plunger attachment and I-bar retainer, J Prosthet Dent 68:492-499, 1992.

Berg TE, Caputo AA: Load transfer by a maxillary distal-extension removable partial denture with extracoronal attachments, J Prosthet Dent 68:784-789, 1992.

Bezzon OL et al: Surveying removable partial dentures: the importance of guiding planes and path of insertion for stability, J Prosthet Dent 78(4):412-418, 1997.

Bridgeman JT et al: Comparison of titanium and cobalt-chromium removable partial denture clasps, J Prosthet Dent 78(2):187-193, 1997.

Browning JD, Eick JD, McGarrah HE: Abutment tooth movement measured in vivo by using stereophotogrammetry, J Prosthet Dent 57:323-328, 1987.

Brudvik JS, Morris HF: Stress-relaxation testing. Part III: Influence of wire alloys, gauges, and lengths on clasp behavior, J Prosthet Dent 46:374-379, 1981.

Cecconi BT: Effect of rest design on transmission of forces to abutment teeth, J Prosthet Dent 32:141-151, 1974.

Cecconi BT, Asgar K, Dootz E: The effect of partial denture clasp design on abutment tooth movement, J Prosthet Dent 25:44-56, 1971.

Cecconi BT, Asgar K, Dootz E: Removable partial denture abutment tooth movement as affected by inclination of residual ridges and types of loading, J Prosthet Dent 25:375-381, 1971.

Cecconi BT, Asgar K, Dootz E: Clasp assembly modifications and their effect on abutment tooth movement, J Prosthet Dent 27:160-167, 1972.

Chou TM et al: Photoelastic analysis and comparison of force-transmission characteristics of intracoronal attachments with clasp distal-extension removable partial dentures, J Prosthet Dent 62:313-319, 1989.

Chou TM et al: Stereophotogrammetric analysis of abutment tooth movement in distal-extension removable partial dentures with intracoronal attachments and clasps, J Prosthet Dent 66:343-349, 1991.

Clayton JA, Jaslow C: A measurement of clasp forces on teeth, J Prosthet Dent 25:21-43, 1971.

Craig RG, Farah JW: Stresses from loading distal extension removable partial dentures, J Prosthet Dent 39:274-277, 1978.

DeVan MM: The nature of the partial denture foundation: suggestions for its preservation, J Prosthet Dent 2:210-218, 1952.

el Charkawi HG et al: The effect of the resilient-layer distal-extension partial denture on movement of the abutment teeth: a new methodology, J Prosthet Dent 60:622-630, 1988.

Fisher RL: Factors that influence the base stability of mandibular distal-extension removable partial dentures: a longitudinal study, J Prosthet Dent 50:167-171, 1983.

Frank RP, Nicholls JI: A study of the flexibility of wrought-wire clasps, J Prosthet Dent 45:259-267, 1981.

Frechette AR: The influence of partial denture design on distribution of force to abutment teeth, J Prosthet Dent 6:195-212, 1956.

Goodkind RJ: The effects of removable partial dentures on abutment tooth mobility, J Prosthet Dent 30:139-146, 1973.

Goodman JJ, Goodman HW: Balance of force in precision free-end restorations, J Prosthet Dent 13:302-308, 1963.

Hall WA: Variations in registering interarch transfers in removable partial denture construction, J Prosthet Dent 30:548-553, 1973.

Harrop J, Javid N: Reciprocal arms of direct retainers in removable partial dentures, J Can Dent Assoc 4:208-211, 1976.

Henderson D, Seward TE: Design and force distribution with removable partial dentures: a progress report, J Prosthet Dent 17:350-364, 1967.

Henriques GE et al: Soldering and remelting influence on fatigue strength of cobalt-chromium alloy, J Prosthet Dent 78(2):146-152, 1997.

Hindels GW: Stress analysis in distal extension partial dentures, J Prosthet Dent 7:197-205, 1957.

Iwama CY et al: Cobalt-chromium-titanium alloy for removable partial dentures, Int J Prosthodont 10(4):309-317, 1997.

Johnson DL, Stratton RJ, Duncanson MGJ: The effect of single plane curvature on half-round cast clasps, J Dent Res 62:833-836, 1983.

Kaires AK: Partial denture design and its relation to force distribution and masticatory performance, J Prosthet Dent 6:672-683, 1956.

Knowles LE: The biomechanics of removable partial dentures and its relationship to fixed prosthesis, J Prosthet Dent 8:426-430, 1958.

Kratochvil FJ: Influence of occlusal rest position and clasp design on movement of abutment teeth, J Prosthet Dent 13:114-124, 1963.

Kratochvil FJ, Caputo AA: Photoelastic analysis of pressure on teeth and bone supporting removable partial dentures, J Prosthet Dent 3:52, 1975.

Kratochvil FJ, Thompson WD, Caputo AA: Photoelastic analysis of stress patterns on teeth and bone with attachment retainers for removable partial dentures, J Prosthet Dent 46:21-28, 1981.

Lofbers PG, Ericson G, Eliasson S: A clinical and radiographic evaluation of removable partial dentures retained by attachments to alveolar bars, J Prosthet Dent 47:126-132, 1982.

Lowe RD, Kydd WL, Smith DE: Swallowing and resting forces related to lingual flange thickness in removable partial dentures, J Prosthet Dent 23:279-288, 1970.

MacGregor AR, Miller TPG, Farah JW: Stress analysis of partial dentures, J Dent 6:125-132, 1978.

Marei MK: Measurement (in vitro) of the amount of force required to dislodge specific clasps from different depths of undercut, J Prosthet Dent 74:258-263, 1995.

Maroso DJ, Schmidt JR, Blustein R: A preliminary study of wear of porcelain when subjected to functional movements of retentive clasp arms, J Prosthet Dent 45:14-17, 1981.

Matheson GR, Brudvik JS, Nicholls JI: Behavior of wrought-wire clasps after repeated permanent deformation, J Prosthet Dent 55:226-231, 1986.

Maxfield JB, Nicholls JI, Smith DE: The measurement of forces transmitted to abutment teeth of removable partial dentures, J Prosthet Dent 41:134, 1979.

McCartney JW: Motion vector analysis of an abutment for a distal-extension removable partial denture, J Prosthet Dent 43:15-21, 1980.

McDowell GC: Force transmission by indirect retainers during unilateral loading, J Prosthet Dent 39:616-621, 1978.
McDowell GC, Fisher RL: Force transmission by indirect retainers when a unilateral dislodging force is applied, J Prosthet Dent 47:360-365, 1982.
McLeod NS: An analysis of the rotational axes of semiprecision and precision distal-extension removable partial dentures, J Prosthet Dent 48:130-134, 1982.
Morris HF, Asgar K, Tillitson E: Stress-relaxation testing. I. A new approach to the testing of removable partial denture alloys, wrought-wires, and clasp behavior, J Prosthet Dent 46:133-141, 1981.
Morris HF, Brudvik JS: Influence of polishing on cast clasp properties, J Prosthet Dent 55:75-77, 1986.
Morris HF et al: Stress-relaxation testing. IV. Clasp pattern dimensions and their influence on clasp behavior, J Prosthet Dent 50:319-326, 1983.
NaBadalung DP et al: Comparison of bond strengths of denture base resins to nickel-chromium-beryllium removable partial denture alloy, J Prosthet Dent 78(6):566-573, 1997.
NaBadalung DP et al: Frictional resistance of removable partial dentures with retrofitted resin composite guide planes, Int J Prosthodont 10(2):116-122, 1997.
NaBadalung DP et al: Laser welding of a cobalt-chromium removable partial denture alloy, J Prosthet Dent 79(3):285-290, 1998.
Ogata K, Shimigu K: Longitudinal study of forces transmitted from denture base to retainers of free-end saddle dentures with Akers clasps, J Oral Rehabil 18:471-480, 1991.
Plotnick IJ, Beresin VE, Simkins AB: The effects of variations in the opposing dentition on changes in the partially edentulous mandible, J Prosthet Dent; I, 33:278-286, 1975; II, 33:403-406, 1975; III, 33:529-534, 1975.
Sansom BP et al: Rest seat designs for inclined posterior abutments: a photoelastic comparison, J Prosthet Dent 58:57-62, 1987.
Shohet H: Relative magnitudes of stress on abutment teeth with different retainers, J Prosthet Dent 21:267-282, 1969.
Smith BH: Changes in occlusal face height with removable partial dentures, J Prosthet Dent 34:278-285, 1975.
Smith BJ, Turner CH: The use of crowns to modify abutment teeth of removable partial dentures, J Dent 7:52-56, 1979.
Smyd ES: Biomechanics of prosthetic dentistry, J Prosthet Dent 4:368-383, 1954.
Stern WJ: Guiding planes in clasp reciprocation and retention, J Prosthet Dent 34:408-414, 1975.
Swoope CC, Frank RP: Stress control and design. In Clark JW, ed: Clinical dentistry, vol 5, New York, 1976, Harper & Row.
Taylor DT, Pflushoeft FA, McGivney GP: Effect of two clasping assemblies on arch integrity as modified by base adaptation, J Prosthet Dent 47:120-125, 1982.
Tebrock OC et al: The effect of various clasping systems on the mobility of abutment teeth for distal-extension removable partial dentures, J Prosthet Dent 41:511, 1979.
Thomspon WD, Kratochvil FJ, Caputo AA: Evaluation of photoelastic stress patterns produced by various designs of bilateral distal-extension removable partial dentures, J Prosthet Dent 38:261, 1977.
Toth RW et al: Shear strength of lingual rest seats prepared in bonded composite, J Prosthet Dent 56:99-104, 1986.
Vallittu PK: Comparison of the in vitro fatigue resistance of an acrylic resin removable partial denture reinforced with continuous glass fibers or metal wires, J Prosthodont 5(2):115-121,1996.
Villittu PK: Deflection fatigue of cobalt-chromium, titanium, and gold alloy cast denture clasp, J Prosthet Dent 74(4):412-419, 1995.
Waldmeier MD et al: Bend testing of wrought-wire removable partial denture alloys, J Prosthet Dent 76(5):559-565, 1996.
Wills DJ, Manderson RD: Biomechanical aspects of the support of partial dentures, J Dent 5:310-318, 1977.
Yurkstas A, Fridley HH, Manly RS: A functional evaluation of fixed and removable bridgework, J Prosthet Dent 1:570-577, 1951.
Zoeller GN, Kelly WJ Jr: Block form stability in removable partial prosthodontics, J Prosthet Dent 25:515-519, 1971.

CLASSIFICATION

Applegate OC: The rationale of partial denture choice, J Prosthet Dent 10:891-907, 1960.
Avant WE: A universal classification for removable partial denture situations, J Prosthet Dent 16:533-539, 1966.
Bailyn M: Tissue support in partial denture construction, Dent Cosmos 70:988-997, 1928.
Beckett LS: The influence of saddle classification on the design of partial removable restoration, J Prosthet Dent 3:506-516, 1953.
Costa E: A simplified system for identifying partially edentulous arches, J Prosthet Dent 32:639-645, 1974.
Cummer WE: Partial denture service. In Anthony LP, ed: American textbook of prosthetic dentistry, Philadelphia, 1942, Lea & Febiger.
Friedman J: The ABC classification of partial denture segments, J Prosthet Dent 3:517-524, 1953.
Godfrey RJ: Classification of removable partial dentures, J Am Coll Dent 18:5-13, 1951.
Kennedy E: Partial denture construction, Dental Items of Interest, pp 3-8, 1928.
Mensor MC Jr: Classification and selection of attachments, J Prosthet Dent 29:494-497, 1973.
Miller EL: Systems for classifying partially dentulous arches, J Prosthet Dent 24:25-40, 1970.
Skinner CN: A classification of removable partial dentures based upon the principles of anatomy and physiology, J Prosthet Dent 9:240-246, 1959.

CLEFT PALATE

Aram A, Subtelny JD: Velopharyngeal function and cleft palate prostheses, J Prosthet Dent 9:149-158, 1959.
Baden E: Fundamental principles of orofacial prosthetic therapy in congenital cleft palate, J Prosthet Dent 4: 420-433, 1954.

Bixler D: Heritability of clefts of the lips and palate, J Prosthet Dent 33:100-108, 1975.
Buckner H: Construction of a denture with hollow obturator, lid and soft acrylic lining, J Prosthet Dent 31:95-99, 1974.
Calvan J: The error of Gustan Passavant, Plast Reconstr Surg 13:275-289, 1954.
Cooper HK: Integration of service in the treatment of cleft lip and cleft palate, J Am Dent Assoc 47:27-32, 1953.
Dalston RM: Prosthodontic management of the cleft palate patient: a speech pathologist's view, J Prosthet Dent 37:327-329, 1978.
Ettinger RL: Use of teeth with a poor prognosis in cleft palate prosthodontics, J Am Dent Assoc 94:10-914, 1977.
Fox A: Prosthetic correction of a severe acquired cleft palate, J Prosthet Dent 8:542-546, 1958.
Gibbons P, Bloomer H: A supportive-type prosthetic speech aid, J Prosthet Dent 8:362-369, 1958.
Graber TM: Oral and nasal structures in cleft palate speech, J Am Dent Assoc 53:693-706, 1956.
Harkins CS: Modern concepts in the prosthetic rehabilitation of cleft palate patients, J Oral Surg 10:298-312, 1952.
Harkins CS, Ivy RH: Surgery and prosthesis in the rehabilitation of cleft palate patients, J South Calif Dent Assoc 19:16-24, 1951.
Immekus JE, Aramany MA: A fixed-removable partial denture for cleft palate patients, J Prosthet Dent 34:286-291, 1975.
Landa JS: The prosthodontist views the rehabilitation of the cleft palate patient, J Prosthet Dent 6:421-427, 1956.
Lavelle WE, Zach GE: The tissue bar and Ceka anchor as aids in cleft palate rehabilitation, J Prosthet Dent 30:321-325, 1973.
Lloyd RS, Pruzansky S, Subtelny JD: Prosthetic rehabilitation of a cleft palate patient subsequent to multiple surgical and prosthetic failures, J Prosthet Dent 7:216-230, 1957.
Merkeley HJ: Cleft palate prosthesis, J Prosthet Dent 9:506-513, 1959.
Minsley GE, Warren DW, Hairfield WM: The effect of cleft palate speech aid prostheses on the nasopharyngeal airway and breathing, J Prosthet Dent 65:122-126, 1991.
Nidiffer TJ, Shipmon TH: The hollow-bulb obturator for acquired palatal openings, J Prosthet Dent 7:126-134, 1957.
Olinger NA: Cleft palate prosthesis rehabilitation, J Prosthet Dent 2:117-135, 1952.
Rosen MS: Prosthetics for the cleft palate patient, J Am Dent Assoc 60:715-721, 1960.
Rothenberg LIA: Overlay dentures for the cleft-palate patient, J Prosthet Dent 37:190-195, 1977.
Schneiderman CR, Maun MB: Air flow and intelligibility of speech of normal speakers and speakers with a prosthodontically repaired cleft palate, J Prosthet Dent 39:193-199, 1978.
Sharry JJ: The meatus obturator in cleft palate prosthesis, Oral Surg 7:852-855, 1954.
Sharry JJ: Meatus obturator in particular and pharyngeal impressions in general, J Prosthet Dent 8:893-896, 1958.
Tautin FS, Schaaf NA: Superiorly based obturator, J Prosthet Dent 33:96-99, 1975.
Walter JD: Palatopharyngeal activity in cleft palate subjects, J Prosthet Dent 63:187-192, 1990.

COMPLETE MOUTH AND OCCLUSAL REHABILITATION

Brewer AA, Fenton AH: The overdenture, Dent Clin North Am 17:723-746, 1973.
Bronstein BR: Rationale and technique of biomechanical occlusal rehabilitation, J Prosthet Dent 4:352-367, 1954.
Cohn LA: Occluso-rehabilitation, principles of diagnosis and treatment planning, Dent Clin North Am 6:281, 1962.
Curtis SR: Integrating fixed and removable provisional restorations, J Prosthet Dent 70:374-377, 1993.
Dubin NA: Advances in functional occlusal rehabilitation, J Prosthet Dent 6:252-258, 1956.
Ferencz JL: Splinting, Dent Clin North Am 31:383-393, 1987.
Kazis H: Functional aspects of complete mouth rehabilitation, J Prosthet Dent 4:833-841, 1954.
Kornfeld M: The problem of function in restorative dentistry, J Prosthet Dent 5:670-676, 1955.
Landa JS: An analysis of current practices in mouth rehabilitation, J Prosthet Dent 5:527-537, 1955.
Lang BR: Complete denture occlusion, Dent Clin North Am 40(1):85-101, 1996.
Mann AW, Pankey LD: Oral rehabilitation utilizing the Pankey-Mann instrument and a functional bite technique, Dent Clin North Am, pp 215-230, March 1959.
Mann AW, Pankey LD: Oral rehabilitation. I: Use of the P-M instrument in treatment planning and restoring the lower posterior teeth, J Prosthet Dent 10:135-150, 1960.
Mann AW, Pankey LD: Oral rehabilitation. II: Reconstruction of the upper teeth using a functionally generated path technique, J Prosthet Dent 10:151-162, 1960.
McCartney JW: Occlusal reconstruction and rebase procedure for distal extension removable partial dentures, J Prosthet Dent 43:695-698, 1980.
Schuyler CH: An evaluation of incisal guidance and its influence on restorative dentistry, J Prosthet Dent 9:374-378, 1959.
Schweitzer JM: Open bite from the prosthetic point of view, Dent Clin North Am 1:269-283, 1957.

CROWNS AND FIXED PARTIAL DENTURES

Alexander PC: Analysis of the cuspid protective occlusion, J Prosthet Dent 13:309-317, 1963.
Bader JD et al: Effect of crown margins on periodontal conditions in regularly attending patients, J Prosthet Dent 65:75-79, 1991.
Beeson PE: The use of acrylic resins as an aid in the development of patterns for two types of crowns, J Prosthet Dent 13:493-498, 1963.
Binkley TK, Binkley C: Porcelain-fused-to-metal crowns as replacements for denture teeth in removable partial denture construction, J Prosthet Dent 58:124-125, 1987.
Blackman R, Baeg R, Barghi N: Marginal accuracy and geometry of cast titanium copings, J Prosthet Dent 67:435-440, 1992.
Budtz-Jorgenson E, Isidor F: A five-year longitudinal study of cantilever fixed partial dentures compared with removable partial dentures in a geriatric population, J Prosthet Dent 64:42-47, 1990.

Caplan J: Maintenance of full coverage fixed-abutment bridges, J Prosthet Dent 5:852-854, 1955.
Cheug SP, Dimmer A: Management of worn dentition with resin-bonded cast metal lingual veneering, J Prosthet Dent 63:122-123, 1990.
Coelho DH: Criteria for the use of fixed prosthesis, Dent Clin North Am 1:299-311, 1957.
Cooper TM et al: Effect of venting on cast gold full crowns, J Prosthet Dent 26:621-626, 1971.
Cowgen GT: Retention, resistance and esthetics of the anterior three-quarter crown, J Am Dent Assoc 62:167-171, 1961.
Culpepper WD, Moulton PS: Considerations in fixed prosthodontics, Dent Clin North Am 23:21-35, 1979.
Dental technology standards: J Dent Technol 14(5):26-31, 1997.
Ekfeldt A et al: Changes of masticatory movement characteristics after prosthodontic rehabilitation of individuals with extensive tooth wear, Int J Prosthodont 9(6):539-546, 1996.
Elledge DA, Schorr BL: A provisional and new crown to fit with a clasp of an existing removable partial denture, J Prosthet Dent 63:541-544, 1990.
Felton DA et al: Effect of in vivo crown margin discrepancies on periodontal health, J Prosthet Dent 65:357-364, 1991.
Glantz PO et al: The devitalized tooth as an abutment in dentitions with reduced but healthy periodontium, Periodontol 2000 4:52-57, 1994.
Goldberg A, Jones RD: Constructing cast crowns to fit existing removable partial denture clasps, J Prosthet Dent 36:382-386, 1976.
Goodacre CJ et al: The prosthodontic management of endodontically treated teeth: a literature review. Part I: Success and failure data, treatment concepts, J Prosthodont 3(4):243-250, 1994.
Guyer SE: Nonrigid subocclusal connector for fixed partial dentures, J Prosthet Dent 26:433-436, 1971.
Hansen CA, Cook PA, Nelson DF: Pin-modified facial inlay to enhance retentive contours on a removable partial denture abutment, J Prosthet Dent 55:480-481, 1986.
Henderson D et al: The cantilever type of posterior fixed partial dentures: a laboratory study, J Prosthet Dent 24:47-67, 1970.
Johnson EA Jr: Combination of fixed and removable partial dentures, J Prosthet Dent 14:1099-1106, 1964.
Johnston JF et al: Construction and assembly of porcelain veneer gold crowns and pontics, J Prosthet Dent 12:1125-1137, 1962.
Kapur KK et al: Veterans Administration Cooperation Dental Implant Study: Comparisons between fixed partial dentures supported by blade-vent implants and removable partial dentures. Part IV. Comparisons of patient satisfaction between two treatment modalities, J Prosthet Dent 66:517-530, 1991.
Kapur KK et al: Veterans Administration Cooperative Dental Implant Study: Comparisons between fixed partial dentures supported by blade-vent implants and removable partial dentures. Part II: Comparison of success rates and periodontal health between two treatment modalities, J Prosthet Dent 62:685-703, 1992.
Kunisch WH, Dodd J: A conversion alternative to ceramics in a crown-and-sleeve coping prosthesis, J Prosthet Dent 49:581-582, 1983.
Leff A: New concepts in the preparation of teeth for full coverage, J Prosthet Dent 5:392-400, 1955.
Leff A: Reproduction of tooth anatomy and positional relationship in full cast or veneer crowns, J Prosthet Dent 6:550-557, 1956.
Libby G et al: Longevity of fixed partial dentures, J Prosthet Dent 78(2):127-131, 1997.
Malson TS: Anatomic cast crown reproduction, J Prosthet Dent 9:106-112, 1959.
Marinello CP, Scharer P: Resin-bonded etched cast extracoronal attachments for removable partial dentures: clinical experiences, Int J Periodont Res Dent 7:36-49, 1987.
McArthur DR: Fabrication of full coverage restorations for existing removable partial dentures, J Prosthet Dent 51:574-576, 1984.
Mojon P et al: Relationship between prosthodontic status, caries and periodontal disease in a geriatric population, Int J Prosthodont 26(6):564-571, 1995.
Morris HF et al: Department of Veterans Affairs Cooperative Studies Project No. 242: quantitative and qualitative evaluation of the marginal fit of cast ceramic, porcelain-shoulder, and cast metal full crown margins, J Prosthet Dent 67:198-204, 1992.
Moulding MB, Holland GA, Sulik WD: An alternative orientation of nonrigid connectors in fixed partial dentures, J Prosthet Dent 6:236-238, 1992.
Mueninghoff LA, Johnson MH: Fixed-removable partial dentures, J Prosthet Dent 48:547-550, 1982.
Palmquist S et al: Multivariate analyses of factors influencing the longevity of fixed partial dentures, retainers and abutments, J Prosthet Dent 71(3): 245-250, 1994.
Patur B: The role of occlusion and the periodontium in restorative procedures, J Prosthet Dent 21:371-379, 1969.
Pezzoli M et al: Magnetizable abutment crowns for distal-extension removable partial dentures, J Prosthet Dent 55:475-480, 1986.
Phillips RW, Biggs DH: Distortion of wax patterns as influenced by storage time, storage temperature, and temperature of wax manipulation, J Am Dent Assoc 41:28-37, 1950.
Phillips RW, Price RR: Some factors which influence the surface of stone dies poured in alginate impressions, J Prosthet Dent 5:72-79, 1955.
Phillips RW, Swartz ML: A study of adaptation of veneers to cast gold crowns, J Prosthet Dent 7:817-822, 1957.
Pound E: The problem of the lower anterior bridge, J Prosthet Dent 5:543-545, 1955.
Preston JD: Preventing ceramic failures when integrating fixed and removable prostheses, Dent Clin North Am 23:37-52, 1979.
Pruden KC: A hydrocolloid technique for pinledge bridge abutments, J Prosthet Dent 6:65-71, 1956.
Pruden WH: Full coverage, partial coverage, and the role of pins, J Prosthet Dent 26:302-306, 1971.
Rhoads JE: The fixed-removable partial denture, J Prosthet Dent 48:122-129, 1982.

Rubin MK: Full coverage: the provisional and final restorations made easier, J Prosthet Dent 8:664-672, 1958.

Schorr BL, Peregrina AM, Elledge DA: Alternatives to posterior complete crowns: integrating foundations with cuspal protection, J Prosthet Dent 69:165-170, 1993.

Seals RR Jr, Stratton RJ: Surveyed crowns: a key for integrating fixed and removable prosthodontics, Quintessence Dent Technol 11:43-49, 1987.

Sheets CE: Dowel and core foundations, J Prosthet Dent 23:58-65, 1970.

Shooshan ED: The reverse pin-porcelain facing, J Prosthet Dent 9:284-301, 1959.

Smith GP: The marginal fit of the full cast shoulderless crown, J Prosthet Dent 7:231-243, 1957.

Smith GP: Objectives of a fixed partial denture, J Prosthet Dent 11:463-473, 1961.

Staffanou RS, Thayer KE: Reverse pin-porcelain veneer and pontic technique, J Prosthet Dent 12:1138, 1145, 1962.

Thurgood BW, Thayer KE, Lee RE: Complete crowns constructed for an existing partial denture, J Prosthet Dent 29:507-512, 1973.

Treppo KW, Smith FW: A technique for restoring abutments for removable partial dentures, J Prosthet Dent 40:398-401, 1978.

Troxell RR: The polishing of gold castings, J Prosthet Dent 9:668-675, 1959.

Turner KA, Messirlian DM: Restoration of the extremely worn dentition, J Prosthet Dent 52:464-474, 1984.

Wagman SS: Tissue management for full cast veneer crowns, J Prosthet Dent 15:106-117, 1965.

Wagner AW, Burkhart JW, Fayle HE Jr: Contouring abutment teeth with cast gold inlays for removable partial dentures, J Prosthet Dent 201:330-334, 1968.

Wallace FH: Resin transfer copings, J Prosthet Dent 8:289-292, 1958.

Wang CJ, Millstein PL, Nathanson D: Effects of cement, cement space, marginal design, seating aid materials, and seating force on crown cementation, J Prosthet Dent 67:786-790, 1992.

Welsh SL: Complete crown construction for a clasp-bearing abutment, J Prosthet Dent 34:320-323, 1975.

Wheeler RC: Complete crown form and the periodontium, J Prosthet Dent 11:722-734, 1961.

Yalisove IL: Crown and sleeve-coping retainers for removable partial prostheses, J Prosthet Dent 16:1069-1085, 1966.

DENTAL LABORATORY PROCEDURES

Asgar K, Peyton FA: Casting dental alloys to embedded wires, J Prosthet Dent 15:312-321, 1965.

Becker CM, Smith EE, Nicholls JI: The comparison of denture-base processing techniques. I: Material characteristics, J Prosthet Dent 37:330-338, 1977.

Berg E et al: Mechanical properties of laser-welded cast and wrought titanium, J Prosthet Dent 74:250-257, 1995.

Blanchard CH: Filling undercuts on refractory casts with investment, J Prosthet Dent 3:417-418, 1953.

Bolouri A, Hilger TC, Gowrylok MD: Modified flasking technique for removable partial dentures, J Prosthet Dent 34:221-223, 1975.

Brudvik JS, Nicholls JI: Soldering of removable partial dentures, J Prosthet Dent 49:762-765, 1983.

Burnett CA et al: Sprue design in removable partial denture casting, J Dent 24(1-2):99-103, 1996.

Calverley MJ, Moergeli JR Jr: Effect on the fit of removable partial denture frameworks when master casts are treated with cyanoacrylate resin, J Prosthet Dent 58:327-329, 1987.

Casey DM, Crowther DS, Lauciello FR: Strengthening abutment or isolated teeth on removable partial denture master casts, J Prosthet Dent 46:105-106, 1981.

Dirksen LC, Campagna SJ: Mat surface and rugae reproduction for upper partial denture castings, J Prosthet Dent 4:67-72, 1954.

Dootz ER, Craig RG, Peyton FA: Influence of investments and duplicating procedures on the accuracy of partial denture castings, J Prosthet Dent 15:679-690, 1965.

Dootz ER, Craig RG, Peyton FA: Simplification of the chrome-cobalt partial denture casting procedure, J Prosthet Dent 17:464-471, 1967.

Elbert CA, Ryge G: The effect of heat treatment on hardness of a chrome-cobalt alloy, J Prosthet Dent 15:873-879, 1965.

Elliott RW: The effects of heat on gold partial denture castings, J Prosthet Dent 13:688-698, 1963.

Enright CM: Dentist-dental laboratory harmony, J Prosthet Dent 11:393-394, 1961.

Fiebiger GE, Parr GR, Goldman BM: Remount casts for removable partial dentures, J Prosthet Dent 48:106-107, 1982.

Firtell DN, Muncheryan AM, Green AJ: Laboratory accuracy in casting removable partial denture frameworks, J Prosthet Dent 54:856-862, 1985.

Fowler JA Jr, Kuebker WA, Escobedo JJ: Laboratory procedures for the maintenance of a removable partial overdenture, J Prosthet Dent 50:121-126, 1983.

Garver DG: Updated laboratory procedure for the subpontic clasping system, J Prosthet Dent 48:734-735, 1982.

Gay WD: Laboratory procedures for fitting removable partial denture frameworks, J Prosthet Dent 40:227-229, 1978.

Gilson TD, Asgar K, Peyton FA: The quality of union formed in casting gold to embedded attachment metals, J Prosthet Dent 15:464-473, 1965.

Grunewald AH, Paffenbarger GC, Dickson G: The effect of molding processes on some properties of denture resins, J Am Dent Assoc 44:269-284, 1952.

Grunewald AH, Paffenbarger GC, Dickson G: Dentist, dental laboratory, and the patient, J Prosthet Dent 8:55-60, 1958.

Grunewald AH, Paffenbarger GC, Dickson G: The role of the dental technician in a prosthetic service, Dent Clin North Am 4:359-370, 1960.

Hanson JG et al: Effect on dimensional accuracy when reattaching fractured lone standing teeth of a cast, J Prosthet Dent 47:488-492, 1982.

Infection control recommendations for the dental office and the dental laboratory: ADA Council on Scientific Affairs and ADA Council on Dental Practice, J Am Dent Assoc 11(3):395-399, 1996.

Johnson HB: Technique for packing and staining complete or partial denture bases, J Prosthet Dent 6:154-159, 1956.

Jones DW: Thermal analysis and stability of refractory investments, J Prosthet Dent 18:234-241, 1967.
Jordan RD, Turner KA, Taylor TD: Multiple crowns fabricated for an existing removable partial denture, J Prosthet Dent 48:102-105, 1982.
Kazanoglu A, Smith EH: Replacement technique for a broken occlusal rest, J Prosthet Dent 48:621-623, 1982.
Krand M et al: Study on the surface of resins that burn without residues in the lost-wax procedure, J Prosthodont 5(4):259-265, Dec 1996.
Lanier BR, Rudd KD, Strunk RR: Making chromium-cobalt removable partial dentures: a modified technique, J Prosthet Dent 25:197-205, 1971.
Lauciello FR: Technique for remounting removable partial dentures opposing maxillary complete dentures, J Prosthet Dent 45:336-340, 1981.
Mahler DB, Ady AB: The influence of various factors on the effective setting expansion of casting investments, J Prosthet Dent 13:365-373, 1963.
Maxson BB et al: Quality assurance for the laboratory aspects of prosthodontic treatment, J Prosthodont 6(3):204-209, 1997.
May KB, Razzoog ME: Silane to enhance the bond between polymethyl methacrylate and titanium, J Prosthet Dent 73:428-431, 1995.
McCartney JW: The acrylic resin base maxillary removable partial denture: technical considerations, J Prosthet Dent 43:467-468, 1980.
Mohammed H et al: Button versus buttonless castings for removable partial denture frameworks, J Prosthet Dent 72(4):433-444, 1994.
Moreno de Delgado M, Garcia LT, Rudd KD: Camouflaging partial denture clasps, J Prosthet Dent 55:656-660, 1986.
Mori T et al: Titanium for removable dentures. I: Laboratory procedures, J Oral Rehabil 24(5):238-341, 1997.
Morris HF et al: The influence of heat treatments on several types of base-metal removable partial denture alloys, J Prosthet Dent 41:388-395, 1979.
NaBadalung DP et al: Comparison of bond strengths of denture base resins to nickel-chromium-beryllium removable partial denture alloy, J Prosthet Dent 78(6):566-573, 1997.
NaBadalung DP et al: Effectiveness of adhesive systems for Co-Cr removable partial denture alloy, J Prosthet Dent 7(3):17-25, Mar 1998.
Nelson DR et al: Expediting the fabrication of a nickel-chromium casting, J Prosthet Dent 55:400-403, 1986.
Nelson DR, von Gonten AS, Kelly TW Jr: The cast round RPA clasp, J Prosthet Dent 54:307-309, 1985.
Palmer BL, Coffey KW: Investing and packing removable partial denture bases to minimize vertical processing error, J Prosthet Dent 56:123-124, 1986.
Parr FR, Gardner LK: The removable partial denture design template, Compendium 8:594, 596, 598-600, 1987.
Perry CK: Transfer base for removable partial dentures, J Prosthet Dent 31:582-584, 1974.
Peyton FA, Anthony DH: Evaluation of dentures processed by different techniques, J Prosthet Dent 13:269-281, 1963.
Quinlivan JT: Fabrication of a simple ball-socket attachment, J Prosthet Dent 32:222-225, 1974.
Radue JT, Unser JW: Constructing stable record bases for removable partial dentures, J Prosthet Dent 46:463, 1981.
Rantanen T, Eerikainen E: Accuracy of the palatal plate of removable partial dentures, and influence of laboratory handling of the investment on the accuracy, Dent Mater 2:28-31, 1986.
Raskin ER: An indirect technique for fabricating a crown under an existing clasp, J Prosthet Dent 50:580-581, 1983.
Ring M: Rest seats in existing crowns, Dent Lab Rev 60:24-25, 1985.
Ryge G, Kozak SF, Fairhurst CW: Porosities in dental gold castings, J Am Dent Assoc 54:746-754, 1957.
Sarnat AE, Klugman RS: A method to record the path of insertion of a removable partial denture, J Prosthet Dent 46:222-223, 1981.
Scandrett FR, Hanson JG, Unsicker RL: Layered silicone rubber technique for flasking removable partial dentures, J Prosthet Dent 40:349-350, 1978.
Schmidt AH: Repairing chrome-cobalt castings, J Prosthet Dent 5:385-387, 1955.
Schmitt SM, Chance DA, Cronin RJ: Refining cast implant-retained restorations by electrical discharge machining, J Prosthet Dent 73:280-283, 1995.
Schneider RL: Custom metal occlusal surfaces for acrylic resin denture teeth, J Prosthet Dent 46:98-101, 1981.
Schneider RL: Adapting ceramometal restorations to existing removable partial dentures, J Prosthet Dent 49: 279-281, 1983.
Schneider R: Metals used to fabricate removable partial denture frameworks, J Dent Technol 13(2):35-42, 1996.
Schwalm CA, LaSpina FY: Fabricating swinglock removable partial denture frameworks, J Prosthet Dent 45:216-220, 1981.
Schwedhelm ER et al: Fracture strength of type IV and type V die stone as a function of time, J Prosthet Dent 78(6):554-559, 1997.
Shay JS, Mattingly SL: Technique for the immediate repair of removable partial denture facings, J Prosthet Dent 47:104-106, 1982.
Smith GP: The responsibility of the dentist toward laboratory procedures in fixed and removable partial denture prostheses, J Prosthet Dent 13:295-301, 1963.
Smith RA: Clasp repair for removable partial dentures, J Prosthet Dent 29:231-234, 1973.
Stade EH et al: Influence of fabrication technique on wrought-wire clasp flexibility, J Prosthet Dent 54:538-543, 1985.
Stankewitz CG: Acrylic resin blockout for interim removable partial dentures, J Prosthet Dent 40:470-471, 1978.
Swoope CC, Frank RP: Fabrication procedures. In Clark JW, ed: Clinical dentistry, vol 5, New York, 1976, Harper & Row.
Sykora O: A new tripoding technique, J Prosthet Dent 44:463-464, 1980.
Sykora O: Removable partial denture design by Canadian laboratories: a retrospective study, J Can Dent Assoc 61(7):615-621, 1995.
Tambasco J et al: Laser welding in the dental laboratory: an alternative to soldering, J Dent Technol 13(4):23-31, May 1996.

Teppo KW, Smith FW: A method of immediate clasp repair, J Prosthet Dent 30:77-80, 1975.
Tran CD, Sherraden DR, Curtis TA: A review of techniques of crown fabrication for existing removable partial dentures, J Prosthet Dent 55:671-673, 1986.
Tuccillo JJ, Nielsen JP: Compatibility of alginate impression materials and dental stones, J Prosthet Dent 25:556-566, 1971.
Ulmer FC, Ward JE: Simplified technique for production of a distal-extension removable partial denture remounting cast, J Prosthet Dent 41:473-474, 1979.
von Gonten AS, Nelson DR: Laboratory pitfalls that contribute to embrasure clasp failure, J Prosthet Dent 53:136-138, 1985.
Williams HN, Falkler WA Jr, Hasler JF: Acinetobacter contamination of laboratory dental pumice, J Dent Res 62:1073-1075, 1983.
Zalkind M, Avital R, Rehany A: Fabrication of a replacement for a broken attachment, J Prosthet Dent 51: 714-716, 1984.

DENTURE ESTHETICS: TOOTH SELECTION AND ARRANGEMENT

Askinas SW: Facings in removable partial dentures, J Prosthet Dent 33:633-636, 1975.
Culpepper WD: A comparative study of shade-matching procedures, J Prosthet Dent 24:166-173, 1971.
DeVan MM: The appearance phase of denture construction, Dent Clin North Am 1:255-268, 1957.
Engelmeier RL: Complete-denture esthetics, Dent Clin North Am 40(1):71-84, 1996.
Fields H Jr, Birtles JT, Shay J: Combination prosthesis for optimum esthetic appearance, J Am Dent Assoc 101:276-279, 1980.
French FA: The selection and arrangement of the anterior teeth in prosthetic dentures, J Prosthet Dent 1:587-593, 1951.
Frush JP, Fisher RD: Introduction to dentogenic restorations, J Prosthet Dent 5:586-595, 1955.
Frush JP, Fisher RD: How dentogenic restorations interpret the sex factor, J Prosthet Dent 6:160-172, 1956.
Frush JP, Fisher RD: How dentogenics interprets the personality factor, J Prosthet Dent 6:441-449, 1956.
Hughes GA: Facial types and tooth arrangement, J Prosthet Dent 1:82-95, 1951.
Krajicek DD: Natural appearance for the individual denture patient, J Prosthet Dent 10:205-214, 1960.
Lang BR: Complete denture occlusion, Dent Clin North Am 40(1):85-101, 1996.
Levin EI: Dental esthetics and the golden proportion, J Prosthet Dent 40:244-252, 1978.
Lombardi RE: Factors mediating against excellence in dental esthetics, J Prosthet Dent 38:243-248, 1977.
Myerson RL: The use of porcelain and plastic teeth in opposing complete dentures, J Prosthet Dent 7:625-633, 1957.
Payne AGL: Factors influencing the position of artificial upper anterior teeth, J Prosthet Dent 26:26-32, 1971.
Pound E: Lost—fine arts in the fallacy of the ridges, J Prosthet Dent 4:6-16, 1954.
Pound E: Recapturing esthetic tooth position in the edentulous patient, J Am Dent Assoc 55:181-191, 1957.
Pound E: Applying harmony in selecting and arranging teeth, Dent Clin North Am 6:241-258, 1962.
Roraff AR: Instant photographs for developing esthetics, J Prosthet Dent 26:21-25, 1971.
Smith BJ: Esthetic factors in removable partial prosthodontics, Dent Clin North Am 23:53-63, 1979.
Sykora O: Fabrication of a posterior shade guide for removable partial dentures, J Prosthet Dent 50:287-288, 1983.
Tillman EJ: Molding and staining acrylic resin anterior teeth, J Prosthet Dent 5:497-507, 1955; Dent Abstr 1:111, 1956.
Van Victor A: Positive duplication of anterior teeth for immediate dentures, J Prosthet Dent 3:165-177, 1953.
Van Victor A: The mold guide cast: its significance in denture esthetics, J Prosthet Dent 13:406-415, 1963.
Vig RG: The denture look, J Prosthet Dent 11:9-15, 1961.
Wallace DH: The use of gold occlusal surfaces in complete and partial dentures, J Prosthet Dent 14:326-333, 1964.
Weiner S, Krause AS, Nicholas W: Esthetic modification of removable partial denture teeth with light-cured composites, J Prosthet Dent 57:381-384, 1987.
Wolfson E: Staining and characterization of acrylic teeth, Dent Abstr 1:41, 1956.
Young HA: Denture esthetics, J Prosthet Dent 6:748-755, 1956.
Zarb GA, MacKay HF: Cosmetics and removable partial dentures: the Class IV partially edentulous patient, J Prosthet Dent 46:360-368, 1981.

DIAGNOSIS AND TREATMENT PLANNING

Academy of Prosthodontics: Principles, concepts and practices in prosthodontics, J Prosthet Dent 73:73-94, 1995.
Applegate OC: Evaluating oral structures for removable partial dentures, J Prosthet Dent 11:882-885, 1961.
Bartels JC: Diagnosis and treatment planning, J Prosthet Dent 7:657-662, 1957.
Bezzon OL et al: Surveying removable partial dentures: the importance of guiding planes and path of insertion for stability, J Prosthet Dent 78(4):412-418, 1997.
Blatterfein L, Kaufman EG: Prevention of problems with removable partial dentures: Council on Dental Materials, Instruments, and Equipment, J Am Dent Assoc 100:919-921, 1980.
Bolender CL, Swenson RD, Yamane C: Evaluation of treatment of inflammatory papillary hyperplasia of the palate, J Prosthet Dent 15:1013-1022, 1965.
Budtz-Jorgensen E: Restoration of the partially edentulous mouth: a comparison of overdentures, removable partial dentures, fixed partial dentures and implant treatment, J Dent 24(4):237-244, July 1996.
Casey DM, Lauciello FR: A review of the submerged-root concept, J Prosthet Dent 43:128-132, 1980.
Contino RM, Stallard H: Instruments essential for obtaining data needed in making a functional diagnosis of the human mouth, J Prosthet Dent 7:66-77, 1957.
Dreizen S: Nutritional changes in the oral cavity, J Prosthet Dent 16:1144-1150, 1966.

Dummer PMH, Cidden J: The upper anterior sectional denture, J Prosthet Dent 41:146-152, 1979.
Dunn BW: Treatment planning for removable partial dentures, J Prosthet Dent 11:247-255, 1961.
Faine MP: Dietary factors related to preservation of oral and skeletal bone mass in women, J Prosthet Dent 73:65-72, 1995.
Foster TD: The use of the face-bow in making permanent study casts, J Prosthet Dent 9:717-721, 1959.
Frechette AR: Partial denture planning with special reference to stress distribution, J Prosthet Dent 1:700-707 (disc, 208-209), 1951.
Friedman S: Effective use of diagnostic data, J Prosthet Dent 9:729-737, 1959.
Garver DC et al: Vital root retention in humans: a preliminary report, J Prosthet Dent 40:23-28, 1978.
Garver DC, Fenster RK: Vital root retention in humans: a final report, J Prosthet Dent 43:368-373, 1980.
Guyer SE: Selectively retained vital roots for partial support of overdentures: a patient report, J Prosthet Dent 33:258-263, 1975.
Harvey WL: A transitional prosthetic appliance, J Prosthet Dent 14:60-70, 1964.
Heintz WD: Treatment planning and design: prevention of errors of omission and commission, Dent Clin North Am 23:3-12, 1979.
Henderson D, Hickey JC, Wehner PJ: Prevention and preservation: the challenge of removable partial denture service, Dent Clin North Am 9:459-473, 1965.
House MM: The relationship of oral examination to dental diagnosis, J Prosthet Dent 8:208-219, 1958.
Kabcenell JL: Planning for individualized prosthetic treatment, J Prosthet Dent 34:405-407, 1975.
Kaldahl WB, Becher CM: Prosthetic contingencies for future tooth loss, J Prosthet Dent 54:1-6, 1985.
Kayser AF: Limited treatment goals: shortened dental arches, Periodontol 2000 4:7-14, 1994.
Killebrew RF: Crown construction and splinting of mobile partial denture abutments, J Am Dent Assoc 70:334-338, 1965.
Krikos AA: Preparing guide planes for removable partial dentures, J Prosthet Dent 34:152-155, 1975.
Lambson GO: Papillary hyperplasia of the palate, J Prosthet Dent 16:636-645, 1966.
Langer Y et al: Modalities of treatment for the combination syndrome, J Prosthodont 4(2):76-81, June 1995.
Lopes I, Norlau LA: Specific mechanics for abutment uprighting, Aust Dent J 25:273-278, 1980.
McCracken WL: Differential diagnosis: fixed or removable partial dentures, J Am Dent Assoc 63:767-775, 1961.
McGill WJ: Acquiring space for partial dentures, J Prosthet Dent 17:163-165, 1967.
Miller EL: Planning partial denture construction, Dent Clin North Am 17:571-584, 1973.
Miller EL: Critical factors in selecting removable prosthesis, J Prosthet Dent 34:486-490, 1975.
Mopsik ER et al: Surgical intervention to reestablish adequate intermaxillary space before fixed or removable prosthodontics, J Am Dent Assoc 95:957-960, 1977.
Moulton GH: The importance of centric occlusion in diagnosis and treatment planning, J Prosthet Dent 10: 921-926, 1960.
Nassif J, Blumenfeld WL: Joint consultation services by the periodontist and prosthodontist, J Prosthet Dent 29:55-60, 1973.
Nassif J, Blumenfeld WL, Tarsitano JT: Dialogue—a treatment modality, J Prosthet Dent 33:696-700, 1975.
Payne SH: Diagnostic factors which influence the choice of posterior occlusion, Dent Clin North Am 1:203-213, 1957.
Rudd KD, Dunn BW: Accurate removable partial dentures, J Prosthet Dent 18:559-570, 1967.
Saunders TR, Gillis RE, Desjardins RP: The maxillary complete denture opposing the mandibular bilateral distal-extension partial denture: treatment considerations, J Prosthet Dent 41:124-128, 1979.
Sauser CW: Pretreatment evaluation of partially edentulous arches, J Prosthet Dent 11:886-893, 1961.
Seiden A: Occlusal rests and rest seats, J Prosthet Dent 8:431-440, 1958.
Silverman SI: Differential diagnosis: fixed or removable prosthesis, Dent Clin North Am 31:347-362, 1987.
Swoope CC, Frank RP: Removable partial dentures indications and planning. In Clark JE, ed: Clinical dentistry, vol 5, New York, 1976, Harper & Row.
Turner CE, Shaffer FW: Planning the treatment of the complex prosthodontic case, J Am Dent Assoc 97:992-993, 1978.
Uccellani EL: Evaluating the mucous membranes of the edentulous mouth, J Prosthet Dent 15:295-303, 1965.
Vahidi F: The provisional restoration, Dent Clin North Am 31:363-381, 1987.
Wagner AG: Instructions for the use and care of removable partial dentures, J Prosthet Dent 26:481-490, 1971.
Waldron CA: Oral leukoplakia, carcinoma, and the prosthodontist, J Prosthet Dent 15:367-376, 1965.
Welker WA, Kramer DC: Claspless chrome-cobalt transitional removable partial dentures, J Am Dent Assoc 96:814-818, 1978.
Wright P, Hellyer PH: Gingival recession related to removable partial dentures in older patients, J Prosthet Dent 74:602-607, 1995.
Young HA: Diagnostic survey of edentulous patients, J Prosthet Dent 5:5-14, 1955.

IMPRESSION MATERIALS AND METHODS: THE PARTIAL DENTURE BASE

Akerly WB: A combination impression and occlusal registration technique for extension-base removable partial dentures, J Prosthet Dent 39:226-229, 1978.
Appleby DC et al: The combined reversible hydrocolloid/irreversible hydrocolloid impression system: clinical application, J Prosthet Dent 46:48-58, 1981.
Applegate OC: The partial denture base, J Prosthet Dent 5:636-648, 1955.
Applegate OC: An evaluation of the support for the removable partial denture, J Prosthet Dent 10:112-123, 1960.
Bailey LR: Rubber base impression techniques, Dent Clin North Am 1:156-166, 1957.
Bauman R, DeBoer J: A modification of the altered cast technique, J Prosthet Dent 47:212-213, 1982.

Beaumont AJ: Sectional impression for maxillary Class I removable partial dentures and maxillary immediate dentures, J Prosthet Dent 49:438-441, 1983.

Berkey D, Berg R: Geriatric oral health issues in the United States, Internatl Dent J 51:254-264, 2001.

Beyerle MP et al: Immersion disinfection of irreversible hydrocolloid impressions. Part I: Microbiology, Int J Prosthodont 7(3):234-238, May 1994.

Birnbach S: Impression technique for maxillary removable partial dentures, J Prosthet Dent 51:286, 1984.

Blatterfein L, Klein IE, Miglino JC: A loading impression technique for semiprecision and precision removable partial dentures, J Prosthet Dent 43:9-14, 1980.

Boretti G, Bickel M, Geering AH: A review of masticatory ability and efficiency, J Prosthet Dent 74:400-403, 1995.

Carlsson GE: Masticatory efficiency: the effect of age, the loss of teeth and prosthetic rehabilitation. Int Dent Jour 34:93-97, 1984.

Chaffee NR et al: Dimensional accuracy of improved dental stone and epoxy resin die materials. Part I: Single die, J Prosthet Dent 77(2):131-135, 1997.

Chaffee NR et al: Dimensional accuracy of improved dental stone and epoxy resin die materials. Part II: Complete arch form, J Prosthet Dent 77(3):235-238, 1997.

Chai J et al: Clinically relevant mechanical properties of elastomeric impression materials, Int J Prosthodont 11(3):219-223, 1998.

Chase WW: Adaptation of rubber-base impression materials to removable denture prosthetics, J Prosthet Dent 10:1043-1050, 1960.

Chau VB et al: In-depth disinfection of acrylic resin, J Prosthet Dent 74:309-313, 1995.

Chen MS et al: An altered-cast impression technique that eliminates conventional cast dissecting and impression boxing, J Prosthet Dent 57:471-474, 1987.

Cho GC et al: Tensile bond strength of polyvinyl siloxane impressions bonded to a custom tray as a function of drying time. Part I, J Prosthet Dent 73(5):419-423, 1995.

Chong MP et al: The tear test as a means of evaluating the resistance to rupture of alginate impression materials, Aust Dent J 16:145-151, 1971.

Clark RJ, Phillips RW: Flow studies of certain dental impression materials, J Prosthet Dent 7:259-266, 1957.

Cohen BI et al: Dimensional accuracy of three different alginate impression materials, J Prosthodont 4(3):195-199, 1995.

Corso M et al: The effect of temperature changes on the dimensional stability of polyvinyl siloxane and polyether impression materials, J Prosthet Dent 79(6):626-631, 1998.

Cserna A et al: Irreversible hydrocolloids: a comparison of antimicrobial efficacy, J Prosthet Dent 71(4):387-389, 1994.

Davidson CL, Boere G: Liquid-supported dentures. Part I: Theoretical and technical considerations, J Prosthet Dent 68:303-306, 1990.

Davidson CL, Boere G: Liquid-supported dentures. Part II: Clinical study: a preliminary report, J Prosthet Dent 68:434-436, 1990.

Davis BA et al: Effect of immersion disinfection on properties of impression materials, J Prosthodont 3(1):31-34, 1994.

DeFreitas JF: Potential toxicants in alginate powders, Aust Dent J 25:224-228, 1980.

Dixon DL, Breeding LC, Ekstrand KG: Linear dimensional variability of three denture base resins after processing and in water storage, J Prosthet Dent 68:196-200, 1992.

Dixon DL, Ekstrand KG, Breeding LC: The transverse strengths of three denture base resins, J Prosthet Dent 66:510-513, 1991.

Dootz ER: Fabricating non-precious metal bases, Dent Clin North Am 24:113-122, 1980.

Dootz ER, Craig RG: Comparison of the physical properties of eleven soft denture liners, J Prosthet Dent 67:707-712, 1992.

Douglas CW, Shih A, Ostry L: Will there be a need for complete dentures in the United States in 2020? J Prosthet Dent 87:5-8, 2002.

Douglas CW, Watson AJ: Future needs for fixed and removable partial dentures in the United States. J Prosthet Dent 87:9-14, 2002.

Drennon DG, Johnson GH: The effect of immersion disinfection of elastomeric impressions on the surface detail reproduction of improved gypsum casts, J Prosthet Dent 63:233-241, 1990.

Fitzloff RA: Functional impressions with thermoplastic materials for reline procedures, J Prosthet Dent 52:25-27, 1984.

Frank RP: Analysis of pressures produced during maxillary edentulous impression procedures, J Prosthet Dent 22:400-403, 1969.

Fusayama T, Nakazato M: The design of stock trays and the retention of irreversible hydrocolloid impressions, J Prosthet Dent 21:136-142, 1969.

Gelbard S et al: Effect of impression materials and techniques on the marginal fit of metal castings, J Prosthet Dent 71(1):1-6, 1994.

Gilmore WH, Schnell RJ, Phillips RW: Factors influencing the accuracy of silicone impression materials, J Prosthet Dent 9:304-314, 1959.

Hans S, Gunne J: Masticatory efficiency and dental state: a comparison between two methods, Acta Odont Scand 43:139-146, 1985.

Harris WT Jr: Water temperature and accuracy of alginate impressions, J Prosthet Dent 21:613-617, 1969.

Harrison JD: Prevention of failures in making impressions and dies, Dent Clin North Am 23:13-20, 1979.

Heartwell CM Jr et al: Comparison of impressions made in perforated and nonperforated rimlock trays, J Prosthet Dent 27:494-500, 1972.

Helkimo E, Carlsson GE, Helkimo M: Chewing efficiency and state of the dentition, Acta Odont Scand 36:33-41, 1978.

Herfort TW et al: Viscosity of elastomeric impression materials, J Prosthet Dent 38:396-404, 1977.

Hesby RM et al: Effects of radiofrequency glow discharge on impression material surface wettability, J Prosthet Dent 77(4):414-422, 1997.

Holmes JB: Influence of impression procedures and occlusal loading on partial denture movement, J Prosthet Dent 15:474-481, 1965.

Hondrum SO et al: Effects of long-term storage on properties of an alginate impression material, J Prosthet Dent 77(6):601-606, 1997.

Hudson WC: Clinical uses of rubber impression materials and electroforming of casts and dies in pure silver, J Prosthet Dent 8:107-114, 1958.

Huggett R et al: Dimensional accuracy and stability of acrylic resin denture bases, J Prosthet Dent 68:634-640, 1992.

Iglesias A et al: Accuracy of wax, autopolymerized, and light-polymerized resin pattern materials, J Prosthodont 5(3):193-200, 1996.

Ivanovski S et al: Disinfection of dental stone casts: antimicrobial effects and physical property alterations, Dent Mater 11(1):19-23, 1995.

James JS: A simplified alternative to the altered-cast impression technique for removable partial dentures, J Prosthet Dent 53:598, 1985.

Jasim FA, Brudvik JS, Nicholls JI: Impression distortion from abutment tooth inclination in removable partial dentures, J Prosthet Dent 54:532-538, 1985.

Johnson GH et al: Dimensional stability and detail reproduction of irreversible hydrocolloid and elastomeric impressions disinfected by immersion, J Prosthet Dent 79(4):446-453, 1998.

Johnston JF, Cunningham DM, Bogan RG: The dentist, the patient, and ridge preservation, J Prosthet Dent 10: 288-295, 1960.

Jones RH et al: Effect of provisional luting agents on polyvinyl siloxane impression materials, J Prosthet Dent 75(4):360-363, 1996.

Kawamura Y: Recent concepts of the physiology of mastication. Adv Oral Biol 1:77-109, 1964.

Kawano F et al: Comparison of bond strength of six soft denture liners to denture base resin, J Prosthet Dent 68:368-371, 1992.

Koran A III: Impression materials for recording the denture bearing mucosa, Dent Clin North Am 24:97-111, 1980.

Kramer HM: Impression technique for removable partial dentures, J Prosthet Dent 11:84-92, 1961.

Landesman HM, Wright WE: A technique for making impressions on patients requiring complete and removable partial dentures, CDA J 14(6):20-24, 1986.

Langenwalter EM, Aquilino SA: The dimensional stability of elastomeric impression materials following disinfection, J Prosthet Dent 63:270-276, 1990.

Leach CD, Donovan TE: Impression technique for maxillary removable partial dentures, J Prosthet Dent 50:283-286, 1983.

Leake JL, Hawkins R, Locker D: Social and functional impact of reduced posterior dental units in older adults, J Oral Rehab 21:1-10, 1994.

Lee IK et al: Evaluation of factors affecting the accuracy of impressions using quantitative surface analysis, Oper Dent 20(6):246-252, 1995.

Lee RE: Mucostatics, Dent Clin North Am 24:81-96, 1980.

Lepe X et al: Accuracy of polyether and addition silicone after long-term immersion disinfection, J Prosthet Dent 78(3):245-249, 1997.

Leupold RJ: A comparative study of impression procedures for distal extension removable partial dentures, J Prosthet Dent 16:708-720, 1966.

Leupold RJ, Flinton RJ, Pfeifer DL: Comparison of vertical movement occurring during loading of distal-extension removable partial denture bases made by three impression techniques, J Prosthet Dent 68:290-293, 1992.

Leupold RJ, Kratochvil FJ: An altered-cast procedure to improve support for removable partial dentures, J Prosthet Dent 15:672-678, 1965.

Liedberg B, Spiechowicz E, Owall B: Mastication with and without removable partial dentures: An intraindividual study. Dysphagia 10:107-112, 1995.

Loh PL et al: An evaluation of microwave-polymerized resin bases for removable partial dentures, J Prosthet Dent 79(4):389-392, 1998.

Lucas W, Luke H: The processes of selection and breakage in mastication, Arch Oral Biol 28:813-818, 1983.

Lund PS, Aquilino SA: Prefabricated custom impression trays for the altered cast technique, J Prosthet Dent 66:782-783, 1991.

Manly RS, Vinton P: A survey of the chewing ability of denture wearers. J Dent Res 30:314-321, 1951.

Matis BA et al: The effect of the use of dental gloves on mixing vinyl polysiloxane putties, J Prosthodont 6(3):189-192, 1997.

Millar BJ et al: The effect of surface wetting agent on void formation in impressions, J Prosthet Dent 77(1):54-56, 1997.

Millar BJ et al: In vitro study of the number of surface defects in monophase and two-phase addition silicone impressions, J Prosthet Dent 80:32-35, 1998.

Mitchell JV, Damele JJ: Influence of tray design upon elastic impression materials, J Prosthet Dent 23:51-57, 1970.

Mitchener RW, Omori MD: Putty materials for stable removable partial denture bases, J Prosthet Dent 53:435-436, 1985.

Morrow RM et al: Compatibility of alginate impression materials and dental stones, J Prosthet Dent 25:556-566, 1971.

Myers GE: Electroformed die technique for rubber base impressions, J Prosthet Dent 8:531-535, 1958.

Myers GE, Wepfer GG, Peyton FA: The Thiokol rubber base impression materials, J Prosthet Dent 8:330-339, 1958.

Nishigawa G et al: Efficacy of tray adhesives for the adhesion of elastomer rubber impression materials to impression modeling plastics for border molding, J Prosthet Dent 79(2):140-144, 1998.

O'Brien WJ: Base retention, Dent Clin North Am 24:123-130, 1980.

Olin PS et al: The effects of sterilization on addition silicone impressions in custom and stock metal trays, J Prosthet Dent 71(4):625-630, 1994.

Oosterhaven SP et al: Social and psychological implications of missing teeth for chewing ability, Comm Dent Oral Epid 16:79-82, 1988.

Parker MH et al: Comparison of occlusal contacts in maximum intercuspation for two impression techniques, J Prosthet Dent 78(3):255-259, 1997.

Pfeiffer KA: Clinical problems in the use of alginate hydrocolloid, Dent Abstr 2:82, 1957.

Phillips RW: Factors influencing the accuracy of reversible hydrocolloid impressions, J Am Dent Assoc 43:1-17, 1951.

Phillips RW: Factors affecting the surface of stone dies poured in hydrocolloid impressions, J Prosthet Dent 2:390-400, 1952.

Phillips RW: Physical properties and manipulation of rubber impression materials, J Am Dent Assoc 59:454-458, 1959.

Pratten DH, Covey DA, Sheats RD: Effect of disinfectant solutions on the wettability of elastomeric impression materials, J Prosthet Dent 63:223-227, 1990.

Prinz JF, Lucas PW: Swallow thresholds in human mastication, Arch Oral Biol 40:401-403, 1995.

Prieskel HW: Impression techniques for attachment retained distal extension removable partial dentures, J Prosthet Dent 25:620-628, 1971.

Rapuano JA: Single tray dual-impression technique for distal extension partial dentures, J Prosthet Dent 24:41-46, 1970.

Redford M et al: Denture use and the technical quality of dental prostheses among persons 18-74 years of age: United States, 1988-1991, J Dent Res 75:714-725, 1996.

Render PJ: An impression technique to make a new master cast for an existing removable partial denture, J Prosthet Dent 67:488-490, 1992.

Rudd KD et al: Comparison of effects of tap water and slurry water on gypsum casts, J Prosthet Dent 24:563-570, 1970.

Rudd KD, Morrow RM, Bange AA: Accurate casts, J Prosthet Dent 21:545-554, 1969.

Rudd KD, Morrow RM, Strunk RR: Accurate alginate impressions, J Prosthet Dent 22:294-300, 1969.

Samadzadeh A et al: Fracture strength of provisional restorations reinforced with plasma-treated woven polyethylene fiber, J Prosthet Dent (5):447-450, 1997.

Scott GK et al: Check bite impressions using irreversible alginate/reversible hydrocolloid combination, J Prosthet Dent 77(1):83-85, 1997.

Sherfudhin H et al: Preparation of void-free casts from vinyl polysiloxane impressions, J Dent 24(1-2):95-98, 1996.

Silver M: Impressions and silver-plated dies from a rubber impression material, J Prosthet Dent 6:543-549, 1956.

Smith RA: Secondary palatal impressions for major connector adaptation, J Prosthet Dent 24:108-110, 1970.

Steffel VL: Relining removable partial dentures for fit and function, J Prosthet Dent 4:496-509, 1954; J Tenn Dent Assoc 36:35-43, 1956.

Taylor TD, Morton TJ Jr: Ulcerative lesions of the palate associated with removable partial denture castings, J Prosthet Dent 66:213-221, 1991.

Thompson GA et al: Effects of disinfection of custom tray materials on adhesive properties of several impression material systems, J Prosthet Dent 72(6):651-656, 1994.

Tjan AH et al: Marginal fidelity of crowns fabricated from six proprietary provisional materials, J Prosthet Dent 77(5):482-485, 1997.

Vahidi F: Vertical displacement of distal-extension ridges by different impression techniques, J Prosthet Dent 40:374-377, 1978.

Vandewalle KS et al: Immersion disinfection of irreversible hydrocolloid impressions with sodium hypochlorite. Part II: Effect on gypsum, Int J Prosthodont 7(4):315-322, 1994.

van Waas M, et al: Relationship between wearing a removable partial denture and satisfaction in the elderly. Comm Dent Oral Epid 22:315-318, 1994.

Verran J et al: Microbiological study of selected risk areas in dental technology laboratories, J Dent 24(1-2):77-80, 1996.

Wang HY et al: Vertical distortion on distal extension ridges and palatal area of casts made by different techniques, J Prosthet Dent 75(3):302-308, 1996.

Wang RR, Nguyen T, Boyle AM: The effect of tray material and surface condition on the shear bond strength of impression materials, J Prosthet Dent 74:449-454, 1995.

Wilson JH: Partial dentures: relining the saddle supported by the mucosa and alveolar bone, J Prosthet Dent 3:807-813, 1953.

Young JM: Surface characteristics of dental stone: impression orientation, J Prosthet Dent 33:336-341, 1975.

Yurkstas AA: The masticatory act, J Prosthet Dent 15:248-260, 1965.

Zinner ID: Impression procedures for the removable component of a combination fixed and removable prosthesis, Dent Clin North Am 31:417-440, 1987.

MAXILLOFACIAL PROSTHESIS

Adams D: A cantilevered swinglock removable partial denture design for the treatment of the partial mandibulectomy patient, J Oral Rehabil 12:113-118, 1985.

Ackerman AJ: Maxillofacial prosthesis, Oral Surg 6:176-200, 1953.

Ackerman AJ: The prosthetic management of oral and facial defects following cancer surgery, J Prosthet Dent 5:413-432, 1955.

Brown KE: Fabrication of a hollow-bulb obturator, J Prosthet Dent 21:97-103, 1969.

Brown KE: Reconstruction considerations for severe dental attrition, J Prosthet Dent 44:384-388, 1980.

Cantor R et al: Methods for evaluating prosthetic facial materials, J Prosthet Dent 21:324-332, 1969.

Curtis TA, Cantor R: The forgotten patient in maxillofacial prosthetics, J Prosthet Dent 31:662-680, 1974.

Desjardins RP: Prosthodontic management of the cleft palate patient, J Prosthet Dent 33:655-665, 1975.

Firtell DN, Curtis TA: Removable partial denture design for the mandibular resection patient, J Prosthet Dent 48:437-443, 1982.

Firtell DN, Grisius RJ: Retention of obturator: removable partial dentures: a comparison of buccal and lingual retention, J Prosthet Dent 43:211-217, 1980.

Gay WD, King GE: Applying basic prosthodontic principles in the dentulous maxillectomy patient, J Prosthet Dent 43:433-435, 1980.

Goll G: Design for maximal retention of obturator prosthesis for hemimaxillectomy patients (letter), J Prosthet Dent 48:108-109, 1982.

Immekus JE, Aramy M: Adverse effects of resilient denture liners in overlay dentures, J Prosthet Dent 32:178-181, 1974.

Kelley EK: Partial denture design applicable to the maxillofacial patient, J Prosthet Dent 15:168-173, 1965.

King GE, Martin JW: Cast circumferential and wire clasps for obturator retention, J Prosthet Dent 49:799-802, 1983.

Metz HH: Mandibular staple implant for an atrophic mandibular ridge: solving retention difficulties of a denture, J Prosthet Dent 32:572-578, 1974.

Monteith GG: The partially edentulous patient with special problems, Dent Clin North Am 23:107-115, 1979.

Moore DJ: Cervical esophagus prosthesis, J Prosthet Dent 30:442-445, 1973.
Myers RE, Mitchell DL: A photoelastic study of stress induced by framework design in a maxillary resection, J Prosthet Dent 61:590-594, 1989.
Nethery WJ, Delclos L: Prosthetic stent for gold-grain implant to the floor of the mouth, J Prosthet Dent 23:81-87, 1970.
Shifman A, Lepley JB: Prosthodontic management of post-surgical soft tissue deformities associated with marginal mandibulectomy. Part I: Loss of the vestibule, J Prosthet Dent 48:178-183, 1982.
Smith EH Jr: Prosthetic treatment of maxillofacial injuries, J Prosthet Dent 5:112-128, 1955.
Strain JC: A mechanical device for duplicating a mirror image of a cast or moulage in three dimensions, J Prosthet Dent 5:129-132, 1955.
Toremalm NG: A disposable obturator for maxillary defects, J Prosthet Dent 29:94-96, 1973.
Weintraub GS, Yalisove IL: Prosthodontic therapy for cleidocranial dysostosis: report of case, J Am Dent Assoc 96:301-305, 1978.
Wright SM, Pullen-Warner EA, LeTissier DR: Design for maximal retention of obturator prosthesis for hemimaxillectomy patients, J Prosthet Dent 47:88-91, 1982.
Young JM: The prosthodontist's role in total treatment of patients, J Prosthet Dent 27:399-412, 1972.

MISCELLANEOUS

Abere DJ: Post-placement care of complete and removable partial dentures, Dent Clin North Am 23:143-151, 1979.
Academy of Denture Prosthetics: principles, concepts and practices in prosthodontics, J Prosthet Dent 61:88-109, 1989.
Adisman IK: What a prosthodontist should know, J Prosthet Dent 21:409-416, 1969.
American Association of Dental Schools: Curricular guidelines for removable prosthodontics, J Dent Educ 44:343-346, 1980.
Applegate OC: Conditions which may influence the choice of partial or complete denture service, J Prosthet Dent 7:182-196, 1957.
Applegate OC: Factors to be considered in choosing an alloy, Dent Clin North Am 4:583-590, 1960.
Asgar K, Techow BO, Jacobson JM: A new alloy for partial dentures, J Prosthet Dent 23:36-43, 1970.
Atwood DA: Practice of prosthodontics: past, present, and future, J Prosthet Dent 21:393-401, 1970.
Augsburger RH: Evaluating removable partial dentures by mathematical equations, J Prosthet Dent 22:528-543, 1969.
Backenstose WM, Wells JG: Side effects of immersion-type cleansers on the metal components of dentures, J Prosthet Dent 37:615-621, 1977.
Baker CR: Difficulties in evaluating removable partial dentures, J Prosthet Dent 17:60-62, 1967.
Baker CR: Occlusal reactive prosthodontics, J Prosthet Dent 17:566-569, 1967.
Barrett DA, Pilling LO: The restoration of carious clasp-bearing teeth, J Prosthet Dent 15:309-311, 1965.
Bates JF: Studies related to fracture of partial dentures, Br Dent J 120:79-83, 1966.
Beck HO: A clinical evaluation of the arcon concept of articulation, J Prosthet Dent 9:409-421, 1959.
Beck HO: Alloys for removable partial dentures, Dent Clin North Am 4:591-596, 1960.
Beck HO, Morrison WE: Investigation of an arcon articulator, J Prosthet Dent 6:359-372, 1956.
Becker CM, Bolender CL: Designing swinglock partial dentures, J Prosthet Dent 46:126-132, 1981.
Bergman B, Hugoson A, Olsson CO: Caries, periodontal and prosthetic findings in patients with removable partial dentures: a ten-year longitudinal study, J Prosthet Dent 48:506-514, 1982.
Blanco-Dalmau L: The nickel problem, J Prosthet Dent 48:99-101, 1982.
Blatterfein L, Pearce RL, Jackota JT: Minimum acceptable procedures for satisfactory removable partial denture service, J Prosthet Dent 27:84-87, 1972.
Bolender CL, Becker CM: Swinglock removable partial dentures: where and when, J Prosthet Dent 45:4-10, 1981.
Boucher CO: Writing as a means for learning, J Prosthet Dent 27:229-234, 1972.
Budtz-Jorgensen E, Isidor F: Cantilever bridges or removable partial dentures in geriatric patients: a two-year study, J Oral Rehabil 14:239-249, 1987.
Cavalaris CJ: Pathologic considerations associated with partial dentures, Dent Clin North Am 17:585-600, 1973.
Chandler JA, Brudvik JS: Clinical evaluation of patients eight to nine years after placement of removable partial dentures, J Prosthet Dent 51:736-743, 1984.
Chen MS et al: Simplicity in interim tooth-supported removable partial denture construction, J Prosthet Dent 54:740-744, 1985.
Cotmore JM et al: Removable partial denture survey: clinical practice today, J Prosthet Dent 49:321-327, 1983.
Coy RE, Arnold PD: Survey and design of diagnostic casts for removable partial dentures, J Prosthet Dent 32:103-106, 1974.
Cunningham DM: Comparison of base metal alloys and type IV gold alloys for removable partial denture frameworks, Dent Clin North Am 17:719-722, 1973.
Diaz-Arnold AM, Langenwalter EM, Hatch LK: Cast restorations made to existing removable partial dentures, J Prosthet Dent 61:414-417, 1989.
Dukes BS, Fields H Jr: Comparison of disclosing media used for adjustment of removable partial denture frameworks, J Prosthet Dent 45:380-382, 1981.
Elliott RW: The effects of heat on gold partial denture castings, J Prosthet Dent 13:688-698, 1963.
Ettinger RL: The acrylic removable partial denture, J Am Dent Assoc 95:945-949, 1977.
Ettinger RL, Beck JD, Jakobsen J: Removable prosthodontic treatment needs: a survey, J Prosthet Dent 51:419-427, 1984.
Ewing JE: The construction of accurate full crown restorations for an existing clasp by using a direct metal pattern technique, J Prosthet Dent 15:889-899, 1965.
Farah JW, MacGregor AR, Miller TPG: Stress analysis of disjunct removable partial dentures, J Prosthet Dent 42:271-275, 1979.

Federation of Prosthodontic Organizations: Guidelines for evaluation of completed prosthodontic treatment for removable partial dentures, J Prosthet Dent 27:326-328, 1972.

Fenton AH, Zarb GA, MacKay HF: Overdenture oversights, Dent Clin North Am 23:117-130, 1979.

Fields H, Campfield RW: Removable partial prosthesis partially supported by an endosseous blade implant, J Prosthet Dent 31:273-278, 1974.

Firtell DN, Kouyoumdjian JH, Holmes JB: Attitudes toward abutment preparation for removable partial dentures, J Prosthet Dent 55:131-133, 1986.

Fish SF: Partial dentures, Br Dent J 128:243-246, 289-293, 339-344, 398-402, 446-453, 495-502, 547-551, 590-592, 1970.

Fisher R: Relation of removable partial denture base stability to sex, age, and other factors, J Dent Res (IADR abstract 613) 59:entire issue, 1980.

Frank RP: Evaluating refractory cast wax-ups for removable partial dentures, J Prosthet Dent 35:388-392, 1976.

Girardot RL: The physiologic aspects of partial denture restorations, J Prosthet Dent 3:689-698, 1953.

Gordon SR: Measurement of oral status and treatment need among subjects with dental prostheses: are the measures less reliable than the prostheses? Part I: Oral status in removable prosthodontics, J Prosthet Dent 65:664-668, 1991.

Harrison WM, Stansbury BE: The effect of joint surface contours on the transverse strength of repaired acrylic resin, J Prosthet Dent 23:464-472, 1970.

Heintz WD: Principles, planning, and practice for prevention, Dent Clin North Am 17:705-718, 1973.

Helel KS, Graser GN, Featherstone JD: Abrasion of enamel and composite resin by removable partial denture clasps, J Prosthet Dent 52:389-397, 1984.

Henderson CW et al: Evaluation of the barrier system: an infection control system for the dental laboratory, J Prosthet Dent 58:517-521, 1987.

Izikowitz L: A long-term prognosis for the free-end saddle-bridge, J Oral Rehabil 12:247-262, 1985.

Jankelson BH: Adjustment of dentures at time of insertion and alterations to compensate for tissue changes, J Am Dent Assoc 64:521-531, 1962.

Jones RR: The lower partial denture, J Prosthet Dent 2:219-229, 1952.

Kaaber S: Twelve year changes in mandibular bone level in free end saddle denture wearers, J Dent Res (IADR abstract 1367) 60:entire issue, 1981.

Kaires AK: A study of partial denture design and masticatory pressures in a mandibular bilateral distal extension case, J Prosthet Dent 8:340-350, 1958.

Kelly E: Fatigue failure in denture base polymers, J Prosthet Dent 21:257-266, 1969.

Kelly E: Changes caused by a mandibular removable partial denture opposing a maxillary complete denture, J Prosthet Dent 27:140-150, 1972.

Kelly EK: The physiologic approach to partial denture design, J Prosthet Dent 3:699-710, 1953.

Kessler B: An analysis of the tongue factor and its functioning areas in dental prosthesis, J Prosthet Dent 5:629-635, 1955.

Klein IE, Blatterfein L, Kaufman EG: Minimum clinical procedures for satisfactory complete denture, removable partial denture, and fixed partial denture services, J Prosthet Dent 22:4-10, 1969.

Kratochvil FJ: Maintaining supporting structures with a removable partial prosthesis, J Prosthet Dent 25:167-174, 1971.

Kratochvil FJ, Caputo AA: Photoelastic analysis of pressure on teeth and bone supporting removable partial dentures, J Prosthet Dent 32:52-61, 1974.

Kratochvil FJ, Davidson PN, Guijt J: Five-year survey of treatment with removable partial dentures. Part I, J Prosthet Dent 48:237-244, 1982.

Landa JS: The troublesome transition from a partial lower to a complete lower denture, J Prosthet Dent 4:42-51, 1954.

Lanser A: Tooth-supported telescope restorations, J Prosthet Dent 45:515-520, 1981.

Lechner SK: A longitudinal survey of removable partial dentures. I: Patient assessment of dentures, Aust Dent J 30:104-111, 1985.

Lechner SK: A longitudinal survey of removable partial dentures. II: Clinical evaluation of dentures, Aust Dent J 30:194-197, 1985.

Lechner SK: A longitudinal survey of removable partial dentures. III, Tissue reactions to various denture components, Aust Dent J 30:291-295, 1985.

Lee MW et al: O-ring coping attachments for removable partial dentures, J Prosthet Dent 74:235-241, 1995.

Lewis AJ: Failure of removable partial denture castings during service, J Prosthet Dent 39:147-149, 1978.

Lewis AJ: Radiographic evaluation of porosities in removable partial denture castings, J Prosthet Dent 39:278-281, 1978.

Lopuck SE, Reitz PV, Altadonna J: Hinge for a unilateral maxillary arch prosthesis, J Prosthet Dent 45:446-448, 1981.

Lorton L: A method of stabilizing removable partial denture castings during clinical laboratory procedures, J Prosthet Dent 39:344-345, 1978.

MacEntee MI, Hawbolt EB, Zahel JI: The tensile and shear strength of a base metal weld joint used in dentistry, J Dent Res 60:154-158, 1981.

Maetani T et al: Effect of TFE coating on plaque accumulation on dental castings, J Dent Res (IADR abstract 1359) 60:entire issue, 1981.

Maison WG: Instructions to denture patients, J Prosthet Dent 9:825-831, 1959.

Makrauer FL, Davis JS: Gastroscopic removal of a partial denture, J Am Dent Assoc 94:904-906, 1977.

Marcus SE et al: The retention and tooth loss in the permanent dentition of adults: United States, 1988-1991, J Dent Res 75:684-695, 1996.

Martone AL: The fallacy of saving time at the chair, J Prosthet Dent 7:416-419, 1957.

Martone AL: The challenge of the partially edentulous mouth, J Prosthet Dent 8:942-954, 1958.

Massler M: Geriatric nutrition: the role of taste and smell in appetite, J Prosthet Dent 32:247-250, 1980.

McCracken WL: A comparison of tooth-borne and tooth-tissue-borne removable partial dentures, J Prosthet Dent 3:375-381, 1953.

McCracken WL: Auxiliary uses of cold-curing acrylic resins in prosthetic dentistry, J Am Dent Assoc 47:298-304, 1953.

McCracken WL: A philosophy of partial denture treatment, J Prosthet Dent 13:889-900, 1963.
Means CR, Flenniken IE: Gagging: a problem in prosthetic dentistry, J Prosthet Dent 23:614-620, 1970.
Mehringer EJ: The saliva as it is related to the wearing of dentures, J Prosthet Dent 4:312-318, 1954.
Michell DL, Wilke ND: Articulators through the years. I: Up to 1940, J Prosthet Dent 39:330-338, 1978; II, from 1940, 39:451-458, 1978.
Miller EL: Clinical management of denture-induced inflammations, J Prosthet Dent 38:362-365, 1977.
Mohamed SE, Schmidt JR, Harrison JD: Articulators in dental education and practice, J Prosthet Dent 36:319-325, 1976.
Morris HF, Asgar K: Physical properties and microstructure of four new commercial partial denture alloys, J Prosthet Dent 33:36-46, 1975.
Neufeld JO: Changes in the trabecular pattern of the mandible following the loss of teeth, J Prosthet Dent 8:685-697, 1958.
Oatlund SG: Saliva and denture retention, J Prosthet Dent 10:658-663, 1960.
Ogle RE, Sorensen SE, Lewis EA: A new visible light-cured resin system applied to removable prosthodontics, J Prosthet Dent 56:497-506, 1986.
Osborne J, Lammie GA: The bilateral free-end saddle lower denture, J Prosthet Dent 4:640-652, 1954.
Overton RG, Bramblett RM: Prosthodontic services: a study of need and availability in the United States, J Prosthet Dent 27:329-339, 1972.
Pascoe DF, Wimmer J: A radiographic technique for the detection of internal defects in dental castings, J Prosthet Dent 39:150-157, 1978.
Phillips RW, Leonard LJ: A study of enamel abrasion as related to partial denture clasps, J Prosthet Dent 6:657-671, 1956.
Plainfield S: Communication distortion: the language of patients and practitioners of dentistry, J Prosthet Dent 22:11-19, 1969.
Prieskel HW: The distal extension prosthesis reappraised, J Dent 5:217-230, 1977.
Ramsey WO: The relation of emotional factors to prosthodontic service, J Prosthet Dent 23:4-10, 1970.
Raybin NH: The polished surface of complete dentures, J Prosthet Dent 13:236-239, 1963.
Removable prosthodontics, Dent Clin North Am 28:entire issue, 1984.
Renggli HH, Allet B, Spanauf AJ: Splinting of teeth with fixed bridges: biological effect, J Oral Rehabil 11:535-537, 1984.
Reynolds JM: Crown construction for abutments of existing removable partial dentures, J Am Dent Assoc 69:423-426, 1964.
Rissen L et al: Effect of fixed and removable partial dentures on the alveolar bone of abutment teeth, J Dent Res (IADR abstract 1368) 60:entire issue, 1981.
Rissen L et al: Six-year report of the periodontal health of fixed and removable partial denture abutment teeth, J Prosthet Dent 54:461-467, 1985.
Rothman R: Phonetic considerations in denture prosthesis, J Prosthet Dent 11:214-223, 1961.
Rudd KD, Dunn BW: Accurate removable partial dentures, J Prosthet Dent 18:559-570, 1967.
Rushford CB: A technique for precision removable partial denture construction, J Prosthet Dent 31:377-383, 1974.
Ruyter IE, Svendsen SA: Flexural properties of denture base polymers, J Prosthet Dent 43:95-104, 1980.
Sadig W, Fahmi F: The modified swing-lock: a new approach, J Prosthet Dent 74:428-431, 1995.
Savage RD, MacGregor AR: Behavior therapy in prosthodontics, J Prosthet Dent 24:126-132, 1970.
Schabel RW: Dentist-patient communication: a major factor in treatment prognosis, J Prosthet Dent 21:3-5, 1969.
Schabel RW: The psychology of aging, J Prosthet Dent 27:569-573, 1972.
Schmitt SM: Combination syndrome: a treatment approach, J Prosthet Dent 54:307-309, 1985.
Schole ML: Management of the gagging patient, J Prosthet Dent 9:578-583, 1959.
Schopper AF: Removable appliances for the preservation of the teeth, J Prosthet Dent 4:634-639, 1954.
Schopper AF: Loss of vertical dimension: causes and effects: diagnosis and various recommended treatments, J Prosthet Dent 9:428-431, 1959.
Schulte JK, Smith DE: Clinical evaluation of swinglock removable partial dentures, J Prosthet Dent 44:595-603, 1980.
Schuyler CH: Stress distribution as the prime requisite to the success of a partial denture, J Am Dent Assoc 20:2148-2154, 1963.
Schwarz WD, Barsby MJ: Design of partial dentures in dental practice, J Dent 6:166-170, 1978.
Sears VH: Comprehensive denture service, J Am Dent Assoc 64:531-552, 1962.
Skinner EW, Gordon CC: Some experiments on the surface hardness of dental stones, J Prosthet Dent 6:94-100, 1956.
Skinner EW, Jones PM: Dimensional stability of self-curing denture base acrylic resin, J Am Dent Assoc 51:426-431, 1955.
Smith DE: Removable prosthodontics research—quo vadis? J Prosthet Dent 62:707-711, 1989.
Smith FW, Applegate OC: Roentgenographic study of bone changes during exercise stimulation of edentulous areas, J Prosthet Dent 11:1086-1097, 1961.
Stendahl CG, Grob DJ: Detection of binding areas on removable partial denture frameworks, Dent Clin North Am 23:101-106, 1979.
Swoope CC, Frank RP: Insertion and post-insertion care. In Clark J, ed: Clinical dentistry, vol 5, New York, 1976, Harper & Row.
Sykora O: Extracoronal removable partial denture service in Canada, J Prosthet Dent 39:37-41, 1978.
Sykora O: Definitive immediate cast removable partial dentures, Can Dent Assoc J 51:767-769, 1985.
Tallgren A: Alveolar bone loss in denture wearers as related to facial morphology, Acta Odontol Scand 28:251-270, 1970.
Taylor TD et al: Prosthodontic survey. I: Removable prosthodontic laboratory survey, J Prosthet Dent 52:598-601, 1984.
Taylor TD et al: Prosthodontic survey. II: Removable prosthodontic curriculum survey, J Prosthet Dent 52:747-749, 1984.
Teppo KW, Smith FW: A method of immediate clasp repair, J Prosthet Dent 34:77-80, 1975.

Trainor JE, Elliott RW Jr: Removable partial dentures designed by dentists before and after graduate level instruction: a comparative study, J Prosthet Dent 27:509-514, 1972.

von Gonten AS, Nelson DR: Laboratory pitfalls that contribute to embrasure clasp failure, J Prosthet Dent 53:136-138, 1985.

von Gonten AS, Palik JF: Tooth preparation guide for embrasure clasp designs, J Prosthet Dent 53:281-282, 1985.

Wagner AG: Maintenance of the partially edentulous mouth and care of the denture, Dent Clin North Am 17:755-768, 1973.

Wagner AG, Forgue EG: A study of four methods of recording the path of insertion of removable partial dentures, J Prosthet Dent 35:267-272, 1976.

Wallace DH: The use of gold occlusal surfaces in complete and partial dentures, J Prosthet Dent 14:326-333, 1964.

Walter JD: Partial denture technique. I: Introduction, Br Dent J 147:241-243, 1979; II: The purpose of the denture: choice of material, 147:302-304, 1979; III: Supporting the denture, 148:13-16, 1980; IV. Guide planes, 148:70-72, 1980.

Weaver RE, Goebel WM: Reactions to acrylic resin dental prostheses, J Prosthet Dent 43:138-142, 1980.

Whitsitt JA, Battle LW, Jarosz CJ: Enhanced retention for the distal extension-base removable partial denture using a heat-cured resilient soft liner, J Prosthet Dent 52:447-448, 1984.

Williams EO, Hartman GE: Instructional aid for teaching removable partial denture design, J Prosthet Dent 48:222, 1982.

Wise HB, Kaiser DA: A radiographic technique for examination of internal defects in metal frameworks, J Prosthet Dent 42:594-595, 1979.

Young HA: Factors contributory to success in prosthodontic practice, J Prosthet Dent 5:354-360, 1955.

Young L Jr: Try-in of the removable partial denture framework, J Prosthet Dent 46:579-580, 1981.

Zach GA: Advantages of mesial rests for removable partial dentures, J Prosthet Dent 33:32-35, 1975.

Zerosi C: A new type of removable splint: its indications and function, Dent Abstr 1:451-452, 1956.

Zurasky JE, Duke ES: Improved adhesion of denture acrylic resins to base metal alloys, J Prosthet Dent 57:520-524, 1987.

MOUTH PREPARATIONS

Alexander JM, Van Sickels JE: Posterior maxillary osteotomies: an aid for a difficult prosthodontic problem, J Prosthet Dent 41:614-617, 1979.

Atwood DA: Reduction of residual ridges in the partially edentulous patient, Dent Clin North Am 17:745-754, 1973.

Axinn S: Preparation of retentive areas for clasps in enamel, J Prosthet Dent 34:405-407, 1975.

Belinfante LS, Abney JM Jr: A teamwork approach to correct a severe prosthodontic problem, J Am Dent Assoc 91:357-359, 1975.

Dixon DL, Breeding LC, Swift EJ: Use of a partial coverage porcelain laminate to enhance clasp retention, J Prosthet Dent 63:55-58, 1990.

Glann GW, Appleby RC: Mouth preparations for removable partial dentures, J Prosthet Dent 10:698-706, 1960.

Johnston JF: Preparation of mouths for fixed and removable partial dentures, J Prosthet Dent 11:456-462, 1961.

Jones RM: Dentin exposed and decay incidence in removable partial denture rest seats, Int J Prosthodont 5:227-236, 1992.

Kahn AE: Partial versus full coverage, J Prosthet Dent 10:167-178, 1960.

Kapur KK et al: A randomized clinical trial of two basic removable partial denture designs. Part I: Comparisons of five-year success rates and periodontal health, J Prosthet Dent 72(3):268-282, 1994.

Laney WR, Desjardins RP: Comparison of base metal alloys and type IV gold alloys for removable partial denture framework, Dent Clin North Am 17:611-630, 1973.

Lorey RE: Abutment considerations, Dent Clin North Am 24:63-79, 1980.

Marquardt GL: Dolder bar joint mandibular overdenture: a technique for nonparallel abutment teeth, J Prosthet Dent 36:101-111, 1976.

McArthur DR, Turvey TA: Maxillary segmental osteotomies for mandibular removable partial denture patients, J Prosthet Dent 41:381-387, 1979.

McCarthy JA, Moser JB: Mechanical properties of tissue conditioners. I: Theoretical considerations, behavioral characteristics and tensile properties, J Prosthet Dent 40:89-97, 1978.

McCarthy JA, Moser JB: Mechanical properties of tissue conditioners. II: Creep characteristics, J Prosthet Dent 40:334-342, 1978.

McCracken WL: Mouth preparations for partial dentures, J Prosthet Dent 6:39-52, 1956.

Mills M: Mouth preparation for removable partial denture, J Am Dent Assoc 60:154-159, 1960.

Mopsik ER et al: Surgical intervention to reestablish adequate intermaxillary space before fixed or removable prosthodontics, J Am Dent Assoc 95:957-960, 1977.

Nishimura RD: Etched metal cingulum rest retainer, J Am Dent Assoc 112:177-179, 1986.

Phillips RJ Jr: Design sequence and mouth preparation for the removable partial denture, J Calif Dent Assoc 25(5):363-370, 1997.

Phillips RW: Report of the Committee on Scientific Investigation of the Academy of Restorative Dentistry, J Prosthet Dent 13:515-535, 1963.

Schorr L, Clayman LH: Reshaping abutment teeth for reception of partial denture clasps, J Prosthet Dent 4:625-633, 1954.

Stamps JT, Tanquist RA: Restoration of removable partial denture rest seats using dental amalgam, J Prosthet Dent 41:224-227, 1979.

Stern WJ: Guiding planes in clasp reciprocation and retention, J Prosthet Dent 34:408-414, 1975.

Swoope CC, Frank RP: Mouth preparation. In Clark JW, ed: Clinical dentistry, vol 5, New York, 1976, Harper & Row.

Tiege JD et al: In vitro investigation of the wear of resin composite materials and cast direct retainers during removable partial denture placement and removal, Int J Prosthodont 5:145-153, 1992.

Tucker KM, Heget HS: The incidence of inflammatory papillary hyperplasia, J Am Dent Assoc 93:610-613, 1976.

Wong R, Nicholls JI, Smith DE: Evaluation of prefabricated lingual rest seats for removable partial dentures, J Prosthet Dent 48:521-526, 1982.

OCCLUSION, JAW RELATION RECORDS, TRANSFER METHODS

Applegate OC: Loss of posterior occlusion, J Prosthet Dent 4:197-199, 1954.

Baraban DJ: Establishing centric relation and vertical dimension in occlusal rehabilitation, J Prosthet Dent 12:1157-1165, 1962.

Bauman R: Minimizing postinsertion problems: a procedure for removable partial denture placement, J Prosthet Dent 42:381-385, 1979.

Beck HO: A clinical evaluation of the arcon concept of articulation, J Prosthet Dent 9:409-421, 1959.

Beck HO: Selection of an articulator and jaw registration, J Prosthet Dent 10:878-886, 1960.

Beck HO: Choosing the articulator, J Am Dent Assoc 64:468-475, 1962.

Beckett LS: Accurate occlusal relations in partial denture construction, J Prosthet Dent 4:487-495, 1954.

Berke JD, Moleres I: A removable appliance for the correction of maxillomandibular disproportion, J Prosthet Dent 17:172-177, 1967.

Berman MH: Accurate interocclusal records, J Prosthet Dent 10:620-630, 1960.

Beyron HL: Occlusal relationship, Int Dent J 2:467-496, l952.

Beyron HL: Characteristics of functionally optimal occlusion and principles of occlusal rehabilitation, J Am Dent Assoc 48:648-656, 1954.

Beyron HL: Occlusal changes in adult dentition, J Am Dent Assoc 48:674-686, 1954.

Block LS: Preparing and conditioning the patient for intermaxillary relations, J Prosthet Dent 2:599-603, 1952.

Block LS: Tensions and intermaxillary relations, J Prosthet Dent 4:204-207, 1954.

Boos RH: Occlusion from rest position, J Prosthet Dent 2:575-588, l952.

Boos RH: Basic anatomic factors of jaw position, J Prosthet Dent 4:200-203, 1954.

Boos RH: Maxillomandibular relations, occlusion, and the temporomandibular joint, Dent Clin North Am, 6:19-35, 1962.

Borgh O, Posselt U: Hinge axis registration: experiments on the articulator, J Prosthet Dent 8:35-40, 1958.

Boucher CO: Occlusion in prosthodontics, J Prosthet Dent 3:633-656, 1953.

Braly BV: Occlusal analysis and treatment planning for restorative dentistry, J Prosthet Dent 27:168-171, 1972.

Breeding LC et al: Accuracy of three interocclusal recording materials used to mount a working cast, J Prosthet Dent 71(3):265-270, 1994.

Cerveris AR: Vibracentric equilibration of centric occlusion, J Am Dent Assoc 63:476-483, 1961.

Christensen PB: Accurate casts and positional relation records, J Prosthet Dent 8:475-482, 1958.

Clayton JA, Kotowicz WE, Zahler JM: Pantographic tracings of mandibular movements and occlusion, J Prosthet Dent 25:389-396, 1971.

Cohn LA: Factors of dental occlusion pertinent to the restorative and prosthetic problem, J Prosthet Dent 9:256-257, 1959.

Collett HA: Balancing the occlusion of partial dentures, J Am Dent Assoc 42:162-168, 1951.

Colman AJ: Occlusal requirements for removable partial dentures, J Prosthet Dent 17:155-162, 1967.

D'Amico A: Functional occlusion of the natural teeth of man, J Prosthet Dent 11:899-915, 1961.

Draper DH: Forward trends in occlusion, J Prosthet Dent 13:724-731, 1963.

Emmert JH: A method for registering occlusion in semiedentulous mouths, J Prosthet Dent 8:94-99, 1958.

Farmer JB, Connelly ME: Treatment of open occlusions with onlay and overlay removable partial dentures, J Prosthet Dent 51:300-303, 1984.

Fedi PF: Cardinal differences in occlusion of natural teeth and that of artificial teeth, J Am Dent Assoc 62:482-485, 1926.

Fountain HW: Seating the condyles for centric relation records, J Prosthet Dent 11:1050-1058, 1961.

Freilich MA, Altieri JW, Wahle JJ: Principles of selecting interocclusal records for articulation of dentate and partially dentate casts, J Prosthet Dent 68:361-367, 1992.

Gilson TD: Theory of centric correction in natural teeth, J Prosthet Dent 8:468-474, 1958.

Granger ER: The articulator and the patient, Dent Clin North Am 4:527-539, 1960.

Hansen CA et al: Simplified procedure for making gold occlusal surfaces on denture teeth, J Prosthet Dent 71(4):413-416, 1994.

Hausman M: Interceptive and pivotal occlusal contacts, J Am Dent Assoc 66:165-171, 1963.

Henderson D: Occlusion in removable partial prosthodontics, J Prosthet Dent 27:151-159, 1971.

Hindels GW: Occlusion in removable partial denture prosthesis, Dent Clin North Am 6:137-146, 1962.

Hughes GA, Regli CP: What is centric relation? J Prosthet Dent 11:16-22, 1961.

Ivanhoe JR, Vaught RD: Occlusion in the combination fixed removable prosthodontic patient, Dent Clin North Am 31:305-322, 1987.

Jankelson B: Considerations of occlusion on fixed partial dentures, Dent Clin North Am 3:187-203, 1959.

Jeffreys FE, Platner RL: Occlusion in removable partial dentures, J Prosthet Dent 10:912-920, 1960.

Kapur KK et al: A randomized clinical trial of two basic removable partial denture designs. Part I: Comparisons of five-year success rates and periodontal health, J Prosthet Dent 72(3):268-282, 1994.

Lang BR: Complete denture occlusion, Dent Clin North Am 40(1):85-101, 1996.

Lauritzen AG, Bodner GH: Variations in location of arbitrary and true hinge axis points, J Prosthet Dent 11:224-229, 1961.

Lay LS et al: Making the framework try-in, altered cast impression and occlusal registration in one appointment, J Prosthet Dent 75(4):446-448, Apr 1996.

Lindblom G: Balanced occlusion with partial reconstructions, Int Dent J 1:84-98, 1951.

Lindblom G: The value of bite analysis, J Am Dent Assoc 48:657-664, 1954.

Long JH Jr: Location of the terminal hinge axis by intraoral means, J Prosthet Dent 23:11-24, 1970.
Lucia VO: Centric relation theory and practice, J Prosthet Dent 10:849-956, 1960.
Lucia VO: The gnathological concept of articulation, Dent Clin North Am, 6:183-197, 1962.
Lundquist DO, Fiebiger GE: Registration for relating the mandibular cast to the maxillary cast based on Kennedy's classification system, J Prosthet Dent 35:371-375, 1976.
Mann AW, Pankey LD: The PM philosophy of occlusal rehabilitation, Dent Clin North Am 7:621-636, 1963.
McCollum BB: The mandibular hinge axis and a method of locating it, J Prosthet Dent 10:428-435, 1960.
McCracken WL: Functional occlusion in removable partial denture construction, J Prosthet Dent 8:955-963, 1958.
McCracken WL: Occlusion in partial denture prosthesis, Dent Clin North Am 6:109-119, 1962.
Mehta JD, Joglekar AP: Vertical jaw relations as a factor in partial dentures, J Prosthet Dent 21:618-625, 1969.
Meyer FS: The generated path technique in reconstruction dentistry: I and II, J Prosthet Dent 9:354-366, 432-440, 1959.
Millstein PL, Kronman JH, Clark RE: Determination of the accuracy of wax interocclusal registrations, J Prosthet Dent 25:189-196, 1971.
Moore AW: Ideal versus adequate dental occlusion, J Am Dent Assoc 55:51-56, 1957.
Moulton GH: The importance of centric occlusion in diagnosis and treatment planning, J Prosthet Dent 10:921-926, 1960.
Nayyar A, Bill JA Jr, Twiggs SW: Comparison of interocclusal recording materials for mounting a working cast, J Dent Res (IADR abstract 1216) 60:entire issue, 1981.
Nuttall EB: Establishing posterior functional occlusion for fixed partial dentures, J Am Dent Assoc 66:341-348, 1963.
O'Leary TJ, Shanley DB, Drake RB: Tooth mobility in cuspid-protected and group-function occlusions, J Prosthet Dent 27:21-25, 1972.
Olsson A, Posselt U: Relationship of various skull reference lines, J Prosthet Dent 11:1045-1049, 1961.
Reitz PV: Technique for mounting removable partial dentures on an articulator, J Prosthet Dent 22:490-494, 1969.
Reynolds JM: Occlusal wear facets, J Prosthet Dent 24:367-372, 1970.
Ricketts RM: Occlusion: the medium of dentistry, J Prosthet Dent 21:39-60, 1969.
Robinson MJ: Centric position, J Prosthet Dent 1:384-386, 1951.
Scaife RR Jr, Holt JE: Natural occurrence of cuspid guidance, J Prosthet Dent 22:225-229, 1969.
Scandrett FR, Hanson JC: Technique for attaching the master cast to its split mounting index, J Prosthet Dent 40:467-469, 1978.
Schireson S: Grinding teeth for masticatory efficiency and gingival health, J Prosthet Dent 13:337-345, 1963.
Schuyler CH: Fundamental principles in the correction of occlusal disharmony: natural and artificial (grinding), J Am Dent Assoc 22:1193-1202, 1935.
Schuyler CH: Factors of occlusion applicable to restorative dentistry, J Prosthet Dent 3:772-782, 1953.
Schuyler CH: An evaluation of incisal guidance and its influence in restorative dentistry, J Prosthet Dent 9:374-378, 1959.
Schuyler CH: Factors contributing to traumatic occlusion, J Prosthet Dent 11:708-715, 1961.
Sears VH: Occlusion: the common meeting ground in dentistry, J Prosthet Dent 2:15-21, 1952.
Sears VH: Occlusal pivots, J Prosthet Dent 6:332-338, 1956.
Sears VH: Centric and eccentric occlusions, J Prosthet Dent 10:1029-1036, 1960.
Sears VH: Mandibular equilibration, J Am Dent Assoc 65:45-55, 1962.
Shanahan TEJ, Leff A: Interocclusal records, J Prosthet Dent 10:842-848, 1960.
Silverman MM: Determination of vertical dimension by phonetics, J Prosthet Dent 6:465-471, 1956; Dent Abstr 2:221, 1957.
Skurnik H: Accurate interocclusal records, J Prosthet Dent 21:154-165, 1969.
Stuart CE: Accuracy in measuring functional dimensions and relations in oral prosthesis, J Prosthet Dent 9:220-236, 1959.
Teteruck WR, Lundeen HC: The accuracy of an ear face-bow, J Prosthet Dent 16:1039-1046, 1966.
Trushkowsky RD, Guiv B: Restoration of occlusal vertical dimension by means of a silica-coated onlay removable partial denture in conjunction with dentin bonding: a clinical report, J Prosthet Dent 66:283-286, 1991.
Wagner AG: A technique to record jaw relations for distally edentulous dental arches, J Prosthet Dent 29:405-407, 1973.
Weinberg LA: The transverse hinge axis: real or imaginary, J Prosthet Dent 9:775-787, 1959.
Weinberg LA: An evaluation of the face-bow mounting, J Prosthet Dent 11:32-42, 1961.
Weinberg LA: An evaluation of basic articulators and their concepts: I and 11, J Prosthet Dent 13:622-863, 1963.
Weinberg LA: Arcon principle in the condylar mechanism of adjustable articulators, J Prosthet Dent 13:263-268, 1963.

PARTIAL DENTURE DESIGN

Akagawa Y, Seo T, Ohkawa S, Tsuru H: A new telescopic crown system using a soldered horizontal pin for removable partial dentures, J Prosthet Dent 69:228-231, 1993.
Antos EW Jr, Tenner RP, Foerth D: The swinglock partial denture: an alternative approach to conventional removable partial denture service, J Prosthet Dent 40:257-262, 1978.
Avant EW: Indirect retention in partial denture design, J Prosthet Dent 16:1103-1110, 1966.
Axinn S, O'Connor RP Jr, Kopp EN: Immediate removable partial denture frameworks, J Am Dent Assoc 95:583-585, 1977.
Beaumont AJ Jr, Bianco HJ: Microcomputer-aided removable partial denture design: the next evolution, J Prosthet Dent 62:551-556, 1989.
Becker CM, Kaiser DA, Goldfogel MH: Evolution of removable partial denture design, J Prosthodont 3:158-166, 1994.

Becker CW, Bolender CL: Designing swinglock partial dentures, J Prosthet Dent 46:126-132, 1981.

Ben-Ur Z et al: Designing clasps for the asymmetric distal extension removable partial denture, Int J Prosthodont 9(4):374-378, July 1996.

Ben-Ur Z et al: Rigidity of major connectors when subjected to bending and torsion forces, J Prosthet Dent 62:557-562, 1989.

Berg E: Periodontal problems associated with use of distal extension removable partial dentures: a matter of construction? J Oral Rehabil 12:369-379, 1985.

Berg T Jr: I-bar: myth and counter-myth, Dent Clin North Am 23:65-75, 1979.

Berg T Jr, Caputo AA: Anterior rests for maxillary removable partial dentures, J Prosthet Dent 39:139-146, 1978.

Blatterfein L: A systematic method of designing upper partial denture bases, J Am Dent Assoc 46:510-525, 1953.

Blatterfein L: The use of the semiprecision rest in removable partial dentures, J Prosthet Dent 22:301-306, 1969.

Bolouri A: Removable partial denture design for a few remaining natural teeth, J Prosthet Dent 39:346-348, 1978.

Breeding L, Dixon DL: Prosthetic restoration of the anterior edentulous space, J Prosthet Dent 67:144-148, 1992.

Bridgeman JT et al: Comparison of titanium and cobalt-chromium removable partial denture clasps, J Prosthet Dent 78(2):187-193, 1997.

Brown DT, Desjardins RP, Chao EY: Fatigue failure in acrylic resin retaining minor connectors, J Prosthet Dent 58:329-335, 1987.

Browning JD et al: Effect of positional loading of three removable partial denture clasp assemblies on movement of abutment teeth, J Prosthet Dent 55:347-351, 1986.

Browning JD, Meadors LW, Eick JD: Movement of three removable partial denture clasp assemblies under occlusal loading, J Prosthet Dent 55:69-74, 1986.

Brudvik J, Reimers D: The tooth-removable partial denture interface, J Prosthet Dent 68:924-927, 1992.

Budtz-Jorgensen E et al: Alternate framework designs for removable partial dentures, J Prosthet Dent 80(1):58-66, July 1998.

Burns DR, Ward JE, Nance GL: Removable partial denture design and fabrication survey of the prosthodontic specialist, J Prosthet Dent 62:303-307, 1989.

Campbell LD: Subjective reactions to major connector designs for removable partial dentures, J Prosthet Dent 36:507-516, 1977.

Campbell SD, Weiner H: The hinged-clasp assembly removable partial denture, J Prosthet Dent 63:59-61, 1990.

Casey DM, Lauciello FR: A method for marking the functional depth of the floor of the mouth, J Prosthet Dent 43:108-111, 1980.

Cecconi BT et al: The component partial: a new RPD construction system, J Calif Dent Assoc 25(5):363-370, 1997.

Cecconi BT: Lingual bar design, J Prosthet Dent 28:635-639, 1973.

Cowles KR: Partial denture design: a simple teaching aid, J Prosthet Dent 47:219, 1982.

Davenport JC et al: The acquisition and validation of removable partial denture design knowledge: I: Methodology and overview, J Oral Rehabil 23(3):152-157, 1996.

Davenport JC et al: The acquisition and validation of removable partial denture design knowledge: II: Design rules and expert reaction, J Oral Rehabil 23(12):811-824, 1996.

Demer WJ: An analysis of mesial rest-I-bar clasps designs, J Prosthet Dent 36:243-253, 1976.

Dunny JA, King GE: Minor connector designs for anterior acrylic resin bases: a preliminary study, J Prosthet Dent 34:496-497, 1975.

Eick JD et al: Abutment tooth movement related to fit of a removable partial denture, J Prosthet Dent 57:66-72, 1987.

Ettinger RL: The acrylic removable partial denture, J Am Dent Assoc 85:945-949, 1977.

Farmer JB et al: Interim removable partial dentures: a modified technique, Quintessence Dent Technol 8:511-516, 1985.

Feingold FM, Grant AA, Johnson W: The effect of partial denture design on abutment tooth and saddle movement, J Oral Rehabil 13:549-557, 1986.

Firtell DN: Effect of clasp design upon retention of removable partial dentures, J Prosthet Dent 20:43-52, 1968.

Firtell DN, Grisius RJ, Muncheryan AM: Reaction of the anterior abutment of a Kennedy Class II removable partial denture to various clasp arm designs: an in vitro study, J Prosthet Dent 53:77-82, 1985.

Fisher RL, Jaslow C: The efficiency of an indirect retainer, J Prosthet Dent 33:24-30, 1975.

Fisher RL, McDowell GC: Removable partial denture design and potential stress to the periodontium, Int J Periodont Restor Dent 4:34-47, 1984.

Frank RP: An investigation of the effectiveness of indirect retainers, J Prosthet Dent 38:494-506, 1977.

Frank RP: Direct retainers for distal-extension removable partial dentures, J Prosthet Dent 56:562-567, 1986.

Frantz WR: Variations in a removable maxillary partial denture design by dentists, J Prosthet Dent 34:625-633, 1975.

Ghamrawy E: Oral ecologic response caused by removable partial dentures, J Dent Res (IADR abstract 2898) 61:entire issue, 1982.

Ghamrawy E: Plaque formation and crevicular temperature relation to minor connector position, J Dent Res (IADR abstract 387) 61:entire issue, 1982.

Giradot RL: History and development of partial denture design, J Am Dent Assoc 28:1399-1408, 1941.

Hansen CA: Metal minibases in removable prosthodontics, J Prosthet Dent 54:442-446, 1985.

Hansen CA, Campbell DJ: Clinical comparison of two mandibular major connector designs: the sublingual bar and the lingual plate, J Prosthet Dent 54:805-809, 1985.

Henderson D: Major connectors for mandibular removable partial dentures, J Prosthet Dent 30:532-548, 1973.

Henderson D: Major connectors: united it stands, Dent Clin North Am 17:661-668, 1973.

Hero H et al: Ductility and structure of some cobalt-base dental casting alloys, Biomaterials 5:201-208, 1984.

Highton R, Caputo AA, Rhodes S: Force transmission and retentive capabilities utilizing labial and palatal I-bar partial dentures, J Dent Res (IADR abstract 1214) 60:entire issue, 1981.

Iwama CY et al: Cobalt-chromium-titanium alloy for removable partial dentures, Int J Prosthodont 10(4):309-317, 1997.

Jacobson TE, Krol AJ: Rotational path removable partial denture design, J Prosthet Dent 48:370-376, 1982.

Jacobson TE: Rotational path partial denture design: a 10-year clinical follow-up: Parts I and II, J Prosthet Dent 71(3):271-282, 1994.

Jordan LG: Designing removable partial dentures with external attachments (clasps), J Prosthet Dent 2:716-722, 1952.

Kapur KK et al: A randomized clinical trial of two basic removable partial denture designs. Part I: comparisons of five-year success rates and periodontal health, J Prosthet Dent 72(3):268-282, 1994.

Kelly EK: The physiologic approach to partial denture design, J Prosthet Dent 3:699-710, 1953.

King GE: Dual-path design for removable partial dentures, J Prosthet Dent 39:392-395, 1978.

King GE, Barco MT, Olson RJ: Inconspicuous retention for removable partial dentures, J Prosthet Dent 39:505-507, 1978.

Knodle JM: Experimental overlay and pin partial denture, J Prosthet Dent 17:472-478, 1967.

Ko SH, McDowell GC, Kotowicz WE: Photoelastic stress analysis of mandibular removable partial dentures with mesial and distal occlusal rests, J Prosthet Dent 56:454-460, 1986.

Krikos AA: Artificial undercuts for teeth which have unfavorable shapes for clasping, J Prosthet Dent 22:301-306, 1969.

Lanser A: Telescope retainers for removable partial dentures, J Prosthet Dent 45:37-43, 1981.

Latta GH et al: Wear of visible light-cured restorative materials and removable partial denture direct retainers, J Prosthodont 6(2):104-109, 1997.

LaVere AM, Smith RC, Serka RJ: Cross-arch bar splint, J Prosthet Dent 67:82-84, 1992.

LaVere AM, Freda AL: A simplified procedure for survey and design of diagnostic casts, J Prosthet Dent 37:680-683, 1977.

LaVere AM, Krol AJ: Selection of a major connector for the extension base removable partial denture, J Prosthet Dent 30:102-105, 1973.

Lindquist TJ et al: Effectiveness of computer-aided partial denture design, J Prosthodont 6(2):122-127, 1997.

Lorencki SF: Planning precision attachment restorations, J Prosthet Dent 21:506-508, 1969.

Luk K et al: Unilateral rotational path removable partial dentures for tilted mandibular molars, J Prosthet Dent 78(1):102-105, 1997.

Marxkors R: Mastering the removable partial denture. Part I: basic reflections about construction, J Dent Technol 14(1):34-39, 1997.

Marxkors R: Mastering the removable partial denture. Part II: connection of partial dentures to the abutment teeth, J Dent Technol 14(2):24-30, 1997.

Maxfield JB, Nicholls JE, Smith DE: The measurement of forces transmitted to abutment teeth of removable partial dentures, J Prosthet Dent 41:134-142, 1979.

McCartney JW: Lingual plating for reciprocation, J Prosthet Dent 42:624-625, 1979.

McCracken WL: Contemporary partial denture designs, J Prosthet Dent 8:71-84, 1958.

McCracken WL: Survey of partial denture designs by commercial dental laboratories, J Prosthet Dent 12:1089-1110, 1962.

McHenry KR, Johansson DE, Christensson LA: The effect of removable partial denture framework design on gingival inflammation: a clinical model, J Prosthet Dent 68:799-803, 1992.

Meeuwissen R, Keltjens HM, Battistugzi PG: Cingulum bar as a major connector for mandibular removable partial dentures, J Prosthet Dent 66:221-223, 1991.

Monteith BD: Management of loading forces on mandibular distal-extension prostheses. I: Evaluation of concepts for design, J Prosthet Dent 52:673-681, 1984.

Monteith BD: Management of loading forces on mandibular distal-extension prostheses. II: Classification for matching modalities to clinical situations, J Prosthet Dent 52:832-836, 1984.

Myers RE et al: A photoelastic study of rests on solitary abutments for distal-extension removable partial dentures, J Prosthet Dent 56:702-707, 1986.

NaBadalung DP et al: Frictional resistance of removable partial dentures with retrofitted resin composite guide planes, Int J Prosthodont 10(2):116-122, 1997.

Naim RI: The problem of free-end denture bases, J Prosthet Dent 16:522-532, 1966.

Navas MTR, del Campo ML: A new free-end removable partial denture design, J Prosthet Dent 70:176-179, 1993.

Pardo-Mindan S, Ruiz-Villandiego JC: A flexible lingual clasp as an esthetic alternative: a clinical report, J Prosthet Dent 69:245-246, 1993.

Perry C: Philosophy of partial denture design, J Prosthet Dent 6:775-784, 1956.

Pipko DJ: Combinations in fixed-removable prostheses, J Prosthet Dent 26:481-490, 1971.

Potter RB, Appleby RC, Adams CD: Removable partial denture design: a review and a challenge, J Prosthet Dent 17:63-68, 1967.

Radford DR, Walter JD: A variation in minor connector design for partial denture, Int J Prosthet 6:50-53, 1993.

Russell MD, Tumer P: A three-part sectional design for an upper removable partial denture with an anterior modification, Br Dent J 162:24-26, 1987.

Rybeck SA Jr: Simplicity in a distal extension partial denture, J Prosthet Dent 4:87-92, 1954.

Schmidt AH: Planning and designing removable partial dentures, J Prosthet Dent 3:783-806, 1953.

Schuyler CH: The partial denture as a means of stabilizing abutment teeth, J Am Dent Assoc 28:1121-1125, 1941.

Schwartz RS, Murchison DG: Design variations of the rotational path removable partial denture, J Prosthet Dent 58:336-338, 1987.

Seals RR Jr, Schwartz IS: Successful integration of fixed and removable prosthodontics, J Prosthet Dent 53:763-766, 1985.

Shifman A: Use of an Adam's clasp for a cast unilateral removable partial denture, J Prosthet Dent 61:703-705, 1989.

Shohet H: Relative magnitudes of stress on abutment teeth with different retainers, J Prosthet Dent 21:267-282, 1969.

Steffel VL: Simplified clasp partial dentures designed for maximum function, J Am Dent Assoc 32:1093-1100, 1945.
Steffel VL: Fundamental principles involved in partial denture design, J Am Dent Assoc 42:534-544, 1951.
Sykora O, Calikkocaoglu S: Maxillary removable partial denture designs by commercial dental laboratories, J Prosthet Dent 22:633-640, 1970.
Sykora O: Removable partial denture design by Canadian dental laboratories: a retrospective study, J Can Dent Assoc 61(7):615-621, 1995.
Tautin FS: Abutment stabilization using a nonresilient gingival bar connector, J Am Dent Assoc 99:988-998, 1979.
Thompson WD, Kratochvil FJ, Caputo AA: Evaluation of photoelastic stress patterns produced by various designs of bilateral distal-extension removable partial dentures, J Prosthet Dent 38:261-273, 1977.
Tsao DH: Designing occlusal rests using mathematical principles, J Prosthet Dent 23:154-163, 1970.
Unger JW, Badr SE: Esthetic placement of bar-clasp direct retainers, J Prosthet Dent 56:381-382, 1986.
Vallittu PK: Comparison of the in vitro fatigue resistance of an acrylic resin removable partial denture reinforced with continuous fibers or metal wires. J Prosthodont 5(2):115-121, 1996.
Vofa M, Kotowicz WE: Plaque retention with lingual bar and lingual plate major connectors, J Dent Res (AADR abstract 609) 59:entire issue, 1980.
Wagner AC, Traweek FC: Comparison of major connectors for removable partial dentures, J Prosthet Dent 47:242-245, 1982.
Waller NI: The root rest and the removable partial denture, J Prosthet Dent 33:16-23, 1975.
Walter JD: Alternative major connectors for mandibular partial dentures, Restorative Dent 2(4):80, 82-84, 1986.
Warren AB, Caputo AA: Load transfer to alveolar bone as influenced by abutment design for tooth supported dentures, J Prosthet Dent 33:137-148, 1975.
Weinberg LA: Lateral force in relation to the denture base and clasp design, J Prosthet Dent 6:785-800, 1956.
Williams RJ et al: Use of a cast flexible plate as a hinge substitute in a hinge-lock design removable partial denture, J Prosthet Dent 80(8):220-223, 1998.
Zach GA: Advantages of mesial rests for removable partial dentures, J Prosthet Dent 33:32-35, 1975.
Zoller GN et al: Technique to improve surveying in confined areas, J Prosthet Dent 73(2):223-224, 1995.

PERIODONTAL CONSIDERATIONS

Amsterdam M, Fox L: Provisional splinting: principles and technics, Dent Clin North Am 3:73-99, 1959.
App GR: Periodontal treatment for the removable partial prosthesis patient. Another half century, Dent Clin North Am 17:601-610, 1973.
Applegate OC: The interdependence of periodontics and removable partial denture prosthesis, J Prosthet Dent 8:269-281, 1958.
Aydinlik E, Dayangac B, Celik E: Effect of splintings on abutment tooth movement, J Prosthet Dent 49:477-480, 1983.
Bates JF, Addy M: Partial dentures and plaque accumulation, J Dent 6:285-293, 1978.
Bazirgan MK, Bates JF: Effect of clasp design on gingival health, J Oral Rehabil 14:271-281, 1987.
Becker CM, Kaldahl WB: Using removable partial dentures to stabilize teeth with secondary occlusal traumatism, J Prosthet Dent 47:587-594, 1982.
Berg TE, Caputo AA: Maxillary distal extension removable partial denture abutments with reduced periodontal support, J Prosthet Dent 70:245-250, 1993.
Bergman B: Periodontal reactions related to removable partial dentures: a literature review, J Prosthet Dent 58:454-458, 1987.
Bergman B, Ericson G: Cross-sectional study of the periodontal status of removable partial denture patients, J Prosthet Dent 61:208-211, 1989.
Brill N et al: Ecologic changes in the oral cavity caused by removable partial dentures, J Prosthet Dent 38:138-148, 1977.
Clarke NG: Treatment planning for fixed and removable partial dentures: a periodontal view, J Prosthet Dent 36:44-50, 1976.
Dello Russo NM: Gingival autografts as an adjunct to removable partial dentures, J Am Dent Assoc 104:179-181, 1982.
Erperstein H: The role of the prosthodontist in the treatment of periodontal disease, Int Dent J 36(1):18-29, 1986.
Fisher RL, McDowell GC: Removable partial denture design and potential stress to the periodontium, Int J Periodont Res Dent 4:34-47, 1984.
Garfield RE: A prosthetic solution to the periodontally compromised/furcation involved abutment tooth: I, Quintessence Int 15:805-813, 1984.
Gilson CM: Periodontal considerations, Dent Clin North Am 24:31-44, 1980.
Gomes BC et al: A clinical study of the periodontal status of abutment teeth supporting swinglock removable partial dentures: a pilot study, J Prosthet Dent 46:7-13, 1981.
Gomes BC, Renner RP, Bauer PN: Periodontal considerations in removable partial dentures, J Am Dent Assoc 101:496-498, 1980.
Hall WB: Periodontal preparation of the mouth for restoration, Dent Clin North Am 24:195-213, 1980.
Hirschfeld Z et al: New sustained release dosage form of chlorhexidine for dental use: use for plaque control in partial denture wearers, J Oral Rehabil 11:477-482, 1984.
Isidor F, Budtz-Jorgensen E: Periodontal conditions following treatment with cantilever bridges or removable partial dentures in geriatric patients: a 2-year study, Gerodontics 3(3):117-121, 1987.
Ivancie GP: Interrelationship between restorative dentistry and periodontics, J Prosthet Dent 8:819-830, 1958.
Jacobson TE: Periodontal considerations in removable partial denture design, Compendium 8:530-534, 536-539, 1987.
Jordan LG: Treatment of advanced periodontal disease by prosthodontic procedures, J Prosthet Dent 10:908-911, 1960.
Kimball HD: The role of periodontia in prosthetic dentistry, J Prosthet Dent 1:286-294, 1951.
Krogh-Poulsen W: Partial denture design in relation to occlusal trauma in periodontal breakdown, Int Dent J 4:847-867, 1954; also Acad Rev 3:18-23, 1955.

McKenzie JS: Mutual problems of the periodontist and prosthodontist, J Prosthet Dent 5:37-42, 1955.
Morris ML: Artificial crown contours and gingival health, J Prosthet Dent 12:1146-1155, 1962.
Nevin RB: Periodontal aspects of partial denture prosthesis, J Prosthet Dent 5:215-219, 1955.
Orban BS: Biologic principles in correction of occlusal disharmonies, J Prosthet Dent 6:637-641, 1956.
Overby GE: Esthetic splinting of mobile periodontally involved teeth by vertical pinning, J Prosthet Dent 11:112-118, 1961.
Perel ML: Periodontal consideration of crown contours, J Prosthet Dent 26:627-630, 1971.
Picton DCA, Wills DJ: Viscoelastic properties of the periodontal ligament and mucous membrane, J Prosthet Dent 40:263-272, 1978.
Rissin L et al: Effect of age and removable partial dentures on gingivitis and periodontal disease, J Prosthet Dent 42:217-223, 1979.
Rudd KD, O'Leary TJ: Stabilizing periodontally weakened teeth by using guide plane removable partial dentures: a preliminary report, J Prosthet Dent 16:721-727, 1966.
Schuyler CH: The partial denture and a means of stabilizing abutment teeth, J Am Dent Assoc 28:1121-1125, 1941.
Schwalm CA, Smith DE, Erickson JD: A clinical study of patients 1 to 2 years after placement of removable partial dentures, J Prosthet Dent 38:380-391, 1977.
Seibert JS, Cohen DW: Periodontal considerations in preparation for fixed and removable prosthodontics, Dent Clin North Am 31:529-555, 1987.
Spiekermann H: Prosthetic and periodontal considerations of free-end removable partial dentures, Int J Periodont Restor Dent 6:148-163, 1986.
Sternlicht HC: Prosthetic treatment planning for the periodontal patient, Dent Abstr 2:81-82, 1957.
Stipho HDK, Murphy WM, Adams D: Effect of oral prostheses on plaque accumulation, Br Dent J 145:47-50, 1978.
Talkov L: Survey for complete periodontal prosthesis, J Prosthet Dent 11:124-131, 1961.
Tebrock OC et al: The effect of various clasping systems on the mobility of abutment teeth for distal-extension removable partial dentures, J Prosthet Dent 41:511-516, 1979.
Thayer HH, Kratochvil FJ: Periodontal considerations with removable partial dentures, Dent Clin North Am 24:195-213, 1980.
Thomas BOA, Gallager JW: Practical management of occlusal dysfunctions in periodontal therapy, J Am Dent Assoc 46:18-31, 1953.
Trapozzano VR, Winter CR: Periodontal aspects of partial denture design, J Prosthet Dent 2:101-107, 1952.
Waerhaug J: Justification for splinting in periodontal therapy, J Prosthet Dent 22:201-208, 1969.
Ward HL, Weinberg LA: An evaluation of periodontal splinting, J Am Dent Assoc 63:48-54, 1961.

PHYSIOLOGY: MANDIBULAR MOVEMENT

Brekke CA: Jaw function I: Hinge rotation, J Prosthet Dent 9:600-606, 1959; II: Hinge axis, hinge axes, 9:936-940, 1959; III: Condylar placement and condylar retrusion. 10:78-85, 1960.
Brotman DN: Contemporary concepts of articulation, J Prosthet Dent 10:221-230, 1960.
Budtz-Jorgensen E: Restoration of the occlusal face height by removable partial dentures in elderly patients, Gerodontics 2(2):67-71, 1986.
Emig GE: The physiology of the muscles of mastication, J Prosthet Dent 1:700-707, 1951.
Fountain HW: The temporomandibular joints: a fulcrum, J Prosthet Dent 25:78-84, 1971.
Gibbs CH et al: Functional movements of the mandible, J Prosthet Dent 26:604-620, 1971.
Jankelson B: Physiology of human dental occlusion, J Am Dent Assoc 50:664-680, 1955.
Jemt T, Hedegard B, Wickberg K: Chewing patterns before and after treatment with complete maxillary and bilateral distal-extension mandibular removable partial dentures, J Prosthet Dent 50:566-569, 1983.
Kurth LE: Mandibular movement and articulator occlusion, J Am Dent Assoc 39:37-46, 1949.
Kurth LE: Centric relation and mandibular movement, J Am Dent Assoc 50:309-315, 1955.
McMillen LB: Border movements of the human mandible, J Prosthet Dent 27:524-532, 1972.
Messerman T: A concept of jaw function with a related clinical application, J Prosthet Dent 13:130-140, 1963.
Naylor JG: Role of the external pterygoid muscles in temporomandibular articulation, J Prosthet Dent 10:1037-1042, 1960.
Plotnick IJ, Beresin VE, Simkins AB: The effects of variations in the opposing dentition on changes in the partially edentulous mandible. I: Bone changes observed in serial radiographs, J Prosthet Dent 33: 278-286, 1975.
Plotnick IJ, Beresin VE, Simkins AB: The effects of variations in the opposing dentition on changes in the partially edentulous mandible. III: Tooth mobility and chewing efficiency with various maxillary dentitions, J Prosthet Dent 33:529-534, 1975.
Posselt U: Studies in the mobility of the human mandible, Acta Odontol Scand 10:19-160, 1952.
Posselt U: Movement areas of the mandible, J Prosthet Dent 7:375-385, 1957.
Posselt U: Terminal hinge movement of the mandible, J Prosthet Dent 7:787-797, 1957.
Saizar P: Centric relation and condylar movement, J Prosthet Dent 26:581-591, 1971.
Schweitzer JM: Masticatory function in man, J Prosthet Dent 11:625-647, 1961.
Shanahan TEJ: Dental physiology for dentures: the direct application of the masticatory cycle to denture occlusion, J Prosthet Dent 2:3, 1952.
Shore NA: Educational program for patients with temporomandibular joint dysfunction (ligaments), J Prosthet Dent 23:691-695, 1970.
Sicher H: Positions and movements of the mandible, J Am Dent Assoc 48:620-625, 1954.
Skinner CN: Physiology of the occlusal coordination of natural teeth, complete dentures, and partial dentures, J Prosthet Dent 17:559-565, 1967.
Sostenbo HR: CE Luce's recordings of mandibular movement, J Prosthet Dent 11:1068-1073, 1961.

Tallgren A, Mizutani H, Tryda G: A two-year kinesiograph, study of mandibular movement patterns in denture wearers, J Prosthet Dent 62:594-600, 1989.

Ulrich J: The human temporomandibular joint: kinematics and actions of the masticatory muscles, J Prosthet Dent 9:399-406, 1959.

Vaughan HC: The external pterygoid mechanism, J Prosthet Dent 5:80-92, 1955.

REBASING AND RELINING

Blatterfein L: Rebasing procedures for removable partial dentures, J Prosthet Dent 8:441-467, 1958.

Breeding LC, Dixon DL, Lund TS: Dimensional changes of processed denture bases after relining with three resins, J Prosthet Dent 66:650-656, 1991.

Bolouri A et al: A procedure for relining a complete or removable partial denture without the use of wax, J Prosthet Dent 79(5):604-606, May 1998.

Grady RD: Objective criteria for relining distal-extension removable partial dentures: a preliminary report, J Prosthet Dent 49:178-181, 1983.

McGivney GP: A reline technique for extension base removable partial dentures. In Lefkowitz W, ed: Proceedings of the Second International Prosthodontic Congress, St Louis, 1979, Mosby.

Steffel VL: Relining removable partial dentures for fit and function, J Prosthet Dent 4:496-509, 1954.

Turck MD, Richards MW: Microwave processing for denture relines, repairs, and rebases, J Prosthet Dent 69:340-343, 1993.

Wilson JH: Partial dentures: relining the saddle supported by the mucosa and alveolar bone, J Prosthet Dent 3:807-813, 1953.

Yasuda N et al: New adhesive resin to metal in removable prosthodontics field, J Dent Res (IADR abstract 213) 59:entire issue, 1980.

STRESS-BREAKER DESIGNS

Bartlett AA: Duplication of precision attachment partial dentures, J Prosthet Dent 16:1111-1115, 1966.

Bickley RW: Combined splint-stress breaker removable partial denture, J Prosthet Dent 21:509-512, 1969.

Cecconi BT, Kaiser C, Rahe A: Stress-breakers and the removable partial denture, J Prosthet Dent 34:145-151, 1975.

Hansen CA, Singer MT: The segmented framework removable partial denture, J Prosthet Dent 47:765-768, 1987.

Hirschtritt E: Removable partial dentures with stress-broken extension bases, J Prosthet Dent 7:318-324, 1957.

James AC: Stress-breakers which automatically return the saddle to rest position following displacement: mandibular distal extension partial dentures, J Prosthet Dent 4:73-81, 1954.

Kabcenell JL: Stress-breaking for partial dentures, J Am Dent Assoc 63:593-602, 1961.

Kane BE: Buoyant stress equalizer, J Prosthet Dent 14:698-704, 1964.

Kane BE: Improved buoyant stress equalizer, J Prosthet Dent 17:365-371, 1967.

Levin B: Stress-breakers: a practical approach, Dent Clin North Am 23:77-86, 1979.

Levitch HC: Physiologic stress-equalizer J Prosthet Dent 3:232-238, 1953.

MacGregor AR: Stress-breaking in partial dentures, Aust Prosthodont Soc Bull 16:65-70, 1986.

Marris FN: The precision dowel rest attachment, J Prosthet Dent 5:43-48, 1955.

Neill DJ: The problem of the lower free-end removable partial denture, J Prosthet Dent 8:623-634, 1958.

Plotnik IJ: Stress regulator for complete and partial dentures, J Prosthet Dent 17:166-171, 1967.

Reitz PV, Caputo AA: A photoelastic study of stress distribution by a mandibular split major connector, J Prosthet Dent 54:220-225, 1985.

Reitz PV, Sanders JL, Caputo AA: A photoelastic study of a split palatal major connector, J Prosthet Dent 51:19-23, 1984.

Simpson DH: Considerations for abutments, J Prosthet Dent 5:375-384, 1955.

Terrell WH: Split bar technique applicable to both precision attachment and clasp cases, J South Calif Dent Assoc 9:10-14, 1942.

Zinner ID: A modification of the Thompson Dowel rest for distal-extension removable partial dentures, J Prosthet Dent 61:374-378, 1989.

SURVEYING

Applegate OC: Use of paralleling surveyor in modern partial denture construction, J Am Dent Assoc 27:1317-1407, 1940.

Atkinson HF: Partial denture problems: surveyors and surveying, Aust J Dent 59:28-31, 1955.

Bezzon OL et al: Surveying removable partial dentures: the importance of guiding planes and path of insertion for stability, J Prosthet Dent 78(4):412-418, 1997.

Chestner SC: A methodical approach to the analysis of study cases, J Prosthet Dent 4:622-624, 1954.

Hanson JC: Surveying, J Am Dent Assoc 91:826-828, 1975.

Katulski EM, Appleyard WN: Biological concepts of the use of the mechanical cast surveyor, J Prosthet Dent 7:627-634, 1959.

Knapp JC, Shotwell JL, Kotowicz WE: Technique for recording dental cast-surveyor relations, J Prosthet Dent 41:352-354, 1979.

McCarthy MF: An intraoral surveyor, J Prosthet Dent 61:462-464, 1989.

Solle W: An improved dental surveyor, J Am Dent Assoc 60:727-731, 1960.

Wagner AC, Forque EC: A study of four methods of recording the path of insertion of removable partial dentures, J Prosthet Dent 35:267-272, 1976.

Yilmaz C: Optical surveying of casts for removable partial dentures, J Prosthet Dent 34:292-296, 1975.

Zoller GN et al: Technique to improve surveying in confined areas, J Prosthet Dent 73(2):223-224, Feb 1995.

WORK AUTHORIZATIONS

Brown ET: The dentist, the laboratory technician, and the prescription law, J Prosthet Dent 15:1132-1138, 1965.

Dutton DA: Standard abbreviations (and definitions) for use in dental laboratory work authorizations, J Prosthet Dent 27:94-95, 1972.

Gehl DH: Investment in the future, J Prosthet Dent 18:190-201, 1968.

Henderson D: Writing work authorizations for removable partial dentures, J Prosthet Dent 16:696-707, 1966.

Henderson D, Frazier Q: Communicating with dental laboratory technicians, Dent Clin North Am 14:603-615, 1970.

Leeper SH: Dentist and laboratory: a love-hate relationship, Dent Clin North Am 23:87-99, 1979.

Quinn L: Status of the dental laboratory work authorization, J Am Dent Assoc 79:1189-1190, 1969.

Travaglini EA, Jannetto LB: A work authorization format for removable partial dentures, J Am Dent Assoc 6:429-431, 1978.

INDEX

Page numbers followed by "f" denote figures, "t" denote tables, and "b" denote boxes